Comorbid Conditions in the Treatment of Headache

This book is a practical reference and educational tool that teaches headache specialists and neurologists about the comorbid illnesses they will encounter in their patients.

Headache Medicine is increasingly recognized as a dedicated specialty with an emerging cohort of physicians focused on treating these patients. Given the prevalence of headaches globally, patients often have comorbid conditions, which affect treatment decisions and outcomes in innumerable ways. This easy-to-use reference of comorbid conditions facilitates an understanding of the patient with a headache. Each chapter discusses the longitudinal illnesses organized by body system, in addition to chapters on general internal medicine and the treatment of special populations. Headache clinicians will benefit from building knowledge of general internal medicine topics as an overlay to their headache practice.

This reference book on comorbid conditions supports a holistic approach to the patient with a headache. In addition to headache specialists, it will benefit a wide range of health care providers, including neurologists, primary care physicians, pediatricians, obstetricians, and gynecologists.

Comorbid Conditions in the Treatment of Headache

Edited by
Leon S. Moskatel
Robert P. Cowan

CRC Press
Taylor & Francis Group
Boca Raton London New York

CRC Press is an imprint of the
Taylor & Francis Group, an **informa** business

Designed cover image: Shutterstock, Ilya Lukichev, 1834342792

First edition published 2025
by CRC Press
2385 NW Executive Center Drive, Suite 320, Boca Raton FL 33431

and by CRC Press
4 Park Square, Milton Park, Abingdon, Oxon, OX14 4RN

CRC Press is an imprint of Taylor & Francis Group, LLC

ISBN: 978-1-032-47171-6 (hbk)
ISBN: 978-1-032-87678-8 (pbk)
ISBN: 978-1-003-38489-2 (ebk)

DOI: 10.1201/b23330

Typeset in Times
by SPi Technologies India Pvt Ltd (Straive)

To my parents Barbara and Ira, wife Rebecca (who also authors the Infectious Disease chapter), son Frank, and mentors Dr. Steven Yung and Dr. Paul Han.

Leon Moskatel

To my wife, Mercedes, and my children, Sotera and Sam, without whom this book and my life in general would never have happened.

Robert Cowan

Contents

About the Editors

Leon S. Moskatel, MD, is a Clinical Assistant Professor in the Division of Headache and Facial Pain in the Department of Neurology of the Stanford School of Medicine. He obtained his Bachelor of the Arts from Columbia University *cum laude* and his medical degree at the University of Southern California Keck School of Medicine. He completed his Internal Medicine residency at Scripps Mercy Hospital in San Diego, followed by a Headache Medicine fellowship at Stanford.

He has published 21 peer-reviewed publications in addition to 6 textbook chapters and other additional publications. He received the American Headache Society's 2020 "Frontiers in Headache Research" award and has served on their Education Task Force. He has reviewed manuscripts for the *Annals of Internal Medicine*, *Headache*, *Cephalalgia*, *BMC Neurology*, and *Pain Medicine*.

His research focuses on exploring comorbid conditions associated with headache and health economics. When not practicing medicine, he loves to travel and bake.

Robert P. Cowan, MD, holds the Higgins Family Trust Endowed Professorship in Neurology and Neurosciences at Stanford University School of Medicine. He was the founding Chief of Headache Medicine at the University of Southern California Keck School of Medicine before coming to Stanford as the founding Chief of the Division of Headache and Facial Pain at Stanford University School of Medicine. He stepped down in March of 2023 to devote full time to his research, and his current title is Director of Research in the Division of Headache Medicine.

He is a founding board member and past officer of the Headache Cooperative of the Pacific (HCOP) and the Alliance for Headache Disorders Advocacy (AHDA). Dr. Cowan has over 200 peer-reviewed articles, abstracts, posters, and lectures on headache-related topics nationally and internationally. Additionally, he has authored or edited multiple books and chapters and serves on multiple editorial boards.

His current research focuses on the pathophysiology of migraine and other headache disorders with three active labs (functional imaging, deep phenotyping, and biomarkers of chronification). He is also the principal investigator of ongoing clinical trials and is actively involved in machine learning in headache medicine. He is a co-founder of BonTriage, Inc. and consults for a variety of companies in the Headache and Facial Pain sector. In his spare time, he builds furniture and writes fiction.

Contributors

Shuchi Anand, MD, MS
Department of Nephrology
Stanford University
Stanford, California, USA

Shanthi Aribindi, MD
Department of Anesthesia
Kaiser Permanente South Sacramento Medical
    Center
Sacramento, California, USA

Vamsi Aribindi, MD
Division of Cardiovascular and Thoracic Surgery
Department of Surgery
University of California, San Diego
San Diego, California, USA

Stephanie Bakaysa, MD
Department of Obstetrics and Gynecology
Hartford Healthcare Medical Group
University of Connecticut Health
Hartford, Connecticut, USA

Hailey Baker, MD, MS
Section of Rheumatology, Allergy, and
    Immunology
Yale University School of Medicine
New Haven, Connecticut, USA

Shanley Banaag, DO
Division of Hematology/Oncology
Scripps Clinic
San Diego, California, USA

Marina Basina, MD
Division of Endocrinology, Gerontology, and
    Metabolism
Stanford University Medical Center
Palo Alto, California, USA

Neha Bijjala, DO
Department of Graduate Medical Education
Scripps Mercy Hospital
San Diego, California, USA

Joshua Bilsborrow, MD, MHS
Section of Rheumatology, Allergy, and
    Immunology
Yale University School of Medicine
New Haven, Connecticut, USA

Anne Lynn S. Chang, MD
Stanford Medicine
Palo Alto, California, USA

Brandon K. Chu, MD
Division of Gastroenterology, Hepatology, and
    Nutrition
The Ohio State University Wexner Medical Center
Columbus, Ohio, USA

Fred Cohen, MD
Department of Medicine and Neurology
Icahn School of Medicine at Mount Sinai
Mount Sinai Hospital
New York, New York, USA

Carrie Costantini, MD
Division of Hematology/Oncology
San Diego, California, USA

Melissa Dang, MD
Department of Internal Medicine
Sky Ridge Medical Center
Lone Tree, Colorado, USA

Yensea M. Costas Encarnación, MD
Neurology Department
Epilepsy Division
University of Miami/Jackson
    Memorial Hospital
Miami, Florida, USA

Sarah Erdelyan, MD
Department of Psychiatry
Los Angeles General Medical Center
University of Southern California Keck School of
    Medicine
Los Angeles, California, USA

Jessica Galant-Swafford, MD
Division of Allergy and Clinical Immunology
Department of Medicine
National Jewish Health
Denver, Colorado, USA

John Garrett, PharmD
Division of Pharmacology
Scripps Clinic
San Diego, California, USA

Rahul Gomez, DO
Division of Pulmonary, Critical Care and Sleep
    Medicine
University of California, San Diego
San Diego, California, USA

Sloane Heller, MD
Division of Critical Care and Hospital
    Neurology
Columbia University Irving Medical Center
New York, New York, USA

Khadijah Hussain, MD
Departments of Internal Medicine, Graduate
    Medical Education and Cardiology
Scripps Mercy Hospital
San Diego, California, USA

Jocelyn Jiao, MD
Movement Disorders Division
Stanford University
Palo Alto, California, USA

Amy Johnson, MD
Department of Obstetrics and Gynecology
University of Connecticut Health
Farmington, Connecticut, USA
and
Department of Obstetrics and Gynecology
Hartford Hospital
Hartford, Connecticut, USA

Elisa Karhu, MD
Department of Medicine
Stanford University
Palo Alto, California, USA

Bruce J. Kimura, MD, MACP
Departments of Internal Medicine, Graduate
    Medical Education and Cardiology
Scripps Mercy Hospital
San Diego, California, USA

B.U.K. Li, MD
Department of Pediatrics
Division of Gastroenterology, Hepatology, and
    Nutrition
Medical College of Wisconsin
Milwaukee, Wisconsin, USA

Rebecca Linfield, MD
Division of Infectious Diseases
Department of Medicine
Stanford University
Palo Alto, California, USA

Alexandra Loza, DO, MS
Department of Obstetrics and Gynecology
Hartford Healthcare Medical Group
University of Connecticut Health
Hartford, Connecticut, USA

Diana V. Maslov, MD, MS
Division of Hematology/Oncology
Scripps Clinic
San Diego, California, USA

Nina Massad, MD
Miller School of Medicine
University of Miami, Florida
Miami, Florida, USA

Charisma Mylavarapu, DO
Division of Hematology/Oncology
Scripps Clinic
San Diego, California, USA

Kendra Pham, MD, MPH
Department of Neurology, Division of Headache
    and Neuro-ophthalmology
University of Utah
Salt Lake City, Utah USA

Angela Primbas, MD
Division of Geriatrics
University of California
Los Angeles, California, USA

Pamela Resnikoff, MD, MPH
Departments of Internal Medicine, Pulmonary
Medicine, and Medical Education
Scripps Mercy Hospital
San Diego, California, USA

Susan M. Seav, MD
Division of Endocrinology, Gerontology, and
    Metabolism
Stanford University Medical Center
Palo Alto, California, USA

Quinne Sember, MD
Division of Hematology/Oncology
Scripps Clinic
San Diego, California, USA

Katelyn A. Seward, DO
Departments of Internal Medicine
Graduate Medical Education and Cardiology
Scripps Mercy Hospital
San Diego, California, USA

Andrea Shields, MD, MS
Department of Obstetrics and Gynecology
University of Connecticut Health
Farmington, Connecticut, USA

Twan Sia
Department of Dermatology
Stanford University School of Medicine
Palo Alto, California, USA

Laura J. Silla, MD
Department of Neurology
University of Utah
Salt Lake City, Utah, USA

Liza Smirnoff, MD
Department of Neurology Headache Division
University of Miami
Miami, Florida, USA

Irene Sonu, MD
Division of Gastroenterology and Hepatology
Stanford University
Palo Alto, California, USA

Nivetha Subramanian, MD
Department of Nephrology
Stanford University
Stanford, California, USA

Lisa Surowiec, MD
Neurology Department, Stroke Division
University of Miami
Miami, Florida, USA

Elizabeth Thottacherry, MD
Stanford Health Care
Palo Alto, California, USA

Leticia Tornes, MD
Multiple Sclerosis Division
University of Miami
Miami, Florida, USA

Beverly Tse, MD
Department of Obstetrics and Gynecology
University of Connecticut Health
Farmington, Connecticut, USA

Marianna Vinokur, DO
Department of Neurology
Icahn School of Medicine at Mount Sinai
Mount Sinai Hospital
New York, New York, USA

Introduction to Comorbid Conditions in the Treatment of Headache

1

Leon S. Moskatel and Robert P. Cowan

In 2019, the landmark Chronic Migraine Epidemiology and Outcomes (CaMEO) study outlined an approach to modeling migraine progression based on the association between migraine and a variety of comorbidities.[1] However, the association of migraine with other medical conditions dates back hundreds of years but has remained largely observational. While there have been several recent compendiums that catalogue the various epidemiologic associations, a cohesive approach through which practitioners and patients alike can make sense of these associations has remained elusive.[2-4]

In the current work, we examine comorbid conditions of migraine in the context of shared pathophysiology, epidemiology and treatment of migraine and a myriad of diseases and conditions. We will consider migraine both as the primary condition being treated and as an ongoing chronic condition that needs consideration when other comorbidities require active management.

Before these associations and overlaps can be examined, it is critical to consider why migraine is so frequently comorbid with other conditions. Though its prevalence is high and some degree of overlap is inevitable, it is crucial to consider the greater implications of these connections beyond happenstance; it is instructive to consider this relationship in an evolutionary context. What is the evolutionary advantage, if any, to migraine?[5, 6] After several hundred thousand years of evolution, why are there still a billion people who suffer with migraine? Traits that do not afford an advantage or offer a distinct disadvantage tend to disappear. Yet migraine persists. One proposed theory is that migraine, along with other medical conditions, afford an "early warning system" to the larger group when there is danger in the environment. For example, when the environment is becoming hostile, certain individuals in the group may perceive the threat earlier and alert the group to that danger.

The diagnostic criteria, as set out in the International Classification of Headache Disorders, highlight the features of migraine (nausea, photophobia, phonophobia, vertigo, etc.) that reflect potential environmental threats, be they external (ingestion of toxic substances, dangerous levels of noise or light) or internal (fluctuations in hormones, stress).[7] Moreover, the body's response to migraine is consistent with the response to a perceived environmental threat (vomiting, darkness, silence, rest). Comorbidities, too, suggest that there is a more subtle, long-term threat from the immediate environment. Understanding migraine and possible comorbidities in this context can equip both patients and caregivers alike to better manage these conditions proactively.

DOI: 10.1201/b23330-1

In the following chapters, example upon example of the association between migraine and other medical comorbidities are presented by organ system. It is our hope that these chapters help the headache specialist and the non-specialist to consider their patients' migraine presentation, diagnosis, and treatment in the greater context of their comorbidities to help develop the best patient-centric migraine management strategy.

Thank you for picking up this volume, and we hope it will help improve lives.

REFERENCES

1. Lipton RB, Fanning KM, Buse DC, Martin VT, Hohaia LB, Adams AM, Reed ML, Goadsby PJ. Migraine progression in subgroups of migraine based on comorbidities: Results of the CaMEO Study. *Neurology.* 2019 Dec 10;*93*(24):e2224–36.
2. Caponnetto V, Deodato M, Robotti M, Koutsokera M, Pozzilli V, Galati C, Nocera G, De Matteis E, De Vanna G, Fellini E, Halili G. Comorbidities of primary headache disorders: a literature review with meta-analysis. *J Headache Pain.* 2021 Dec;*22*:1–8.
3. Lal V, Singla M. Migraine comorbidities-a discussion. *J Assoc Physicians India.* 2010 Apr 1;*54*:18–20.
4. Giamberardino MA, Martelletti P. *Comorbidities in headache disorders.* Cham: Springer International Publishing; 2018.
5. Cowan, RP. Toward a Philosophy of Migraine. *Headache.* 2019;*59*(4):481–83.
6. Loder E. What is the Evolutionary Advantage of Migraine? *Cephalalgia.* 2002;*22*(8):624–632. doi:10.1046/j.1468-2982.2002.00437.x
7. Headache Classification Committee of the International Headache Society (IHS). The International Classification of Headache Disorders, 3rd edition. *Cephalalgia.* 2018;*38*(1):1–211.

Primary Headache Disorders

2

Kendra Pham and Laura J. Silla

LEARNING OBJECTIVES

1. Review diagnostic criteria of migraine, tension-type headache, and trigeminal autonomic cephalalgias
2. Review epidemiology of migraine, tension-type headache, and trigeminal autonomic cephalalgias
3. Review pathophysiology of migraine, tension-type headache, and trigeminal autonomic cephalalgias
4. Discuss treatment for migraine, tension-type headache, and trigeminal autonomic cephalalgias
5. Be able to distinguish between different types of primary headache disorders, including among the trigeminal autonomic cephalalgias
6. Gain awareness of other primary headache disorders

MIGRAINE

Case Scenario

A 33-year-old female presents to the clinic for worsening headaches. As a teen, she recalls having headaches with menses that sometimes kept her home from school due to their severity. In college, her headache frequency increased to once per week. She delivered a baby at age 27, with improvement in headache burden during her pregnancy but with a return to her prepregnancy headache baseline shortly after delivery. Her headaches have worsened since then, and by age 31, she is reporting four to five headache days per week. She now has daily sensitivities to light, sound, smell, and nausea with her more severe attacks. Each attack lasts 12–48 hours, and she only has 0–2 headache-free days per month. Two days per month, her most severe attacks are preceded by zigzag lines in the periphery of her vision lasting 20 minutes.

DOI: 10.1201/b23330-2

3

Diagnostic Criteria for Migraine

In the previous scenario, the patient is suffering from chronic migraine and has attacks both with and without aura. According to the *International Classification of Headache Disorders, 3rd Edition (ICHD-3)*, to satisfy criteria for migraine without aura, there must be at least 5 headache attacks lasting between 4 and 72 hours with at least 2 of the following: unilateral pain, pulsating pain, moderate to severe pain intensity, or aggravation by/avoidance of routine physical activity due to the attack, and also at least one of the following: nausea and/or vomiting, or photophobia and phonophobia (1). For migraine with aura, there must be at least 2 attacks with 1 or more fully reversible aura symptoms (visual, sensory, speech, and/or language, motor, brainstem, retinal) and at least 3 of the following characteristics: at least 1 aura symptom spreads gradually over 5 or more minutes, 2 or more aura symptoms occur in succession, each individual aura symptom lasts 5–60 minutes, at least 1 aura symptom is unilateral, at least 1 aura symptom is positive, and the aura is accompanied by or followed within 60 minutes by headache (2). To be considered chronic migraine, criteria must be met not only for migraine without aura and/or migraine with aura but requires attacks to fulfill these criteria on at least 8 or more days per month with 15 or more total headache days per month for at least 3 months (3). Additional details of specific types of aura can be found in the *ICHD-3* (3).

Epidemiology of Migraine

Migraine is a leading cause of disability worldwide (4). The prevalence of migraine is reported at 12% of the US general population (18% of women, 6% of men) (5). Migraine prevalence is higher in prepubescent boys than girls, but the rate of increase is higher in girls after puberty onset (5). The worldwide prevalence of migraine is 14% (19% of women, 10% of men) (4). Migraine prevalence also varies by race when adjusted for socioeconomic status, with the highest prevalence among White women and men (20.4% and 8.6%, respectively), intermediate prevalence in African American women and men (16.2% and 7.2%, respectively), and lowest prevalence in Asian American women and men (9.2% and 4.2%, respectively) (6). Another survey showed migraine prevalence was highest among Whites (21% women, 10% men) compared to Hispanics (20.6% women, 8.4% men) and Blacks (19.6% women, 9.3% men) (7).

The incidence of migraine is reported as 8.1 per 1,000 person-years, with a peak incidence in women between ages 20 and 24 years (18.2 per 1,000 person-years) and in men between ages 15 and 19 years (6.2 per 1,000 person-years) (8, 9).

The global prevalence of chronic migraine is estimated at around 1.4%–2.2%, higher among women than men (10). Estimates are that chronic migraine accounts for 7.7% of all migraine cases, excluding probable migraine (5). The prevalence of chronic migraine is inversely related to household income (10). Chronic migraine is the most prevalent in women 18–49 years old (11). Roughly 2.5%–3.5% of people with episodic migraine go on to meet criteria for chronic migraine in the subsequent year (12). Several factors increase the risk of episodic migraine becoming chronic, including female sex, obesity, snoring, higher baseline frequency of migraine attacks, increased frequency of abortive medication use, lower socioeconomic status, and the presence of cutaneous allodynia (13). When overused, opioids and/or butalbital-containing medications are the most strongly linked to migraine chronification. Triptans and nonsteroidal anti-inflammatory drugs (NSAIDs) used ten or more days per month can also lead to migraine chronification (13). By contrast, when used up to nine days per month, NSAIDs may have a protective effect (13). Of patients with chronic migraine, 26.1% revert to episodic migraine with less than ten headache days per month, 40% transition in and out of chronic and episodic migraine, and only 33.9% have persistent chronic migraine (13). Factors associated with reversion out of chronic migraine are fewer baseline headache days (15–19 vs. 25–31 days per month), preventive medication adherence, exercise, discontinuing overused abortive medications, and absence of allodynia (13).

Pathophysiology of Migraine

A migraine attack is divided into premonitory, aura, headache, and postdrome phases (14). Distinguishing these phases was proposed as a way to better understand the pathophysiology of migraine (15).

During the premonitory phase, patients may experience yawning, polyuria, irritability, mood change, neck pain, food cravings, etc., occurring hours to days prior to the headache phase (16, 17) (Figure 2.1). Patients experiencing sensory sensitivities during the premonitory phase also more readily report light exposure, odors, and certain foods as migraine triggers, perhaps mistaking premonitory symptoms as triggers (17). During this phase, changes in positron emission tomography (PET) studies show increased activity in the occipital cortex correlated with light sensitivity (18). Activation of the rostral dorsal medulla and periaqueductal gray has been seen in PET studies correlating with nausea during the premonitory phase (19). In addition, changes seen in activity and connectivity of the hypothalamus on functional magnetic resonance imaging (fMRI) and PET studies are proposed as potential explanations for polyuria, mood, and appetite changes during this phase (17, 20).

During the aura phase, a visual aura is most commonly reported (i.e., scintillating scotoma), with sensory aura the second most common; however, other aura types can occur, such as language or motor (21). Aura is thought to be due to cortical spreading depolarization (CSD), formerly called cortical spreading depression. Based on mapping models, CSD of visual aura in humans propagates in a more linear and spatially limited manner than previously thought based on rat models where depolarization is more hemispheric and concentric (15). It is hypothesized that CSD may only represent a portion of the nervous system dysfunction seen with migraine (14).

The headache phase is characterized by not only head pain but also associated symptoms. Several neuropeptides have been implicated in its pathophysiology. Migraine is thought to be mediated via trigeminovascular activation. Classic teaching is that trigeminal sensory afferents innervate the meningeal dura, and upon sensitization of these trigeminovascular neurons, a signal is initiated that communicates with second-order neurons in the trigeminal cervical complex found in the brainstem and subsequently activates third-order neurons in the thalamus, which then, via projection of nociceptive impulses to the somatosensory cortex, leads to pain perception (22).

Various neuropeptides are thought to activate this trigeminovascular system. Calcitonin gene-related peptide (CGRP) is released during migraine attacks and remains elevated interictally in patients with chronic migraine but with a return to normal levels with the use of triptans (23–25). Likewise, migraine attacks can be brought on by an infusion of CGRP (26). CGRP is not thought to cross the blood–brain barrier well, suggesting a more peripheral role; CGRP antagonists inhibit activation of trigeminovascular neurons along the trigeminal pathway (15). Pituitary adenylate cyclase-activating polypeptide (PACAP) likely plays a similar role to CGRP, having been shown to trigger migraine attacks in susceptible individuals, and elevated levels are found in patients with migraine during attacks (15, 27). PACAP stimulates G-protein coupled receptors to initiate downstream cyclic adenosine monophosphate in close proximity to cranial vessels, thought to modulate nociceptive neurons in sensory C-fibers and A-fibers in the trigeminal vascular system (27). PACAP is also thought to play a role as a potent vasodilator in peripheral and central sensitization, as well as dural inflammation (27). Vasoactive intestinal peptide, substance P, and substance Y have been studied and have not been shown to elevate during migraine attacks, nor have drug targets blocking substance P been effective at treating migraine attacks in clinical trials (15).

The postdrome phase occurs after the resolution of the headache, often described as the "migraine hangover." Neck pain, often beginning in the premonitory phase, can persist in the postdrome (15).

Determining the exact role of genetics in migraine is ongoing but there is often a familial component. The heritability of migraine in twin studies is 42% (28). Many forms of migraine are polygenic with multiple identified loci, but monogenic forms also exist (28). For example, familial hemiplegic migraine (FHM) follows an autosomal dominant pattern of inheritance with 70%–90% penetrance and variable expressivity (28). Although considered monogenic, there are three main causative genes: FHM1 is due to mutations of the CACNA1A gene at chromosome 19p13, which is also the gene mutation implicated in

THE PHASE OF MIGRAINE: DURATION AND SEVERITY

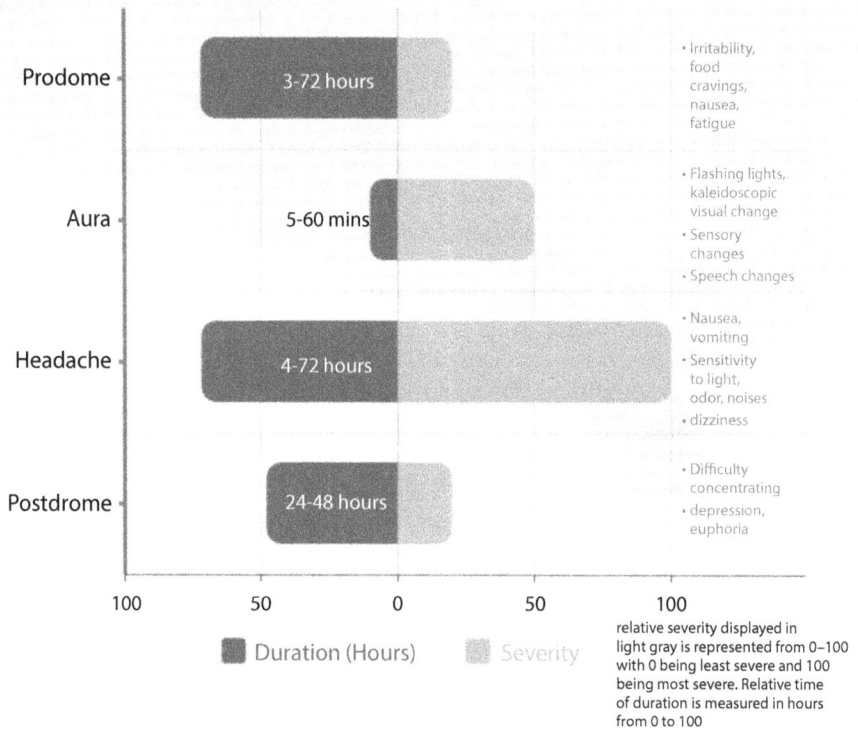

FIGURE 2.1   The Phase of Migraine.

episodic ataxia 2 and spinocerebellar ataxia 6; FHM2 is due to mutations of the ATP1A2 gene at chromosome 1q23, overlapping with epilepsy, alternating hemiplegia of childhood and migraine with brainstem aura, previously called basilar migraine; and FHM3 is due to mutations in the SCN1A gene at chromosome 2q24, overlapping with Dravet syndrome (28). A causal gene is identified in only about 25% of patients with hemiplegic migraine who undergo genetic testing, and while other genes (PPRT2, SLC2A1, PNKD, SLC1A3, and EAAT1) have been proposed, evidence to support them is limited (28).

In a large family with migraine with aura, a mutation of KCNK18 that encodes the TRESK channel was identified (28). In two families, two mutations to the gene encoding casein kinase 1δ, associated with advanced sleep phase syndrome, were found (29). Mice engineered with casein kinase 1δ mutations are more susceptible to CSD and increased pain sensitivity following administration of nitroglycerin (29). Likewise, cerebral autosomal dominant arteriopathy with subcortical infarcts and leukoencephalopathy (CADASIL) is caused by mutations of the NOTCH3 gene (28). Up to 40% of these patients have migraine with aura, which can present decades prior to its other symptoms of stroke and vascular dementia (28).

Pragmatic Approach for Treating Migraine

Treatment of migraine is individualized and may include multimodal therapies; a consistent and predictable lifestyle is the foundation for successful symptom management. Physical activity is important for weight management and improved sleep, and in one study, it was as effective as topiramate in reducing the severity and frequency of migraine attacks (30, 31). The benefit is reported with moderate and intense aerobic exercise (perhaps more tolerable when moderate), and yoga plus standard preventive medications reduced the frequency of attacks compared to preventive medications alone (32). No particular diet is shown to improve migraine; adhering to a healthy balanced diet that contributes to overall health and well-being, in some cases tailored to a patient's medical comorbidities, and eating at regular intervals is also important (30). Likewise, remaining adequately hydrated is associated with reduced headache frequency (30, 32). Sleep disorders (i.e., insomnia and sleep apnea) have a negative impact on migraine and should be screened for and treated (30). Sleep disruption is a proposed premonitory phase symptom (32). Regular caffeine use and/or its withdrawal is associated with worsened headaches, with caffeine and alcohol being the most reported migraine triggers; the likelihood of developing an attack appears largely related to variance from usual consumption (30, 32). Both stress and stress letdown are associated with migraine attacks; mindfulness and stress management strategies can be helpful in managing migraine and its related disability (32, 33). Overall, consistency and predictability in lifestyle are important, as major deviations from someone's normal routine are associated with migraine attacks (33).

Beyond lifestyle modifications, treatments for migraine are divided into two major categories: preventive and acute. Preventive treatments seek to reduce the frequency and severity of attacks and prevent chronification (34). The goal of acute treatments is pain/symptom relief and, if possible, pain/symptom freedom from an acute migraine attack.

Many medications are available, but they can also come with side effects and often require trial and error to find the right treatment; at best, medications shown to be effective have a reduction in headache days by half in 50%–60% of patients (34). This can also be limited by a patient's willingness to take a daily preventive medication, cost, accessibility, and insurance coverage (34). Being upfront about the iterative nature of migraine treatment and providing patients with some autonomy in selecting treatments may help with adherence.

Initiation of preventive therapies is considered when four to six or more headache days occur each month, fewer if severe or highly disabling, medication-overuse headache (MOH) is present, acute treatments are ineffective/contraindicated, and based on patient preference (34). Choosing medications involves consideration of medical comorbidities, avoidance and/or capitalization of potential side effects, and patient preference. Understanding pregnancy and lactation goals, as appropriate, is critical too. An adequate trial, barring intolerable side effects, is at least 8–12 weeks (35). There may be more success in discontinuing/reducing a medication the longer a patient has been headache-free on the preventive medication (34). Table 2.1 outlines available treatments for migraine prevention.

Table 2.2 shows medications available for the acute treatment of migraine. Like preventive medications, acute medications may be selected based on medical comorbidities, side effects, and patient preference. Avoiding acute medication overuse (MO) is important ($\geq$15 days per month for simple analgesics, $\geq$10 days per month for others for 3 months, even if used for other reasons) to prevent MOH (3). MO is seen in 15% of adults with episodic migraine and 50% of adults with chronic migraine using acute treatments in the United States, which can increase headache frequency and reduce productivity and quality of life (36).

Neuromodulation is a relatively new and evolving category of treatment for migraine and other primary headache disorders. Currently, Food and Drug Administration (FDA)–cleared devices include remote electrical stimulation (REN; preventive and acute), noninvasive trigeminal nerve stimulation (eTNS; preventive and acute), noninvasive vagal nerve stimulation (nVNS; preventive and acute), single-pulse transcranial magnetic stimulation (sTMS; preventive), and external combined occipital and trigeminal nerve stimulation (eCOT-NS, preventive and acute). Data exists in favor of neuromodulation devices;

TABLE 2.1 Available Preventive Medications

DRUG CATEGORIES	TYPICAL DOSING	COMMON/SERIOUS SIDE EFFECTS	COMORBIDITY BENEFITS
Antidepressant medications (TCAs, SNRIs)			
Amitriptyline	50 mg nightly	Better tolerated when uptitrated slowly, sedation, weight gain, fatigue; constipation, dry eye, dry mouth more common at higher doses, **acute angle glaucoma (contraindactation)**	Insomnia
Nortriptyline	50 mg daily	Less anticholinergic side effects as amitriptyline	
Venlafaxine	75–225 mg daily	Well tolerated, discontinuation syndrome with abrupt withdrawal	
Duloxetine	60 mg daily	Less prone to discontinuation syndrome than venlafaxine, may be used instead due to another non-headache pain indication	
Antiseizure medications			
Topiramate	100 mg daily (OR 50 mg twice daily)	**Least safe in pregnancy** (cleft palate/lip deformities, intrauterine growth restriction, metabolic acidosis, **nephrolithiasis (contraindication), acute angle glaucoma (contraindactation)**, weight loss, cognitive side effects, appendicular paresthesias	Obesity, frequent migraine aura
Valproic Acid	250–500 mg twice daily (500–1000 mg delayed release daily)	**Least safe in pregnancy** (neural tube defects, craniofacial defects, cardiovascular malformations), thrombocytopenia, hepatotoxicity, weight gain, tremor, cognitive side effect	Frequent migraine aura
Gabapentin	900–3600 mg daily divided 3 times daily	Renal disease may restrict to smaller doses, variable effect and lacking clinical trials despite commonly used, cognitive side effects	
Pregabalin	25–75 mg three times daily	Use if gabapentin is effective but poorly tolerated or stops working	
Keppra	500–1000 mg twice daily	Possible benefit, cognitive side effects	
Antihypertensive medications (Beta-blockers, calcium channel blockers, ACEis/ARBs)		(all antihypertensives contraindicated if hypotensive)	
Propranolol	60 mg once or twice daily	**More safe in pregnancy**, exacerbation of asthma, exercise intolerance, fatigue	Anxiety, hypertension

(Continued)

TABLE 2.1 (Continued) Available Preventive Medications

DRUG CATEGORIES	TYPICAL DOSING	COMMON/SERIOUS SIDE EFFECTS	COMORBIDITY BENEFITS
Metoprolol	50 mg twice daily	Cardioselective (less likely to exacerbate asthma), exercise intolerance, fatigue	Anxiety, hypertension
Verapamil	120–240 mg daily	Generally well tolerated, lack of clinical trial data despite commonly used, fatigue	Hypertension, frequent migraine aura
Lisinopril	10–40 mg daily	**Least safe in pregnancy** (oligohydramina, lung hypoplasia, renal failure, skeletal deformities, hyperkalemia, retal/neonatal death with third trimester exposure), cough	Hypertension
Candesartan	8–16 mg daily	**Least safe in pregnancy** (oligohydramina, lung hypoplasia, renal failure, skeletal deformities, hyperkalemia, retal/neonatal death with third trimester exposure)	Hypertension
OnabotulinumtoxinA (Often requires insurance prior authorization)	155–195 units every 3 months per PREEMT trial	Well tolerated, low side effect profile	
Calcitonin gene-related peptide monoclonal antibodies (Often requires insurance prior authorization)		(half life ranges between 21–31 days)	
Erenumab	70 or 140 mg subcutaneous monthly	**Least safe in pregnancy** (insufficient evidence), constipation, hypertension, injection site reaction	
Fremanezumab	225 mg subcutaneous monthly	**Least safe in pregnancy** (insufficient evidence), constipation less likely, injection site reaction more likely	
Galcanezumab	240 mg subcutaneous loading dose following by 120 mg subcutaneous monthly	**Least safe in pregnancy** (insufficient evidence), constipation less likely, injection site reaction more likely	
Eptinezumab	100–300 mg IV every 3 months	**Least safe in pregnancy** (insufficient evidence)	
Gepants (Often require insurance prior authorization)		(half life ~10 hours)	
Rimegepant	75 mg every other day	**Least safe in pregnancy** (insufficient evidence)	
Atogepant	10, 30, or 60 mg once daily	**Least safe in pregnancy** (insufficient evidence)	

(Continued)

TABLE 2.1   (Continued) Available Preventive Medications

DRUG CATEGORIES	TYPICAL DOSING	COMMON/SERIOUS SIDE EFFECTS	COMORBIDITY BENEFITS
Nutritional/herbal supplements			
Magnesium	400–600 mg daily or 200–300 mg twice daily	**More safe in pregnancy**, diarrhea, nausea	Frequent migraine aura
Riboflavin (Vitamin B2)	400 mg daily	Diarrhea, yellow discoloration of urine, increased urinary frequency	
Coenzyme Q10	300 mg daily	**More safe in pregnancy**, well tolerated	
Feverfew	50–300 mg daily	**Least safe in pregnancy** (uterine contractions, spontaneous abortion), nausea, bloating, avoid if allergies to ragweed or chamomile	
Butterbur		**Not recommended due to risk of hepatotoxicity**	
Melatonin	3 mg nightly	Sedation, fatigue	Insomnia
Other			
Memantine	10 mg twice daily	**More safe in pregnancy**, well tolerated	
Cyproheptadine	4–8 mg once daily or divided twice daily	Sedation, weight gain	

TABLE 2.2   Available Acute Medications

DRUG CATEGORIES	TYPICAL DOSING	SPECIAL CONSIDERATIONS
Analgesics		
Acetaminophen		**More safe in pregnancy**
NSAIDs		
Ibuprofen	Oral 400–800 mg	**Moderately safe for second trimester of pregnancy only** (spontaneous abortion in first trimester, premature closure of ductus arteriosus in third trimester)
Naproxen	Oral 275–825 mg	
Diclofenac	Oral 50 mg	
Celecoxib	Oral solution 120 mg	Boxed warning for serious cardiovascular thrombotic events (myocardial infarction, stroke), increased bleeding risk, gastrointestinal ulceration/perforation, **contraindications: coronary artery bypass graft surgery**
Aspirin	Oral 900–1300 mg	**Avoid for acute treatment of migraine in pregnancy** (premature closure of ductus arteriosus, fetal/neonatal hemorrhage, prenatal mortality, intrauterine growth restriction)

(Continued)

TABLE 2.2   (Continued) Available Acute Medications

DRUG CATEGORIES	TYPICAL DOSING	SPECIAL CONSIDERATIONS
Ketoralac	Intravenous OR intramuscular 30–60 mg	**Contraindications: use of another NSAID within 24 hours, coronary artery bypass graft surgery**; reduced dosing for renal impairment, weight <50 kg or age ≥65, boxed warnings for cardiovascular thrombotic events, GI bleeding
Triptans	*Taken at onset, may repeat in 2 hours if needed (max dose per 24 hours)*	Moderately to more safe in pregnancy (use second line), Contraindications: coronary artery disease, history of stroke, uncontrolled hypertension, peripheral vascular disease
Sumatriptan	Oral 50–100 mg (200 mg) Nasal 5–20 mg (40 mg) Injection 3–6 mg (12 mg)	
Rizatriptan	Oral, Oral disintegrating tablet 5–10 mg (20 mg)	
Eletriptan	Oral 20–40 mg (80 mg)	
Zolmitriptan	Oral, Oral disintegration tablets, nasal 2.5–5 mg (10 mg)	
Naratriptan	Oral 1–2.5 mg (5 mg)	May repeat in 4 hours if needed
Frovatriptan	Oral 2.5 mg (5 mg)	
Almotriptan	Oral 6.25–12.5 mg (25 mg)	
Gepants	*Taken at onset (max dose per 24 hours)*	**Least safe in pregnancy** (insufficient evidence); not known to cause medication overuse headache
Ubrogepant	Oral 50–100 mg, may repeat in 2 hours, maximum dose of 200 mg per day	
Rimegepant	Oral disintigrating tablet 75 mg (75 mg)	
Zavegepant	Nasal 10 mg (10 mg)	
Ditans	*Taken at onset (max dose per 24 hours)*	**Least safe in pregnancy** (insufficient evidence)
Lasmiditan	Oral 50–200 mg (1 dose)	Driving impairment, dizziness and sleepiness, **restrict from driving for 8 hours following use**
Ergotamine/Ergatamine derivatives		
Dyhydroergotamine	Nasal 0.5 mg per spray, may repeat in 15 minutes (4 sprays) Nasal 0.725 mg per spray, may repeat in 1 hour (2 sprays) Intravenous for status migrainosus (Raskin OR Ford protocol)	**Least safe in pregnancy** (intrauterine growth restriction, oxytocic); **contraindications: coronary artery disease, angina pectoris, history of myocardial infarction, coronary vasospasm, uncontrolled hypertension, peripheral vascular disease, severe renal or hepatic disease, use of triptan in past 24 hours**
Anti-emetics/dopamine antagonists		
Metoclopramide	Oral 5–10 mg	**More safe in pregnancy**
Promethazine	Oral 12.5–25 mg	
Prochlorperazine	Oral 5–10 mg	
Butalbital containing medications/ Opioids		Recommended to avoid use

however, studies investigating them are not standardized, some sham-controlled and others compared against standard medications with variability in outcome measures. Devices also receive the much less rigorous FDA clearance, instead of FDA approval. Their current cost and lack of insurance coverage present additional challenges. However, they are reasonable options for some patients (i.e., those who prefer nonpharmacologic management, pregnant or adolescent patients, and patients with medication-limiting medical comorbidities) (37–39).

Behavioral therapies with good evidence include cognitive behavioral therapy, biofeedback, and relaxation training, which can yield a 35%–50% reduction in migraine burden, with home-based behavioral treatments being at least as effective as clinic-based treatments (40). In 10–17-year-olds, outcomes were superior with cognitive behavioral therapy and amitriptyline compared to amitriptyline alone (40, 41). Similar findings are seen in adults with chronic tension-type headache, as discussed later. Emerging behavioral therapies with less data include acceptance and commitment therapy, mindfulness-based interventions, and sleep interventions (40).

Migraine Considerations in Pregnancy

With 21%–28% of women of childbearing age suffering from migraine (4), encountering patients with migraine who either are pregnant or desire pregnancy is likely, and preconception counseling is important. Twenty percent of patients reported avoiding pregnancy due to concerns of worsening migraine symptoms, a more difficult pregnancy, or risk of harm to their baby due to migraine (42). Sixty percent to 90% of patients with migraine without aura report improvement in their symptoms during pregnancy, over 80% with improvement in the second and third trimesters (43). Forty-four percent of women with migraine with aura experience improvement in symptoms during pregnancy, and 3%–6% will experience their first migraine attack during pregnancy (43). Headache frequency often returns to prepregnancy baseline within the first couple of months following delivery, potentially longer in women who are breastfeeding (43).

The rate of secondary headache disorders is higher during pregnancy; as many as 35% of pregnant women presenting acutely to an emergency room (ER) for headache are found to have secondary headache, 51% of which are hypertensive disorders (44). Patients with migraine are at a higher risk for gestational hypertension and preeclampsia compared to those without migraine (45). A higher preconception prevalence of hypertension is reported as an increased risk of pregnancy-associated hypertensive disorders, preeclampsia, and miscarriage in pregnant women with migraine (46). The risk for ischemic stroke in pregnant patients with active migraine is also higher (odds ratio of 7.9–30.7) (45). Risk for other vascular disorders, including acute myocardial infarction, deep vein thrombosis, and pulmonary embolism, is shown to be increased in pregnant women with migraine (45).

Neurologic complications of pregnancy and the postpartum time period may present with headache, including preeclampsia/eclampsia, posterior reversible encephalopathy syndrome (PRES), reversible cerebral vasoconstriction syndrome (RCVS), idiopathic intracranial hypertension (IIH), cerebral venous sinus thrombosis (CVST), subarachnoid hemorrhage (SAH), ischemic stroke, arterial dissection, postdural puncture headache, and pituitary apoplexy (42, 43, 47). Pregnant women with migraine are more likely than pregnant women without migraine to develop a secondary headache; however, lack of a prior history of headache in the presence of hypertension increases the risk of secondary headache in pregnant women presenting acutely for headache (42, 44). Headache due to preeclampsia can present with visual symptoms (i.e., scotoma), which could easily be confused with migraine aura (47). It is no longer thought that a progressively refractory headache presentation can distinguish preeclampsia from migraine; therefore, a low threshold for neuroimaging to look for secondary headache is recommended (47). MRI is preferred, barring emergent situations, in which case the need for computed tomography (CT) and CT angiography studies may outweigh the risks of ionizing radiation to the fetus (42). When MRI studies are used, it is recommended to avoid gadolinium (42).

Medication considerations during pregnancy are noted in Tables 2.1 and 2.2. For example, while there are no animal studies suggesting teratogenic effects of CGRP-targeted therapies, there is limited human data about their use in pregnancy; therefore, it is recommended to avoid these treatments in pregnancy. Due to the long half-life of CGRP-blocking monoclonal antibody-based treatments, discontinuation of these medications is recommended several months prior to trying to conceive (42). Triptans historically have been avoided in pregnancy and are now considered a reasonable second-line acute treatment option for migraine during pregnancy (42, 47).

TENSION-TYPE HEADACHE

Case Scenario

A 40-year-old male presents to clinic with a chief complaint of bilateral headache. He has had headaches on and off throughout his life that have not been particularly bothersome and respond to over-the-counter analgesics. Previously, these would occur at most four to six times per year during stressful days at work. Since recently becoming a father, these headaches have increased to once weekly, and when his baby cries, it bothers him. The headaches last 30 minutes to several days, never longer than 7 days. He denies sensitivity to light, nausea, or worsening of his headaches with physical activity. He does not snore or have insomnia but does wake frequently to tend to his baby. He denies any systemic symptoms. He is concerned about the recent worsening of his headaches.

Diagnostic Criteria for Tension-Type Headache

In the previous scenario, the patient is experiencing frequent tension-type headache (TTH). Previously, he had experienced infrequent TTH. According to the *ICHD-3*, he meets criteria for TTH with at least 10 headaches lasting 30 minutes to 7 days long, meeting at least two of the following: bilateral, pressing or tightening quality that is nonpulsating, symptoms not worsened by physical activity, and mild to moderate in intensity, as well as both of the following: not associated with nausea and no more than one of photophobia and phonophobia (3). TTH is divided into infrequent, frequent, and chronic types based on the number of headache days per month. Infrequent TTH occurs on less than one day per month, no more than 12 days per year, frequent TTH occurs between 1 and 14 days per month for at least 3 months, and chronic TTH occurs 15 or more days per month for at least 3 months (3). Chronic TTH also allows for mild nausea in place of photophobia or phonophobia but not moderate or severe nausea (3). When criteria for both chronic migraine and chronic TTH are met, chronic migraine should be used (3).

Epidemiology of Tension-Type Headache

TTH is the most prevalent headache disorder, with a global prevalence of 38% (2). The prevalence of TTH is higher in Europe compared to Asia and the Americas (80% vs. 20%–30%) (2). The lifelong prevalence of TTH is reported in a Danish population-based study to be 86%, with a majority of the patients having infrequent TTH (59%), 24%–37% having frequent TTH (several times per month), 10% weekly and 3%

were chronic (8). The peak prevalence of TTH is between the ages of 30–39 in men and women, the average age of onset occurs between 25–30 years old, and the male-to-female ratio is 4:5 (2, 8).

The incidence of frequent TTH is reported as 14.2 per 1,000 person-years according to a Danish epidemiologic survey with a 1:3 male-to-female ratio (8). Reported risk factors for TTH include inability to relax after work, limited sleep at nighttime, and poor self-rated health (2). Up to 47% of patients with chronic TTH are reported to achieve remission, and 12% with episodic TTH are reported to develop chronic TTH in one study (8).

Pathophysiology of Tension-Type Headache

The pathophysiology of TTH is less well reported. Both peripheral and central mechanisms have been proposed involving myofascial structures, peripheral nociception of pericranial structures, and dysregulation of pain processing pathways (48–50).

For infrequent TTH, peripheral mechanisms are felt to be predominant; muscle strain and poor posture are considered to physically trigger hyperexcitable peripheral nociceptors (48). Muscle tenderness and increased muscle hardness of the trapezius were reported to correlate with chronic TTH that remained unchanged between days with and without headache (50). Tonic muscle contraction and resultant swelling via chemical mediators, such as serotonin and bradykinin, that have induced headache when administered together but not separately, may sensitize nociceptive nerve endings (50). Neuropeptides such as substance P and CGRP have also been thought to play a potential role in myofascial pain (50).

For chronic TTH, both central and peripheral mediation of pain is proposed (48). Described qualitatively, nociception of the stimulus-response function of pressure versus pain is altered in chronic TTH, where the threshold for detection of a pressure stimulus as painful is lower, and this has been linked to pericranial tenderness (48, 50). Reduced pressure pain tolerance is indicative of allodynia, a clinical correlate of central sensitization (48, 50). One study showed an increase in central nervous system sensitivity to peripheral nociceptive stimuli (50). Pain hypersensitivity is reported with various types of stimuli and is present at both symptomatic cephalic locations and nonsymptomatic extracephalic locations, which is supportive of increased central nervous system sensitivity in chronic TTH, likely modulated at the supraspinal level (50). Central sensitization is thought to occur at the level of the dorsal horn in the trigeminal nucleus caudalis from repeated peripheral nociceptive input from pericranial myofascial tissues (48, 50). The interaction between peripheral and centrally mediated pain has been described as a positive feedback loop where peripheral sensitization occurs later, followed by central sensitization (51).

Imaging studies have also shown altered gray matter density, increased in the anterior cingulate and somatosensory cortices ictally but not interictally in episodic TTH, and decreased in the anterior cingulate and insular cortices in chronic TTH (52, 53). Decreased synchronization of neuronal activity has also been seen in cortical and subcortical areas associated with pain in fMRI studies in patients with TTH (54).

Nitric oxide is shown to increase the response to noxious stimuli at the trigeminal spinal nucleus, leading to headache and inhibition of nitric oxide synthase; subsequently, inhibiting nitric oxide has been shown to reduce pain, pericranial tenderness, and muscle hardness in chronic TTH (51). Several other neuropeptides have been studied without convincing evidence that they play a role in TTH—for example, CGRP is not altered in TTH (55).

Genetics may also play a role in the pathophysiology of TTH. In a Danish study of over 11,000 participants, there was a high concordance between monozygotic twins and episodic TTH (including infrequent and frequent TTH) and also a high concordance among twins without TTH (51). In a smaller study, a three times increased risk was seen for TTH among first-degree relatives relative to nongenetically related spouses (51).

Treatment of Tension-Type Headache

There are published guidelines for the treatment of TTH by the European Federation of Neurological Societies (56). Recommendations are to consider nonpharmacologic therapies such as biofeedback, cognitive behavioral therapy, physical therapy, and acupuncture, although for some of these modalities, evidence may be limited (56). For acute treatment, NSAIDs and simple analgesics are considered first line, with higher doses tending to be more effective but also tending to be less effective with more frequent headaches; combination analgesics are second line with caution to avoid MO, which, despite improved efficacy, may occur more readily with combination analgesics (55, 56). NSAIDs tend to work better than acetaminophen but also have more side effects (56). These guidelines recommend against triptans, muscle relaxants, and opioids for acute treatment of TTH (56). Preventive treatment is recommended in patients with chronic TTH and may be considered in frequent TTH. Amitriptyline is considered first line followed by venlafaxine and mirtazapine (55, 56). A greater reduction in headache burden by about 30% was shown at six months with combined behavioral therapy (stress management therapy) and pharmacotherapy (amitriptyline 75 mg or nortriptyline 50 mg) compared to behavioral therapy or pharmacotherapy alone (40, 57). Mirtazapine 30 mg and venlafaxine 150 mg, both serotonin and norepinephrine reuptake inhibitors, were shown to be about as effective as amitriptyline for prevention of chronic TTH; selective serotonin reuptake inhibitors have not been shown to have a preventive benefit in chronic TTH (56). Weight gain is a potential side effect of both mirtazapine and amitriptyline and should be considered mindfully in patients who already have an elevated body mass index (56). Studies have looked at other medications, such as tizanidine, memantine, and onabotulinumtoxinA, for prevention of chronic TTH but have not shown benefit (56).

Common Medical Comorbidities That Can Worsen Tension-Type Headache

Secondary headache disorders may present similarly to TTH. For example, sleep apnea headache may closely resemble chronic TTH given the bilateral yet featureless characteristics. The presence of other symptoms of sleep apnea may point away from TTH, with polysomnography helping to confirm the presence of sleep apnea (58). Headache attributed to hypothyroidism is another example of a secondary headache that is bilateral and featureless, where the presence of other symptoms of hypothyroidism may illuminate this as a contributor to a patient's headaches rather than TTH alone (58). A bidirectional relationship between TTH and psychiatric comorbidities (i.e., depression and anxiety) has also been reported and is important to identify for adequate treatment of both disorders (58). Likewise, insomnia has been shown to be more prevalent among people with TTH, and, in addition, associated with worsened headache and psychiatric symptoms (59).

TRIGEMINAL AUTONOMIC CEPHALALGIAS

Case Scenario

A 56-year-old female presents as a referral to the neurology clinic with a chief complaint of headache with left ocular itching and discomfort. She notes that she has been having continuous left-sided head pain for the last three years that waxes and wanes in intensity. She reports that sometimes she will have jolt-like stabs of pain superimposed on her existing headache that lasts for a few minutes at a time. She sometimes notices tearing and nasal congestion on the left side. The patient is adamant that her head pain is continuous, has been present for many years, and never fully goes away. Previously, the patient has used oxygen, sumatriptan, and zolmitriptan, all of which have been unhelpful. The neurologist prescribes indomethacin, which relieves her pain completely.

Types of Trigeminal Autonomic Cephalalgias

In the previous case, the patient has findings concerning for a trigeminal autonomic cephalalgia (TAC); in this case, she specifically meets criteria for hemicrania continua (3). There are several types of TACs, including hemicrania continua, cluster headache, paroxysmal hemicrania, and short-lasting unilateral neuralgiform headache attacks (SUNCT/SUNA), which are most easily distinguished by their duration and frequency, as shown in Figure 2.2.

Hemicrania Continua

Diagnostic criteria for hemicrania continua

In the previous case, the patient is having continuous pain with a sawtooth pattern of exacerbation in association with ipsilateral cranial autonomic symptoms. Hemicrania continua (HC), as the name suggests, is a continuous, unilateral headache. Per the *ICHD-3*, there must be at least one cranial autonomic symptom (as mentioned earlier) ipsilateral to the side of the pain or a sense of restlessness, agitation, or exacerbation of the pain by movement, pain lasting for at least the past three months, and pain that is absolutely responsive to indomethacin (3). There are both remitting and unremitting subtypes of HC, with unremitting occurring continuously for at least 1 year without pain freedom lasting more than 24 hours and the remitting subtype allowing for periods of symptom relief for more than 24 hours without the use of medication

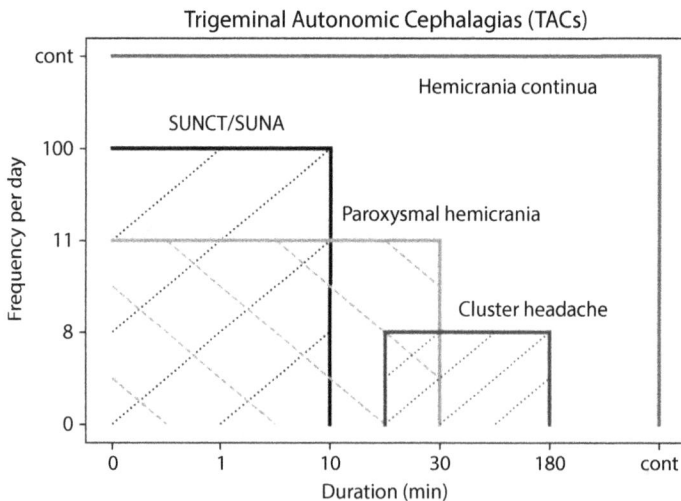

FIGURE 2.2 Trigeminal autonomic cephalalgias by duration and frequency. cluster headaches last 15–180 minutes, with an average frequency of 1–8 times per day. Paroxysmal hemicrania typically latest 2-30 minutes with an average frequency of 11 times a day. SUNCT/SUNA lasts 1–10 minutes and occurs up to 100 times a day. Hemicrania continua will last continuously. (Data source: M Eller, PJ Goadsby, Trigeminal Autonomic Cephalalgias. June 2014. Accessed Online http//doi.org/10.1111/odi.12263).

(3). It is important to note that up to 20% of patients report pain-free periods between days to months (59). HC usually occurs in a unilateral distribution behind the eye, in the forehead, and temporal region. While less severe than that of cluster headaches, the pain in HC can often have overlying attacks superimposed on the continuous pain. These attacks can range from mild to severe in intensity. Patients with HC also frequently report ocular itchiness or pain, called "false foreign body sensation" (59).

Epidemiology of hemicrania continua

It is estimated that HC occurs in approximately 2% of all patients who present to neurology clinics for headache and is found in about 0.8% of all patients presenting for daily headache (60, 61). The male-to-female ratio is 2:1, with onset most typically in the fourth to sixth decades of life (62, 63). Cranial autonomic features may be less pronounced in patients with HC compared with other TACs but also may exhibit more features typical of migraine (62).

Pathophysiology of hemicrania continua

The pathophysiology for TACs is less well understood, with a majority of data coming from research on cluster headache. The pathophysiology of TACs is thought to involve the trigeminal vascular system and autonomic system via the trigeminal autonomic reflex and the hypothalamus; there may also be a role for the vagus nerve in the pathophysiology of TACs (65). Additionally, there is a potential role for molecular signaling, including the involvement of CGRP, substance P, PACAP-38, neurokinin-A, VIP, orexin, and melatonin (65). Cranial autonomic symptoms of TACs are thought to be due primarily to parasympathetic activation, but also sympathetic inactivation mediated by the superior salivatory nucleus and sphenopalatine ganglion (65). PET studies have shown the involvement of the hypothalamus. In HC, activation of the contralateral posterior hypothalamus and ipsilateral rostral pons has been demonstrated and shown to be blocked by intramuscular indomethacin in PET studies (66).

Treatment of hemicrania continua

The response to indomethacin in HC is often so profound that, in some instances, it is reasonable to trial a patient on a three-week course of indomethacin to help differentiate between TACs (67). If there is no response after a one- to two-week trial of indomethacin (at least 75 mg three times daily), the clinician should reconsider the diagnosis of HC (62). In the previous case, the patient failed therapies largely associated with other TACS, and her response to indomethacin helped to secure the diagnosis of HC. More treatments for patients who cannot tolerate indomethacin are discussed later in the chapter.

Paroxysmal Hemicrania

Diagnostic criteria for paroxysmal hemicrania

A close relative of HC, paroxysmal hemicrania (PH) is instead characterized by sudden, brief, unilateral attacks of pain (or "paroxysms") that occur throughout the day. To meet the diagnostic criteria for PH, patients need to have at least 20 attacks of severe, unilateral orbital, supraorbital, or temporal pain lasting 2–30 minutes that must occur more than 5 times a day for more than half of the patient's attack periods, with at least one cranial autonomic symptom or a sense of restlessness. The attacks must also be prevented by therapeutic doses of indomethacin (3). In episodic PH, attacks occur for seven days to one year with remissions of pain lasting at least three months; in chronic PH, remission periods last less than three months (3). PH attacks will often occur frequently, with reports of up to 105 attacks per day, though typically ranging from 6–11 daily attacks (68). The pain is noted to be excruciating, sharp, stabbing, or burning. PH attacks last from 2–30 minutes, with prospective studies showing a duration of up to 10 hours, though on average is 21–26 minutes (3, 69). Alternation of sides of head pain is atypical; pain tends to remain side-locked. The pain is most commonly in the V1 distribution of the trigeminal nerve (CNV) with temporal, orbital, or retro-orbital involvement but has also been reported in the neck, ears, teeth, and even the ipsilateral arm and shoulder (68, 69). Interestingly, some patients can experience migrainous symptoms during attacks of PH, such as photophobia or nausea. In one study, 66% of patients noted that photophobia was unilateral and ipsilateral to the side of pain, a feature that is not typically shared with migraine (70).

Epidemiology of paroxysmal hemicrania

PH is estimated to occur in 1 in 25,000 individuals (68, 71) in a 1:1 male-to-female ratio, though other studies demonstrate a female predominance (72). PH is most likely to occur in the third to fourth decade of life, with 80% of cases being the chronic subtype (65).

Pathophysiology of paroxysmal hemicrania

The pathophysiology of PH is not yet fully understood. However, one proposed mechanism of PH concerns the trigeminovascular pathways, specifically with the involvement of CNV1 (73). PET studies and fMRI have revealed findings suggesting that PH attacks involve the contralateral posterior hypothalamus, dorsal rostral pons, ventrolateral midbrain, and pontomedullary junction (74). It is theorized that PH acts through the release of neuropeptides orexin-A and orexin-B, which are crucial to signal relay in CNV (75).

Treatment of paroxysmal hemicrania

In the patient where PH is suspected, it is imperative to trial oral indomethacin with an initial therapeutic dose of 150 mg daily increased up to 225 mg daily, or 100–200 mg intravenously, as PH will have a profound and absolute response to indomethacin therapy that can take effect in as little as one to two days (76). For this reason, indomethacin can be a helpful diagnostic tool. In fact, an "indotest," which consists of intramuscular indomethacin, may show resolution of symptoms in patients with PH within an average of 11 hours. Unfortunately, IM indomethacin is currently not available in the United States (74, 75).

Patients who cannot take indomethacin

For patients who cannot take indomethacin, such as those with gastrointestinal or kidney dysfunction, melatonin at high doses (9–20 mg nightly) could be offered as an alternative, as several case reports have demonstrated response in patients with HC and cluster headache (67, 102). The effectiveness of melatonin in lieu of indomethacin is likely due to the fact that these two medications share a similar chemical structure (103). For PH and HC, other treatments to consider include verapamil, acetazolamide, topiramate, gabapentin, lamotrigine, cyclooxygenase-2 inhibitors (may have similar limitations to use as indomethacin), and nerve blocks (104–106). OnabotulinumtoxinA has shown clinically significant benefit in some patients with HC in a limited case series with doses ranging between 110–185 units (107).

Boswellia serrata, also known as frankincense, was shown to reduce frequency and severity of attacks in chronic cluster headache in four patients and is occasionally trialed as a treatment for HC given reported benefit and a good tolerability profile (108, 109).

Cluster Headache

Diagnostic criteria for cluster headache

Cluster headache (CH) is a strictly side-locked headache with a range of severe, very severe, and excruciating orbital, supraorbital, or temporal pain lasting 15–180 minutes and occurring every other day up to

8 times per day. This is usually associated with ipsilateral cranial autonomic symptoms and/or a sense of restlessness or agitation (3). Patients will often present with agitation and pacing, and will sometimes even note cutaneous allodynia (3, 78).

Around 80%–90% of patients will present with *episodic* CH, meaning that attacks typically occur in "clusters" present for weeks to months with times of pain-free remission lasting from months to years (3). According to the *ICHD-3*, untreated cluster periods should last between seven days and one year, and periods of pain-free remission at least three months long (3). Other patients, however, have *chronic* CH, with remission of attacks lasting less than three months or pain occurring for a year without remission (3).

Epidemiology of cluster headache

CH is believed to occur three times more frequently in men than women, with a wider range depending on age of onset (79, 80). For onset between the ages of 20–49 years old, the male-to-female ratio is 7.2:1 for episodic CH and 11:1 for chronic CH. For onset after 50 years old, the male-to-female ratio is 2.3:1 for episodic CH and 0.6:1 for chronic CH (79). However, recent studies indicate that the male predominance of CH may be inaccurate due to underdiagnosis of CH in women who were initially misdiagnosed with migraine (80). CH occurs in 0.1% of the population, typically with onset in the second to fourth decade of life (81). In women, the average onset of chronic CH is bimodal, with peaks in the second and sixth decades of life (79). One epidemiological study shows a lifetime prevalence of CH ranging from 0.06% to 0.3% (82). In addition, surveys show that chronic tobacco and secondary exposure to tobacco smoke may be associated with CH (62). Both episodic and chronic CH also have circadian rhythmicity, with attacks most commonly observed in spring and fall (83).

Pathophysiology of cluster headache

The pathophysiology of CH, while better understood than that of other TACs is yet to be fully explored. Thought of as a neurovascular headache, CH is likely due to activation of the trigeminal vascular system and the trigeminal autonomic reflex. This occurs due to increased parasympathetic activity via a trigeminal-hypothalamic pathway with the involvement of trigeminal and facial nerves, and the hypothalamus (65, 79). Ipsilateral activation of the hypothalamus has also been seen in PET and fMRI studies (84, 85). Another proposed mechanism suggests that CH is caused by inflammation in the walls of the cavernous sinus secondary to sympathetic and trigeminal c-fiber injury along the intracranial carotid artery (86). Additionally, the release of CGRP has been demonstrated to occur during CH attacks; likewise, administration of CGRP has been shown to trigger attacks in a patient while in an active disease phase but not during the remission phase, suggesting that CGRP may play a role in the mechanism and subsequent treatment of CH (23, 87). By contrast, CGRP plasma levels have been observed to be lower in patients with chronic CH compared with those with episodic CH in remission (88).

Treatment of cluster headache

Treatment of CH can be divided into acute, preventive, and bridging therapies, which aim to help reduce attack frequency until preventive therapies are optimized. Acute treatment is 100% oxygen delivered at a rate of at least 12 liters per minute via a non-rebreather mask for 20 minutes and/or use of an injectable or intranasal triptan, such as sumatriptan or zolmitriptan, administered at headache onset (83). Subcutaneous sumatriptan is considered more effective than nasal triptans and tends to be more effective at higher doses. Additionally, subcutaneous sumatriptan is more effective in episodic CH than chronic CH (83). Oral triptans are not recommended due to their slower time to onset and CH's shorter duration of attacks (83). Aerosolized ergotamine derivatives could be considered, as they can reduce the severity of attacks, but they have not been shown to reduce the duration of attacks (83). Bridging therapies consist of corticosteroids and can be administered orally, intravenously, or via ipsilateral greater occipital nerve injections (83).

Preventive treatments are used in patients with chronic CH or in those where the duration of the active cluster phase is suspected to be at least four weeks long. Verapamil is a preferred preventive treatment for

CH, often requiring daily doses of 240–480 mg, sometimes as high as 960 mg daily, and requires a baseline electrocardiogram (EKG) and repeat EKG with each 160 mg increase (83). Verapamil is also considered first line to treat CH in pregnancy and lactation (89).

Galcanezumab 300 mg monthly has an FDA indication for the prevention of CH and showed a 52% reduction in attack frequency in the initial three weeks compared to a 27% reduction in attack frequency in the placebo group (83). Other preventive treatments to consider for CH include lithium, topiramate, valproic acid, gabapentin, and melatonin (83). Noninvasive vagal nerve stimulation has also been shown to be effective in the treatment of CH (65). Currently, other therapies under investigation for CH include eptinezumab, onabotulinumtoxinA, pasireotide, ketamine, and psychedelics such as psilocybin and lysergic acid diethylamide (LSD) (83, 90).

Short-Lasting Unilateral Neuralgiform Headache Attacks (SUNCT/SUNA)

Diagnostic criteria for SUNCT/SUNA

Short-lasting unilateral neuralgiform headache attacks include short-lasting unilateral neuralgiform headache attacks with conjunctival injection and tearing (SUNCT) and short-lasting unilateral neuralgiform headache attacks with cranial autonomic symptoms (SUNA). These headaches are characterized by short-lasting, severe attacks of pain, typically in the V1 and V2 distribution but sometimes in the V3 distribution. As the name suggests, patients with SUNCT will show conjunctival injection and tearing. In SUNA, patients can have conjunctival injection or tearing, but *not both*. Outside of this difference, SUNCT and SUNA are quite similar. The patient is required to have had at least 20 attacks of moderate to severe unilateral head, orbital, supraorbital, temporal, or trigeminal pain lasting 1–600 seconds to meet SUNCT's and SUNA's respective diagnostic criteria. These attacks occur as single stabs, a series of stabs, or in a sawtooth pattern with at least one cranial autonomic symptom ipsilateral to the pain and occurring at least once daily (3). SUNCT and SUNA are considered episodic if attacks occur for seven days to one year untreated with remission lasting at least three months; chronic if remission is less than three months (3).

SUNCT/SUNA is often brought on by benign activities such as brushing teeth, talking, washing hair, and even exposure to bright lights, though most attacks occur spontaneously (91). Unilateral exacerbation by benign triggers may lead to SUNCT/SUNA being misdiagnosed as trigeminal neuralgia (TN) due to their shared characteristic of ability to evoke pain from minor stimuli (92). While conjunctival injection and/or tearing can occur in TN, it is typically less profound than seen in SUNCT (93, 94). In addition, patients with TN have noted a refractory period following attacks, whereas patients with SUNCT/SUNA typically do not have a refractory period (91). Another way to differentiate SUNCT/SUNA from TN is that TN tends to favor V2 and V3 distributions of CNV, whereas SUNCT/SUNA seems to favor the V1 distribution (95).

Epidemiology of SUNCT/SUNA

SUNCT and SUNA are considered rare, with a prevalence between 1 to 100 per 100,000, with SUNCT around five times more common than SUNA and a typical age of onset between 40–70 years old (65). A more concrete estimate of prevalence is currently lacking (82, 96). One study found SUNCT/SUNA to be more common in females, with the female-to-male ratio greater in SUNA than SUNCT (2.4:1 and 1.2:1, respectively) (91).

Pathophysiology of SUNCT/SUNA

Currently, the leading hypothesis of the pathophysiology of SUNCT/SUNA concerns the hypothalamus and its regulatory actions on trigeminovascular nociceptive pathways and the trigeminal autonomic reflex, as has been the case for the other TACs as already described (65). fMRI has shown activation in the ipsilateral hypothalamus during pain events (97). A peripheral component has also been proposed due to neurovascular conflict with the trigeminal nerve based on limited case reports (98, 99).

Treatment of SUNCT/SUNA

Lamotrigine is the first line treatment for prevention of SUNCT/SUNA, with two-thirds of patients experiencing improvement, more so with SUNCT than SUNA and episodic than chronic presentations; the best responses are found at 200 mg per day (100). Other potentially beneficial medications include carbamazepine, oxcarbazepine, topiramate, and gabapentin (73, 100). Greater occipital nerve blocks, intravenous lidocaine, and a short course of corticosteroids have been used with variable efficacy as bridging treatments (100). SUNCT/SUNA will typically not respond to indomethacin, oxygen, or sumatriptan, which can help further narrow the diagnosis (101).

OTHER PRIMARY HEADACHE DISORDERS

While migraine, TTH, and TACs are most frequently encountered in practice, there are several other lesser-known types of primary headache disorders with which one may contend. As a general rule, the clinician should always attempt to rule out other more serious causes of headache prior to establishing a diagnosis of a primary headache disorder. According to the *ICHD-3*, there are currently 10 "other" primary headache disorders. A select few are discussed in the following text.

Case Scenario

A 50-year-old businessman presents to the emergency department for a headache. He notes that for the last several months, he has had a small, 2 cm, well-circumscribed, and coin-like area of "pressing" pain on the parietal region of his right scalp. He can elicit this pain with a gentle touch of the area. He denotes the pain as being mild at most, but due to a recent diagnosis of melanoma, he is concerned that the pain may be a result of skin cancer. Upon evaluation, examination of the scalp showed male-patterned baldness without overlying skin lesion or abrasion.

Overview of the Other Primary Headache Disorders

Nummular headache

In the previous example, the patient notes a well-circumscribed region of the scalp where he feels pain. This scenario is indicative of a nummular headache, from the Latin "*nummus*" meaning "coin." Also referred to as the "Harry Potter Headache" (110), nummular headache is best understood as a small, well-defined, and fixed area (usually 1–6 cm in diameter) present on the scalp where the headache is concentrated (3). Thought to be due to focal neuralgia of the trigeminal nerve, this headache type is less common and is noted to occur in 6.4 out of every 100,000 individuals, predominantly in females (111). The key component in diagnosis is that this headache must be well-circumscribed and limited to the scalp area. While the patient can have a variety of sensations, such as throbbing, pressing, or stabbing, other neurological symptoms are absent, and their presence should prompt the clinician to consider an alternate diagnosis (3). There have been reports of nummular headaches, which are often round or elliptical, occurring in two locations on the scalp, though most commonly, they are found in one location on the parietal scalp (112). Symptomatic treatment of nummular headaches may be achieved through the use of oral medications or local injections. In one prospective observational study, over-the-counter (OTC) analgesics have been shown to be effective (greater than 50% reduction in pain) in 72% of patients (113). Another study has demonstrated effectiveness with preventive medications such as gabapentin, amitriptyline, and lamotrigine (114).

If patients do not respond to OTC analgesics or preventive medications, some studies have found that onabotulinumtoxinA can be effective for nummular headache, typically using five units per injection site in the affected area (115). This vignette also demonstrates the importance of a physical exam of the head on initial evaluation; prior to diagnosis, an overlying skin disorder or other pathology should be ruled out.

Headache attributed to sexual activity

Primary headache associated with sexual activity, previously known as coital or orgasmic cephalalgia, is a headache that occurs only in the setting of sexual activity. These headaches will occur either in an explosive fashion immediately prior to or just after orgasm or increase linearly with increasing sexual excitement. In some cases, both of these situations will occur (3). Headaches that develop preorgasm can last anywhere from 1 minute to 180 minutes. In headaches that occur during orgasm or immediately prior, patients have noted a more "explosive" type headache that, while lasting fewer than 15 minutes, has an ensuing throbbing component that persists for hours after the initial explosive-like episode (116). While pre-orgasmic and orgasmic subtypes have previously been differentiated in *ICHD-1* and *ICHD-2*, this is now considered one headache type with varying presentations. The demographics of this headache are not well documented, likely due to reluctance to self-report. Estimates place primary headache attributed to sexual activity occurring in approximately 1% of the population, with a 3:1 male-to-female ratio (117, 118). This headache type has been shown to occur at any age; two-thirds of cases report bilateral head pain that is typically occipital or diffuse and is described as "pressure-like" or "throbbing." Severe symptoms last minutes, whereas a more moderate headache in these patients has been shown to persist for 24 to 72 hours (3, 119, 120)

The pathophysiology of this headache is likely due to excessive contraction of the neck or jaw muscles, as well as trigeminovascular activation that then subsequently results in vasodilation (121, 122).

Upon evaluation of the patient with a sudden and explosive headache, it is prudent for the clinician to rule out other potentially life-threatening causes such as SAH, RCVS, and intracerebral hemorrhage (ICH), among others. Thus, prior to diagnosing headache associated with sexual activity, neuroimaging is highly recommended.

In terms of treatment, triptans are first line for acute therapies. Fifty percent of patients show benefit from zolmitriptan (IN) or sumatriptan (SubQ) (123). However, if these medications are contraindicated in the patient, NSAIDs, such as naproxen, IV/IM ketorolac, IV metoclopramide, or IV prochlorperazine, are also shown to be of benefit and should be selected based on the patient's comorbidities. For preventative treatment, patients may take indomethacin or propranolol as needed 30–60 minutes prior to sexual activity. For those for whom this level of planning is not possible, patients may consider daily indomethacin or propranolol, showing up to 80%–90% efficacy in one case series (124). Luckily, spontaneous remission is high (124).

Primary thunderclap headache

Arguably, the headache necessitating the most urgent evaluation, a thunderclap headache is an excruciatingly painful headache that reaches maximum intensity within one minute of onset (3). The patient presenting with a thunderclap headache must be emergently evaluated, as numerous etiologies for thunderclap headache exist, including RCVS, CVST, SAH, and others. Typically, patients need to undergo extensive workup for primary thunderclap headache, as it is a diagnosis of exclusion and can only be made when all other underlying causes have been ruled out. An underlying cause for thunderclap headache is found in up to 71% of patients (125). Primary thunderclap headache does remain controversial, as retrospective review of some cases reflects evidence of missed diagnoses. In fact, diagnosis of primary thunderclap headache may only be made in the setting of normal brain and vessel imaging, as well as normal lumbar puncture studies (3). The pathophysiology of this disorder is not yet known (126).

SUMMARY

- Headache is cited as the second-most common presenting chief complaint to a neurology clinic.
- The global prevalence of headache is 47%, a majority of which is accounted for by primary headache disorders (2).
- TTH is the most common primary headache disorder, followed by migraine.
- Primary headache disorders are divided into the following categories: migraine, TTH, trigeminal autonomic cephalalgias, and other primary headache disorders.
- Trigeminal autonomic cephalalgias are most easily distinguished by frequency and duration of attacks.
- Treatment varies by headache type, often an iterative process, taking into account medical comorbidities, side effects, and patient preference.

REFERENCES

1. Ahmed ZA, Faulkner LR. Headache education in adult neurology residency: A survey of program directors and chief residents: Headache. *Headache J Head Face Pain*. 2016 May;*56*(5):871–7.
2. Jensen R, Stovner LJ. Epidemiology and comorbidity of headache. *Lancet Neurol*. 2008 Apr;*7*(4):354–61.
3. Headache classification committee of the international headache society (IHS) the international classification of headache disorders, 3rd edition. *Cephalalgia*. 2018 Jan;*38*(1):1–211.
4. Feigin VL, Nichols E, Alam T, Bannick MS, Beghi E, Blake N, et al. Global, regional, and national burden of neurological disorders, 1990–2016: A systematic analysis for the Global Burden of Disease Study 2016. *Lancet Neurol*. 2019 May;*18*(5):459–80.
5. Burch RC, Buse DC, Lipton RB. Migraine. *Neurol Clin*. 2019 Nov;*37*(4):631–49.
6. Stewart WF, Lipton RB, Liberman J. Variation in migraine prevalence by race. *Neurology*. 1996 Jul;*47*(1):52–9.
7. Loder S, Sheikh HU, Loder E. The prevalence, burden, and treatment of severe, frequent, and migraine headaches in US minority populations: Statistics from national survey studies. *Headache J Head Face Pain*. 2015 Feb;*55*(2):214–28.
8. Lyngberg AC, Rasmussen BK, Jørgensen T, Jensen R. Incidence of primary headache: A Danish epidemiologic follow-up study. *Am J Epidemiol*. 2005 Jun 1;*161*(11):1066–73.
9. Stewart W, Wood C, Reed M, Roy J, Lipton R. Cumulative lifetime migraine incidence in women and men. *Cephalalgia*. 2008 Nov;*28*(11):1170–8.
10. Natoli J, Manack A, Dean B, Butler Q, Turkel C, Stovner L, et al. Global prevalence of chronic migraine: A systematic review. *Cephalalgia*. 2010 May;*30*(5):599–609.
11. Buse DC, Manack AN, Fanning KM, Serrano D, Reed ML, Turkel CC, et al. Chronic migraine prevalence, disability, and sociodemographic factors: Results from the American migraine prevalence and prevention study. *Headache J Head Face Pain*. 2012 Nov;*52*(10):1456–70.
12. Bigal ME, Serrano D, Buse D, Scher A, Stewart WF, Lipton RB. Acute migraine medications and evolution from episodic to chronic migraine: A longitudinal population-based study. *Headache J Head Face Pain*. 2008 Sep;*48*(8):1157–68.
13. Schwedt TJ. Chronic migraine. *BMJ*. 2014 Mar 24;*348*(5):g1416–g1416.
14. Charles A. Migraine: A brain state. *Curr Opin Neurol*. 2013 Jun;*26*(3):235–9.
15. Charles A. The pathophysiology of migraine: Implications for clinical management. *Lancet Neurol*. 2018 Feb;*17*(2):174–82.

16. Lampl C, Rudolph M, Deligianni CI, Mitsikostas DD. Neck pain in episodic migraine: premonitory symptom or part of the attack? *J Headache Pain.* 2015 Dec;*16*(1):80.

17. Schulte LH, Jürgens TP, May A. Photo-, osmo- and phonophobia in the premonitory phase of migraine: mistaking symptoms for triggers? *J Headache Pain.* 2015 Dec;*16*(1):14.

18. Maniyar FH, Sprenger T, Schankin C, Goadsby PJ. Photic hypersensitivity in the premonitory phase of migraine - A positron emission tomography study. *Eur J Neurol.* 2014 Sep;*21*(9):1178–83.

19. Maniyar FH, Sprenger T, Schankin C, Goadsby PJ. The origin of nausea in migraine–A PET study. *J Headache Pain.* 2014 Dec;*15*(1):84.

20. Maniyar FH, Sprenger T, Monteith T, Schankin C, Goadsby PJ. Brain activations in the premonitory phase of nitroglycerin-triggered migraine attacks. *Brain.* 2014 Jan;*137*(1):232–41.

21. Viana M, Sances G, Linde M, Ghiotto N, Guaschino E, Allena M, et al. Clinical features of migraine aura: Results from a prospective diary-aided study. *Cephalalgia.* 2017 Sep;*37*(10):979–89.

22. Dominguez-Moreno R, Do TP, Ashina M. Calcitonin gene-related peptide and pituitary adenylate cyclase-activating polypeptide in migraine treatment. *Curr Opin Endocrinol Diabetes Obes.* 2022 Apr;*29*(2):225–31.

23. Goadsby PJ, Edvinsson L, Ekman R. Vasoactive peptide release in the extracerebral circulation of humans during migraine headache. *Ann Neurol.* 1990 Aug;*28*(2):183–7.

24. Cernuda-Morollon E, Larrosa D, Ramon C, Vega J, Martinez-Camblor P, Pascual J. Interictal increase of CGRP levels in peripheral blood as a biomarker for chronic migraine. *Neurology.* 2013 Oct 1;*81*(14):1191–6.

25. Ramón C, Cernuda-Morollón E, Pascual J. Calcitonin gene-related peptide in peripheral blood as a biomarker for migraine. *Curr Opin Neurol.* 2017 Jun;*30*(3):281–6.

26. Ashina M, Hansen JM, Olesen J. Pearls and pitfalls in human pharmacological models of migraine: 30 years' experience. *Cephalalgia.* 2013 Jun;*33*(8):540–53.

27. Amin FM, Hougaard A, Schytz HW, Asghar MS, Lundholm E, Parvaiz AI, et al. Investigation of the pathophysiological mechanisms of migraine attacks induced by pituitary adenylate cyclase-activating polypeptide-38. *Brain.* 2014 Mar;*137*(3):779–94.

28. Sutherland HG, Griffiths LR. Genetics of migraine: Insights into the molecular basis of migraine disorders. *Headache J Head Face Pain.* 2017 Apr;*57*(4):537–69.

29. Brennan KC, Bates EA, Shapiro RE, Zyuzin J, Hallows WC, Huang Y, et al. Casein Kinase Iδ mutations in familial migraine and advanced sleep phase. Sci Transl Med. 2013 May;*5*(183).

30. Varkey E, Cider Å, Carlsson J, Linde M. Exercise as migraine prophylaxis: A randomized study using relaxation and topiramate as controls. *Cephalalgia.* 2011 Oct;*31*(14):1428–38.

31. Agbetou M, Adoukonou T. Lifestyle modifications for migraine management. *Front Neurol.* 2022 Mar 18;*13*:719467.

32. Seng EK, Martin PR, Houle TT. Lifestyle factors and migraine. *Lancet Neurol.* 2022 Oct;*21*(10):911–21.

33. Seng EK, Gosnell I, Sutton L, Grinberg AS. Behavioral management of episodic migraine: Maintaining a healthy consistent lifestyle. *Curr Pain Headache Rep.* 2022 Mar;*26*(3):247–52.

34. Burch R. Preventive migraine treatment. *Contin Lifelong Learn Neurol.* 2021 Jun;*27*(3):613–32.

35. Ailani J, Burch RC, Robbins MS, The board of directors of the American headache society. The American headache society consensus statement: Update on integrating new migraine treatments into clinical practice. *Headache J Head Face Pain.* 2021 Jul;*61*(7):1021–39.

36. Schwedt TJ, Hentz JG, Sahai-Srivastava S, Murinova N, Spare NM, Treppendahl C, et al. Patient-centered treatment of chronic migraine with medication overuse: A prospective, randomized. *Pragmatic Clinical Trial. Neurology.* 2022 Apr 5;*98*(14):e1409–21.

37. Peretz A, Stark-Inbar A, Harris D, Tamir S, Shmuely S, Ironi A, et al. Safety of remote electrical neuromodulation for acute migraine treatment in pregnant women: A retrospective controlled survey-study. *Headache J Head Face Pain.* 2023 Jul;*63*(7):968–70.

38. Hershey AD, Irwin S, Rabany L, Gruper Y, Ironi A, Harris D, et al. Comparison of remote electrical neuromodulation and standard-care medications for acute treatment of migraine in adolescents: A Post Hoc analysis. Pain Med. 2022 Apr 8;*23*(4):815–20.

39. Jicha and Pham (2024) Neuromodulation for primary headache disorders: Advantages and challenges. *Headache 64* (2) 226–228. DOI https://doi.org/10.1111/head.14671

40. Vekhter D, Robbins MS, Minen M, Buse DC. Efficacy and feasibility of behavioral treatments for migraine, headache, and pain in the acute care setting. *Curr Pain Headache Rep.* 2020 Oct;*24*(10):66.

41. Powers SW, Kashikar-Zuck SM, Allen JR, LeCates SL, Slater SK, Zafar M, et al. Cognitive behavioral therapy plus amitriptyline for chronic migraine in children and adolescents: A randomized clinical trial. *JAMA.* 2013 Dec 25;*310*(24):2622.

42. Rayhill M. Headache in pregnancy and lactation. *Contin Lifelong Learn Neurol*. 2022 Feb;*28*(1):72–92.

43. Van Casteren DS, Van Den Brink AM, Terwindt GM. Migraine and other headache disorders in pregnancy. In: Handbook of Clinical Neurology [Internet]. Elsevier; 2020 [cited 2023 Aug 30]. p. 187–99. Available from: https://linkinghub.elsevier.com/retrieve/pii/B9780444642400000118

44. Robbins MS, Farmakidis C, Dayal AK, Lipton RB. Acute headache diagnosis in pregnant women: A hospital-based study. *Neurology*. 2015 Sep 22;*85*(12):1024–30.

45. Wabnitz A, Bushnell C. Migraine, cardiovascular disease, and stroke during pregnancy: Systematic review of the literature. *Cephalalgia*. 2015 Feb;*35*(2):132–9.

46. Skajaa N, Szépligeti SK, Xue F, Sørensen HT, Ehrenstein V, Eisele O, et al. Pregnancy, birth, neonatal, and postnatal neurological outcomes after pregnancy with migraine. *Headache J Head Face Pain*. 2019 Jun;*59*(6):869–79.

47. Burch R. Headache in pregnancy and the puerperium. *Neurol Clin*. 2019 Feb;*37*(1):31–51.

48. Monteith TS, Oshinsky ML. Tension-type headache with medication overuse: Pathophysiology and clinical implications. *Curr Pain Headache Rep*. 2009 Dec;*13*(6):463–9.

49. Jensen R. Mechanisms of tension-type headache. *Cephalalgia*. 2001 Sep;*21*(7):786–9.

50. Bendtsen L. Central sensitization in tension-type headache—Possible pathophysiological mechanisms. *Cephalalgia*. 2000 Jun;*20*(5):486–508.

51. Chen Y. Advances in the pathophysiology of tension-type headache: From stress to central sensitization. *Curr Pain Headache Rep*. 2009 Dec;*13*(6):484–94.

52. Chen WT, Chou KH, Lee PL, Hsiao FJ, Niddam DM, Lai KL, et al. Comparison of gray matter volume between migraine and "strict-criteria" tension-type headache. *J Headache Pain*. 2018 Dec;*19*(1):4.

53. Chen B, He Y, Xia L, Guo LL, Zheng JL. Cortical plasticity between the pain and pain-free phases in patients with episodic tension-type headache. *J Headache Pain*. 2016 Dec;*17*(1):105.

54. Wang P, Du H, Chen N, Guo J, Gong Q, Zhang J, et al. Regional homogeneity abnormalities in patients with tensiontype headache: a resting-state fMRI study. *Neurosci Bull*. 2014 Dec;*30*(6):949–55.

55. Steel SJ, Robertson CE, Whealy MA. Current understanding of the pathophysiology and approach to tension-type headache. *Curr Neurol Neurosci Rep*. 2021 Oct;*21*(10):56.

56. Bendtsen L, Evers S, Linde M, Mitsikostas DD, Sandrini G, Schoenen J. EFNS guideline on the treatment of tension-type headache - Report of an EFNS task force: Guideline for treatment of tension-type headache. *Eur J Neurol*. 2010 Nov;*17*(11):1318–25.

57. Holroyd KA, O'Donnell FJ, Stensland M, Lipchik GL, Cordingley GE, Carlson BW. Management of chronic tension-type headache with tricyclic antidepressant medication, stress management therapy, and their combination: A randomized controlled trial. *JAMA*. 2001 May 2;*285*(17):2208.

58. Sacco S, Ricci S, Carolei A. Tension-type headache and systemic medical disorders. *Curr Pain Headache Rep*. 2011 Dec;*15*(6):438–43.

59. Kim J, Cho SJ, Kim WJ, Yang KI, Yun CH, Chu MK. Insomnia in tension-type headache: a population-based study. *J Headache Pain*. 2017 Dec;*18*(1):95.

60. Cittadini E, Goadsby PJ. Hemicrania continua: a clinical study of 39 patients with diagnostic implications. *Brain*. 2010 Jul 1;*133*(7):1973–86.

61. Al-Khazali HM, Al-Khazali S, Iljazi A, Christensen RH, Ashina S, Lipton RB, et al. Prevalence and clinical features of hemicrania continua in clinic-based studies: A systematic review and meta-analysis. *Cephalalgia*. 2023 Jan;*43*(1):0333d10242211313.

62. Burish M. Cluster headache and other trigeminal autonomic cephalalgias. *Contin Lifelong Learn Neurol*. 2018 Aug;*24*(4):1137–56.

63. Dodick D. Hemicrania continua: Diagnostic criteria and nosologic status. *Cephalalgia*. 2001 Nov;*21*(9):869–72.

64. Peres MFP, Silberstein SD, Nahmias S, Shechter AL, Youssef I, Rozen TD, et al. Hemicrania continua is not that rare. *Neurology*. 2001 Sep 25;*57*(6):948–51.

65. Burish MJ, Rozen TD. Trigeminal autonomic cephalalgias. *Neurol Clin*. 2019 Nov;*37*(4):847–69.

66. Matharu MS, Cohen AS, McGonigle DJ, Ward N, Frackowiak RS, Goadsby PJ. Posterior hypothalamic and brainstem activation in Hemicrania Continua. *Headache J Head Face Pain*. 2004 Sep;*44*(8):747–61.

67. Mendizabal A. Chapter 67: Trigeminal Autonomic *Cephalalgia*. In: *Decision-Making in Adult Neurology*. 1st Edition. Elsevier; 2020.

68. Antonaci F, Sjaastad O. Chronic Paroxysmal Hemicrania (CPH): A review of the clinical manifestations. *Headache J Head Face Pain*. 1989 Nov;*29*(10):648–56.

69. Boes CJ, Dodick DW. Refining the clinical spectrum of chronic paroxysmal hemicrania: A review of 74 patients. *Headache J Head Face Pain*. 2002 Sep;*42*(8):699–708.

70. Irimia P, Cittadini E, Paemeleire K, Cohen A, Goadsby P. Unilateral photophobia or phonophobia in migraine compared with trigeminal autonomic cephalalgias. *Cephalalgia*. 2008 Jun;*28*(6):626–30.

71. Russell MB. Epidemiology and genetics of cluster headache. *Lancet Neurol*. 2004 May;*3*(5):279–83.

72. Cittadini E, Matharu MS, Goadsby PJ. Paroxysmal hemicrania: A prospective clinical study of 31 cases. *Brain*. 2008 Feb 26;*131*(4):1142–55.

73. Eller M, Goadsby P. Trigeminal autonomic cephalalgias. *Oral Dis*. 2016 Jan;*22*(1):1–8.

74. Matharu MS, Cohen AS, Frackowiak RSJ, Goadsby PJ. Posterior hypothalamic activation in paroxysmal hemicrania. *Ann Neurol*. 2006 Mar;*59*(3):535–45.

75. Wei DY, Jensen RH. Therapeutic approaches for the management of trigeminal autonomic cephalalgias. *Neurotherapeutics*. 2018 Apr;*15*(2):346–60.

76. Antonaci F, Sjaastad O. Hemicrania continua. In: Handbook of Clinical Neurology [Internet]. Elsevier; 2010 [cited 2023 Aug 31]. p. 483–7. Available from: https://linkinghub.elsevier.com/retrieve/pii/S0072975210970437

77. Antonaci F, Pareja JA, Caminero AB, Sjaastad O. Chronic paroxysmal hemicrania and hemicrania continua. Parenteral indomethacin: The "Indotest." *Headache J Head Face Pain*. 1998 Feb;*38*(2):122–8.

78. Wilbrink LA, Louter MA, Teernstra OPM, Van Zwet EW, Huygen FJPM, Haan J, et al. Allodynia in cluster headache. *Pain*. 2017 Jun;*158*(6):1113–7.

79. Wei DT, Yuan Ong J, Goadsby P. Cluster headache: Epidemiology, pathophysiology, clinical features, and diagnosis. *Ann Indian Acad Neurol*. 2018;*21*(5):3.

80. Marulanda E, Tornes L. Obstetric and gynecologic disorders and the nervous system. *Contin Lifelong Learn Neurol*. 2023 Jun;*29*(3):763–96.

81. Fischera M, Marziniak M, Gralow I, Evers S. The incidence and prevalence of cluster headache: A meta-analysis of population-based studies. *Cephalalgia*. 2008 Jun;*28*(6):614–8.

82. Sjaastad O, Bakketeig L. Cluster headache prevalence. *Vågå Study of Headache Epidemiology*. *Cephalalgia*. 2003 Sep;*23*(7):528–33.

83. Diener HC, May A. Drug treatment of cluster headache. *Drugs*. 2022 Jan;*82*(1):33–42.

84. Sprenger T, Boecker H, Tolle TR, Bussone G, May A, Leone M. Specific hypothalamic activation during a spontaneous cluster headache attack. *Neurology*. 2004 Feb 10;*62*(3):516–7.

85. Morelli N, Pesaresi I, Cafforio G, Maluccio MR, Gori S, Di Salle F, et al. Functional magnetic resonance imaging in episodic cluster headache. *J Headache Pain*. 2009 Feb;*10*(1):11–4.

86. Hardebo JE. Activation of pain fibers to the internal carotid artery intracranially may cause the pain and local signs of reduced sympathetic and enhanced parasympathetic activity in cluster headache. *Headache J Head Face Pain*. 1991 May;*31*(5):314–20.

87. Carmine Belin A, Ran C, Edvinsson L. Calcitonin Gene-Related Peptide (CGRP) and cluster headache. *Brain Sci*. 2020 Jan 6;*10*(1):30.

88. Snoer A, Vollesen ALH, Beske RP, Guo S, Hoffmann J, Fahrenkrug J, et al. Calcitonin gene-related peptide and disease activity in cluster headache. *Cephalalgia*. 2019 Apr;*39*(5):575–84.

89. Calhoun AH, Peterlin BL. Treatment of Cluster Headache in Pregnancy and Lactation. *Curr Pain Headache Rep*. 2010 Apr;*14*(2):164–73.

90. Schindler EAD. Psychedelics in the Treatment of Headache and Chronic Pain Disorders. In: Barrett FS, Preller KH, editors. Disruptive Psychopharmacology [Internet]. Cham: Springer International Publishing; 2022 [cited 2023 Aug 30]. p. 261–85. (Current Topics in Behavioral Neurosciences; vol. 56). Available from: https://link.springer.com/10.1007/7854_2022_365

91. Lambru G, Rantell K, Levy A, Matharu MS. A prospective comparative study and analysis of predictors of SUNA and SUNCT. *Neurology*. 2019 Sep 17;*93*(12):e1127–37.

92. Lambru G, Rantell K, O'Connor E, Levy A, Davagnanam I, Zrinzo L, et al. Trigeminal neurovascular contact in SUNCT and SUNA: a cross-sectional magnetic resonance study. *Brain*. 2020 Dec 1;*143*(12):3619–28.

93. Sjaastad O, Pareja JA, Zukerman E, Jansen J, Kruszewski P. Trigeminal Neuralgia. Clinical Manifestations of First Division Involvement. *Headache J Head Face Pain*. 1997 Jun;*37*(6):346–57.

94. Goadsby P, Matharu M, Boes C. SUNCT Syndrome or Trigeminal Neuralgia with Lacrimation. *Cephalalgia*. 2001 Mar;*21*(2):82–3.

95. Wei DT, Yuan Ong J, Goadsby P. Overview of trigeminal autonomic cephalalgias: Nosologic evolution, diagnosis, and management. *Ann Indian Acad Neurol*. 2018;*21*(5):39.

96. Williams MH, Broadley SA. SUNCT and SUNA: Clinical features and medical treatment. *J Clin Neurosci*. 2008 May;*15*(5):526–34.

97. May A, Bahra A, Büchel C, Turner R, Goadsby PJ. Functional magnetic resonance imaging in spontaneous attacks of SUNCT: Short-lasting neuralgiform headache with conjunctival injection and tearing. *Ann Neurol*. 1999 Nov;*46*(5):791–4.

98. Rinaldi F, Rao R, Venturelli E, Liberini P, Gipponi S, Pari E, et al. Where SUNCT Contacts TN: A Case Report: *Headache J Head Face Pain*. 2013 Feb;n/a-n/a.

99. Williams M, Bazina R, Tan L, Rice H, Broadley SA. Microvascular decompression of the trigeminal nerve in the treatment of SUNCT and SUNA. *J Neurol Neurosurg Psychiatry*. 2010 Sep 1;*81*(9):992–6.

100. Duggal A, Chowdhury D. SUNCT and SUNA: An Update. *Neurol India*. 2021;*69*(7):144.

101. Cohen AS. Short-lasting unilateral neuralgiform headache attacks with conjunctival injection and tearing (SUNCT) or cranial autonomic features (SUNA)--a prospective clinical study of SUNCT and SUNA. *Brain*. 2006 Jul 15;*129*(10):2746–60.

102. Gelfand AA, Goadsby PJ. The Role of Melatonin in the Treatment of Primary Headache Disorders: The Role of Melatonin in the Treatment of Primary Headache Disorders. *Headache J Head Face Pain*. 2016 Sep;*56*(8):1257–66.

103. Rozen TD. Melatonin Responsive Hemicrania Continua. *Headache J Head Face Pain*. 2006 Jul;*46*(7):1203–4.

104. Paliwal V, Uniyal R. Paroxysmal Hemicrania: An Update. *Neurol India*. 2021;*69*(7):135.

105. Prakash S, Rawat K. Hemicrania Continua: An Update. *Neurol India*. 2021;*69*(7):160.

106. Osman C, Bahra A. Paroxysmal hemicrania. *Ann Indian Acad Neurol*. 2018;*21*(5):16.

107. Miller S, Correia F, Lagrata S, Matharu MS. OnabotulinumtoxinA for Hemicrania Continua: open label experience in 9 patients. *J Headache Pain*. 2015 Dec;*16*(1):19.

108. Lampl C, Haider B, Schweiger C. Long-term efficacy of *Boswellia serrata* in four patients with chronic cluster headache. *Cephalalgia*. 2012 Jul;*32*(9):719–22.

109. Eross, Eric. A comparison of efficacy, tolerability and safety in subjects with Hemicrania continua responding to indomethacin and specialized Boswellia Serrata extract (5250). *Neurology*. 2020;*94*(15 Supplement):5250.

110. Mohen SA, Robbins MS. Harry Potter and Nummular Headache. *Headache J Head Face Pain*. 2012 Feb;*52*(2):323–4.

111. Cuadrado ML. Epicranial headaches part 2: Nummular headache and epicrania fugax. *Cephalalgia*. 2023 Apr;*43*(4):033310242211469.

112. Cuadrado M, Valle B, Fernández C, Barriga F, Pareja J. Bifocal nummular headache: the first three cases. *Cephalalgia*. 2009 May;*29*(5):583–6.

113. Guerrero ÁL, Cortijo E, Herrero-Velázquez S, Mulero P, Miranda S, Peñas ML, et al. Nummular headache with and without exacerbations: Comparative characteristics in a series of 72 patients*. *Cephalalgia*. 2012; Jun *32*(8):649–53.

114. García-Iglesias C, Puledda F, Echavarría-Íñiguez A, González-Osorio Y, Sierra-Mencía Á, Recio-García A, et al. Treatment of primary nummular headache: A Series of 183 Patients from the NUMITOR Study. *J Clin Med*. 2022 Dec 23;*12*(1):122.

115. García-Azorín D, Trigo-López J, Sierra Á, Blanco-García L, Martínez-Pías E, Martínez B, et al. Observational, open-label, non-randomized study on the efficacy of onabotulinumtoxinA in the treatment of nummular headache: The pre-numabot study. *Cephalalgia*. 2019 Dec;*39*(14):1818–26.

116. Lance JW. Headaches related to sexual activity. *J Neurol Neurosurg Psychiatry*. 1976 Dec 1;*39*(12):1226–30.

117. Rasmussen BK, Olesen J. Symptomatic and nonsymptomatic headaches in a general population. *Neurology*. 1992 Jun 1;*42*(6):1225–1225.

118. Frese A, Eikermann A, Frese K, Schwaag S, Husstedt IW, Evers S. Headache associated with sexual activity: Demography, clinical features, and comorbidity. *Neurology*. 2003 Sep 23;*61*(6):796–800.

119. Allena M, Rossi P, Tassorelli C, Ferrante E, Lisotto C, Nappi G. Focus on therapy of the Chapter IV headaches provoked by exertional factors: primary cough headache, primary exertional headache and primary headache associated with sexual activity. *J Headache Pain*. 2010 Dec;*11*(6):525–30.

120. Ari BC, Mayda Domac F, Ulutas S. Primary headache associated with sexual activity: A case series of 13 patients. *J Clin Neurosci*. 2020 Sep;*79*:51–3.

121. Silbert PL, Edis RH, Stewart-Wynne EG, Gubbay SS. Benign vascular sexual headache and exertional headache: Interrelationships and long term prognosis. *J Neurol Neurosurg Psychiatry*. 1991 May 1;*54*(5):417–21.

122. Pascual J, González-Mandly A, Martín R, Oterino A. Headaches precipitated by cough, prolonged exercise or sexual activity: A prospective etiological and clinical study. *J Headache Pain*. 2008 Oct;*9*(5):259–66.

123. Frese A, Gantenbein A, Marziniak M, Husstedt I, Goadsby P, Evers S. Triptans in orgasmic headache. *Cephalalgia*. 2006 Dec;*26*(12):1458–61.

124. Frese A, Rahmann A, Gregor N, Biehl K, Husstedt IW, Evers S. Headache associated with sexual activity: Prognosis and treatment options. *Cephalalgia*. 2007 Nov;*27*(11):1265–70.

125. Landtblom AM, Fridriksson S, Boivie J, Hillman J, Johansson G, Johansson I. Sudden onset headache: A prospective study of features, incidence and causes. *Cephalalgia*. 2002 Jun;*22*(5):354–60.

126. Linn FHH. Primary thunderclap headache. In: *Handbook of Clinical Neurology*. Elsevier; 2010 [cited 2023 Aug 30]. p. 473–81. Available from: https://linkinghub.elsevier.com/retrieve/pii/S0072975210970425

Approach to Secondary Headaches

3

Marianna Vinokur and Fred Cohen

LEARNING OBJECTIVES

1. Understand the differentiation of primary headache disorders from secondary headaches and the clinical relevance of this distinction
2. Be able to identify key "red flags" in patients' history that should alert the provider to investigate for secondary causes of headache
3. Define common vocabulary, such as thunderclap headache, medication-overuse headache
4. Provide overview of key elements of the physical examination and associated features of secondary headaches
5. Overview modalities used in diagnostic workup of secondary headaches

---

This chapter will provide an approach to secondary headache disorders. One of the first distinctions that needs to be made in the diagnosis of headache disorders is differentiating a primary from a secondary etiology of headache. Primary headache disorders exist without an underlying pathologic process, medical condition, or injury. Simply put, they are caused by a misfiring of the nerves responsible for carrying sensory information to the head and neck. Primary headache disorders must be diagnosed based on their individual characteristics and criteria, rather than simply being diagnoses of exclusion of secondary headache disorders. Examples of primary headache disorders include tension-type headache, migraine, and trigeminal autonomic cephalgia, such as cluster headache.

Conversely, secondary headaches are caused by other medical conditions or external factors. An estimated 18% of patients with a headache have a secondary headache disorder.[1] Although most headaches encountered in clinical practice are primary headaches, clinicians must remain vigilant to exclude secondary headaches, as the underlying conditions can lead to morbidity and mortality and may change the course of diagnostic workup and treatment.

The *International Classification of Headache Disorders, 3rd Edition* (*ICHD-3*), the current diagnostic manual for headache disorders, provides criteria for both primary and secondary etiologies of headache.[2] The diagnostic criterion for secondary headache is as follows:

DOI: 10.1201/b23330-3

General Diagnostic Criteria for Secondary Headaches:

A.   Any headache fulfilling criterion C
B.   Another disorder scientifically documented to be able to cause headache has been diagnosed.
     Evidence of causation demonstrated by at least two of the following:
     1.   Headache has developed in temporal relation to the onset of the presumed causative disorder
     2.   Either or both of the following:
          •   Headache has significantly worsened in parallel with worsening of the presumed caus-
              ative disorder
          •   Headache has significantly improved in parallel with improvement of the presumed
              causative disorder
     3.   Headache has characteristics typical for the causative disorder
     4.   Other evidence exists of causation
C.   Not better accounted for by another *ICHD-3* diagnosis

When a patient develops a new headache in close temporal proximity to another clinical diagnosis, such as hypertensive emergency, and especially when headache resolves with treatment of the underlying, it can be concluded that the headache is secondary to the underlying condition, in this case, hypertension. However, the phenotypic description of the symptoms may meet the same or similar criteria for primary headache disorders like migraine, tension-type, or trigeminal autonomic cephalalgia. For example, if a headache is secondary to a hypertensive crisis but has features commonly associated with migraine, such as photophobia, phonophobia, nausea, or vomiting, it is said to have a migrainous phenotype. Additionally, headache is a common symptom; headache can begin at the same time as the onset of another disorder simply by chance, without a direct causal relationship. Therefore, a secondary headache also requires scientific evidence that the disorder can cause headaches.

COMPREHENSIVE MEDICAL HISTORY

Like any medical condition, the keystone of diagnosing secondary headache disorders begins with a comprehensive patient history. Headache clinic notes are often distinguishable by the level of detail in the patient history, as often the crucial key is in the details.

In individuals with a preexisting history of primary headache disorders, the provider must discern whether the presenting headache is

A.   A continuation of their known primary headache disorder with new features (i.e., a new visual
     aura in a patient with a history of migraine without aura),
B.   A comorbid primary headache condition (i.e., new primary stabbing headache in a patient
     with known migraine),
C.   An exacerbation due to another systemic illness (i.e., migraine attack triggered by an upper
     respiratory infection), or
D.   New headache with a secondary cause (i.e., intracranial hypotension due to lumbar puncture).

When obtaining a headache history, it is best to start the encounter with open-ended questions and allow the patient an opportunity to describe their own clinical course. In addition to providing an unbiased first-person record of the condition, letting the patient tell their story nurtures the patient-clinician relationship. Headache disorders are often misunderstood and stigmatized by the general population and medical community. Providing the patient with a safe space to be heard and validated can be therapeutic in and of itself. After the open-ended interview, a clinician can guide the patient to more directed questions to fill in the details to ensure the clinician has a comprehensive understanding of the disease process. A complete history should include onset, precipitating factors, current and past frequency, duration of attacks, location, quality, intensity, and associated symptoms. It is also imperative to review other current and past medical conditions, current medications, allergies, surgical history, and family history.

In people who menstruate, it is important to establish if there is any relationship between their menstrual cycle and headaches. Special attention must be paid regarding the use of exogenous hormones, such as for treatment of contraception, gender-affirming care, active fertility treatments, or menopausal symptoms.

As previously mentioned, one of the first distinctions the clinician should consider is whether the patient is having a primary versus a secondary headache. The history can be filtered to address this question. For example, many patients with migraine carry a positive family history of migraine, pointing to a primary headache disorder.

Onset

It is important to document a clear history of the onset of the headache.

- When did this headache begin?
  - It may be helpful to note the general starting point of the headache as "spring of the year 2024" in addition to a more general, "three months ago," which may help retroactive review of the start of future encounters.
- Did the patient have a prior, even remote, headache history? Or is this truly the onset of a new headache?
  - The patient may downplay a previous headache they have had as "normal" or not clinically significant, causing them to omit it from history. It is important for the clinician to elicit a complete headache history, including the frequency of less severe headaches.
- Can the patient identify an inciting event surrounding the onset, such as head trauma, infection, emotional stress, change in medication?
- Age at onset of headache?
  - Particularly, headaches that begin before age 5 or after age 50 should be highly considered for causes of secondary headache, such as malignancy or infection.
- Has the headache been continuous since onset, or does it come and go?
- Was the onset gradual or sudden?
- If sudden, was the peak intensity of the pain immediately present, or did it increase over time?

Description of Pain

- What does the pain feel like?
  - Common qualifying descriptors can be sharp, needle-like, jabs, electric, burning, jolts, pressure, pulsation/throbbing.
- What is the intensity of pain?
  - Commonly described on a scale of zero to ten, where zero is no pain, and ten is the most severe pain imaginable. Be wary of comparing these numbers between patients as a one for patient A could be a ten for patient B.
- What is the location of the pain? Does it travel, or is it locked to one side or one specific area?
  - Although migraine is classically thought of as a unilateral headache, many patients actually experience holocephalic or traveling pain.

- A location-locked headache may be an indication of an underlying pathology; however, many primary headache disorders also affect the same nerve distribution with each attack.
- Has there been a change in headache patterns or characteristics?
  - This may be an indicator of a new secondary headache disorder in patients with an existing primary headache history.

Frequency

Headache frequency is one of the most prominent features of the history, as treatment decisions are often based on the number of the patients' monthly headache days. For example, if a migraine patient has four headache days or fewer per month, they may be able to treat simply with effective acute medication. In contrast, patients with more than 15 headache days per month may require more than one simultaneous preventive treatment. An accurate frequency should include all headache days, including mild or background pain rather than just severe episodes. Patients may focus on their most severe episodes but, upon further questioning, reveal a low baseline pain daily with more severe exacerbations. As memory is often unreliable, keeping a headache diary may allow for a more accurate record of headaches.

- What is the frequency of the headache?
  - How many total headache days?
  - How many of those are severe/disabling headache days per month?
  - If a headache is constant at baseline with exacerbations, it may be more prudent to ask instead about the frequency and duration of the headache-free periods.

Duration

Headaches can often be broken down into the following categorizations based on their duration.

- **Acute headaches** typically last for a short duration, from a few minutes to a few hours. Common inciting events are alcohol consumption, stressful events, or dehydration. However, depending on severity, acute new-onset headaches may also be dangerous in etiology, such as a thunderclap headache.
- **Subacute headaches** usually last several hours or days. Common causes include viral infections, sinusitis, cervical muscle spasm, and caffeine withdrawal.
- **Chronic headaches** last for an extended period, typically more than 15 days a month for three months or longer. Common causes include consumption of excessive abortive medications, and space-occupying lesions.
- **Episodic headaches** occur sporadically but may have a recurring pattern. This is a common pattern of some primary headache disorders, such as episodic migraine, but can also occur in secondary headache disorders, such as idiopathic intracranial hypertension, which worsens at night when patient is supine, and remits during the day when patient is upright.

Other important questions:

- Is it continuous, or does it occur in recurrent attacks?
- How long does each headache episode typically last?
- Are they consistent in duration, or do they vary?
- Will symptoms fluctuate through the duration of the attack?
- Is the general trend that it is improving or worsening with time?

Inciting and Remitting Factors

The context in which the headache occurs can give clues to the etiology. Headache diaries can be one of the best ways to assess comorbid influences, such as triggers. For example, does the headache only occur at the onset of menses or with ovulation? Is it elicited by exercise or exertion?

- What exacerbates the pain and what remits it?
- Are there clear triggers or eliciting maneuvers?
- Are there comorbid conditions for the headache? For example, the presence of inflammatory arthropathies or autoimmune conditions? Difficulty chewing? Sleep disorders? Vascular conditions?
- Is the headache positional?

The **positionality** of a headache may be a clue to intracranial pressure abnormalities. For example, headaches that happen upon awakening after sleeping or lying flat may indicate an increased pressure in the intracranial cavity. This contrasts with an orthostatic headache classic of a low-pressure headache, such as in the case of spontaneous intracranial hypotension or postdural puncture headache.

Headaches provoked by coughing, sneezing, orgasm, bearing down, or other Valsalva maneuvers should be investigated with neuroimaging.

Associated Symptoms

The associated features of a headache are some of the most important clinical indicators and occasionally and occasionally can be more disabling than the pain itself.

Common associated symptoms of headache:

- Sensitivity to light (photophobia) and sound (phonophobia)
- Nausea and/or Vomiting
- Tension or pain in the neck, trapezius, sternocleidomastoid
- Autonomic Symptoms: nasal congestion, conjunctival injection, ptosis, miosis, rhinorrhea, facial swelling
- Visual Disturbances: In addition to auras, headaches associated with visual disturbances might include bilaterally blurred vision, temporary blindness or partial vision loss
- Vertigo
- Hearing loss or tinnitus
- Pulsatile tinnitus

Red Flag Symptoms

"SNOOP" is one of the most common mnemonics in headache medicine. It is a collection of warning signs and symptoms to alert a clinician that a headache may be secondary in nature or contain dangerous features, which may prompt more vigilant monitoring and workup. Originally described in 2003 by Dr. David Dodick, this mnemonic was later revised to "SNNOOP10" to include a more comprehensive list of alarming features (Table 3.1).[3, 4]

There are many neurological causes of secondary headaches, many of which may be acutely life-threatening or result in stroke and morbidity. Headache is a common presenting feature of many serious

TABLE 3.1   SNNOOP10 mnemonic

MNEMONIC	SIGN OR SYMPTOM	SECONDARY HEADACHE ETIOLOGY
S	**Systemic** symptoms (fever, hypertension)	Infection, hypertensive emergency, Posterior Reversible Encephalopathy syndrome (PRES)
N	History of **Neoplasm**	Metastatic or primary brain tumor
N	Focal **Neurologic deficit**	Space-occupying lesion, carcinomatosis, infection, autoimmune process (Sjogren's, multiple sclerosis, etc.)
O	Sudden **Onset**	Cerebrovascular emergency such as subarachnoid hemorrhage (SAH), reversible cerebral vasoconstriction syndrome (RCVS)
O	**Older** than 50 years old	Increased risk of giant cell arteritis, neoplasm
P	Change in **Pattern** of headache	Neoplasm, cerebrovascular dysfunction, meningitis in existing headache history (i.e., migraine)
P	**Positional** headache	Idiopathic intracranial hypertension (IIH), space-occupying lesion, spontaneous intracranial hypotension
P	Headache **Precipitated** by cough, sneeze, sex, Valsalva	Posterior fossa space-occupying lesion, Chiari malformation
P	**Papilledema**	IIH, space-occupying lesion
P	**Progressive** or unremitting pattern	Space-occupying lesion
P	**Pregnancy** or **Postpartum**	Pre-eclampsia, cerebral venous thrombosis, postdural puncture headache, intracerebral hemorrage
P	**Post-traumatic** onset	Subdural hematoma, epidural hematoma, SAH, cervical instability, concussion
P	**Pain** medication or new medication use	Medication adaptation headache (aka rebound or medication-overuse headache), adverse effect of headache after initiation of a new drug
P	**Painful** eye with autonomic features	Cavernous sinus pathology such as Tolosa Hunt, infection, Sjogren's disease,
P	**Pathology** of immune system	HIV, immunosuppressive agents causing associated opportunistic infection

cerebrovascular conditions, such as hemorrhagic stroke, SAH, dural venous sinus thrombosis, vertebral artery dissection, RCVS, vasculitis such as primary centrual nervous system angiitis and giant cell arteritis, and many more. It is crucial to recognize the association of headache with these disorders, especially as **thunderclap** or **sentinel headache** is often a common first presenting symptom.

A "sentinel headache" describes a "warning" headache that occurs before a more serious medical event, such as a slow aneurysm leak prior to rupture. It is also characterized as sudden, intense, and persistent and can happen once or multiple times preceding a potentially catastrophic event, most commonly aneurysm rupture resulting in SAH. Sentinel headaches precede rupture by days or weeks and occur in 15%–60% of patients with spontaneous SAH. Although its pathophysiology has not been completely understood, the current consensus is that structural changes in the aneurysm wall or minor bleeding result in the pain.

"Thunderclap headache" refers to the sudden onset of a severe headache that reaches peak intensity within seconds to a minute. It is often described as one of the most intense headaches a person can experience or "worst headache of their life," striking suddenly and fiercely, like a clap of thunder (Table 3.2).

TABLE 3.2   Thunderclap Headache Etiologies

CAUSE	DESCRIPTION
Subarachnoid Hemorrhage	Bleeding into the subarachnoid space (between the arachnoid membrane and the pia mater). Often caused by aneurysm rupture or trauma
Cerebral Venous Sinus Thrombosis	Blood clot in the veins of the brain, causing increased pressure or bleeding in the brain tissue
Carotid or Vertebral Artery Dissection	Tear in the inner lining of an artery, leading to blood clot formation. Can be traumatic from chiropractic manipulation
RCVS	Sudden vasoconstriction of brain blood vessels, often from medication
Meningitis	Inflammation of brain and spinal cord membranes secondary to viral, bacterial, or fungal infection
Intracerebral Hemorrhage	Bleeding within brain tissue itself
Hypertensive Emergency	Often causes focal neurologic deficits or AMS in addition to headache. Causes include sympathomimetic drugs, pheochromocytoma
Spontaneous Intracranial Hypotension	Cerebrospinal fluid leak causing low intracranial pressure
Ischemic Stroke	Clot causing abrupt cessation in blood flow to the brain
Pituitary Apoplexy	Bleeding into or impaired blood supply to the pituitary gland
Ruptured Arteriovenous Malformation (AVM)	Abnormal connection between arteries and veins, prone to bleeding
PRES (Posterior Reversible Encephalopathy Syndrome)	Brain swelling often due to high blood pressure or other causes
Idiopathic Thunderclap Headache	Some cases of thunderclap headache may have no identifiable cause

Notably absent from the discussion is perhaps the most well-known cerebrovascular disease, ischemic stroke, and transient ischemic attack (TIA). In the setting of ischemic stroke, there is permanent damage to the brain parenchyma being fed by the occluded vessel, in contrast to a TIA, when the blood flow resumes before permanent damage can occur. Ischemic stroke affects approximately 800,000 individuals annually in the United States and accounts for 1 in every 20 deaths.[5] Stroke generally presents with acute onset focal neurologic deficits such as hemi-body weakness, numbness, decreased consciousness, vertigo, vision loss, dysarthria, or aphasia.

The general thought among emergency physicians and neurologists is that headache is not one of the main presenting features of ischemic stroke. A study evaluating 2,196 patients experiencing ischemic stroke or TIA found that 27% of patients experienced headache at stroke onset. Based on a systematic review and meta-analysis, headaches occurred in 6%–44% of the ischemic stroke population, and most of those headaches had tension-type features, were moderate to severe, and became chronic in nature.[6] Interestingly, ischemic strokes affecting the posterior circulation—namely, the cerebellum, were more likely to result in headache. It is important to note that exact statistics vary widely, and headache is not generally considered a universal or common symptom of ischemic stroke.

If any of the aforementioned conditions are suspected, it is important to direct your patient to seek emergency evaluation. This will often initiate activation of a neuro or stroke alert system by Emergency Medical Services (EMS) or within an institution, resulting in timely evaluation by appropriate clinicians, expedited imaging, and decision-making regarding treatment, thus preventing potentially devastating neurological consequences. The most common initial studies done for the evaluation of cerebrovascular causes of headache are computed tomography (CT) head and CT angiography of the head and neck. Based on the symptoms and findings of these studies, further urgent workup such as magnetic resonance imaging (MRI), cerebral angiography, or lumbar puncture may be appropriate.

Lastly, it is important to note that all the aforementioned conditions can occur in patients who carry a diagnosis of a primary headache disorder. In patients who have known migraine or tension-type headache, sudden onset of new symptoms, thunderclap headache, or a change in headache sensation or intensity should prompt urgent evaluation for vascular conditions.

Medication-Overuse Headache

When a patient presents for evaluation for headache in a primary care setting, one of the first orders of action is to ask the patient what they are currently using to treat their headache and specify the exact dosage and frequency of use. Often, patients will have tiers to their abortive plans, such as hydrating, lying down in a dark, quiet room, or ice. If that fails, they may move on to common over-the-counter medication, such as acetaminophen and nonsteroidal anti-inflammatory medications. Frequent or excessive use of pain-relieving medications can result in one of the most common secondary headache disorders known as medication-overuse headache (MOH). This condition has had many names throughout the years, such as rebound headache and the newer and less stigmatizing term medication adaptation headache (MAH). This paradoxical condition, in which the perceived treatment may worsen the overall disease, is a common culprit in headaches becoming more frequent, severe, and refractory over time. MOH can develop as a result of using various types of pain-relief medications, including over-the-counter pain relievers, opioids, and headache-targeted prescription medications.

Common offending agents of medication adaptation headache include:

- NSAIDS: naproxen, ibuprofen, diclofenac, etodolac, celecoxib, nabumetone, etc.
- Acetaminophen
- Triptans medications: prescription medications used to treat migraine and cluster headache. The mechanism of action is agonism of select serotonin receptors (5-HT_{1B} and 5-HT_{1D})
  - Examples: sumatriptan, rizatriptan, zolmitriptan, eletriptan, naratriptan, almotriptan, and zolmitriptan
- Dihydroergotamine (DHE): a prescription medication used to treat migraine and cluster headache. It is available in a variety of formulations, including nasal spray, intramuscular and intravenous injection, suppository
- Opioids such as oxycodone, hydrocodone, morphine, codeine, fentanyl, hydromorphone, or tramadol
- Combination formations such as caffeine/acetaminophen/aspirin, triptan/NSAID, and butalbital/acetaminophen/caffeine

NEUROLOGICAL EXAM

When conducting a neurological exam to assess a patient's headache, the process should be systematic and thorough. The assessment should include testing mental status, motor and sensory functions, cranial nerve functions, coordination, reflexes, and gait. It is crucial in the evaluation of a patient with headache to thoroughly investigate and exclude any secondary causes, as many neurological disorders can manifest primarily through headaches.

It is common to start a neurological assessment with an eye evaluation, as the lights need to be dimmed to allow the pupils to dilate for adequate view of the optic discs. Table 3.3 details each cranial nerve (CN), its function, and how to assess it. CN I (olfactory) can be difficult to assess in a clinical setting, but you can ask the patient if they have difficulty smelling or notice any changes in taste. CN II can be assessed by checking the patients' visual fields. CN III, IV, and VI can be assessed by having

TABLE 3.3 Cranial nerve function and assessment

CRANIAL NERVE	FUNCTION	ASSESSMENT METHOD
I. Olfactory	Sense of Smell	Ask the patient to identify different smells with each nostril separately.
II. Optic	Visual Acuity and Visual Field	Test visual acuity with a Snellen chart and assess visual fields by confrontation.
III. Oculomotor	Eye Movement, Pupil Constriction	Check pupil response to light, eyelid elevation, and eye movements in all directions.
IV. Trochlear	Downward, Inward Eye Movement	Ask the patient to follow an object downward and toward the nose.
V. Trigeminal	Facial Sensation, Jaw Movement	Test facial sensation with light touch and check jaw muscles for strength and symmetry.
VI. Abducens	Lateral Eye Movement	Have the patient follow an object to each side.
VII. Facial	Facial Expressions, Taste on Anterior Two-Thirds Tongue	Assess facial symmetry, ask the patient to frown, smile, puff cheeks, and identify tastes.
VIII. Vestibulocochlear	Hearing, Balance	Perform a hearing test and assess balance and coordination.
IX. Glossopharyngeal	Swallowing, Taste on Posterior One-Third Tongue	Evaluate gag reflex, ability to swallow, and taste perception.
X. Vagus	Palate Elevation, Gag Reflex, Speech	Check for symmetrical palate elevation, gag reflex, and clarity of speech.
XI. Accessory	Shoulder Shrug, Head Turn	Test strength of trapezius muscles and ability to turn head against resistance.
XII. Hypoglossal	Tongue Movement	Ask the patient to protrude and move the tongue in all directions.

the patient's eyes move in all directions. CN V can be assessed by testing for facial sensation on both sides (and if they are equal). CN VII can be assessed by asking to patient to frown, smile, move their mouth, and puff their cheeks. CN VIII can be assessed by checking if the patient has hearing difficulties (such as rubbing your fingers by their ears). CN IX and CN X can be assessed by checking for symmetrical palate elevation. CN XI can be assessed by testing the strength of the patient's trapeziuses by asking them to shrug their shoulders. And CN XII can be assessed by having the patient stick out their tongue and move in all directions.

After assessing CN functions, the next area of the neurological exam would be assessing motor and sensory functions in all extremities. This can be achieved with the upper extremities by having the patient raise and push their arms and hands against the examiner. For the lower extremities, have the patient raise their thigh and kick their leg against the provider. Biceps, brachioradialis, patellar, and ankle reflexes should be assessed. If there are signs of corticospinal tract dysfunction, such as ipsilateral paralysis, paresis, or hypertonia, Hoffman's sign and Babinski's sign should be checked. To assess for Hoffman's test, sharply flick the nail of the patient's middle finger and look for involuntary thumb and index finger flexion, while for Babinski's sign, gently stroke the lateral sole of the foot from heel to toe and watch for the big toe to extend and other toes to fan out, both indicating positive signs.

To assess cerebellar dysfunction, conduct coordination tests such as the finger-to-nose and heel-to-shin tests, observing for dysmetria or uncoordinated movements. Rapid alternating movements, like pronation-supination of hands and tapping of feet, help evaluate for any cerebellar ataxia or dysdiadochokinesia. Gait should always be assessed, which can easily be accomplished by observing the patient as they enter the examination room. Additionally, assess a patient's ability to walk heel to toe to assess for ataxia or imbalance.

PHYSICAL EXAM

Head

It is always paramount during the physical examination while evaluating a headache to ensure there are no signs of head trauma (commonly documented as normocephalic atraumatic [NCAT]). Signs of head trauma can include Battle's sign (bruising behind the ears), raccoon eyes (bruising around the eyes), confusion, disorientation, uneven pupil size, and clear or bloody fluid draining from the nose or ears.[7] It is pertinent during a review of systems to ask about any history of trauma. Post-concussion syndrome can present similarly to migraine, characterized by symptoms including headaches, dizziness, fatigue, sleep disturbances, difficulty with concentrating and remembering, and sensitivity to noise and light.

Ophthalmologic

The eye examination is one of the most crucial components of the physical exam during a headache evaluation. Equal and reactive pupils should always be checked with a light source (such as a penlight). An ophthalmologic exam can reveal various signs and findings, especially with changes in intracranial pressure and CN compressions.[8] Careful observation is essential in an eye examination, as even slight variations in the following presentations could suggest an underlying condition related to the brain or skull.

Papilledema

Papilledema is swelling of the optic disc, which is where the optic nerve enters the posterior eye. This swelling is typically a result of increased intracranial pressure. Papilledema is one of the earliest signs of increased intracranial pressure.[9] Increased intracranial pressure can be the result of various conditions such as IIH, hydrocephalus, abscesses, and brain tumors. If left unchecked and untreated, this swelling can result in permanent vision loss. Findings related to papilledema can also be observed on MR imaging. [10, 11]

Abnormal eye movements

Extraocular movements should be evaluated, as any irregularities might point to a range of intracranial issues.[12] For example, if a patient is unable to abduct their left eye, it could suggest a problem with their left sixth CN. This could be the result of conditions such as CN palsy or a lesion pressing on the nerve. Additionally, movements like nystagmus (involuntary eye movement) or strabismus (misaligned eyes) should be carefully evaluated.

Pupil changes and irregularities

Changes in pupil size and reaction can indicate intracranial pathology.[13] For instance, an unresponsive or abnormally dilated pupil may be a sign of increased pressure or damage to the cranial nerves, often associated with traumatic brain injury or a mass in the brain. Pupillary changes using a light (such as a penlight) should always be conducted during an eye examination.

Visual field defects

Changes in the visual field (the area one can see while looking straight ahead) can indicate problems in specific parts of the brain.[14] For example, a pituitary tumor can lead to a specific pattern of vision loss known as bitemporal hemianopsia (this could also present with diplopia). Visual field defects can present in one eye (monocular) or both eyes (binocular).

Retinal exudates or hemorrhages

Retinal exudates, which are deposits that can appear on the retina, can be the result of several conditions. Age-related macular degeneration (AMD), diabetic retinopathy inflammatory diseases (such as uveitis or retinitis), and infectious processes (such as cytomegalovirus [CMV]) cause retinal exudates.[15] Retinal hemorrhages can be the result of hypertensive retinopathy, as well as diabetic retinopathy.

Ears

Tinnitus can be a common symptom that comes up during a review of systems during a headache evaluation.[16] In addition to evaluating for decreasing hearing, an otologic examination should be conducted. The examination of the tympanic membrane is crucial, as a blood-stained membrane may suggest trauma, whereas a bulging or reddened membrane could be indicative of infection or inflammation.[17]

Nose

Sinus and nasal issues are frequently observed in individuals with migraines, to the extent that sinus headaches are often mistakenly diagnosed as migraine attacks.[18] Nevertheless, nasal causes of headaches exist and should be assessed during a physical examination. Additional nasal causes of headaches may include chronic sinusitis, allergic and nonallergic rhinitis, and upper respiratory infections (URIs). Structural abnormalities in the nasal passages, such as nasal polyps, turbinate hypertrophy, and sinus neoplasms, can also cause headaches, though these conditions typically necessitate a nasal endoscopy for proper visualization.[19]

Neck

The neck's suppleness should always be evaluated, noting any tenderness or pain upon palpation or movement. In cases where a headache is accompanied by fever and a stiff neck, meningitis should be considered. Cervicogenic headaches are a frequent cause of head pain, and cervicalgia is often found in those with migraine.[20, 21] The muscles typically involved in these conditions include the occipitalis, sternocleidomastoid, semispinalis capitis, splenius capitis, and the upper trapezius.

Pulmonary

While the pulmonary examination may be overlooked during a headache evaluation, there are certain key findings that should never be missed when considering a differential diagnosis. An oxygen saturation level should always be obtained while collecting vital signs to rule out hypoxemia. Additionally, patients should be asked whether they experience rapid or shallow breathing. Hypoxemia can be caused by a myriad of conditions; common ones to always be vigilant for are pulmonary embolism, respiratory infections, and carbon monoxide.[22] Always ask if the patient's home is outfitted with a working carbon monoxide detector, even more so during months with cold weather.

Even though a patient might not be presenting with any pulmonary findings, it is important to ask about any history of difficult or abnormal breathing. For example, asking if a patient wakes up in the night trying to catch their breath. This could be a sign of obstructive sleep apnea, which can certainly lead to headaches.[23]

Cardiovascular

Similar to the pulmonary exam, the cardiovascular exam could be overlooked during a headache evaluation. Postural orthostatic tachycardia syndrome (POTS) is the most common disorder of the autonomic nervous system and has a high prevalence with migraine.[24] Common symptoms of POTS include dizziness, weakness, rapid heartbeat, and palpitations, and therefore, it is important to assess these during a review of systems.[25] Additionally, individuals experiencing palpitations should undergo a detailed cardiac evaluation to check for arrhythmias, including conditions like premature ventricular contractions, atrial fibrillation/flutter, and sinus node dysfunction.[26] Patients should be asked about chest pain during headache attacks to assess for the possibility of cardiac cephalgia.[27] In the presence of cardiovascular risk factors, including hypertension, elevated cholesterol, or diabetes, the physical exam should include an assessment for carotid bruits.

Endocrine

Signs and symptoms of hypothyroidism and hyperthyroidism should be assessed during a review of systems, for these conditions have a prevalence of 10.5% and 1.3%, respectively.[28] Abnormal reflexes are among the initial symptoms of these two conditions, with hyporeflexia occurring in hypothyroidism and hyperreflexia in hyperthyroidism.[29] When thyroid dysfunction is suspected, it's important to palpate the thyroid gland during the examination to check for the presence of nodules and goiter (Table 3.4).

Gastrointestinal

Migraine and gastrointestinal (GI) symptoms often share a complex and bidirectional relationship, where the occurrence of one can influence the other. Many individuals with migraines report accompanying GI symptoms such as nausea, vomiting, and abdominal pain.[30] This relationship is further supported by the prevalence of GI disorders like irritable bowel syndrome (IBS), gastroparesis, and

TABLE 3.4   Signs and symptoms of hypothyroidism and hyperthyroidism

HYPOTHYROIDISM	HYPERTHYROIDISM
Fatigue	Weight loss
Weight gain	Increased appetite
Cold intolerance	Heat intolerance
Dry skin	Sweating
Hair loss	Tremor
Constipation	Frequent bowel movements
Depression	Nervousness, anxiety
Muscle weakness	Muscle weakness
Slow heart rate	Rapid heart rate

functional dyspepsia in people with migraine. Therefore, it is pertinent to ask GI related questions during the review of systems.

Skin

The skin, which is the largest organ in the body, is commonly overlooked during the physical examination. It is important to inquire about skin lesions when evaluating a new headache. For example, urticaria coinciding with headaches could indicate mast cell activation syndrome (MCAS).[31] Additionally, vesicles, particularly around the face, eyes, and ears, might suggest a herpes zoster infection.[32] Therefore, assessing skin lesions is an essential part of examining the head.

DIAGNOSTIC WORKUP

Apart from a complete history and physical exam, additional diagnostic tests may help in the assessment of secondary causes of headache. The specific tests depend on each patient's unique presentation, as discussed earlier, and must be chosen on an individual basis. Often, history and physical exam are enough to deduce etiology or rule out more sinister causes of headache. For example, a headache secondary to bruxism or temporomandibular joint (TMJ) disorder can be diagnosed on the basis of history and exam alone and does not warrant further imaging. However, if a patient presents with an acute change to their headache pattern or displays the red flag signs previously discussed, further workup may be critical to reducing morbidity and mortality. It is also important to consider the goal and utility of ordering further workup, as iatrogenic harm to the patient may result in the process. For example, many patients are claustrophobic and cannot tolerate MRIs. Lumbar puncture can result in its own secondary headache condition called postdural puncture headache. CT imaging subjects the patient to, albeit small, quantities of radiation.

Imaging

CT Head: CT head without contrast is often used in an emergency setting as initial imaging for evaluation of acute causes of headaches, such as intracerebral bleeds, stroke, hydrocephalus, or traumatic brain injury. It can also be helpful in diagnosis of sinus infection or inflammation. CT scans are often quick, taking five minutes or fewer, and are generally easier to obtain on an emergent basis. Typically, a CT head is ordered without contrast for evaluation of acute intracranial pathologies, although there are instances in which contrast can be helpful, such as in the case of a patient with a suspected brain mass who cannot undergo MRI.

    MRI Brain: MRI provides the most detailed look at structural abnormalities; however, it is also a more time-consuming study and can take upward of one to two hours to complete. For this reason, MRI is most often obtained in the outpatient setting, although on occasion can be ordered in the emergency department (ED) to further work up findings seen on initial CT or with high suspicion for a specific diagnosis. Gadolinium is a heavy metal agent used as contrast in MRI. Contrast enhancement is a critical finding on MRI, identifying areas of active blood–brain breakdown and can indicate an area of demyelination, infection, or malignancy. For this reason, unless otherwise specified, MRI brain with and without contrast should be ordered when working up a possible secondary headache. Masses and associated edema are best characterized by MRI, as well are intracranial pressure abnormalities. Imaging stigmata of IIH include empty sella, flattened optic globes, and optic nerve sheath distention. Imaging stigmata of spontaneous intracranial hypotension (SIH), such as pachymeningeal enhancement, venous engorgement, subdural hygromas or hematomas, and cerebellar tonsillar sag.

Vessel Imaging

Vessel imaging is useful in the workup of vascular abnormalities such as RCVS, aneurysms, fibromuscular dysplasia, dissections, arteriovenous malformations (AVM), and venous sinus thrombosis.

- **Magnetic Resonance Angiography (MRA) and Computed Tomography Angiography (CTA):** CTA is done with iodinated contrast, whereas MRA can often be done without contrast, instead using a technique called "time of flight" to capture blood flow. While both are vessel imaging techniques, each modality is superior in certain situations. For example, MRA is better at imaging vascular abnormalities at the skull base or near bony structures, whereas artifacts from bony structures can obscure CTA. In contrast, CTA is often better at imaging very tortuous vessels.
- **CT Venography (CTV)/MR Venography (MRV):** As the name suggests, while MRA and CTA focus on arterial structures, MRV and CTV are venous imaging modalities. Some rudimentary venous structures may be visualized on MRA; however, if suspicion is high for a venous thrombus, a dedicated venous study is recommended. MRV is generally considered more sensitive and specific than CTV for detecting dural venous sinus thrombosis.

MRI Cervical Spine: MRI can be useful in identifying structural abnormalities of the cervical spine, such as disc herniation, degenerative changes, spinal stenosis, and many other pathologies that may result in a cervicogenic headache.

Lumbar Puncture (LP): Evaluation of cerebrospinal fluid (CSF) can be used to evaluate for infectious and aseptic meningitis, SAH, malignancy, neuro-inflammatory and demyelinating conditions. Please note that prior to performing an LP brain imaging, a CT head or MR brain must be performed to evaluate for space-occupying lesions and to minimize the risk of herniation. An opening pressure must be obtained in the lateral recumbent, with legs extended, to allow for accurate pressure measurements in the diagnostic evaluation of low and high intracranial pressure etiologies. Intracranial hypotension is formally diagnosed with opening pressure of <6 cm H_2O, whereas IIH is diagnosed at >25.0 cm H_2O.

Blood Tests: Blood tests can be helpful in the diagnosis of infections, inflammation, metabolic disorders, and various systemic conditions. Some useful and commonly ordered tests are complete blood count (CBC), electrolyte panel, erythrocyte sedimentation rate (ESR), C-reactive protein (CRP), and other specialized tests based on suspected causes like autoimmune conditions or infections. ESR and CRP are critical in evaluation of temporal arteritis in patients over 50 years old with new-onset temporal headache.

Less common modalities:

- **Digital subtraction angiography (DSA)** is an invasive imaging technique that involves the injection of contrast dye into the intracranial blood vessels under X-ray imaging to capture vessel flow in real time. This is the gold standard modality for diagnosis of vascular malformations such as aneurysms, AVMs, or RCVS. However, it is usually done after CTA or MRA, which are less invasive.
- **Transcranial Doppler ultrasound** helps assess blood flow velocities in the brain's arteries and can detect abnormalities or changes in vascular tone due to conditions such as vasospasm after SAH, ischemic and hemorrhagic stroke, and cerebral blood flow monitoring after cardiac arrest.
- **Electroencephalogram (EEG)** measures the electrical activity of the brain. It can detect phases of sleep/wake cycles and is critical in diagnosing seizure disorders. While EEG is not a routine part of a secondary headache workup, it may be useful in certain clinical situations. Both new-onset headaches and new-onset seizures may be the first presenting symptoms of an underlying space-occupying lesion. Certain seizure conditions can present with headaches as a symptom. Additionally, headaches can occur in tandem with transient focal neurologic deficits, such as in migraine aura, transient ischemic attacks, or focal aware seizures. EEG is routinely used in the workup of these common but often challenging cases.

CHAPTER SUMMARY

- Secondary headache disorders are those caused by an underlying medical condition or external factors.
- The keystone of diagnosing secondary headache disorders begins with a comprehensive patient history. Key clinical features include onset, frequency, a precipitating event, description of pain, associated symptoms, etc.
- It is important to remain vigilant for "red flags" in the history and physical exam, such as those outlined in the SNNOOP10 mnemonic, which could indicate an alarming etiology, prompting immediate medical evaluation.
- This chapter provides an overview of key elements of a focused physical exam and considerations for selecting the optimal diagnostic modality if necessary.

Case 1

A 41-year-old woman with a history of acid reflux, seasonal environmental allergies, osteoarthritis of the knee, and episodic migraine presents to the neurology resident clinic with the chief complaint of daily headaches of six months duration. The headaches are a near constant, bitemporal pressure or squeezing sensation and fluctuate between a 4 and 6/10 in severity. When asked what she is currently taking to treat the headaches, she reports alternating acetaminophen and ibuprofen about three times daily because she cannot function with the headache. With these medications, the severity improves to 3–4/10 to the point where she can complete her activities of daily living. She also usually runs out of rizatriptan, which she is prescribed for migraine in the first week after picking up her monthly prescription. She is otherwise healthy and does not use any other medications on a regular basis apart from an antacid for acid reflux. She has an IUD. Clinical evaluation reveals no significant neurological abnormalities. The neurology resident astutely diagnoses the patient with MOH, also known as MAH or rebound headache. The treatment plan involves counseling the patient regarding the secondary headache disorder, addressing the psychological aspect of the medication dependence, and explaining that other medical problems may arise from chronically using nonsteroidal anti-inflammatory medications. The patient and clinician formulate a plan for discontinuation of the overused medications alongside initiation of preventive therapy for migraine with a topiramate taper. All of the patient's questions are answered, and a close follow-up appointment is scheduled.

Case 2

A 25-year-old woman presents to the neurology clinic for follow-up after an ED visit one week prior. The patient presented to the ED clinic with an intractable headache of two weeks duration, which became so severe that it prompted her to be evaluated. She has a history of headaches for the past year, which have been progressively worsening. Headaches are holocranial and pressure sensation and appear to be positional, worsened with lying down. On review of systems, she also endorses pulsatile tinnitus and transient visual obscurations. On examination, the patient is lying in a dark, quiet room and appears uncomfortable with the head of the bed elevated to 45 degrees. Physical exam is notable for bilateral papilledema on fundoscopy, BMI is 31, but vital signs were stable, and neurologic exam is otherwise unremarkable. Lab work was benign. MRI brain and MRV were done and were remarkable for a partially empty sella and stenosis of the right transverse sinus without dural venous thrombosis. LP was performed with an opening pressure of 32 and otherwise benign CSF studies. The patient wants to better understand her diagnosis now that she is past the most severe pain. The resident explains that she has IIH, counsels on lifestyle modifications and the correlation of weight loss and improvement in IIH symptoms, and prescribes acetazolamide. She refers the patient for prompt ophthalmology follow-up and visual field testing.

REFERENCES

1. Ravishankar K. Which headache to investigate, when, and how? *Headache.* 2016;*56*(10):1685–1697.
2. International Committee on the Classification of Headache. The International Classification of Headache Disorders, 3rd edition. *Cephalalgia.* 2018;*38*(1):1–211
3. Dodick DW. Clinical clues and clinical rules: primary vs secondary headache. *Adv Stud Med* 2003;*3*:87–92.
4. Do TP, Remmers A, Schytz HW, Schankin C, Nelson SE, Obermann M, Hansen JM, Sinclair AJ, Gantenbein AR, Schoonman GG. Red and orange flags for secondary headaches in clinical practice: SNNOOP10 list. *Neurology.* 2019 Jan 15;*92*(3):134–144.
5. Benjamin EJ, Blaha MJ, Chiuve SE, et al.. Heart disease and stroke statistics: 2017 update: a report from the American Heart Association. *Circulation* 2017;*135*:e146–e603.
6. Harriott AM, Karakaya F, Ayata C. Headache after ischemic stroke: A systematic review and meta-analysis. *Neurology.* 2020 Jan 7;*94*(1):e75–e86. doi: 10.1212/WNL.0000000000008591. Epub 2019 Nov 6. PMID: 31694924; PMCID: PMC7011689.
7. Pretto Flores L, De Almeida CS, Casulari LA. Positive predictive values of selected clinical signs associated with skull base fractures. *J Neurosurg Sci.* 2000 Jun;*44*(2):77–82; discussion 82–3. PMID: 11105835.
8. Kumar V. Eye is the Window to the Brain Pathology. *Curr Adv Ophthalmol.* 2018 Aug;*1*(1):3–4. doi: 10.29199/2638-9940/CAOP-101013. Epub 2017 Nov 15. PMID: 31123726; PMCID: PMC6528662.
9. Bellur S, Thomasian J, Hacopian A, Vilar N. Papilledema as the initial presenting clinical sign of subdural hemorrhage. *J Neuroophthalmol.* 2023 Dec 1;*43*(4):e154–e155. doi: 10.1097/WNO.0000000000001376. Epub 2021 Aug 18. PMID: 37974366.
10. Schirmer CM, Hedges TR 3rd. Mechanisms of visual loss in papilledema. *Neurosurg Focus.* 2007;*23*(5):E5. doi: 10.3171/FOC-07/11/E5. PMID: 18004967.
11. Passi N, Degnan AJ, Levy LM. MR imaging of papilledema and visual pathways: effects of increased intracranial pressure and pathophysiologic mechanisms. *AJNR Am J Neuroradiol.* 2013 May;*34*(5):919–924. doi: 10.3174/ajnr.A3022. Epub 2012 Mar 15. PMID: 22422187; PMCID: PMC7964659.
12. Froment Tilikete C. How to assess eye movements clinically. *Neurol Sci.* 2022 May;*43*(5):2969–2981. doi: 10.1007/s10072-022-05981-5. Epub 2022 Mar 3. PMID: 35239052.
13. Spector RH. The Pupils. In: Walker HK, Hall WD, Hurst JW, editors. *Clinical Methods: The History, Physical, and Laboratory Examinations.* 3rd edition. Boston: Butterworths; 1990. Chapter 58.
14. Cooper SA, Metcalfe RA. Assess and interpret the visual fields at the bedside. *Pract Neurol.* 2009 Dec;*9*(6):324–334. doi: 10.1136/jnnp.2009.193920. PMID: 19923112.
15. Venkatramani J, Mitchell P. Ocular and systemic causes of retinopathy in patients without diabetes mellitus. *BMJ.* 2004 Mar 13;*328*(7440):625–9. doi: 10.1136/bmj.328.7440.625. PMID: 15016695; PMCID: PMC381138.
16. Nowaczewska M, Wiciński M, Straburzyński M, Kaźmierczak W. The prevalence of different types of headache in patients with subjective tinnitus and its influence on tinnitus parameters: A prospective *Clinical Study. Brain Sci.* 2020 Oct 24;*10*(11):776. doi: 10.3390/brainsci10110776. PMID: 33114375; PMCID: PMC7694111.
17. Hakimi AA, Lalehzarian SP, Lalehzarian AS, Azhdam AM, Boodaie BD, Walner DL. Development and evaluation of an objective tympanic membrane visualization assessment technique. *Ann Otol Rhinol Laryngol.* 2020 Aug;*129*(8):767–771. doi: 10.1177/0003489420912438. Epub 2020 Mar 8. PMID: 32148067.
18. Robblee J, Secora KA. Debunking myths: Sinus headache. *Curr Neurol Neurosci Rep.* 2021 Jun 20;*21*(8):42. doi: 10.1007/s11910-021-01127-w. PMID: 34148140.
19. La Mantia I, Grillo C, Andaloro C. Rhinogenic contact point headache: Surgical treatment versus medical treatment. *J Craniofac Surg.* 2018 May;*29*(3):e228–e230. doi: 10.1097/SCS.0000000000004211. PMID: 29283946.
20. Davis LE, Katzman JG. Chronic daily headache: when to suspect meningitis. *Curr Pain Headache Rep.* 2008 Jan;*12*(1):50–55. doi: 10.1007/s11916-008-0010-9. PMID: 18417024.

21. Sollmann N, Schandelmaier P, Weidlich D, Stelter J, Joseph GB, Börner C, Schramm S, Beer M, Zimmer C, Landgraf MN, Heinen F, Karampinos DC, Baum T, Bonfert MV. Headache frequency and neck pain are associated with trapezius muscle T2 in tension-type headache among young adults. *J Headache Pain.* 2023 Jul 12;*24*(1):84.

22. Henig NR, Pierson DJ. Mechanisms of hypoxemia. *Respir Care Clin N Am.* 2000 Dec;*6*(4):501–521. doi: 10.1016/s1078-5337(05)70087-3. PMID: 11172576.

23. Błaszczyk B, Martynowicz H, Więckiewicz M, Straburzyński M, Antolak M, Budrewicz S, Staszkiewicz M, Kopszak A, Waliszewska-Prosół M. Prevalence of headaches and their relationship with obstructive sleep apnea (OSA) - Systematic review and meta-analysis. *Sleep Med Rev.* 2023 Dec 1;*73*:101889. doi: 10.1016/j.smrv.2023.101889. Epub ahead of print. PMID: 38056382.

24. Mueller BR, Robinson-Papp J. Postural orthostatic tachycardia syndrome and migraine: A narrative review. *Headache.* 2022 Jul;*62*(7):792–800. doi: 10.1111/head.14365. Epub 2022 Jul 19. PMID: 35852052.

25. Fedorowski A. Postural orthostatic tachycardia syndrome: clinical presentation, aetiology and management. *J Intern Med.* 2019 Apr;*285*(4):352–366. doi: 10.1111/joim.12852. Epub 2018 Nov 23. PMID: 30372565.

26. Abbott AV. Diagnostic approach to palpitations. *Am Fam Physician.* 2005 Feb 15;*71*(4):743–750. PMID: 15742913.

27. Torres-Yaghi Y, Salerian J, Dougherty C. Cardiac cephalgia. *Curr Pain Headache Rep.* 2015 Apr;*19*(4):14. doi: 10.1007/s11916-015-0481-4. PMID: 25819974.

28. Strikić Đula I, Pleić N, Babić Leko M, Gunjača I, Torlak V, Brdar D, Punda A, Polašek O, Hayward C, Zemunik T. Epidemiology of hypothyroidism, hyperthyroidism and positive thyroid antibodies in the Croatian population. *Biology (Basel).* 2022 Mar 2;*11*(3):394. doi: 10.3390/biology11030394. PMID: 35336768; PMCID: PMC8945477.

29. Everts ME. Effects of thyroid hormones on contractility and cation transport in skeletal muscle. *Acta Physiol Scand.* 1996 Mar;*156*(3):325–333. doi: 10.1046/j.1365-201X.1996.203000.x. PMID: 8729693.

30. Aurora SK, Shrewsbury SB, Ray S, Hindiyeh N, Nguyen L. A link between gastrointestinal disorders and migraine: Insights into the gut-brain connection. *Headache.* 2021 Apr;*61*(4):576–589. doi: 10.1111/head.14099. Epub 2021 Apr 1. PMID: 33793965; PMCID: PMC8251535.

31. Frieri M. Mast cell activation syndrome. *Clin Rev Allergy Immunol.* 2018 Jun;*54*(3):353–365. doi: 10.1007/s12016-015-8487-6. PMID: 25944644.

32. Lee HL, Yeo M, Choi GH, Lee JY, Kim JS, Shin DI, Lee SS, Lee SH. Clinical characteristics of headache or facial pain prior to the development of acute herpes zoster of the head. *Clin Neurol Neurosurg.* 2017 Jan;*152*:90–94. doi: 10.1016/j.clineuro.2016.12.004. Epub 2016 Dec 8. PMID: 27978460.

Allergy/Immunology Comorbidities in the Treatment of Headache

Jessica Galant-Swafford and Melissa Dang

LEARNING OBJECTIVES

1. Identify the allergy/immunology comorbidities that play a role in the treatment of head-ache, including rhinosinusitis, asthma, atopic dermatitis, urticaria, systemic mastocytosis, and immunodeficiency
2. Describe hypothesized mechanisms linking atopic disorders and headache, including the potential role of mast cells and histamine
3. Understand that dedicated evaluation for and treatment of headache disorders is critically important, as they can be misdiagnosed as allergic diseases

---

INTRODUCTION

Patients with headache disorders can present to their primary care provider, neurologist, or allergist with concomitant allergic/immunologic symptoms. Observational cohort studies have demonstrated that individuals with headache syndromes are more likely to have atopic disorders and vice versa.[1] In one study, atopic disorders were 21.6% more common in migraine with aura compared to migraine without aura and tension-type headaches.[2] The most significant atopic disorders were found to be conjunctivitis, rhinitis, and asthma.[2] In this chapter, we will review the most common allergic/immunologic comorbidities associated with headache and provide a summary of the diagnosis and treatment of these disorders (Table 4.1 and Figure 4.1), which we hope will assist providers in their management of these patients.

DOI: 10.1201/b23330-4

TABLE 4.1 Allergy immunology comorbidities in the treatment of headache

- Rhinitis
  - Allergic rhinitis
  - Nonallergic rhinitis
- Sinusitis
  - Acute sinusitis
  - Chronic rhinosinusitis with nasal polyps
  - Chronic rhinosinusitis without nasal polyps
- Eosinophilic diseases
  - Eosinophilic granulomatosis with polyangiitis
- Chronic urticaria with or without angioedema
- Atopic dermatitis
- Adverse food reactions (not including food allergy or anaphylaxis)
- Mast cell disorders
  - Systemic mastocytosis
  - Mast cell activation syndrome
- Immunodeficiency
  - Primary antibody deficiency (especially those on immunoglobulin replacement therapy)

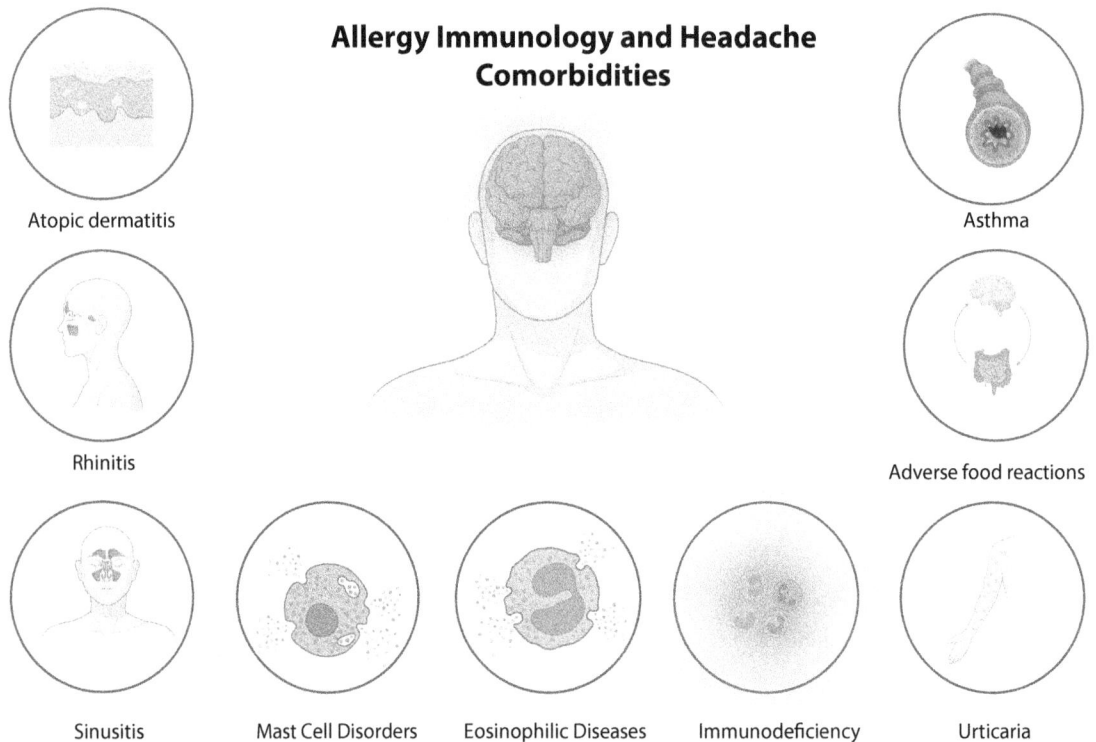

FIGURE 4.1 Overview of allergic and immunologic comorbidities in the treatment of headache.

THE ROLE OF MAST CELLS AND HISTAMINE IN ATOPIC DISEASE AND HEADACHE

Inquiry into a potential linking mechanism between allergic disease and headache and whether treatment of one disease has an impact on the other has been ongoing for decades. Histamine is a monoamine known to play a significant role in anaphylaxis and allergic disease in the skin, nose, and airways. Histamine has three primary sources in humans: mast cells and basophils, gastric enterochromaffin-like cells, and the central nervous system. There are multiple histamine receptor subtypes. Within the syndrome of anaphylaxis and other allergic states, signaling through the H1 receptor mediates vascular permeability, leading to urticaria and angioedema, and signaling through the H2 receptor mediates mucous secretion. H3 is the receptor that dominates in the brain. Histamine in the brain is synthesized by neurons in the posterior basal hypothalamus and, more specifically, the tuberomammillary nucleus.[3] This region is a suspected locus in several primary headache disorders. The histaminergic system in the brain plays an important role in the sleep-wake cycle, and activation of both H3 and H4 receptors inhibits neurons and neurologic inflammation, promoting sleep and reducing the sensation of pain. Increased levels of histamine have been found in migraine.[4] However, this increase in histamine may be a secondary phenomenon relative to other primary signaling processes, as histamine does not penetrate the blood–brain barrier. As well, most antihistamines have been shown to be ineffective as abortive migraine medications, outside of two potent H1 receptor antagonists, cinnarizine (quite nonspecific) and cyproheptadine[5] (also inhibits the serotonin receptor); however, evidence is limited. There are currently no ongoing clinical trials for migraine prophylaxis or treatment targeting the H3 or H4 receptors.

Unlike histamine, mast cells residing in peripheral tissues can penetrate the blood–brain barrier and may be found in the dura mater close to trigeminal afferent nerves. These mast cells may secrete proinflammatory and vasodilatory molecules, which can contribute to migraine. One study in rats showed that mast cells degranulate in response to meningeal nociceptors, a process that may be mediated by substance P via the neurokinin-1 receptor.[6] However, no elevation of substance P has been shown in migraine, and antagonists of substance P have not been effective in treating migraine. In contrast, calcitonin gene-related peptide (CGRP), a vasoactive peptide with similar properties to substance P, which can also induce degranulation of dural mast cells, has been found elevated in the plasma during migraine,[7] and many CGRP antagonists have been shown to be effective in treating migraine.[8] Of note, CGRP and its receptor complex are expressed by type-2 innate lymphoid cells (ILC2).[9] Whether CGRP antagonists that are used in migraine affect ILC2 function is unknown.

> **Clinical Case #1**
>
> A 54-year-old woman with chronic rhinitis with nasal polyposis who has been treated for migraine has presented to the clinic for further management. She has had a 30-year history of dull headaches in temporal relation to rhinosinusitis, which waxes and wanes with the degree of sinus congestion, exacerbated by pressure over her sinuses with sneezing with associated facial pain and hyposmia. She has had minimal improvement with nasal steroid sprays. Her vital signs are 98.7, BP 132/74, HR 68 beats/min. On physical exam she has sinus tenderness but no visualized nasal polyps. What is the next step?

ALLERGIC AND NONALLERGIC RHINITIS

Allergic and nonallergic rhinitis are common presentations to a primary care and allergists' office. Rhinitis can be defined as inflammation found in the nasal mucosa, with common symptoms manifesting as nasal congestion, sneezing, rhinorrhea, and pruritus. The prevalence in the United States ranges from

15% to 30% by physician and patient self-report, respectively.[10] Allergic rhinitis (AR) typically manifests in childhood, with more than 80% starting before the second decade of life.[11] In AR, allergens are responsible for triggering these symptoms through immunoglobulin E (IgE)-mediated pathways. When an allergen bound to a specific serum IgE binds to FcεRI receptors on target cells, including mast cells and eosinophils; these cells in turn release cytokines, eicosanoids, and their secretory granules that lead to allergic inflammation.

In contrast, nonallergic rhinitis (NAR) lacks an associated allergenic component and can be attributed to vasomotor, infectious, occupational, hormone, and drug-induced causes. NAR may have an innate form of inflammation, and both AR and NAR can coexist. Both disease processes can significantly affect quality of life, including sleep and school performance, as well as lead to a large economic burden on society.[12] However, readily available treatments such as nasal corticosteroids, antihistamines, and nasal irrigation exist that can treat chronic inflammation in the nasal mucosa and lead to an improvement in symptoms and improved quality of life.

Various studies have shown a link between migraine and AR. Patients with AR have been found to have a higher chance of developing migraine compared to NAR patients, with some studies showing up to 14.4 times higher incidence, with greater frequency in the mixed rhinitis, both AR and NAR, group.[13–15] This relationship exists across age groups, with AR and migraine frequently occurring together in childhood.[16] Collectively, these studies demonstrate a clinical association between migraine and rhinitis; however, whether this is due to a shared mechanism or another mediating demographic or comorbid factor is unknown. Whether the dual presence of AR/NAR and migraine could suggest a particular endotype of disease and therefore warrant a more specific treatment strategy is also not known and a topic for further research.

Observational studies have suggested that the character of headaches can differ in patients with AR vs. NAR. Allergic subjects tended to develop headaches in the morning compared to nonallergic subjects who developed headaches in the evening with no significant difference in allergic and nonallergic patients between migraine duration, frequency of attacks, or location of pain.[16]

The potential benefit of treatments for AR and NAR helping to prevent migraine attacks is unknown. Intranasal topical therapies are the mainstay of therapy for both AR and NAR, which include intranasal corticosteroid sprays (i.e., fluticasone, triamcinolone), intranasal muscarinic antagonist sprays (i.e., ipratropium bromide), and intranasal mast cell stabilizing sprays (i.e., azelastine). In one study, the treatment of migraine associated with AR with intranasal corticosteroids and oral antihistamines was studied over three months with a notable decline in the prevalence and frequency of migraine.[17] Another study examined anti-asthmatic and anti-allergic therapies and found that nasal corticosteroids, inhaled corticosteroids, and antihistamines significantly reduced migraine in children and adolescents.[18]

Allergen immunotherapy (AIT) has been shown over many decades to improve symptoms in AR. Subcutaneous immunotherapy has been found to significantly reduce clinical symptoms in moderate to severe cases of AR by desensitizing individuals to their allergens.[19] Sublingual immunotherapy is also now available, and there are now four Food and Drug Administration (FDA)–approved tablets to treat sensitization to various aeroallergens.[20] A study of AR patients investigated the relationship between immunotherapy and headache prevalence, frequency, and disability.[21] Compared to individuals not on AIT, AIT was correlated with a decreased prevalence of migraine, but only in populations younger than age 40.[21] Within the immunotherapy groups, individuals over age 40 had a higher prevalence of migraine.[21] When examining migraine frequency and disability in those with a lesser burden of atopic disease, they found that those with less allergic sensitization had decreased migraine frequency and disability, while a higher burden of atopic disease was associated with more allergic sensitization and higher frequency of migraine.[21] In patients below 45 years of age, less migraine frequency and disability were associated with immunotherapy.[21] In summary, more studies examining the link between the benefit of immunotherapy and headache in AR are needed, given that AIT may be a preferable treatment strategy in this group.

RHINOSINUSITIS AND NASAL POLYPS

Rhinosinusitis is a common reported condition in any primary care office, defined as inflammation in the nasal and sinus cavities, further separated into acute rhinosinusitis (ARS), chronic rhinosinusitis (CRS), and chronic rhinosinusitis with nasal polyps (CRSwNP).[22] The prevalence of ARS can be up to 6%–15%, while CRS has been found to impact 12% of the US population.[22]

ARS is diagnosed by a clinical history with symptoms that include purulent nasal discharge, facial pain, cough, fever, and tooth pain. These symptoms last for fewer than four weeks. Most cases of ARS are viral and resolve in ten days or fewer, while bacterial ARS fails to improve or exhibits a worsening of symptoms. The most common bacterial pathogens involved are *Streptococcus pneumoniae, Haemophilus influenzae, Moraxella catarrhalis, Staphylococcus aureus*, and *anaerobes*, while common viruses include rhinovirus and coronavirus.[23, 24]

In contrast, CRS is defined as symptoms lasting longer than 12 weeks. The clinical history combined with a sinus CT scan or nasal endoscopy shows sinonasal inflammation. CRS can be associated with fungal disease (both infectious and allergic). Treatment strategies vary from oral and nasal steroids to irrigation, antibiotics, and, less commonly, surgical intervention.

Nasal polyps are benign growths in the sinus cavities reflective of specific subtypes/endotypes of chronic inflammation. While males are more likely to get nasal polyps compared to their female counterparts, no environmental or genetic link has been found to have a strong association.[25] Contributory factors in disease have been hypothesized to be related to exposures to colonized bacteria and pathogens, host immune system dysregulation, and dysfunction of the sinonasal epithelial barrier.[25]

Nasal polyps are associated with distinct inflammatory syndromes. Aspirin-, or NSAID-, exacerbated respiratory disease (AERD) is defined by the clinical triad of asthma, nasal polyposis, and aspirin or NSAID hypersensitivity involving provoked symptoms of the upper and lower airways including nasal congestion and shortness of breath, wheeze, or cough suggestive of bronchospasm. AERD is considered an endotype of asthma in which intrinsic overproduction of cysteinyl leukotrienes predisposes individuals to bronchial inflammation and hyperresponsiveness as a consequence of the deficiency of the protective prostaglandin E2 with COX-1 inhibition. Eosinophilic granulomatosis with polyangiitis (EGPA) is a small vessel vasculitis involving eosinophilic infiltration into tissues. In the airways, EGPA clinically presents with asthma, pulmonary infiltrations, and nasal polyposis, and outside of the airways can involve rash, neuropathy, gastrointestinal disease, and even cardiomyopathy. Lastly, cystic fibrosis is also associated with nasal polyposis and thick sinonasal secretions.

Headache and facial pain have been reported to be as high as 16%–67% in those with nasal polyps, with endoscopic surgery relieving pain in 80% of patients.[26] In contrast, other studies have found a negative association of migraine with nasal polyps.[27]

The term "sinus headache" has often been used as a vague term to describe facial pain and pressure in those with headaches.[28] Misdiagnosis of primary headache disorder as sinus headaches has been found to be between 50% and 80%.[29] More accurately, the term "rhinogenic" headache refers to secondary headache that originates from mucosal contact points in nasal cavities. These headaches do not have notable inflammatory signs of hyperplastic mucosa or purulent discharge. It has been hypothesized that the anatomic or mechanical obstruction points are what leads to headache symptoms.[30] Before examining rhinogenic headache, it is crucial for the clinician to rule out primary headache disorders such as cluster, tension-type, and migraine, as these are more common (Figure 4.2).

There is controversy in the literature regarding the association between chronic headache and CRS. One group examined the association between chronic headache and CRS in a population of 30,000 individuals aged 30 to 44 years and found that those with CRS had at least a nine-fold increased risk of chronic headache. A follow-up 36 months later showed treatment with nasal surgery, steroids, and discontinuation of headache medications and decongestants improved headaches associated with CRS.[31] Conversely, some studies have suggested an overdiagnosis of headaches in rhinosinusitis.[32] Although primary headache

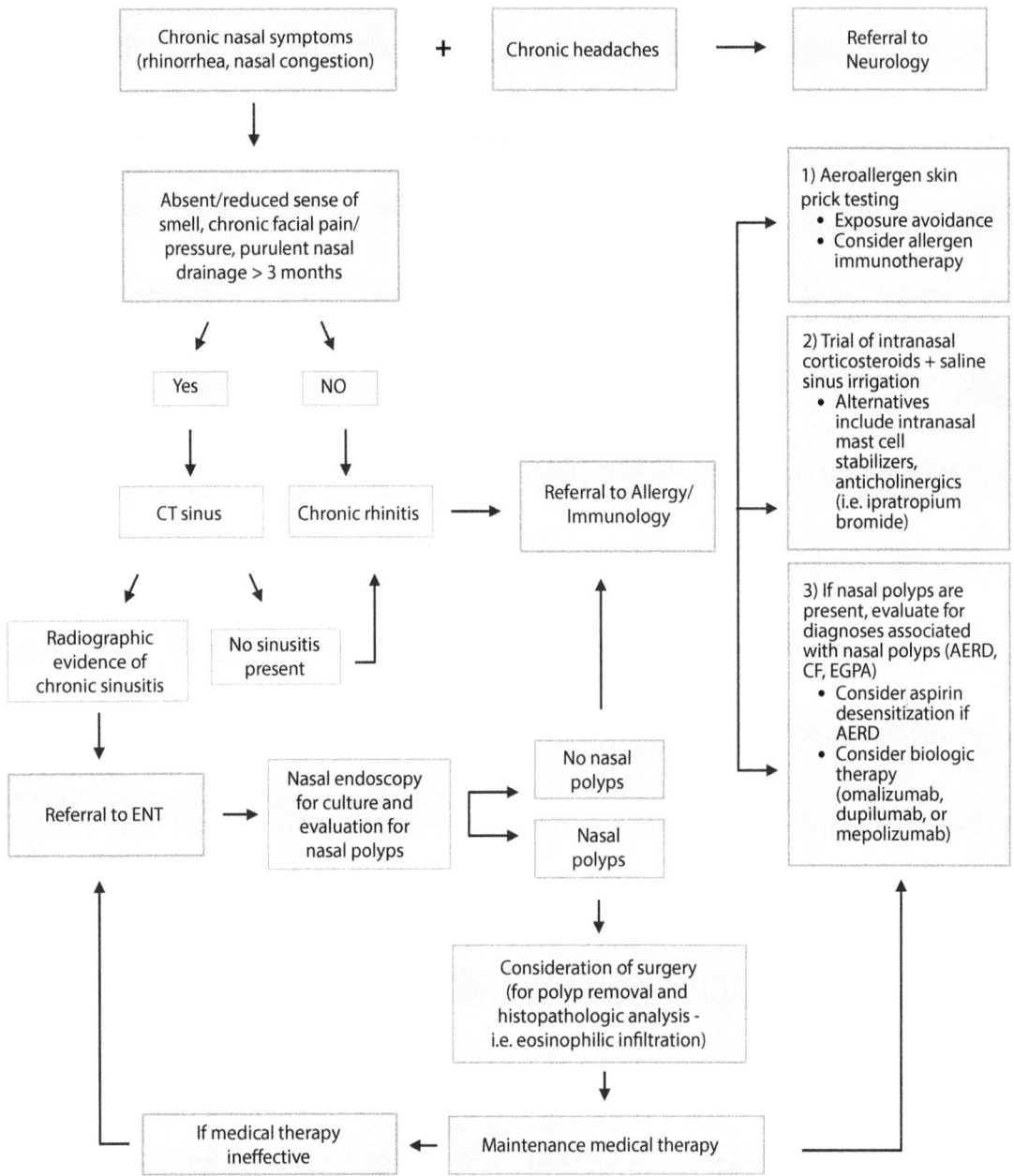

FIGURE 4.2 Diagnostic algorithm in patients with rhinosinusitis and headache. (AERD: Aspirin exacerbated respiratory disease; CF: Cystic Fibrosis; EGPA: Eosinophilic granulomatosis with polyangiitis.)

disorders and rhinosinusitis may coexist, these studies suggest headache from rhinosinusitis is uncommon. Migraine presentation may mimic rhinosinusitis with activation of parasympathetic nerves, leading to autonomic symptoms found in both disorders.[33] Even more, pain was not found to be an accurate prognostic factor in headaches.[34] Even though the diagnostic criteria for CRS can include pain, there was a noted poor correlation between pain, headache, and paranasal sinus inflammation on imaging.[35] In another study called the Sinus, Allergy, and Migraine Study (SAMS), 100 patients were examined who had a self-diagnosis of sinus headache, and the investigators found the majority of these patients had migraine or likely migraine. Misdiagnosis was due in part to triggers and location of pain.[36]

There are three biologic agents FDA-approved for the treatment of CRS with nasal polyposis. Dupilumab is a monoclonal antibody that binds to and blocks the alpha subunit of the interleukin-4 receptor (IL-4Rα), thereby blocking signaling through both IL-4 and interleukin 13 pathways, which results in the release of proinflammatory cytokines, chemokines, and IgE. Dupilumab is also FDA-approved for atopic dermatitis, asthma, eosinophilic esophagitis, and prurigo nodularis. Omalizumab is a monoclonal antibody that binds to free IgE, thereby reducing allergic inflammation by downregulating activating FcεRI receptors on basophils and mast cells. In addition to nasal polyposis, omalizumab is also FDA-approved for chronic urticaria, allergic asthma, and most recently IgE-mediated food allergies. Lastly, mepolizumab is a monoclonal antibody that blocks interleukin-5 (IL-5), the cytokine responsible for the maturation, proliferation, and activation of eosinophils. To date, no studies suggest treatment with these various biologics has helped improve headache symptoms but rather note headache as a potential side effect (reference?). However, if treatment aims to address headaches from nasal polyps, patients may find symptomatic relief. Additional studies are required to investigate this association.

In summary, a careful multidisciplinary and personalized approach by primary care physicians, allergists, neurologists, and otolaryngologists is needed in complex cases of sinus disease, facial pain/pressure, and headache.

Answer to Clinical Case #1

It is important for clinicians to rule out a primary headache before considering rhinogenic causes. Rhinogenic headaches may stem from referred pain from mucosal contact or nasal polyp proliferation, leading to continued pressure. Even if there are negative results from previous exams, including rhinoscopy, this does not rule out sinus etiologies. Referrals to otolaryngology may be justified. Otolaryngologists may perform nasal endoscopies and imaging, such as computed tomography of the paranasal sinuses, as part of their evaluation. Depending on these findings, this patient would be a candidate for endoscopic sinus surgery. Biologics, such as dupilumab, mepolizumab, or omalizumab, are another modality aimed to reduce the need for repeated surgical intervention of CRS with nasal polyposis. These are novel treatment approaches that may be suitable for a certain patient population.

ALLERGIC EYE DISEASES

Allergic conjunctivitis (AC) is characterized by the conjunctiva's inflammatory response to an allergen with subsequent bilateral ocular redness, pruritus, and tearing. To date, there is limited evidence for a relationship between AC and migraine, but some notable findings exist. In a population-based cohort study, the incidence of migraine in the AC cohort was 1.92-fold higher compared to the nonallergic conjunctivitis (NAC) cohort. The timing of developing migraine was four to five years after a diagnosis of AC.[37] As well, individuals with AC have been found to have an increased risk of migraine development.[38, 39] Many topical ophthalmic agents for AC, such as azelastine, emedastine, ketotifen fumarate, loteprednol, nedocromil, and olopatadine, have headache listed as a potential side effect ranging from 5% to 11%.[40] Therefore, clinicians should note allergic eye disease as a consideration in their diagnosis of migraine.

Clinical Case #2

A 36-year-old woman with a prior history of asthma presents to her primary care physician with reports of increased frequency and severity of headaches. Symptoms started after the birth of her third child. The headaches meet criteria for migraine with aura. She reports that she has also been experiencing increased chest tightness, limiting her physical exertion and cough, particularly in

the springtime, where usually she would only have a mild runny nose and itchy eyes that were controlled with as-needed antihistamines in the past. She has a prescription for albuterol that she has been using about twice per day, which helps her exertional symptoms but wears off quickly; currently, she is waking up at night at least three times per week coughing and feeling the need to use her inhaler. Moreover, she reports that she had one emergency room visit this year when she caught a cold from her toddler, and she had persistent wheezing and coughing two weeks later. She was treated with azithromycin and a taper of prednisone, her first such course in many years.

Asthma is a chronic heterogeneous obstructive airway disease affecting more than 300 million people worldwide and is a leading cause of school absenteeism in children, with socioeconomically disadvantaged and minority individuals having worse outcomes (PMID: 30055181, H. S. Zahran, C. M. Bailey, S. A. Damon, P. L. Garbe, P. N. Breysse Vital signs: Asthma in children—United States, 2001–2016 Morb Mortal Wkly Rep, 67 (2018), pp. 149–155).

Asthma is characterized by chronic airway inflammation, reversible airflow limitation, and airway hyperresponsiveness that leads to symptoms of cough, chest tightness, and shortness of breath. It ranges in severity from mild, intermittent to severe, persistent with exacerbations of disease that can be triggered by allergen exposure, natural weather events including wildfires and thunderstorms, air pollutants, exercise, and respiratory viruses. Left untreated or undercontrolled, asthma can result in airway remodeling with fixed airflow obstruction, increased mucus production, higher rate of lower respiratory infections, reduced exercise tolerance, and poor quality of life.

Migraine is a frequent comorbidity identified in individuals with asthma and vice versa. In one meta-analysis, migraine was associated with an increased prevalence of asthma (OR: 1.54; 95% CI: 1.34–1.77) and individuals with asthma had an increased risk for migraine (pooled RR: 1.42, 95% CI: 1.26–1.60).[41] One cohort study found that asthma was a risk factor in the progression of episodic migraine to chronic migraine, and this was associated with the severity of respiratory symptoms.[42] Headache frequency and headache pain intensity were also found to be associated with comorbid asthma.[43]

The reason for the bidirectional relationship between asthma and migraine is unknown and likely multifactorial, including underlying immunologic mechanisms and shared genetic or environmental factors, with the relative contributions of these factors varying in individual patients (Figure 4.3). As previously discussed, proinflammatory and vasodilatory mediators can be released from mast cells in the dura, including neuropeptides such as substance P. However, the relationship between the cytokines and signaling molecules discussed in the various endotypes of asthma have not been specifically studied in migraine. Air pollution may play a role in the connection between the two disorders; increased levels of $PM_{2.5}$, PM_{10}, NO_2, O_3, and CO have been found to significantly increase the risk of migraine[44] and are known contributors to asthma severity and exacerbations.[45–47]

Parasympathetic stimulation is thought to be a linking mechanism in asthma and migraine as well. Increased cholinergic tone is implicated in asthma, leading to increased airway mucous secretion with airway smooth muscle hyperreactivity and thickening.[48] In migraine, acetylcholine can activate the trigeminal pain pathway and trigger degranulation of dural mast cells.[49] Activation of transient receptor potential vanilloid subfamily member 1 (TRPV1) is also relevant in both asthma and migraine. TRPV1 is expressed on trigeminal nociceptors, and when activated by chemical substances, including acid and heat, it results in the release of various neuropeptides, potentially leading to the generation of migraine.[50] Activation of TRPV1 in airway C-fiber afferent neurons endogenously or by inhaled irritants has been demonstrated in patients with asthma.[51]

Hormonal factors may also connect asthma and headache. Cyclical changes in estrogens are known to provoke migraine in migraine-prone individuals.[52] In asthma, the relationship between sex and disease severity is complex.[53] In contrast to children where asthma is more common in males, adult women have an increased prevalence of asthma compared to men, a switch that coincides with puberty.[54] Studies have also shown worsening of asthma symptoms during the premenstrual and menstrual cycles.[55] Changes in asthma severity and symptoms have also been reported by women during pregnancy and menopause, though whether the disease worsens, is stable, or improves through these physiologic changes may depend on the endotype of the disease and the existing asthma therapy in each patient.[56, 57]

Key features:
- Chronic airway inflammation
- Reversible airflow limitation
- Airway hyperresponsiveness

Neurology and allergy/immunology comanagement

Key features:
- Without aura: hours, typically unilateral, pulsating, moderate to severe, photophobia, phonophobia
- With aura: minutes, unilateral symptoms: visual, sensory, speech, motor impairments
- Physical activity can exacerbate symptoms

ASTHMA ⟷ MIGRAINE

Symptoms:
- Cough
- Chest tightness
- Shortness of breath

Multifactorial linking mechanisms:
- Underlying immunologic mechanisms
- Shared genetic or environmental factors
- Air pollution
- Parasympathetic stimulation
- Hormones
- estrogen

Triggers:
- Stress
- Diet
- Light
- Hormones
- Medications
- Odors
- estrogen

Triggers:
- Allergen exposure
- Exercise
- Viruses

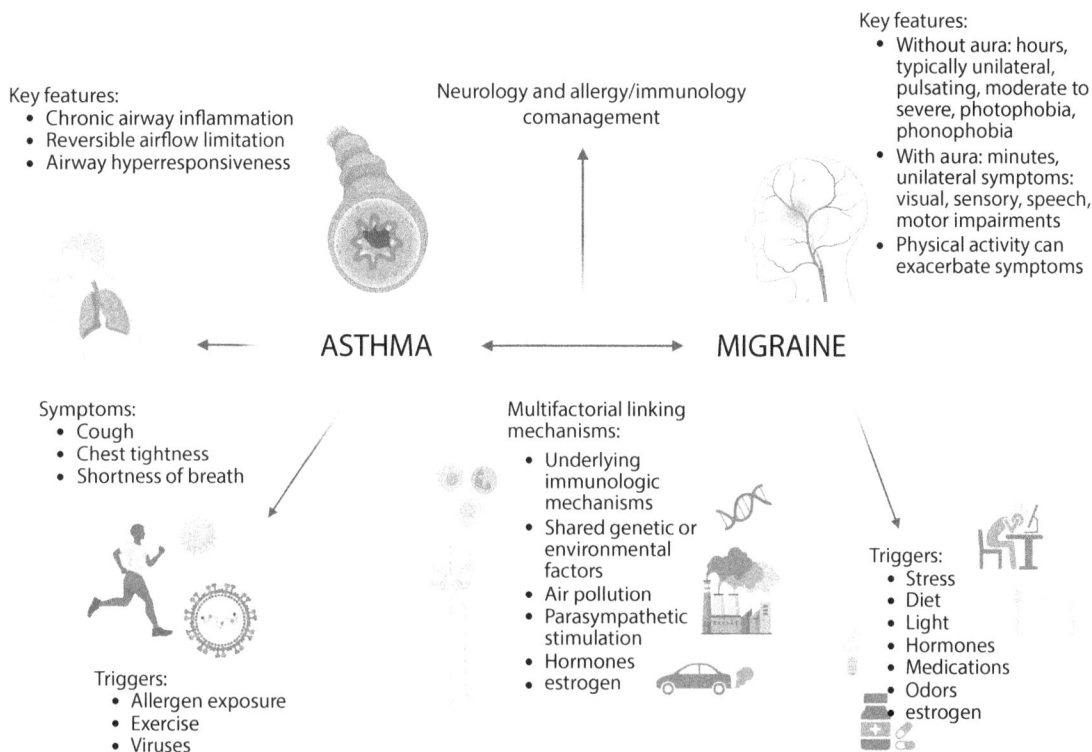

FIGURE 4.3 Bidirectional relationship of asthma and migraine.

Over the past 20 years, significant advancements in understanding the pathophysiology of asthma have focused on endotypes of disease defined by specific systemic and airway inflammatory pathways in each patient. Two broad categories have been identified: type 2 high asthma, which includes allergic asthma and separately eosinophilic asthma, and type 2 low asthma. The identification of these endotypes has led to more personalization of asthma therapy. In brief, allergic asthma, often starting in childhood, involves specific binding of aeroallergens (e.g., house dust mite, animal dander, or pollen) to resident dendritic cells in the airway, which then present these particles to tissue-resident memory CD4+ type 2–helper T (Th2) lymphocytes triggering a signaling cascade, which leads to allergic inflammation in the airways. Type 2–innate lymphoid cells are another important source of type 2 cytokines in asthma. Eosinophilic asthma is a specific subtype of type 2 asthma and is characterized by endogenous overproduction of type 2 cytokines interleukin-4, interleukin-5, and interleukin-13. Together, these cytokines lead to mucous hypersecretion, bronchoconstriction, and increased eosinophilic airway inflammation. Type 2 low asthma includes paucigranulocytic asthma and neutrophilic asthma, with the absence of allergic or eosinophilic inflammation. This type of asthma relies on type 1 helper T (Th1) and type 17 helper T (TH17) CD4+ lymphocytes, which stimulate neutrophilic inflammation via inflammatory molecules, such as tumor necrosis factor alpha (TNF-a), interferon-gamma, interleukin-6, interleukin-17A, and the alarmin thymic stromal lymphopoietin.

Asthma therapy depends on the severity (frequency of symptoms) and degree of control (number of exacerbations requiring systemic corticosteroids). There are many different factors that affect the severity of asthma in an individual: these include disease-specific factors (genetics, disease endotype, response to corticosteroids, comorbid conditions including rhinosinusitis, gastroesophageal reflux disease, cardiovascular disease, and vocal cord dysfunction) and also socio-economic factors including race/ethnicity, air quality, school and home location, and access to health care. There is a stepwise escalation of therapy for difficult-to-treat asthma with updated guidelines as of 2020.[58] The mainstay of therapy is daily inhaled corticosteroid therapy along with short-acting bronchodilator on-demand therapy to reduce airway inflammation and provide relief as needed. Long-acting bronchodilator therapy (beta agonist or muscarinic antagonist) can be added to the inhaled corticosteroid for improved symptomatic relief. Additional therapies include leukotriene receptor antagonist therapy (montelukast). For difficult-to-control asthma, there are now six FDA-approved biologic agents: omalizumab for allergic asthma (anti-IgE); reslizumab, mepolizumab, and benralizumab for eosinophilic asthma, dupilumab for steroid-dependent; and the newer tezepelumab, which has no biomarker requirement, being utilized for refractory asthma.

Importantly, it is not known whether particular endotypes of asthma may be more or less correlated with headache or migraine. Future research may shed light on more optimal treatments for asthma in individuals with headache disorders and vice versa. For instance, propranolol, which is widely used for migraine prophylaxis, should be avoided in individuals with severe asthma, as propranolol is a nonselective beta-blocker that can worsen bronchospasm. Further research will lead to more personalized approaches in patients with both diagnoses.

Answer to Clinical Case #2

The patient has symptoms that suggest both migraine and uncontrolled asthma. The hormonal shift following childbirth could be linked to the worsening of these two diseases. Her asthma would be classified as moderate persistent, given that she describes nocturnal awakenings multiple times per week and symptoms that limit her activity level nearly every day, with one exacerbation requiring an emergency room visit and systemic corticosteroids within the past 12 months. Uncontrolled AR is an important comorbidity that has likely led to worsening respiratory symptoms. In addition to a neurology referral, she will benefit from evaluation by an allergy/immunology specialist. Aeroallergen skin testing, pulmonary function testing, and escalation of her rhinitis and asthma treatment regimens are recommended. She can start a once daily antihistamine along with an intranasal steroid spray to help reduce nasal inflammation and resulting mucous drainage to the lower airway. Based on asthma treatment guidelines, her disease is undertreated with the use of a short-acting bronchodilator as needed; she will benefit from starting a controller agent starting with either an inhaled corticosteroid or inhaled corticosteroid plus long-acting, beta-agonist combination to improve daily symptoms and prevent exacerbations.

ANAPHYLAXIS AND FOOD ALLERGY

Anaphylaxis is a severe, life-threatening allergic reaction. Foods and stinging insect venom are the leading causes of anaphylaxis in children and adolescents, while medication and stinging insect venom are the most common triggers in adults. An updated 2020 consensus definition for anaphylaxis includes (1) acute onset of an illness (minutes to hours) with involvement of the skin, mucosal tissue, or both with either respiratory involvement or reduced blood pressure and/or associated symptoms of end-organ dysfunction; or (2) two or more of the following that occur rapidly after exposure to a likely allergen for the patient, including (i) involvement of skin-mucosal tissue, (ii) respiratory involvement, (iii) reduced blood pressure, or (iv) gastrointestinal symptoms; or (3) reduced blood pressure as a result of exposure to a known allergen trigger.[59] Cutaneous symptoms include flushing, urticaria, and angioedema; upper respiratory symptoms include rhinorrhea and laryngospasm, lower respiratory symptoms include bronchoconstriction leading to cough, wheeze, dyspnea, and hypoxemia; and digestive symptoms include nausea/vomiting and abdominal pain. Cardiovascular symptoms driven by vasodilatation include hypotension, tachycardia, and syncope; in its most severe form, it creates a distributive shock that can occur in the absence of involvement of other organ symptoms. Histamine is a critical contributor to these pathophysiological changes; however, other important mediators have been identified, including cysteinyl leukotrienes (CysLTs), anaphylatoxins, and platelet-activating factor (PAF).[60] Antigen-specific IgE antibodies and FcepsilonR1-bearing effector cells (e.g., basophils, mast cells) play a dominant role; however, other non-IgE-mediated mechanisms have been identified, including complement activation via anaphylatoxins C3a, C4a, and C5a[61] and activation of a mast-cell-specific receptor called Mas-related G protein-coupled receptor X2 (MRGPRX2) which can cause similar syndrome without immune priming.[62] The first-line treatment of anaphylaxis is intramuscular epinephrine, which reverses the life-threatening physiologic changes driven by vasodilatation within minutes. Early recognition of anaphylaxis and treatment with epinephrine is lifesaving and can prevent adverse outcomes.

Headache and migraine are not considered symptoms of anaphylaxis, though there has been inquiry into this connection for many years.[63] As previously discussed, the role of histamine in migraine pathophysiology is undefined, and the use of antihistamines to prevent migraine is limited by a lack of randomized controlled trials (RCTs) or medications specifically targeting H3 or H4 receptors in the central nervous system (CNS). In general, the role of vasodilatation in the pathophysiology of migraine is debated and may represent an epiphenomenon, though many vasoactive peptides are implicated in migraine, including CGRP, pituitary adenylate cyclase-activating polypeptide (PACAP-38), and nitric oxide (NO).[64] Platelet hyperactivity is a common finding in migraine, and the release of CysLTs, a byproduct of arachidonic acid metabolism, along with prostaglandins, has been suggested as a possible mediator but has been incompletely investigated with one study demonstrating that during the headache phase of migraine, both LTC4 and LTB4 were present in the peripheral blood.[65] There has been one open-label study of montelukast, a leukotriene receptor antagonist, in the prophylaxis of migraine, with 53% of 17 patients showing a reduction of > 50% in the frequency of severe attacks after three months on therapy[66]; however, there have not been follow-up, double-blinded, placebo-controlled studies. Epinephrine has not been used in the treatment of migraine; in fact, propranolol, an FDA-approved therapy for migraine prophylaxis, is a beta-blocker that works via the precise opposite mechanism of epinephrine.

Many foods are known to be self-reported triggers of migraine; however, there has been no concrete evidence that this is immunologic or allergic. The mechanism is unknown; however, gut microbial interactions with neuropeptides in a so-called gut-brain axis may play a role.[67] Food allergy testing is, therefore, not recommended in the evaluation of migraine. The few studies that suggest a connection between food-specific IgG and migraine are lacking in scientific rigor.[68] Food-specific IgG testing has not been validated as a clinical test for any disease state and is not recommended in allergic disease or in the evaluation of migraine. If there are food intolerances that are suspected as triggers of migraine, a strict avoidance strategy followed by reintroduction to evaluate for the recurrence of symptoms is recommended.

URTICARIA

Chronic urticaria (CU) is a common inflammatory condition defined by the onset of transient pruritic wheals (hives) lasting typically less than 24 hours but recurring for longer than 6 weeks. CU is further divided into chronic spontaneous urticaria (CSU) and chronic inducible urticaria (CIU). CIU involves hives that develop in response to physical triggers (cold, heat, pressure, sun, vibration) or nonphysical stimuli (cholinergic and aquagenic urticaria). The most common age of onset is age 30–50, and it is more common in women. Many patients with urticaria also have angioedema; however, angioedema can occur in the absence of urticaria, and other mechanisms of angioedema exist—namely, swelling triggered by the bradykinin-pathway in hereditary angioedema (HAE) syndromes. The pathophysiology of CU is complex; many different mechanisms, cell types, and molecules play a role in the disease, including IgE, mast cells, basophils, and eosinophils. As well, distinct endotypes of CU have been described; for example, chronic autoimmune spontaneous urticaria is now a recognized subset reflecting an antibody-mediated, cell-stimulating reaction that can accompany other autoimmune and rheumatologic diseases (i.e., Hashimoto's thyroiditis, systemic lupus erythematosus).[69] CU can profoundly affect a patient's quality of life, work productivity, and emotional well-being. Headache has been identified as an important factor that can impair the quality of life in individuals with CU.[70] However, patients with CSU do not necessarily experience headache or migraine at an increased rate compared to those without CSU, though further research is warranted.[71] In contrast, comorbid atopic, autoimmune, and psychiatric disorders are more prevalent in patients with CSU. These related disorders can potentially be associated with headache; therefore, the association with CSU could be indirect. Headache may be correlated with CSU due to potential side effects of therapy. Headache has also been described as a side effect of antihistamines and increased by up-dosing, though most individuals tolerate up-dosing without issues.[72]

Chronic daily antihistamine therapy with second-generation H1-receptor targeted antihistamines (e.g. cetirizine, fexofenadine) is the cornerstone of therapy for CU, and dosing can be escalated to fourfold the licensed dose as tolerated to achieve clinical improvement. In the past ten years, the introduction of biologic therapy for CSU has been a considerable advance in the field. Omalizumab, a humanized IgG1 monoclonal antibody that binds to free IgE in the blood and interstitial fluid, was FDA-approved for CSU in 2014 for those >12 years and older who have failed H1-antihistamine therapy and has significantly improved the quality of life for those with CSU inducing clinical remission in many individuals. However, there are individuals who do not respond. Headache has been reported more frequently in omalizumab treatment groups compared to placebo;[73] however, it is unclear whether this relates to the underlying disease or the therapy itself and few patients report this side effect in clinical practice. Other therapies include cyclosporine, mycophenolate mofetil, and other immunosuppressants. The identification of improved biomarkers that predict response to particular therapies in CSU is an active area of research.

EOSINOPHILIC DISORDERS

Eosinophilic disorders represent a spectrum of diseases characterized by eosinophilic infiltration into tissues that can be organ specific (eosinophilic asthma, eosinophilic gastrointestinal diseases, such as eosinophilic esophagitis) or systemic (eosinophilic granulomatosis with polyangiitis, hypereosinophilic syndromes). Currently, there is limited information investigating the link between eosinophilic disorders and migraine.

Hypereosinophilic syndrome (HES), a myeloproliferative disorder defined by a peripheral blood absolute eosinophil count greater than 1,500 eosinophils per microliter on at least two occasions at least one month apart. In this condition, eosinophils proliferate in various organs throughout the body and lead to inflammation and organ dysfunction including the skin, gastrointestinal tract, nervous system, cardiac, and pulmonary tracts. HES is a heterogeneous clinical entity representing a number of distinct diseases depending on the pathophysiology of the excess proliferation of eosinophils (e.g myeloproliferative HES, T cell lymphocytic HES). In rare instances, hypereosinophilic syndromes have been described to be complicated by central sinovenous thrombosis, which can lead to headache.[75, 76] Studies have investigated the association between headache and gastrointestinal (GI) symptoms, but not eosinophilic gastrointestinal diseases specifically.[74] For instance, a higher prevalence of headache has been identified in individuals with reflux, diarrhea, constipation, and nausea. However, in this analysis, there were no major differences in character of GI symptoms in those with migraine and no migraine. Overall, further research is needed to correlate eosinophilic disorders and headache/migraine syndromes.

ATOPIC DERMATITIS

Atopic dermatitis (AD), or eczema, is a chronic, relapsing, pruritic, inflammatory skin condition that is the most common chronic inflammatory skin disease in children. The prevalence ranges from 8.7%

to 18.1% in the United States to 10%–20% worldwide.[84–86] Genetic factors influence the prevalence of AD, as parents with atopy usually have children with atopic disease, and genetic alterations in filaggrin, an epidermal protein, have been associated with AD predisposing to impairment in skin barrier function (PMID: 35628125). Environmental factors, like weather and household allergens, have also been found to influence the prevalence of AD.

AD can manifest throughout life, with 60% of cases classified as early onset atopic dermatitis before the first year of life, however adult-onset and senile onset AD have also been described.[86] Physical examination findings of AD are variable depending on age, with children developing skin manifestations with papules and plaques on the face, scalp, and extensor surfaces, and adults presenting with lichenified lesions on hand and flexural surfaces.

Studies have investigated the link between eczema and increased risk of headaches. In a multivariate analysis, the link between childhood eczema and headaches in the United States was examined, with more severe eczema leading to more headache development.[87] The relationship may be indirect as the study also examined the relationship between sleep disturbances in eczema and development of headaches, and found that sleep disturbances in children with or without AD had an increased propensity for headaches. Although eczema-predicting headache prevalence in the United States was low, there was still an increase in headaches in childhood eczema at all ages, even more in those with atopic disease, fatigue, and sleep disturbances.[87]

Various studies have explored with the potential linkage between eczema and migraine across the lifespan. In the pediatric population, those with AD, mental health comorbidities, and sleep disturbances have been found to have a higher incidence of headaches.[88] A significant association was found in adolescents with AD and migraine, while a study of individuals over age 20 found more atopic disorders lead to higher risk of migraine.[1, 89] In adults, those with eczema were 89% more likely to have a concomitant diagnosis of migraine.[90]

The mechanism between AD and headache remains unknown, but many studies have examined the expression of different cytokines during headaches and migraine. For example, increased IL-10 expression and decreased IL-4 and IL-5, were found in migraine.[91] Treatment with sumatriptan decreased IL-10 and increased IL-4 and IL-5.[91] Those with migraine were found to have higher Th2 inflammation,[91] while those with tension headaches have been found to have increased IL-13 expression.[92]

In the evaluation of headache and migraine, the clinician should consider comorbid conditions like AD. Biologics such as dupilumab and tralokinumab have been studied in AD, but an endpoint to observe efficacy in headaches has not been established. Notably, these biologics have a side effect of headache in some patients.[93, 94] Further research is needed to understand the mechanism of headaches and eczema in order to develop better prevention and treatment modalities.

MAST CELL DISORDERS

Mast cell diseases (MCDs) include both mastocytosis and mast cell activation disorders (MCAD), including mast cell activation syndrome (MCAS).

Mastocytosis is a rare disease defined as a hematologic neoplasm resulting from the expansion of mast cells in the skin (cutaneous mastocytosis) or in multiple organs (systemic mastocytosis), including bone marrow, gastrointestinal tract, lymph organs (spleen and lymph nodes), and liver. Systemic mastocytosis (SM) is defined by dense aggregates of spindle-shaped mast cells (>15 mast cells) in bone marrow biopsies or other organs but can also be defined if >25% of all mast cells in the BM are atypical if a KIT-activating mutation is present, or if mast cells express certain surface markers, including CD3, CD25, or CD30.[95] A large subset of patients with SM have a gain-of-function mutation (D816V) in the mast cell c-KIT receptor which results in premature mast cell activation. SM is further divided into indolent SM, smoldering SM, and aggressive SM.

MCAD are defined broadly by inappropriate mast cell activation, whereas MCAS is defined as severe, episodic, and recurrent symptoms induced by MC mediators (i.e., including histamine, prostaglandin D2, PAF, cysteinyl leukotrienes). The definition of MCAS involves three diagnostic criteria[96]: (1) typical MCA-related symptoms, (2) event-related increase in baseline serum tryptase (sBT) above an individual's baseline according to the formula sBT + 20% of sBT (= 120% of sBT = sBT × 1.2) plus 2 ng/mL, and (3) response to therapeutics directed against MCA—for example, antihistamines (first and second generation), H2 receptor antagonists, and leukotriene receptor antagonists. MCA-related symptoms include clinically acute episodes involving at least two organ systems. These include cutaneous (flushing, urticaria, angioedema), respiratory (wheezing, shortness of breath, rhinorrhea), gastrointestinal, and cardiovascular.[97] Patients with MCDs may be at risk for anaphylaxis. Specifically, patients with clonal mast cell disorders, including SM and elevated serum tryptase, are at higher risk of anaphylaxis from Hymenoptera stings.[98]

Comorbidities, including disease-modifying genetic traits such as hereditary alpha-tryptasemia (HaT), defined by the increased copy number of the *TPSAB1* gene encoding alpha tryptase, IgE-mediated allergies to foods, aeroallergens, and medications, and non-IgE-mediated hypersensitivity disorders, can be important modifiers in MCDs.

Headache is not part of the clinical criteria for MCDs; however, many patients with MCDs report headache along with flairs of their disease and headache is identified by patients as a cause for morbidity in mastocytosis.[99–101] Other neurologic symptoms, including cognitive dysfunction and neuropathy are also reported in these individuals. Case series have demonstrated an increased frequency of headache in patients with SM compared to the general population.[102] In an observational survey-based study of 64 individuals with SM, 56.2% reported headache, 25% with chronic daily headache, 37.5% with migraine (25% with aura, 12.5% without aura, 17.2% episodic, 20.3% chronic), and 17.2% tension-type headache.[103] Patients experiencing headache with mastocytosis flairs were more likely to be male, have itching and runny nose, and have unilateral cranial autonomic features. As previously discussed, there is a possible pathophysiologic relationship between mast cell dysfunction and migraine through the activation of mediators, such as histamine and cysteinyl leukotrienes; however, more research is needed to establish this association.

Clinical Case #3

A 50-year-old man with a history of migraine on CRGP antagonist therapy presents to an allergy/ immunology clinic after being referred by his oncologist. He was treated for non-Hodgkin's lymphoma five years ago with a regimen including rituximab. He has had an increase in the number of respiratory infections over the past year. In the office, he denies fevers or worsening frequency or severity or changes in the character of his headaches in the past six months. He has had pneumonia twice in the past year. One of these episodes of pneumonia required hospitalization and intensive care unit admission; during this admission, sputum cultures grew Strep pneumoniae. He received the PPSV23 pneumonia vaccination four years ago and the PCV13 vaccination one year later. He was found to have hypogammaglobulinemia with IgG level 300mg/dL (reference 700– 1200 mg/dL), IgA level 20 (ref 70–300), and normal IgM. *Streptococcus pneumoniae* vaccination titers six weeks following a PPSV23 booster vaccination are nonprotective. The decision is made to start immunoglobulin replacement therapy (IGRT) with intravenous immunoglobulin (IVIG). He is concerned about IVIG worsening his headaches and asks what can be done to prevent this.

Answer to Clinical Case #3

This gentleman presents with acquired antibody deficiency secondary to the rituximab therapy he received in the past for lymphoma. Rituximab is an anti-CD20 monoclonal antibody that selectively targets a subset of B cells. It is FDA-approved for a number of diagnoses, including hematologic malignancies and autoimmune diseases. In most individuals, B cells will recover within six months of rituximab therapy; however, in some cases, B cells may not recover, leading to hypogammaglobulinemia, poor vaccine responses, and subsequent increased risk of infections, specifically bacterial upper and lower respiratory infections. IGRT involves regular infusions of purified polyclonal IgGs from healthy donors and is used to prevent infections in individuals with

functional antibody defects. One of the most common side effects of this IGRT includes headache. Pretreatment of each infusion with medications such as NSAIDs, aspirin, acetaminophen, triptans, propranolol, and/or systemic corticosteroids have been shown to help mitigate the side effects of headache. Importantly, slowing down the rate of infusion has also been found to be helpful as well. Escalating baseline preventative migraine therapy is also indicated. If symptoms are refractory to preventive and acute therapies, one could consider switching from IVIG to subcutaneous Ig, which is associated with reduced side effects due to the lower dose with each infusion and more steady IgG levels over time. Close communication between the immunologist and neurologist is important to choose the optimal strategy to help the patient better tolerate infusions.

IMMUNODEFICIENCY

The differential diagnosis and evaluation for headache in individuals with disorders of immunity is broad and includes infection, autoimmunity, and malignancy. There are two main categories of immunodeficiency: primary immune deficiency (PID), which implies a genetic (known or unknown) cause of the impaired immunity, and secondary immune deficiency, in which the defect of the immune function is acquired—for example, by infection (e.g., HIV), hematologic malignancy, malnutrition, protein-losing process (e.g., enteropathy, nephropathy), liver disease, or most commonly by immunomodulating agents and chemotherapeutics.[104] Within the category of PID, there have now been 485 inborn errors of immunity (IEI) described in which a monogenic defect has been identified affecting immune system function.[105] These diagnoses have been made possible by advances in immunodiagnostics and genetic sequencing. While most of these diagnoses are made in childhood, more patients are being diagnosed as adults. Treatment in most cases includes hematopoietic stem cell transplantation (HSCT); however, novel therapeutics, including immunomodulatory therapy and gene therapy are in development for many of these conditions.[106–107]

The precise immunologic compartment that is compromised dictates the possible differential for headache in these patients—for example, broadly speaking, T cell defects can increase the risk of fungal and viral infections, B cell deficiency leading to antibody defects can predispose to bacterial infections, and innate immune defects or phagocytic disorders can predispose to disseminated infection and/or deep abscesses.[108] Immunosuppressants associated with reduced T cell function include mycophenolate mofetil and azathioprine, whereas rituximab and belimumab are associated with B cell and antibody deficiency, and chemotherapeutics such as cyclophosphamide and prolonged systemic corticosteroids can result in combined T and B cell deficiency.[109] Importantly, these immunologic defects do not always improve with time. Therefore, a detailed past medical history with attention to immunosuppressive medications used in the present and past is critical to considering a differential for headache in these patients.

Infectious CNS disease should be considered in any individual with an immunodeficiency, fever, and headache, and should prompt examination for meningeal signs and immediate referral to an emergency department. Organisms include viral meningoencephalitis (adenovirus, HSV, cytomegalovirus (CMV)), enteroviruses (including echovirus, poliomyelitis, varicella, and west nile), bacterial meningitis (*Streptococcus pneumoniae, Neisseria meningitidis, Haemophilus influenzae*) fungal meningitis and brain abscess (histoplasmosis, cryptococcus, aspergillus). Progressive multifocal leukoencephalopathy and encephalitis due to BK virus should be considered, especially for solid-organ transplant recipients on immunosuppression. Autoimmune and autoinflammatory CNS disease can be associated with headache, including multiple sclerosis, myasthenia gravis, optic neuritis, myelitis, CNS vasculitis, limbic encephalitis, granulomatous disease, and chronic inflammatory demyelinating polyneuropathy. Neurologic neoplasms can also occur, including pituitary adenomas and acoustic neuromas. CNS lymphoma should also be considered in the immunocompromised patient.

Independent of these causes, individuals with disorders of immunity also report primary headache syndromes with greater frequency. In one study, upwards of 80% of individuals with common variable immune deficiency (CVID), one of the most common immune deficiency syndromes characterized by recurrent bacterial infections, hypogammaglobulinemia, and poor vaccine responses as well as autoimmune and lymphoproliferative sequelae in a subset of patients, reported headache affecting their quality of life.[110–112] Sleep disturbances are also very common in this group of patients, which can exacerbate headaches as well.[113]

Headache is also associated with treatments for immunologic disorders, most notably IGRT. IGRT involves pooled and purified immunoglobulin G that is infused either intravenously (IV) or subcutaneously to correct hypogammaglobulinemia and antibody deficiencies. Headache is reported in up to half of patients receiving IGRT.[114–115] The mechanism is unknown and likely varies depending on the patient but may relate to hyperviscosity or a reaction to stabilizers or vascular mediators. Headache with IGRT is worse in patients with higher doses of immunoglobulin, faster infusion rates, and those with underlying migraine. A rare complication of IGRT is aseptic meningitis, which should be considered in patients with severe headache and meningeal signs during or shortly after their infusions and is also more likely to occur in patients with a prior history of migraine.[116] Lumbar puncture is required for diagnosis, and cerebral spinal fluid (CSF) will demonstrate increased levels of nucleated cells and high protein content with negative cultures. Prophylactic treatments prior to infusion include acetaminophen and NSAIDs, propranolol, triptans, and corticosteroids; however, the most efficacious medication is unknown.[117] A slow-rate escalation protocol has been associated with reduced rates of migraine and headache with IVIG.[117] Therefore, when starting on immunoglobulin therapy, immunologists, oncologists, and rheumatologists should query patients about their headache history and work with their neurologist to optimally manage their disease.

CONCLUSION

Individuals with atopic diseases, including AR, asthma, CU, and mastocytosis, have been found to have increased frequencies of migraine and headache. A shared pathophysiologic mechanism potentially involving mast cells and their mediators possibly links the two disorders; however, this association has not been firmly established, and further research is necessary. As well, there is a paucity of clinical trials examining the prevention or treatment of acute migraine with agents targeting allergic inflammation. Linking comorbidities may be more relevant to the association between atopic disease and headache, including disturbed sleep, poor air quality, and hormonal fluctuations. Importantly, primary headache disorders can be missed and should be directly evaluated by a neurologist in individuals presenting with atopic disease who are linking particular exposures to their headaches. An interdisciplinary approach with good communication between the allergy/immunologist and neurologist, and often also otolaryngologist, is necessary to improve the quality of life for individuals with atopic disease and headache.

In summary:

1. Individuals with AR and nonallergic rhinitis are more likely to report comorbid migraine than the general population. While the impact of specific treatments for rhinitis on migraine is unknown, allergen immunotherapy may be associated with reduced frequency and severity of migraine, though more research is needed to confirm this association.
2. Dedicated headache evaluation is important in patients with rhinosinusitis and headache, as migraine disorders are often misdiagnosed as "sinus headaches."
3. Asthma is a chronic heterogeneous disease of airway inflammation that is common in the general population. Patients with asthma are more likely to have comorbid headaches and vice versa. Air quality and hormonal fluctuations may be linking mediators of disease.
4. AD has been linked to an increased risk of headaches with more severe disease leading to more headache development. Sleep disturbances in children with or without AD have been shown to have an increased likelihood of headache.
5. Foods can be self-reported triggers of headache; however, headache is not an established symptom of food allergy or anaphylaxis. In individuals with headache related to the ingestion of

certain foods in the absence of features of anaphylaxis (urticaria, angioedema, shortness of breath, hypotension, etc.), food allergy testing is not indicated, a food and headache diary with a trial of elimination and reintroduction of suspect foods, and referral to a neurologist for dedicated headache evaluation are the next best steps.

6. Patients with CU and SM report that headaches can affect their quality of life; therefore, screening for headache disorders and referral to a neurologist is important for these individuals.

7. Immune deficiency includes primary genetic disease or secondary/acquired disease, the latter most frequently due to hematologic malignancy and immunosuppressive therapies. The differential diagnosis is broad for individuals with headache and immune deficiency and includes infection and autoimmunity. Fever in these individuals should prompt immediate referral to the emergency department for appropriate evaluation, including lumbar puncture.

8. Headache is a common side effect of IGRT. Pretreatment with analgesics or abortive headache agents or slowing down the rate of infusion are strategies to reduce the frequency of this side effect.

REFERENCES

1. Han JH, Lee HJ, Yook HJ, Han K, Lee JH, Park YM. Atopic Disorders and Their Risks of Migraine: A Nationwide Population-Based Cohort Study. *Allergy Asthma Immunol Res.* 2023;*15*(1):55–66. doi:10.4168/aair.2023.15.1.55

2. Özge A, Öksüz N, Ayta S, et al. Atopic disorders are more common in childhood migraine and correlated headache phenotype. *Pediatr Int.* 2014;*56*(6):868–872. doi:10.1111/ped.12381

3. Alstadhaug KB. Histamine in migraine and brain. *Headache.* 2014;*54*(2):246–259. doi:10.1111/head.12293

4. Heatley R V, Denburg JA, Bayer N, Bienenstock J. Increased plasma histamine levels in migraine patients. *Clin Allergy.* 1982;*12*(2):145–149. doi:10.1111/j.1365-2222.1982.tb01633.x

5. Rao BS, Das DG, Taraknath VR, Sarma Y. A double blind controlled study of propranolol and cyproheptadine in migraine prophylaxis. *Neurol India.* 2000;*48*(3):223–226.

6. Li WW, Guo TZ, Liang De-yong, Sun Y, Kingery WS, Clark JD. Substance P signaling controls mast cell activation, degranulation, and nociceptive sensitization in a rat fracture model of complex regional pain syndrome. *Anesthesiology.* 2012;*116*(4):882–895. doi:10.1097/ALN.0b013e31824bb303

7. Goadsby PJ, Edvinsson L, Ekman R. Vasoactive peptide release in the extracerebral circulation of humans during migraine headache. *Ann Neurol.* 1990;*28*(2):183–187. doi:10.1002/ana.410280213

8. Olesen J, Diener HC, Husstedt IW, et al. Calcitonin gene-related peptide receptor antagonist BIBN 4096 BS for the acute treatment of migraine. *N Engl J Med.* 2004;*350*(11):1104–1110. doi:10.1056/NEJMoa030505

9. Wallrapp A, Burkett PR, Riesenfeld SJ, et al. Calcitonin Gene-Related Peptide Negatively Regulates Alarmin-Driven Type 2 Innate Lymphoid Cell Responses. *Immunity.* 2019;51(4):709–723.e6. doi:10.1016/j.immuni.2019.09.005

10. Salo PM, Calatroni A, Gergen PJ, et al. Allergy-related outcomes in relation to serum IgE: results from the National Health and Nutrition Examination Survey 2005–2006. *J Allergy Clin Immunol.* 2011;*127*(5):1226–35. doi:10.1016/j.jaci.2010.12.1106

11. Gershwin ME, Maguwa S. *Allergy & Immunology Secrets.* 2nd ed. Elsevier Inc.; 2001.

12. Schuler IV CF, Montejo JM. Allergic Rhinitis in Children and Adolescents. *Immunol Allergy Clin North Am.* 2021;*41*(4):613–625. doi:10.1016/j.iac.2021.07.010

13. Graif Y, Shohat T, Machluf Y, Farkash R, Chaiter Y. Association between asthma and migraine: A cross-sectional study of over 110 000 adolescents. *Clin Respir J.* 2018;*12*(10):2491–2496. doi:10.1111/crj.12939

14. Ku M, Silverman B, Prifti N, Ying W, Persaud Y, Schneider A. Prevalence of migraine headaches in patients with allergic rhinitis. *Ann Allergy Asthma Immunol.* 2006;*97*(2):226–230. doi:10.1016/S1081-1206(10)60018-X

15. Martin VT, Fanning KM, Serrano D, et al. Chronic rhinitis and its association with headache frequency and disability in persons with migraine: results of the American Migraine Prevalence and Prevention (AMPP) Study. *Cephalalgia.* 2014;*34*(5):336–348. doi:10.1177/0333102413512031

16. Passali FM, Spinosi MC, Mignacco G, Cingi C, Rodriguez HA, Passali D. Influence of allergic rhinitis in children and adolescents with recurrent headache. *Otolaryngol Pol.* 2018;*72*(2):50–59. doi:10.5604/01.3001.0011.7252

17. Zittoon RF, Ahmed DI, Iskander NM, Madian YT. Allergic rhinitis patients associated with migraine: effect of treatment of allergic rhinitis on migrainous attack. *The Egyptian Journal of Otolaryngology.* 2021;*37*(1):14. doi:10.1186/s43163-021-00077-x

18. Aupiais C, Wanin S, Romanello S, et al. Association Between Migraine and Atopic Diseases in Childhood: A Potential Protective Role of Anti-Allergic Drugs. *Headache.* 2017;*57*(4):612–624. doi:10.1111/head.13032

19. Sohn MH. Efficacy and Safety of Subcutaneous Allergen Immunotherapy for Allergic Rhinitis. *Allergy Asthma Immunol Res.* 2018;*10*(1):1–3. doi:10.4168/aair.2018.10.1.1

20. Sivam A, Tankersley M, American College of Allergy A and II and DC. Perception and practice of sublingual immunotherapy among practicing allergists in the United States: A follow-up survey. *Ann Allergy Asthma Immunol.* 2019;*122*(6):623–629.e2. doi:10.1016/j.anai.2019.03.023

21. Martin VT, Taylor F, Gebhardt B, et al. Allergy and immunotherapy: are they related to migraine headache? *Headache.* 2011;*51*(1):8–20. doi:10.1111/j.1526-4610.2010.01792.x

22. Fokkens WJ, Lund VJ, Hopkins C, et al. European Position Paper on Rhinosinusitis and Nasal Polyps 2020. *Rhinology.* 2020;*58*(Suppl S29):1–464. doi:10.4193/Rhin20.600

23. Anon JB, Jacobs MR, Poole MD, et al. Antimicrobial treatment guidelines for acute bacterial rhinosinusitis. *Otolaryngol Head Neck Surg.* 2004;*130*(1 Suppl):1–45. doi:10.1016/j.otohns.2003.12.003

24. Louie JK, Hacker JK, Gonzales R, et al. Characterization of viral agents causing acute respiratory infection in a San Francisco University Medical Center Clinic during the influenza season. *Clin Infect Dis.* 2005;*41*(6):822–828. doi:10.1086/432800

25. Stevens WW, Schleimer RP, Kern RC. Chronic Rhinosinusitis with Nasal Polyps. *J Allergy Clin Immunol Pract.* 2016;*4*(4):565–572. doi:10.1016/j.jaip.2016.04.012

26. Nguyen DT, Felix-Ravelo M, Sonnet MH, et al. Assessment of facial pain and headache before and after nasal polyposis surgery with the DyNaChron questionnaire. *Eur Ann Otorhinolaryngol Head Neck Dis.* 2016;*133*(5):301–305. doi:10.1016/j.anorl.2016.04.007

27. Derbarsegian A, Adams SM, Phillips KM, Sedaghat AR. The Burden of Migraine on Quality of Life in Chronic Rhinosinusitis. *Laryngoscope.* Published online March 27, 2023. doi:10.1002/lary.30662

28. Patel ZM, Kennedy DW, Setzen M, Poetker DM, DelGaudio JM. "Sinus headache": rhinogenic headache or migraine? An evidence-based guide to diagnosis and treatment. *Int Forum Allergy Rhinol.* 2013;*3*(3):221–230. doi:10.1002/alr.21095

29. Bernichi J V, Rizzo VL, Villa JF, Santos RF, Caparroz FA. Rhinogenic and sinus headache - Literature review. *Am J Otolaryngol.* 2021;*42*(6):103113. doi:10.1016/j.amjoto.2021.103113

30. La Mantia I, Grillo C, Andaloro C. Rhinogenic Contact Point Headache: Surgical Treatment Versus Medical Treatment. *J Craniofac Surg.* 2018;*29*(3):e228–e230. doi:10.1097/SCS.0000000000004211

31. Aaseth K, Grande RB, Kvaerner K, Lundqvist C, Russell MB. Chronic rhinosinusitis gives a ninefold increased risk of chronic headache. The Akershus study of chronic headache. *Cephalalgia.* 2010;*30*(2):152–160. doi:10.1111/j.1468-2982.2009.01877.x

32. Ceriani CE, Silberstein SD. Headache and rhinosinusitis: A review. *Cephalalgia.* 2021;*41*(4):453–463. doi:10.1177/0333102420959790

33. Cady RK, Schreiber CP. Sinus headache or migraine? Considerations in making a differential diagnosis. *Neurology.* 2002;*58*(9 Suppl 6):S10–4. doi:10.1212/wnl.58.9_suppl_6.s10

34. Jones NS. Sinus headaches: avoiding over- and mis-diagnosis. *Expert Rev Neurother.* 2009;*9*(4):439–444. doi:10.1586/ern.09.8

35. Pipolo C, Saibene AM, Felisati G. Prevalence of pain due to rhinosinusitis: a review. *Neurol Sci.* 2018;*39*(Suppl 1):21–24. doi:10.1007/s10072-018-3336-z

36. Eross E, Dodick D, Eross M. The Sinus, Allergy and Migraine Study (SAMS). *Headache.* 2007;*47*(2):213–224. doi:10.1111/j.1526-4610.2006.00688.x

37. Wang IC, Tsai JD, Shen TC, Lin CL, Li TC, Wei CC. Allergic Conjunctivitis and the Associated Risk of Migraine Among Children: A Nationwide Population-based Cohort Study. *Ocul Immunol Inflamm.* 2017;*25*(6):802–810. doi:10.1080/09273948.2016.1178303

38. Wei CC, Lin CL, Shen TC, Chen AC. Children with allergic diseases have an increased subsequent risk of migraine upon reaching school age. *J Investig Med.* 2018;*66*(7):1064–1068. doi:10.1136/jim-2018-000715

39. Bielory L, Katelaris CH, Lightman S, Naclerio RM. Treating the ocular component of allergic rhinoconjunctivitis and related eye disorders. *MedGenMed.* 2007;*9*(3):35.

40. Hayashi T. Asthma and migraine--is asthma a part of acephalgic migraine? A hypothesis. *Ann Allergy.* 1988;*60*(4):374.

41. Wang L, Deng ZR, Zu MD, Zhang J, Wang Y. The Comorbid Relationship Between Migraine and Asthma: A Systematic Review and Meta-Analysis of Population-Based Studies. *Front Med (Lausanne).* 2020;*7*:609528. doi:10.3389/fmed.2020.609528

42. Martin VT, Fanning KM, Serrano D, Buse DC, Reed ML, Lipton RB. Asthma is a risk factor for new onset chronic migraine: Results from the American migraine prevalence and prevention study. *Headache.* 2016;*56*(1):118–131. doi:10.1111/head.12731

43. Buse DC, Reed ML, Fanning KM, et al. Comorbid and co-occurring conditions in migraine and associated risk of increasing headache pain intensity and headache frequency: results of the migraine in America symptoms and treatment (MAST) study. *J Headache Pain.* 2020;*21*(1):23. doi:10.1186/s10194-020-1084-y

44. Lee H, Myung W, Cheong HK, et al. Ambient air pollution exposure and risk of migraine: Synergistic effect with high temperature. *Environ Int.* 2018;*121*(Pt 1):383–391. doi:10.1016/j.envint.2018.09.022

45. Bowatte G, Lodge C, Lowe AJ, et al. The influence of childhood traffic-related air pollution exposure on asthma, allergy and sensitization: a systematic review and a meta-analysis of birth cohort studies. *Allergy.* 2015;*70*(3):245–256. doi:10.1111/all.12561

46. D'Amato G, Holgate ST, Pawankar R, et al. Meteorological conditions, climate change, new emerging factors, and asthma and related allergic disorders. A statement of the World Allergy Organization. *World Allergy Organ J.* 2015;*8*(1):25. doi:10.1186/s40413-015-0073-0

47. Guarnieri M, Balmes JR. Outdoor air pollution and asthma. *Lancet.* 2014;*383*(9928):1581–1592. doi:10.1016/S0140-6736(14)60617-6

48. Gosens R, Gross N. The mode of action of anticholinergics in asthma. *Eur Respir J.* 2018;*52*(4). doi:10.1183/13993003.01247-2017

49. Shelukhina I, Mikhailov N, Abushik P, Nurullin L, Nikolsky EE, Giniatullin R. Cholinergic Nociceptive Mechanisms in Rat Meninges and Trigeminal Ganglia: Potential Implications for Migraine Pain. *Front Neurol.* 2017;*8*:163. doi:10.3389/fneur.2017.00163

50. Meents JE, Neeb L, Reuter U. TRPV1 in migraine pathophysiology. *Trends Mol Med.* 2010;*16*(4):153–159. doi:10.1016/j.molmed.2010.02.004

51. Kim JH. The Emerging Role of TRPV1 in Airway Inflammation. *Allergy Asthma Immunol Res.* 2018;*10*(3):187–188. doi:10.4168/aair.2018.10.3.187

52. Brandes JL. The influence of estrogen on migraine: a systematic review. *JAMA.* 2006;*295*(15):1824–1830. doi:10.1001/jama.295.15.1824

53. Yung JA, Fuseini H, Newcomb DC. Hormones, sex, and asthma. *Ann Allergy Asthma Immunol.* 2018;*120*(5): 488–494. doi:10.1016/j.anai.2018.01.016

54. Vink NM, Postma DS, Schouten JP, Rosmalen JGM, Boezen HM. Gender differences in asthma development and remission during transition through puberty: the TRacking Adolescents' Individual Lives Survey (TRAILS) study. *J Allergy Clin Immunol.* 2010;*126*(3):498–504.e1-6. doi:10.1016/j.jaci.2010.06.018

55. Eliasson O, Scherzer HH, DeGraff AC. Morbidity in asthma in relation to the menstrual cycle. *J Allergy Clin Immunol.* 1986;*77*(1 Pt 1):87–94. doi:10.1016/0091-6749(86)90328-3

56. Schatz M, Harden K, Forsythe A, et al. The course of asthma during pregnancy, post partum, and with successive pregnancies: a prospective analysis. *J Allergy Clin Immunol.* 1988;*81*(3):509–517.

57. Triebner K, Johannessen A, Puggini L, et al. Menopause as a predictor of new-onset asthma: A longitudinal Northern European population study. *J Allergy Clin Immunol.* 2016;*137*(1):50–57.e6. doi:10.1016/j.jaci.2015.08.019

58. Expert Panel Working Group of the National Heart L and BI (NHLBI) administered and coordinated NAE and PPCC (NAEPPCC), Cloutier MM, Baptist AP, et al. 2020 Focused Updates to the Asthma Management Guidelines: A Report from the National Asthma Education and Prevention Program Coordinating Committee Expert Panel Working Group. *J Allergy Clin Immunol.* 2020;*146*(6):1217–1270. doi:10.1016/j.jaci.2020.10.003

59. Shaker MS, Wallace D V, Golden DBK, et al. Anaphylaxis-a 2020 practice parameter update, systematic review, and Grading of Recommendations, Assessment, Development and Evaluation (GRADE) analysis. *J Allergy Clin Immunol.* 2020;*145*(4):1082–1123. doi:10.1016/j.jaci.2020.01.017

60. Reber LL, Hernandez JD, Galli SJ. The pathophysiology of anaphylaxis. *J Allergy Clin Immunol.* 2017;*140*(2):335–348. doi:10.1016/j.jaci.2017.06.003

61. Brown SGA, Stone SF, Fatovich DM, et al. Anaphylaxis: clinical patterns, mediator release, and severity. *J Allergy Clin Immunol.* 2013;*132*(5):1141–1149.e5. doi:10.1016/j.jaci.2013.06.015

62. McNeil BD. MRGPRX2 and Adverse Drug Reactions. *Front Immunol.* 2021;*12*:676354. doi:10.3389/fimmu.2021.676354

63. Lubbers HA. Migraine And Anaphylaxis. *J Nerv Ment Dis.* 1923;*58*(2):174.

64. Mason BN, Russo AF. Vascular Contributions to Migraine: Time to Revisit? *Front Cell Neurosci.* 2018;*12*:233. doi:10.3389/fncel.2018.00233

65. LaMancusa R, Pulcinelli FM, Ferroni P, et al. Blood leukotrienes in headache: correlation with platelet activity. *Headache.* 1991;*31*(6):409–414. doi:10.1111/j.1526-4610.1991.hed3106409.x

66. Sheftell F, Rapoport A, Weeks R, Walker B, Gammerman I, Baskin S. Montelukast in the prophylaxis of migraine: a potential role for leukotriene modifiers. *Headache.* 2000;*40*(2):158–163. doi:10.1046/j.1526-4610.2000.00022.x

67. Arzani M, Jahromi SR, Ghorbani Z, et al. Gut-brain Axis and migraine headache: a comprehensive review. *J Headache Pain.* 2020;*21*(1):15. doi:10.1186/s10194-020-1078-9

68. Arroyave Hernández CM, Echavarría Pinto M, Hernández Montiel HL. Food allergy mediated by IgG antibodies associated with migraine in adults. *Rev Alerg Mex.* 2007;*54*(5):162–168.

69. Konstantinou GN, Riedl MA, Valent P, Podder I, Maurer M. Urticaria and Angioedema: Understanding Complex Pathomechanisms to Facilitate Patient Communication, Disease Management, and Future Treatment. *J Allergy Clin Immunol Pract.* 2023;*11*(1):94–106. doi:10.1016/j.jaip.2022.11.006

70. Filiz S, Kutluk MG, Uygun DFK. Headache deteriorates the quality of life in children with chronic spontaneous urticaria. *Allergol Immunopathol (Madr).* 2019;*47*(3):254–259. doi:10.1016/j.aller.2018.09.002

71. Papapostolou N, Xepapadaki P, Katoulis A, Makris M. Comorbidities of Chronic Urticaria: A glimpse into a complex relationship. *Frontiers in allergy.* 2022;*3*:1008145. doi:10.3389/falgy.2022.1008145

72. Iriarte Sotés P, Armisén M, Usero-Bárcena T, et al. Efficacy and Safety of Up-dosing Antihistamines in Chronic Spontaneous Urticaria: A Systematic Review of the Literature. *J Investig Allergol Clin Immunol.* 2021;*31*(4):282–291. doi:10.18176/jiaci.0649

73. Maurer M, Rosén K, Hsieh HJ. Omalizumab for chronic urticaria. *N Engl J Med.* 2013;*368*(26):2530. doi:10.1056/NEJMc1305687

74. Aamodt AH, Stovner LJ, Hagen K, Zwart JA. Comorbidity of headache and gastrointestinal complaints. The Head-HUNT Study. *Cephalalgia.* 2008;*28*(2):144–151. doi:10.1111/j.1468-2982.2007.01486.x

75. Sakuta R, Tomita Y, Ohashi M, Nagai T, Murakami N. Idiopathic hypereosinophilic syndrome complicated by central sinovenous thrombosis. *Brain Dev.* 2007;*29*(3):182–184. doi:10.1016/j.braindev.2006.08.004

76. Song XH, Xu T, Zhao GH. Hypereosinophilia with cerebral venous sinus thrombosis and intracerebral hemorrhage: A case report and review of the literature. *World J Clin Cases.* 2021;*9*(28):8571–8578. doi:10.12998/wjcc.v9.i28.8571

77. Choung RS, Alexander JA, Katzka DA, Murray JA. Management of eosinophilic esophagitis and celiac disease. *Curr Opin Pharmacol.* 2017;*37*:118–125. doi:10.1016/j.coph.2017.10.007

78. Gorchakov LG, Belyanko NE. The questionnaire–as a method for examining endocrine morbidity genealogy with children. *Sante Publique (Bucur).* 1987;*30*(1):31–34.

79. Cámara-Lemarroy CR, Rodriguez-Gutierrez R, Monreal-Robles R, Marfil-Rivera A. Gastrointestinal disorders associated with migraine: A comprehensive review. *World J Gastroenterol.* 2016;*22*(36):8149–8160. doi:10.3748/wjg.v22.i36.8149

80. Fanaeian MM, Alibeik N, Ganji A, Fakheri H, Ekhlasi G, Shahbazkhani B. Prevalence of migraine in adults with celiac disease: A case control cross-sectional study. *PLoS One.* 2021;*16*(11):e0259502. doi:10.1371/journal.pone.0259502

81. Dimitrova AK, Ungaro RC, Lebwohl B, et al. Prevalence of migraine in patients with celiac disease and inflammatory bowel disease. *Headache.* 2013;*53*(2):344–355. doi:10.1111/j.1526-4610.2012.02260.x

82. Hom GL, Hom BL, Kaplan B, Rothner AD. A Single Institution's Experience of Primary Headache in Children With Celiac Disease. *J Child Neurol.* 2020;*35*(1):37–41. doi:10.1177/0883073819873751

83. Ameghino L, Farez MF, Wilken M, Goicochea MT. Headache in Patients with Celiac Disease and Its Response to the Gluten-Free Diet. *J Oral Facial Pain Headache.* 2019;*33*(3):294–300. doi:10.11607/ofph.2079

84. Shaw TE, Currie GP, Koudelka CW, Simpson EL. Eczema prevalence in the United States: data from the 2003 National Survey of Children's Health. *J Invest Dermatol.* 2011;*131*(1):67–73. doi:10.1038/jid.2010.251

85. Leung R, Wong G, Lau J, et al. Prevalence of asthma and allergy in Hong Kong schoolchildren: an ISAAC study. *European Respiratory Journal.* 1997;*10*(2):354–360. doi:10.1183/09031936.97.10020354

86. Kolb LFBSJ. Atopic Dermatitis. StatPearls Publishing.

87. Silverberg JI. Association between childhood eczema and headaches: An analysis of 19 US population-based studies. *J Allergy Clin Immunol.* 2016;*137*(2):492–499.e5. doi:10.1016/j.jaci.2015.07.020

88. Manjunath J, Silverberg JI. Association between atopic dermatitis and headaches throughout childhood and adolescence-A longitudinal birth cohort study. *Pediatr Dermatol.* 2021;*38*(4):780–786. doi:10.1111/pde.14607

89. Shreberk-Hassidim R, Hassidim A, Gronovich Y, Dalal A, Molho-Pessach V, Zlotogorski A. Atopic Dermatitis in Israeli Adolescents from 1998 to 2013: Trends in Time and Association with Migraine. *Pediatr Dermatol.* 2017;*34*(3):247–252. doi:10.1111/pde.13084

90. Fan R, Leasure AC, Damsky W, Cohen JM. Migraine among adults with atopic dermatitis: a cross-sectional study in the All of Us research programme. *Clin Exp Dermatol.* 2023;*48*(1):24–26. doi:10.1093/ced/llac004

91. Munno I, Marinaro M, Bassi A, Cassiano MA, Causarano V, Centonze V. Immunological aspects in migraine: increase of IL-10 plasma levels during attack. *Headache*. 2001;*41*(8):764–767. doi:10.1046/j.1526-4610.2001.01140.x

92. Boćkowski L, Smigielska-Kuzia J, Sobaniec W, Zelazowska-Rutkowska B, Kułak W, Sendrowski K. Anti-inflammatory plasma cytokines in children and adolescents with migraine headaches. *Pharmacol Rep*. 2010;*62*(2):287–291. doi:10.1016/s1734-1140(10)70268-1

93. Kelly KA, Perche PO, Feldman SR. Therapeutic Potential of Tralokinumab in the Treatment of Atopic Dermatitis: A Review on the Emerging Clinical Data. *Clin Cosmet Investig Dermatol*. 2022;*15*:1037–1043. doi:10.2147/CCID.S267217

94. Wu S, Wang H. Efficacy and safety of dupilumab in the treatment of moderate-to-severe atopic dermatitis: a meta-analysis of randomized controlled trials. *Postepy Dermatol Alergol*. 2022;*39*(3):601–610. doi:10.5114/ada.2022.117740

95. Valent P, Akin C, Hartmann K, et al. Updated Diagnostic Criteria and Classification of Mast Cell Disorders: A Consensus Proposal. *Hemasphere*. 2021;*5*(11):e646. doi:10.1097/HS9.0000000000000646

96. Valent P, Akin C, Bonadonna P, et al. Proposed Diagnostic Algorithm for Patients with Suspected Mast Cell Activation Syndrome. *J Allergy Clin Immunol Pract*. 2019;*7*(4):1125–1133.e1. doi:10.1016/j.jaip.2019.01.006

97. Gülen T, Akin C, Bonadonna P, et al. Selecting the Right Criteria and Proper Classification to Diagnose Mast Cell Activation Syndromes: A Critical Review. *J Allergy Clin Immunol Pract*. 2021;*9*(11):3918–3928. doi:10.1016/j.jaip.2021.06.011

98. Bonadonna P, Perbellini O, Passalacqua G, et al. Clonal mast cell disorders in patients with systemic reactions to Hymenoptera stings and increased serum tryptase levels. *J Allergy Clin Immunol*. 2009;*123*(3):680–686. doi:10.1016/j.jaci.2008.11.018

99. Jennings S V, Slee VM, Finnerty CC, Hempstead JB, Bowman AS. Symptoms of mast cell activation: The patient perspective. *Ann Allergy Asthma Immunol*. 2021;*127*(4):407–409. doi:10.1016/j.anai.2021.07.004

100. Smith JH, Butterfield JH, Cutrer FM. Primary headache syndromes in systemic mastocytosis. *Cephalalgia*. 2011;*31*(15):1522–1531. doi:10.1177/0333102411421683

101. Hermine O, Lortholary O, Leventhal PS, et al. Case-control cohort study of patients' perceptions of disability in mastocytosis. *PLoS One*. 2008;*3*(5):e2266. doi:10.1371/journal.pone.0002266

102. Smith JH, Butterfield JH, Pardanani A, DeLuca GC, Cutrer FM. Neurologic symptoms and diagnosis in adults with mast cell disease. *Clin Neurol Neurosurg*. 2011;*113*(7):570–574. doi:10.1016/j.clineuro.2011.05.002

103. Tuano KS, Seth N, Chinen J. Secondary immunodeficiencies: An overview. Ann Allergy Asthma Immunol. 2021 Dec;*127*(6):617–626. doi: 10.1016/j.anai.2021.08.413. Epub 2021 Sep 3. PMID: 34481993.

104. Bousfiha A, Moundir A, Tangye SG, Picard C, Jeddane L, Al-Herz W, Rundles CC, Franco JL, Holland SM, Klein C, Morio T, Oksenhendler E, Puel A, Puck J, Seppänen MRJ, Somech R, Su HC, Sullivan KE, Torgerson TR, Meyts I. The 2022 Update of IUIS Phenotypical Classification for Human Inborn Errors of Immunity. J Clin Immunol. 2022 Oct;*42*(7):1508–1520. doi: 10.1007/s10875-022-01352-z. Epub 2022 Oct 6. PMID: 36198931.

105. Arlabosse T, Booth C, Candotti F. Gene Therapy for Inborn Errors of Immunity. J Allergy Clin Immunol Pract. 2023 Jun;*11*(6):1592–1601. doi: 10.1016/j.jaip.2023.04.001. Epub 2023 Apr 20. PMID: 37084938.

106. Fischer A. Gene therapy for inborn errors of immunity: past, present and future. Nat Rev Immunol. 2023 Jun;*23*(6):397–408. doi: 10.1038/s41577-022-00800-6. Epub 2022 Nov 25. PMID: 36434109.

107. Knight V, Heimall JR, Chong H, Nandiwada SL, Chen K, Lawrence MG, Sadighi Akha AA, Kumánovics A, Jyonouchi S, Ngo SY, Vinh DC, Hagin D, Forbes Satter LR, Marsh RA, Chiang SCC, Willrich MAV, Frazer-Abel AA, Rider NL. A Toolkit and Framework for Optimal Laboratory Evaluation of Individuals with Suspected Primary Immunodeficiency. *J Allergy Clin Immunol Pract*. 2021 Sep;*9*(9):3293–3307.e6. doi: 10.1016/j.jaip.2021.05.004. Epub 2021 May 24. PMID: 34033983.

108. Otani IM, Lehman HK, Jongco AM, Tsao LR, Azar AE, Tarrant TK, Engel E, Walter JE, Truong TQ, Khan DA, Ballow M, Cunningham-Rundles C, Lu H, Kwan M, Barmettler S. Practical guidance for the diagnosis and management of secondary hypogammaglobulinemia: A Work Group Report of the AAAAI Primary Immunodeficiency and Altered Immune Response Committees. J Allergy Clin Immunol. 2022 May;*149*(5):1525–1560. doi: 10.1016/j.jaci.2022.01.025. Epub 2022 Feb 14. PMID: 35176351.

109. Nguyen JTU, Green A, Wilson MR, DeRisi JL, Gundling K. Neurologic Complications of Common Variable Immunodeficiency. *J Clin Immunol*. 2016;*36*(8):793–800. doi:10.1007/s10875-016-0336-8

110. Lee M, Nguyen J, Fuleihan R, Gundling K, Cunningham-Rundles C, Otani IM. Neurologic Conditions and Symptoms Reported Among Common Variable Immunodeficiency Patients in the USIDNET. *J Clin Immunol*. 2020;*40*(8):1181–1183. doi:10.1007/s10875-020-00861-z

111. De Almeida BI, Smith TL, Delic A, et al. Neurologic Manifestations of Common Variable Immunodeficiency: Impact on Quality of Life. *Neurology(R) neuroimmunology & neuroinflammation.* 2023;*10*(3). doi:10.1212/NXI.0000000000200088

112. Punj M, Neshat S, Lee-Mateus AY, Cheung J, Squire J. Assessment of Sleep Disturbances and Sleep Disordered Breathing in Primary Immunodeficiency Disorders. *Clinical Immunology.* 2023;*250*:109511. doi:10.1016/j.clim.2023.109511

113. Guo Y, Tian X, Wang X, Xiao Z. Adverse Effects of Immunoglobulin Therapy. *Front Immunol.* 2018;*9*:1299. doi:10.3389/fimmu.2018.01299

114. Brannagan TH, Nagle KJ, Lange DJ, Rowland LP. Complications of intravenous immune globulin treatment in neurologic disease. *Neurology.* 1996;*47*(3):674–677. doi:10.1212/wnl.47.3.674

115. Bharath V, Eckert K, Kang M, Chin-Yee IH, Hsia CC. Incidence and natural history of intravenous immunoglobulin-induced aseptic meningitis: a retrospective review at a single tertiary care center. *Transfusion (Paris).* 2015;*55*(11):2597–2605. doi:10.1111/trf.13200

116. Thornby KA, Henneman A, Brown DA. Evidence-based strategies to reduce intravenous immunoglobulin-induced headaches. *Ann Pharmacother.* 2015;*49*(6):715–726. doi:10.1177/1060028015576362

117. Geng B, Clark K, Evangelista M, Wolford E. Low rates of headache and migraine associated with intravenous immunoglobulin infusion using a 15-minute rate escalation protocol in 123 patients with primary immunodeficiency. *Front Immunol.* 2022;*13*:1075527. doi:10.3389/fimmu.2022.1075527

Headache and the Cardiovascular Patient

5

Katelyn A. Seward, Khadijah Hussain, and Bruce J. Kimura

> *Mr. D is a 70-year-old man with a chronic history of migraine without aura that typically respond to triptan therapy or CGRP inhibitors. Prophylaxis with divalproex and CGRP inhibitors have greatly reduced episodes. During treatment for suspected angina, a bitemporal headache occurred after an initial dose of isosorbide mononitrate and was resistant to acetaminophen but responded to his CGRP inhibitor. He believes the nitrates triggered this and wants to stop this medication.*

HEADACHE SECONDARY TO COMMON CARDIOVASCULAR MEDICATIONS

Headache is a common adverse effect of many medications. Non-life threatening/non-serious adverse drug reactions are less studied and not quantified with the same accuracy as reactions that are considered serious (1, 2). Failing to detect headache as an adverse drug reaction can prolong patient anxiety and suffering, decreased adherence and come with a cost of unnecessary prescriptions, testing, and consults (3). Although most cardiovascular medications are well tolerated, there are several common prescriptions that can induce headache as an adverse effect, usually attributed to their vasodilatory properties.

Nitroglycerin and Nitrate Therapy

Nitrates are effective anti-anginal and anti-ischemic agents that act as potent dilators of vascular smooth muscle (4). From its discovery, nitroglycerin has been observed to reliably induce headache (5–10). Nitroglycerin was first synthesized in 1846 by Italian chemist Ascanio Sobrero who noted a "violent headache" lasting several hours when minute quantities were placed on the tongue. In the early 1900s, severe headaches were a common occurrence amongst workers in the formative days of handling nitroglycerin as dynamite. Nitroglycerin was first used as treatment for angina pectoris in 1879 by English physician William Murrell and has since been widely used in both acute chest pain and chronic angina presentations.

DOI: 10.1201/b23330-5

Today, headache remains one of the most common side effects of nitrates and up to 10% of patients are unable to tolerate any nitrate therapy due to headache (4).

All nitric oxide (NO) donors can cause headache (11). Interestingly, in the treatment of acute chest pain, sublingual nitroglycerin has been observed to cause significantly more headaches in patients with little or no coronary artery disease compared to those with obstructive coronary artery disease, 73% vs. 23%, respectively (12). Typically, nitrate therapy induces two types of headaches: immediate or delayed. Immediate headache after NO has been observed in healthy subjects, regardless of any history of headache (7, 11). Onset of headache occurs within minutes, is usually pulsatile, fronto-temporal in location, but usually does not fulfill the full diagnostic criteria for migraine and spontaneously resolves (13). Delayed onset headache typically occurs in patients with history of migraine, tension, or cluster type headache, develops 3–6 hours after exposure, and usually involves severe, long-lasting symptoms that resemble the patient's primary headache (2, 6, 7, 11, 14). Patients with a history of migraine typically develop a more severe immediate headache that requires anti-migraine therapy when placed on nitrates as in the case presented. Unfortunately, triptan therapy should be avoided in patients with migraine who have a history of ischemic heart disease, ischemic stroke, or uncontrolled hypertension (15, 16).

The exact relationship between NO and headaches remains unclear. Generally, headache from nitrates has been attributed to vasodilation, which is the main biological role of NO. However, there has been controversial evidence suggesting that vasodilation is not the only mechanism involved, especially in delayed-onset migraines induced by nitrates. Immediate and transient vasodilation of the cerebral and meningeal vasculature has been well documented during NO donor administration and may be related to the immediate headache experienced within minutes of administration. However, in nitroglycerin-induced delayed-onset migraine, human 3T magnetic resonance angiography has demonstrated no association with cerebral or meningeal blood vessel dilation (17), which contradicts previous beliefs of vasodilation being key to the headache phase of migraine. Nitroglycerin-induced migraine is one of the most studied human migraine models due to considerable similarities with spontaneous migraine attacks (3, 13). More recently, the neurotransmitter CGRP (calcitonin gene-related peptide) is thought to play a pivotal role in migraine pain, and elevated levels of CGRP have been found in patients during both spontaneous and nitroglycerin-induced migraine, suggesting that a migraine attack is a result of trigeminovascular activation (7).

The phenomenon of nitrate tolerance is incompletely understood, but generally develops in 5–7 days. This was observed by industry in the 1800s and led to the development of the term "Monday disease" as workers handling nitroglycerin throughout the week developed tolerance that subsequently wore off over the weekend, leading to return of headache with re-exposure on Monday (5). In the therapeutic use of nitrates, tolerance commonly leads to the resolution of headache as a side effect (11). Nitric oxide donor isosorbide dinitrate undergoes very high first past metabolism resulting in the major metabolite isosorbide-5-mononitrate (5-ISMN) which has anti-anginal effects for at least 12 hours. Because of this pathway, a much longer lasting headache due to the slow release of NO can occur. The strategy of starting at low doses of nitrates is associated with both reduced frequency and severity of headache without reducing the beneficial anti-anginal effect (18). Such concepts of pharmacologic tolerance, central sensitization, and "rebound" have been considered in the medication overuse headache phenomenon (19, 20).

Other Cardiovascular Medications

Many cardiovascular drugs with either direct or indirect vasodilation properties have been found to cause headache as an adverse reaction (Table 5.1). Most headaches caused by cardiovascular medications are classified as a Type A adverse drug reaction producing a headache that is predictable, related to the principal pharmacological action of the drug, and dose-dependent. The mechanisms of how headache occurs due to simple vasodilation, in patients with and without migraines, are not fully understood and can be confounded by inflammation, hypertension and its treatment. *In the case of Mr. D, discontinuation of nitrate therapy and empiric trials of alternative antianginal therapies may need to be considered.*

TABLE 5.1   Cardiovascular classes and more commonly used drugs associated with headache

DRUGS	% OF HA	MECHANISM OF HA
Calcium Channel Blockers[a]		
Nifedipine	3–6	Vasodilation
Nicardipine	3.8–12.6	
Diltiazem	4	
Verapamil	1.7	
Beta-Blockers[a]		
Bisoprolol	10.9	Highest incidence in non-selective beta-blockers with
Propranolol	<10	vasodilating properties
Metoprolol	<10	
Atenolol	<10	
ACE Inhibitor[a,c]		
Benazepril	6.2	Vasodilation. Accumulation of bradykinin, a potent
Enalapril	2.9–5.2	vasodilator
Lisinopril	3.8	
Nitrates[a,b,c]		
Nitroglycerin	45	Vasodilation via NO induced increased cGMP.
Isosorbide dinitrate	11–38	Proposed mechanism leading to migraine involves
Isosorbide mononitrate	23–42	CGRP or changes in ion channel function mediated by cGMP
Phosphodiesterase inhibitors[a,b]		
Dipyridamole	2.3	Inhibition of phosphodiesterase leading to increase of cAMP/cGMP and subsequent vasodilation
Alpha-2 adrenergic agonist		
Clonidine		Vasodilation, associated with headache after discontinuation of drug/withdrawal headache
Angiotensin receptor blockers[a]		
Valsartan	9.8	Angiotensin II is potent vasoconstrictor, mechanism of headache may be related to vasodilation
Alpha-1 adrenergic blockers		
Doxazosin	4	Vasodilation
Prazosin[c]	7.8	

Source: Ferrari 2006 (2). Headache: One of the most common and troublesome adverse reactions to drugs. *Curr Drug Saf.* 2006 Jan; 1(1):43–58.

Note:
[a] All drugs in class associated with headache.
[b] Drug associated with migraine headache.
[c] Headache has been reported to cause discontinuation of the drug.

SUMMARY

- Many cardiovascular medications can cause headache presumably through vasomotor effects. Nitrate therapy can induce immediate headache, likely related to vasodilation, and delayed long-lasting headache in patients already with a primary headache disorder.
- The immediate nitrate-induced headache can be a model of a pure vasodilatory triggers for cephalgia.

Ms. J is a 74-year-old woman who presents to the emergency department with severe headache and changes in vision. She reports left parietal headaches that have worsened since last week. She has had intermittent fevers of 100.6°F and over the past day, has noted two episodes of transient visual loss in the right upper quadrant of her right eye that lasted for five minutes. The patient's fundoscopic exam was unremarkable but the left parietal area was notably tender to palpation. ESR and CRP were elevated. What is the next step in the evaluation of her symptoms?

HEADACHE AND VASCULAR DISORDERS

Headaches secondary to vasculopathies can lead to significant morbidity and mortality. Temporal arteritis, also known as giant cell arteritis (GCA), is the most common vasculitis affecting adults older than 50 years (Table 5.2). It is a systemic autoimmune vasculitis causing chronic vascular inflammation in medium and large cranial arteries, often affecting the temporal and ophthalmic arteries (21, 22). Involvement of the aorta, carotid, subclavian, and axillary arteries is seen in 30–80% of cases (23, 24). GCA is associated with polymyalgia rheumatica (PMR) which occurs in 40–50% of GCA patients, while 15–20% of patients with PMR have GCA. Symptom onset is often insidious and presents with new headache, visual disturbances and jaw claudication. Non-specific symptoms such as chest pain, abdominal pain, malaise and fevers also manifest, making it a difficult diagnosis to promptly and accurately suspect (25).

Over two-thirds of GCA patients experience headaches that may also be associated with scalp tenderness. Headaches are bilateral and classically located over the temples but may also be frontal, occipital or generalized. They may be continuous or progress, wax and wane, or subside temporarily.

Cranial vasculature and the meninges are richly innervated by nociceptor fibers from the trigeminal system and contain the neuropeptides calcitonin gene-related peptide (CGRP) and substance P. Endothelial damage and inflammation lead to increased nerve growth factor (NGF) production by the blood vessel which can act via its high-affinity trk A receptor to release CGRP and substance P from nerve terminals and induce neurogenic edema and hyperalgesia (21, 26). This mechanism of nociception is supported by Saldanha et al (26) in a post-mortem analysis of temporal arteries in GCA that demonstrated increased NGF in inflamed tissues and markedly decreased CGRP immunoreactivity in nerve fibers in regions of inflamed blood vessels, suggesting CGRP secretion from nerve terminals (Figure 5.1). As such, scalp tenderness reflects inflammation in the affected arteries or subcutaneous tissue (27, 28). In contrast to scalp tenderness, inflammation of the dura may explain internal headaches. Dural enhancement has been seen on contrast MRI due to the "leaky" inflamed arteries supplying the dura in the presence of inflammation (27, 29, 30).

Anemia, thrombocytosis, elevated erythrocyte sedimentation rate, C-reactive protein and liver enzymes support the diagnosis. Temporal artery biopsy remains the gold standard of diagnosis and demonstrates transmural inflammatory infiltrates with lymphocytes, macrophages, and giant cell granulomas. Noninvasive techniques are being explored including color doppler ultrasound (CDUS), high-resolution MRI/MRA, and FDG-PET/CT. Studies on CDUS have demonstrated about 55–69% sensitivity and 82–94% specificity (31, 32) and can be operator-dependent. MRA helps identify vessel wall edema and has demonstrated sensitivity and specificity of 73% and 88%, respectively (33). FDG-PET is useful in evaluating large vessels but limited in intracranial arteries due to high FDG uptake in the brain (34).

It is imperative that diagnostics not delay treatment because rapid, irreversible bilateral vision loss due to impaired blood flow to the optic nerve (s) can ensue. Thus, an urgent ophthalmology referral should

TABLE 5.2 Vascular disorders that cause headaches

CONDITION	EPIDEMIOLOGY	HEADACHE CHARACTERISTICS	OTHER CLINICAL FEATURES	DIAGNOSIS	MANAGEMENT
GCA (22, 25, 34, 37–39)	– Age >50, average onset age 70 – Women>Men – 20/100,000	– New or worsening headache (>66%) – Bilateral, temporal – Scalp tenderness	– Visual changes; high risk of rapid irreversible vison loss that can be partial, unilateral or bilateral – Jaw claudication – Generalized pain, malaise, fevers – Associated with polymyalgia rheumatica – Elevated ESR, CRP, LFTs	– Temporal artery biopsy* – Color doppler ultrasound – MRI/MRA – FDG-PET for large vessels	– Prednisone 40–60 mg/day – Preceded by intravenous methylprednisolone 500 or 1000 mg/day for 3 days if threatened or established vision loss – Tocilizumab (interleukin-6 receptor antagonist) – Methotrexate (second line)
Cerebrovascular FMD (40, 41)	– 90% women in adult cases – Mean age at diagnosis: 52	– Headaches (70%) – Migraines (30%) – Pulsatile tinnitus	– High prevalence of carotid or vertebral dissection – Intracranial aneurysms – TIA, ischemic stroke – Carotid bruit – Strong association with SCAD – Unclear contribution of hormones, genetics	– Angiography: "String of beads" vs concentric stenosis	– One-time, head-to-pelvic, cross-sectional imaging when newly diagnosed – Daily low dose aspirin – Smoking cessation
PACNS (42–44)	– Median age 50 – Men>Women – 700 cases worldwide	– Subacute onset headache	– Progressive course with long prodromal period – Neurologic deficits from tissue ischemia; recurrent strokes in patients without cardiovascular risk factors – Cognitive impairment, seizures, altered consciousness, affective changes	– Biopsy* (Sn=75%) – MRI – CSF analysis: aseptic meningitis pattern – Cerebral angiography: beading of blood vessels	– Prednisone 1 mg/kg per day to max of 80 mg/day in combination with oral cyclophosphamide 1.5–2 mg/kg per day or monthly IV – Rituximab (limited data)
RCVS (21, 28, 45–50)	– Women>Men – True incidence unknown	– Sudden onset "thunderclap" headache	– Ischemic or hemorrhagic strokes – Vasoactive substance use – Postpartum state – Associated with migraines	– CSF analysis: normal – Angiography: beading of vessels, reversible in 1–3 months	– Nimodipine – Recommend avoiding glucocorticoids

* = gold standard

GCA = giant cell arteritis; ESR = erythrocyte sedimentation rate; CRP = C-reactive protein; LFT = liver function tests; MRI = magnetic resonance imaging; MRA = magnetic resonance angiography; FDG-PET = fludeoxyglucose positron emission tomography; FMD = fibromuscular dysplasia; TIA = transient ischemic attack; SCAD = spontaneous coronary artery dissection; Sn = sensitivity; PACNS = primary angiitis of the central nervous system; RCVS = reversible vasoconstriction syndrome; CSF = cerebrospinal fluid

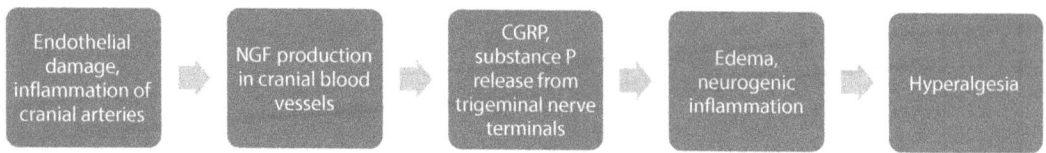

| Endothelial damage, inflammation of cranial arteries | ⇒ | NGF production in cranial blood vessels | ⇒ | CGRP, substance P release from trigeminal nerve terminals | ⇒ | Edema, neurogenic inflammation | ⇒ | Hyperalgesia |

FIGURE 5.1 Possible mechanism of cerebral nociception. (NGF = nerve growth factor; CGRP = calcitonin gene-related peptide.)

be made when the diagnosis is suspected. Per guidelines, biopsy should be completed within two weeks of starting treatment with at least 1 cm sample (limited biopsies can be negative in 30% of GCA patients due to skip lesions) (34–36). Sensitivity of non invasive imaging is too low to "rule out" the diagnosis and further decreases within 5–7 days of treatment initiation. Treatment is initiated with high-dose corticosteroids. Methotrexate and tocilizumab are useful in decreasing steroid doses (34, 37, 38). Patients report a dramatic improvement in symptoms within 24–48 hours of treatment, with almost all responding within 1–7 days (21, 39).

Other disorders of the vessel wall also merit mention in the discussion of headache (Table 5.2). Fibromuscular dysplasia (FMD) is a noninflammatory, nonatherosclerotic vascular disorder most often involving the renal, internal carotid, and vertebral arteries, with 65% cases having cerebrovascular disease (40, 41). Possible mechanisms of headaches in FMD include alterations in cerebrovascular flow, dysautonomia, structural injury (such as dissection or microtrauma), or heightened sensitivity to pain. Cerebrovascular FMD affects the carotid artery (often bilaterally) in 95% of cases and the vertebral artery in 60% to 85% of cases (often with co-involvement of the carotid). FMD patients are at risk of artery dissection, with age >50 being an independent risk factor. Mechanical factors such as extension and lateral rotation of the head and neck have been speculated to play a role in dissection by enhancing stretching of the cervical arteries. Primary angiitis of the central nervous system (PACNS) is a rare vasculitis that can present with headaches in 60% and cognitive impairment, seizures, spinal cord lesions, altered consciousness, and affective abnormalities (42–44). Presenting headache is often subacute; PACNS has an insidious course with a long prodromal period. Reversible cerebral vasoconstriction syndrome (RCVS) can mimic vasculitis. It encompasses the various pathologies that result in vasospasm of cerebral vessels and typically presents with thunderclap headaches with or without neurologic deficits (28, 45, 46). About 60% of cases are secondary to exposure to vasoactive substances and postpartum status (21, 47–50). Angiographic findings may demonstrate beading of the affected blood vessels; however, the key feature is reversibility of radiographic findings (21, 28).

There was a high clinical suspicion of GCA in Ms. J's presentation, so she underwent temporal artery biopsy and was discharged on high-dose steroids. Pathology confirmed giant cell arteritis two days later. Steroids were continued for four weeks before being tapered and the patient did not have recurrent symptoms at follow-up visit. Timely and accurate diagnosis was vital, ensuring the right approach and preventing potential complications in her.

SUMMARY

- Recognizing vascular headaches demands an understanding of symptoms, diagnostic methods and appropriate treatments.
- Inflammation of the vessel wall itself may trigger headache, by way of neurotransmitters and nociceptor fibers.

Mrs. K is a 60-year-old female with a history of migraines since age 28. Headaches occur without aura and cause pain in the right temporal region, associated with nausea and photophobia, and are precipitated by stress and hormonal changes. Over the years, she has failed beta-blocker and calcium-channel blocker prophylaxis and has used triptan therapies for acute breakthroughs, which typically occurred twice per month. Currently, she uses a CGRP inhibitor for less frequent, post-menopausal episodes for shorter, monthly episodes. She has never had an echocardiogram. Should she get one to exclude a patent foramen ovale?

MIGRAINE, CARDIOVASCULAR RISK AND PATENT FORAMEN OVALE

Migraine headache is a common and complex neurovascular disease that affects about 15% of the general population (51). Migraine affects women more than men, especially young to middle-aged women, and can be a chronic disabling disorder with socioeconomic burden (52). There is considerable evidence that links migraine, particularly migraine with aura, to cardiovascular events and an increased risk of cardiovascular mortality. Migraine has also been associated with an increased risk of stroke and patent foramen ovale (PFO). In the realm of cardiovascular disorders associated with headache, chronic migraine is also present amongst those with postural orthostatic tachycardia syndrome (POTS) and is associated with a greater degree of autonomic symptoms (53). Although there are still many questions that remain unanswered, the commonality and burden of both migraine and cardiovascular disease in society makes awareness of their association an important topic for all physicians.

The underlying mechanism for increased cardiovascular disease in those with migraine is incompletely understood, likely multifactorial, and rapidly evolving. Patients with migraine, with or without aura, have higher rates of hypertension, hypercholesterolemia, and diabetes (52, 54–56). The risk of cardiovascular disease is further compounded by smoking and use oral contraception pills (56). However, there is still demonstration of increased risk of cardiovascular disease in patients with migraine even after traditional cardiovascular risk factors have been addressed (52, 55).

Migraine with aura has a stronger associated risk of cardiovascular disease, myocardial infarction, stroke and even atrial fibrillation than migraine without aura (52, 54–56). The migraine aura and headache are both linked to the phenomenon of cortical spreading depression (CSD), a self-propagating wave of neuronal depolarization over the cerebral cortex. The activation of the trigeminal vascular system and its subsequent effect is a complex and intricate process that leads to release of key inflammatory peptides, one of which is CGRP which mediates transmission of pain and vasodilation leading to neurogenic inflammation (57, 58). Migraine, especially migraine with aura, is a systemic disease associated with endothelial dysfunction and increased platelet aggregation (52). Peripheral endothelial function has been tested by different methods in patients with migraine and healthy controls, however results have been inconclusive and contradictory (55). Sympathetic nervous system dysfunction and central sensitization has been proposed as a common mechanism in migraine headache and POTS (59). As it currently stands, definitive answers on the relationship between the migraine aura, inflammation, platelet aggregation and cardiovascular disease are still unclear.

The choice of migraine treatments in patients with potential cardiovascular disease deserves thoughtful consideration of the vessel wall. Triptans can cause vasoconstriction and, although based on limited evidence, should be avoided in patients with ischemic heart disease, ischemic stroke, uncontrolled hypertension, or Prinzmetal's angina (60). Conversely, in the preventative treatment of migraine, some medications may have favorable cardiovascular effects. Comorbid cardiovascular disorders can help guide the choice of medication selection for migraine prevention such as a beta-blocker for patients with comorbid atrial fibrillation or calcium channel blockers in patients with hypertension. Antiepileptics such as valproic acid pose little to no concern in the cardiovascular patient, however valproic acid is contraindicated in women of childbearing age due to teratogenic effects (55). Interestingly, statins with vitamin D, a therapy without hemodynamic effects but with possible salutary effects against endothelial dysfunction and inflammation, have shown benefit in migraine prophylaxis (61). The newer CGRP antagonists are effective in both acute and preventative treatment of migraine. There are some recommendations that CGRP antagonists should be avoided in patients with recent ischemic cardiovascular events because of vasomotor effects, however long-term trials to justify this warning are still awaited (62, 63).

Right-to-left Shunt and PFO

Whether a patient should get an echocardiogram is addressed by a potential relationship between migraine and right-to-left cardiac shunt. This mechanism is controversial, yet well documented (64–68). Migraine has been commonly associated with the presence of a patent foramen ovale, an embryonic remnant of fetal circulation that permits inter atrial shunting of blood and persists in 25–30% of normal adults, most remaining asymptomatic. Data is strongest for patients who suffer from migraine with aura and suggests the prevalence of a PFO in migraineurs with aura is as high as 48% (64, 68–69).

Typically, a PFO is found incidentally on echocardiography by the presence of a small abnormal Color Doppler jet crossing the interatrial septum, typically from the left atrium to the right atrium, due to the pressure gradient. However, a transient, or "paradoxical" reversal of the shunt can occur allowing small aliquots of venous blood to bypass the lung's filtering properties and enter the arterial circulation. Although technique-dependent, PFO can be diagnosed with approximate 50% sensitivity and 99% specificity by transthoracic echocardiography with intravenous agitated saline contrast injection revealing a transient right-to-left shunting of bubbles during inspiraton or upon Valsalva maneuver release (69–73) (Figure 5.2). The presence of any bubbles in the left atrium within 3–5 beats of their right atrial presence suggests a PFO, and a longer delay suggests pulmonary passage through a much rarer arterio venous

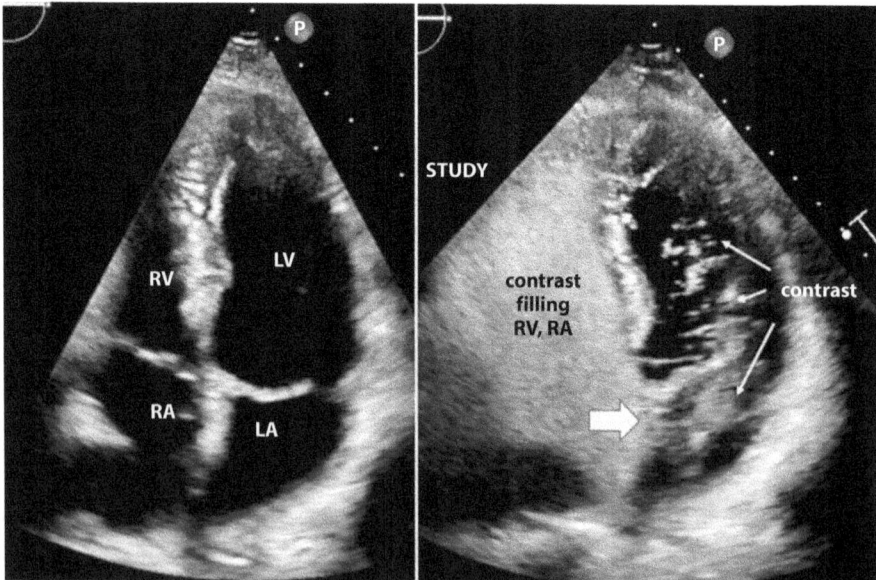

FIGURE 5.2   Agitated saline "bubble" study in patent foramen ovale. (Transthoracic echocardiogram apical view with agitated saline contrast ("bubble") study is positive for PFO with contrast moving from right to left atrium (right panel, yellow arrows). RV, right ventricle; LV, left ventricle; RA, right atrium; LA, left atrium.)

malformation in the lung. Associated risks of paradoxic embolism with PFO include the size of the shunt, as signified by the presence of multiple (>10) bubbles in the left atrium, and the presence of a hypermobile interatrial septum or prominent Eustachian valve in the right atrium (74, 75). These findings relate to the size or frequency of shunting and can be seen with more clarity by transesophageal echocardiography. Transcranial doppler can additionally diagnose the presence of a right-to-left shunt with a higher sensitivity than echocardiography but is less specific as it cannot differentiate between cardiac versus pulmonary shunting (72,73, 76). Larger sized right-to-left shunts and the presence of spontaneous shunting with a PFO has been associated with more persistent migraine with aura (66).

Although a PFO is the most highlighted cause of a right-to-left shunt, increased prevalence and risk for migraine has been found in other types of right-to-left shunt as well. Higher prevalence of migraine has been observed in patients with atrial septal defects. Adults with congenital heart disease have been found to have up to four times higher prevalence of migraine with aura than the general population (77, 78). Noncardiac right-to-left shunts such as pulmonary arteriovenous malformations (PAVM), either isolated or in association with hereditary hemorrhagic telangiectasia, are also associated with migraine headache (79–81). There is some evidence that migraine headaches improve following embolization of PAVM (81).

The exact pathophysiology that links right-to-left shunt to migraine is not completely understood. One common theory involves the passage of serotonin or microemboli, both gaining access to the arterial circulation through right-to-left shunting (68) and thereby avoiding the normal metabolism or filtering by the lung before reaching the cerebral circulation. Facilitation of CSD and trigeminovascular nociceptive pathway activation has been postulated to be in part related to chronic imbalance of serotonin activity and triggered by a sudden rise in serotonin levels (82–86). The majority of peripherally circulating serotonin is stored in platelets and release of serotonin from abnormal platelet aggregation in the circulation has been hypothesized as a pathological bases for migraine headaches (85, 87). Patients with migraine and PFO have been found to have inflammatory and prothrombotic platelet function (87). Shear stress induced platelet aggregation at sites of increased vascular flow, such as shunting through a PFO, has additionally been proposed as a potential mechanism for abnormal platelet behavior (86). Patients with migraine and a PFO treated with aspirin or P2Y12 inhibitors for a prior stroke have been observed to have reduction in migraine symptoms (88–90). Remarkably, both P2Y12 receptor antagonism and percutaneous PFO closure has been observed to not only reduced migraine symptoms but to reverse the prothrombotic platelet function and reduce oxidative stress in migraine-PFO patients (87–90). Venous injection of agitated saline in the presence of permanent right-to-left shunting does have correlation with the precipitation of typical migraine (91–93), presumably through transient ischemic or hypoxic triggers.

PFO Closure as Treatment for Migraine

Although the closure of a PFO has value in certain populations with cryptogenic stroke (70), the role of PFO closure specifically for prevention of migraine headache still remains controversial. Several small observational studies of patients undergoing PFO closure for other comorbid conditions have demonstrated significant reduction and even resolution of migraine after transcutaneous PFO closure (64,65,69,94). However, randomized control trials to assess PFO closure for the prevention of migraine have failed to consistently reproduce the same results (Table 5.3) due to differences in patient populations, the presence or absence of migraine aura, and responsiveness to anti platelet therapies.

Post-hoc analyses seem to suggest that the probability of a PFO being causally related to migraine headache was increased by the presence of migraine aura. A pooled analysis of the PRIMA and PREMIUM trials found a significant reduction in migraine in patients with PFO closure plus medical therapy versus medical therapy alone, and the significance was even greater for migraine with frequent aura (94). Increased prevalence of PFO is found even amongst those who experience migraine aura without any associated migraine headache (95). Additionally, late follow-up on patients after PFO closure for secondary stroke prevention revealed patients with migraine with aura were 4.5x more likely to experience migraine relief than those

TABLE 5.3   Randomized control trials to assess the efficacy of PFO closure for primary prevention of migraine and their major outcomes

TRIAL	DESIGN/CRITERIA	OUTCOMES
Migraine Intervention with STARFlex Technology (MIST) Trial (96), (n=147)	• Prospective, multicenter, double blinded sham-control trial to assess effectiveness of PFO repair for refractory migraine • Selected patients with migraine with aura with moderate to large right-to-left shunts consistent with PFO and frequent migraine attacks despite treatment with 2 or more prophylactic migraine medications	• Confirmed high prevalence of right-to-left shunt in patients with migraine (60.2% of patients with any type of right-to-left shunt, 37.7% with moderated to large PFO) • No significant difference observed of primary end point of migraine cessation between implant and sham groups • No significant difference in secondary end point of reduction in migraine days between implant and sham groups
Percutaneous Closure of Patent Foramen Ovale in Migraine with Aura (PRIMA) Trial (97), (n=107)	• Multicenter, prospective, randomized, open-label international trial • Selected patients with refractory episodic migraine with aura and PFO unresponsive to preventive medications randomized to PFO closure vs medical treatment. Both groups given aspirin for 6 months and clopidogrel for 3 months	• Did not reach primary end point, there was no significant reduction in migraine days per month in PFO closure group vs medical therapy group • Post hoc analysis focusing on migraines with aura revealed that migraine aura days and attacks of migraine with aura was significantly reduced in PFO closure group compared to controls (p = 0.0003)
Prospective, Randomized Investigation to Evaluate Incidence of Headache Reduction in subjects with Migraine and PFO Using the AMPLATZER PFO Occluder to Medical Management (PREMIUM) Trial (98), (n=230)	• Prospective, randomized, double-blind study investigating migraine characteristics for more than 1 year in subjects randomized to medical therapy plus PFO closure vs medical therapy plus sham procedure • Subjects had episodic migraine, with or without aura, failed at least 3 migraine preventative medications, significant right-to-left shunt by TCD	• No difference in primary end point of a >=50% decrease in migraines between PFO closure and control groups (38% vs. 32%, respectively, p=0.3) • PFO closure group had significant reduction in migraine days compared to control (p = 0.025) • 8.5% who underwent PFO closure had migraine remission by 1 year vs 1% in the control group (p = 0.01) • Subjects with frequent aura had significantly greater complete cessation of their migraine attack in the PFO closure group vs control (p = 0.04)

without aura (95). An additional characteristic of pathologic PFO in migraine may be rooted within the abnormal platelet hypothesis. Aspirin-allergic patients with a history of ischemic stroke and PFO treated with thienopyridines (clopidogrel/prasugrel) have been observed to have an unexpected reduction in migraine headache and lasting migraine relief. Off-label PFO closure in patients with migraine in whom relief may have been a result of thienopyridine therapy has been trialed in a small study and resulted in migraine reduction even after discontinuation of thienopyridine therapy (89). Therefore, it seems the presence of migraine aura and response to antiplatelet may be indicators of a pathologic PFO amenable to closure for migraine prevention.

There are no current specific guidelines to reduce the risk of cardiovascular disease in patients with migraine outside of addressing identified modifiable cardiovascular risk factors. Additionally, the current data does not fully support PFO closure for prevention of migraine nor routine screening for PFO in patients with migraine, as there is still much left to be answered on which subgroups may benefit. *As it currently stands, a screening echocardiogram would not be recommended for Mrs. K.*

SUMMARY

- Patients with migraine, especially with aura, have an increased risk for cardiovascular disease. There is a relationship between migraine with aura, right-to-left shunting, and PFO. However, there is no recommendation for screening or closure of a PFO in patients with migraine.
- Migraine with aura may represent the vasomotor and inflammatory mechanisms involving the vessel wall that interact with neuronal hypersensitivity.

Mr. O, a 52-year-old gentleman with hypertension, chronic obstructive pulmonary disease, chronic kidney disease, and type 2 diabetes, had an increase in blood pressure from 150/93 to 182/94 within an hour while in the emergency room. He was given a dose of intravenous antihypertensive therapy. The next morning, his systolic blood pressure rapidly increased by 30mmHg within an hour and he began to experience headaches and blurry vision. Can headache solely be attributed to elevated blood pressure?

HEADACHE AND HYPERTENSION

Elevated arterial blood pressure is often believed to cause headache. Conversely, pain is known to elevate blood pressure. Further, some headache syndromes, such as chronic migraine, are associated with hypertension. This section explores the multifaceted associations between headache and high blood pressure, both in acute crises and in chronic presentations.

HYPERTENSIVE HEADACHES

Commonly, people manifest high blood pressure (BP) with headache. A throbbing headache that occurs upon awakening and gradually subsides in the morning is a well-established feature of hypertension (99). Patients who visited an emergency department with a chief complaint of headache were more likely to have moderately or severely elevated BP than those with other chief complaints (99, 100). However, it is difficult to elucidate whether elevated BP causes the headache or whether pain causes an elevation in blood pressure, as both are phenomena appreciated in the clinical setting. A clear way to delineate these two events has not been defined, however international guidelines establish that headache should be attributed to elevated blood pressure if the systolic BP (SBP) rises quickly to 180 mmHg or higher, or if the diastolic BP (DBP) rises to 120 mmHg or higher, and if the headache resolves with normalization of BP

(101). A hypertensive crisis is defined when systolic blood pressure ≥180 mmHg and/or diastolic blood pressure ≥120 mmHg is present with end-organ damage (102).

Acute elevations in BP can lead to end-organ manifestations including headaches. Mild to moderate increases in BP result in appropriate arterial vasoconstriction to maintain steady tissue perfusion, as dictated by cerebral autoregulation (103). Rapid or marked BP elevation impairs autoregulation leading to increased blood flow and pressure in the vessels, resulting in vascular endothelial damage. In the brain, severe hypertension can break down the blood-brain barrier and cause leakage of intravascular fluid into the parenchyma leading to cerebral edema (Figure 5.3). This may be seen in the setting of primary or malignant hypertension from pheochromocytoma, synergistic drug effects, or other secondary causes. Pressure or flow-mediated vasodilation with impaired cerebrovascular autoregulation, has been implicated in cough, exercise, and sexual headaches (104).

Other studies have not found an association between elevated BP and headaches. The Vobarno study enrolled 301 subjects and demonstrated that in patients with an accurate diagnosis of hypertension from a general population sample, the elevation in office and/or 24-hour BP was not associated with increasing prevalence, frequency, or severity of headache (105). No statistically significant differences in headache prevalence and use of analgesic drugs were observed between hypertensive and normotensive subjects (105). A Brazilian study with 1,763 patients concluded that headache was not associated with moderate-to-severe hypertension in patients attending a hypertension clinic (106). Rather, an inverse association between pulse pressure and headaches was seen. A cross-sectional study of 2,100 subjects in Nepal also demonstrated a negative association between hypertension and headache (107). All headache types were significantly less prevalent among hypertension cases than non-cases.

Tronvik et al. (108) describes a phenomenon called hypertension-associated hypoalgesia as a mechanism for decreased headaches in hypertensive patients. It suggests that increased blood pressure causes stimulation of the baroreflex arch which subsequently inhibits pain transmission at spinal and supraspinal levels, possibly from an interaction of the nociception centers and cardiovascular reflexes in the brainstem. In a large public health HUNT study among 46,901 adults, increasing blood pressure was related to decreased pain in all parts of the body, including musculoskeletal pain, and was not limited to headaches (109). Baroreflex influences various sites in pain modulation; BP changes have been shown to excite neurons of the periaqueductal gray and nucleus raphe magnus.

Epidemiologic data demonstrates an inverse relationship of decreasing prevalence of non-migraine headache with increasing SBP values. For DBP, higher values were also associated with a decreased non-migraine headache prevalence, as was noted in men who used antihypertensives. Increasing pulse pressure was most consistently associated with decreased prevalence of both headache types in both sexes. When stratified, this inverse relationship was significant in participants not using antihypertensives but was lost with therapy (108). Pulse pressure and SBP are related to arterial stiffness and tend to increase with age. The influence of age on the association between headache and blood

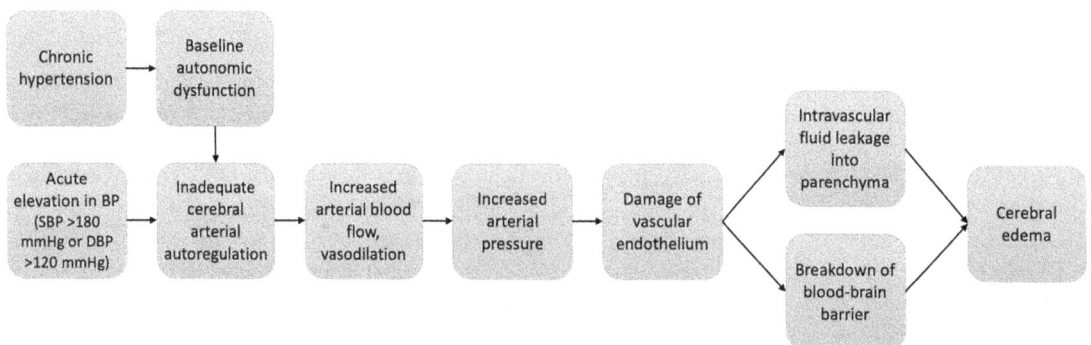

FIGURE 5.3 Possible mechanism of headache in hypertensive emergency. (BP = blood pressure, SBP = systolic blood pressure, DBP = diastolic blood pressure.)

pressure was evaluated by repeating the analyses in subjects older and younger than age 50. The inverse associations remained significant for all groups except male migraineurs older than 50 years. Another large prospective population-based study showed similar findings, with the strongest evidence backing the inverse association between increased pulse pressure and both migraine and tension headaches (110). It is known that increased pulse pressure in healthy middle-aged subjects is associated with reduced baroreflex sensitivity (111). These studies suggest that the modulations of the baroreflex may be associated with pain thresholds, perhaps explaining the inverse relationship between pulse pressure and headache.

Hypertension and Migraine

Hypertension may be a factor in increased frequency and severity of migraine headaches (100, 101, 112, 113). In a large population-based study of 21,537 subjects (114), a one standard deviation increase in DBP increased the probability of having migraine by 30% in women and 14% in men, while a similar increase in SBP decreased the probability of having migraine by 19% in men and 25% in women. In contrast to the previous discussion, migraine patients were found to have lower pulse pressure compared with controls.

People with migraine, with and without aura, are known to have a higher prevalence of hypertension and higher risk of cardiovascular diseases (99–101, 115–118). In one study, subjects with migraine had a 1.4-fold increased risk of hypertension compared to those without migraine (119). Migraine is an independent predictor for hypertension after controlling for various confounding variables (120). Vascular risks may be compounded in migraine with aura, particularly in women (117). The MIRACLES study was a multicenter, cross-sectional, survey that included 2,973 patients with a known diagnosis of hypertension or migraine. It demonstrated that compared to having hypertension or migraine alone, patients with both diseases had a significantly higher prevalence of cerebrovascular events such as stroke and transient ischemic attack (118). Between 40 and 49 years of age, this disparity was five-fold. Cigarette smoking and oral contraceptive use increased these risks further.

Hypertension and migraine share a common pathophysiologic mechanism involving alteration of vascular tone, autonomic dysregulation, and endothelial dysfunction (101, 112, 115). Nitric oxide is a vasodilator and an important molecule in the regulation of intra-arterial blood flow. Hypersensitivity to nitric oxide is thought to be a migraine trigger. Endothelial dysfunction and subsequent impairment of nitric oxide leading to abnormal vasoconstriction is also the suggested mechanism of cardiovascular diseases (121, 122). Additionally, pathologic autonomic cardiovascular regulation in migraineurs manifests with vagal hyperactivity at baseline and a hypersensitivity to catecholamines, leading to platelet aggregation and vasoconstriction with sympathetic activation (123, 124). Platelet serotonin is seen in lower levels in migraineurs at baseline while calcitonin gene-related peptide (CGRP) has vasodilatory effects and tends to be present at higher levels. Given that these neurotransmitters have opposite effects on the vasculature, there may be complex temporal correlations between blood pressure, vascular risk, and migraines (115). CGRP is also suggested to activate meningeal nociceptors (100).

The association of hypertension and migraine is supported by the observation that many antihypertensive medications are effective in migraine prophylaxis such as beta-blockers, angiotensin-converting enzyme (ACE) inhibitors, and angiotensin II receptor blockers (ARBs) (125). The renin-angiotensin-aldosterone system is well-established in the regulation of blood pressure in the body. It is also involved in medullary adrenaline release, vasoconstriction and increased sympathetic activity along with having neuroendocrine effects and stimulating NO production through NF-kb (115). ARBs have been found to restore vasoreactivity, attenuate hyperalgesia via inflammatory and oxidative stress, and regulate nitric oxide synthase expression (126). Furthermore, in a study of 302 subjects (127), a polymorphism in the ACE-D allele (DD genotype) conferred higher plasma ACE activity and was associated with higher frequency of migraines without aura than in those without the polymorphism. The inverse was also true that subjects with migraines showed higher incidence of the DD allele than controls.

Despite a pathologic basis and clinical observations, data surrounding the association between migraine and hypertension is contradictory. Population-based studies have not established this association and some have found inverse effects (128, 129). In a population-based study analyzing cross-sectional data from 1,174 subjects in Brazil (128), migraineurs had lower blood pressure than those without migraine.

Besides population differences, another possible explanation for the disparities among studies include not using the standardized criteria for migraine diagnosis (100). Particularly, the terms *migraine* and *headache* are used interchangeably in these studies when they may represent different conditions. Blood pressure parameters are defined and analyzed differently, as some studies separate SBP, DBP, pulse pressure, mean arterial pressure and degree or rate of elevation for comparison. Age is also a factor that can affect these findings, as migraine and hypertension have opposite age trends (104). A cross-sectional study by Mancia et al established a population in whom migraine started primarily after the age of 30 years, hypertension started before the age of 50 years, and the onset of comorbidity of migraine AND hypertension occurred at about 45 years of age (118). Arterial wall thickness or stiffness with age, as mentioned previously, become a confounding factor between hypertension and migraines (129).

Mr. O was likely experiencing a hypertensive headache given the rapidity with which his blood pressure elevated to SBP >180. He was started on a different anti-hypertensive agent with good effect and his headache subsequently resolved, supporting this clinical suspicion.

SUMMARY

- There are conflicting data supporting the relationship between hypertension and headaches, as a number of studies have also failed to find a positive association and have even established a negative one.
- Cerebral vessel wall compliance under increased pressure or flow may partly explain blood pressure and epidemiologic observations in headache.

Ms. C is a 51-year-old woman with hypertension who presented for acute onset of severe headache, dizziness, and nausea with rapid decline in mentation. Her husband reported that she had been having intermittent episodes of nausea and headaches for the past several weeks, and had an acute episode of severe, worsening headache prior to admission. He worries she is having a stroke.

HEADACHE AND STROKE

Stroke is the second-most common cause of mortality and disability worldwide (130). A cerebrovascular accident is the most feared outcome of the cardiovascular patient presenting with headache. This section will review common classifications of stroke and discuss the prevalence of headache pain and cardiovascular considerations (Table 5.4). In the cardiovascular patient, the risks of cardioembolism and intracranial hemorrhage often co-exist in hypertension, atherosclerosis, structural heart disease, and the use of antiplatelets and anticoagulants.

Hemorrhagic Stroke

A patient claiming to have the sudden onset of the "worst headache of my life" is a classic red flag for sinister etiologies of headache, particularly subarachnoid hemorrhage. About 20% of strokes are hemorrhagic with subarachnoid hemorrhage (SAH) and intracerebral hemorrhage (ICH) each accounting for 10%. Studies suggest that headaches are reported in about 50% of hemorrhagic strokes and over 95% in SAH (131). The prevalence varies based on the type and location of the hemorrhage, with subarachnoid hemorrhages, being arterial, often causing very severe headaches.

Etiology of SAH can be traumatic or nontraumatic; about 85% of nontraumatic cases are secondary to aneurysm rupture, for which hypertension is a major risk factor. Meningismus and focal neurologic deficits may also be present. CT of the head reveals blood in the basal cisterns in the first 12 hours after SAH with approximately 95% sensitivity and specificity. If no blood is seen on CT, a lumbar puncture can be performed to confirm or rule out the diagnosis of SAH (132).

After treatment of aneurysmal subarachnoid hemorrhage, severe headache may last from two weeks up to months (133). The mechanism of this headache is attributable to high intracranial pressure and inflammatory responses to blood breakdown products. The blood-brain barrier has increased permeability after SAH and is exposed to immune cells. Glia cells are activated and secrete pro-inflammatory cytokines and assist in early brain injury after SAH. Pro-inflammatory cytokines concentrations in the CSF including IL-6, IL-1β and TNF-α were closely associated with headache after aneurysmal SAH (133) and IL-6 was associated in nonaneurysmal subarachnoid hemorrhage (134).

Subdural hematoma (SDH) is also a form of hemorrhagic stroke that can cause headache. Due to a lower pressure in the venous circulation, the onset and presenting headache may be more subacute and does not present as distinctly as SAH. Headache in chronic SDH was studied in a group of 1,080 surgically treated patients and headache was present in 22.6% of patients while nausea or vomiting suggesting increased intracranial pressure was noted in 3% (135). Patients with headaches tended to be younger. Midline shift was the most influential factor for headache, suggesting a potential mechanism to be stretching or twisting of the pain-sensitive meninges and meningeal arteries or veins.

The mechanism of headaches in hemorrhagic strokes is multifaceted. The skull has a limited and finite space, thus the accumulation of blood within the brain quickly raises intracranial pressure, compressing surrounding tissues and stimulating pain receptors. Additionally, blood products released during hemorrhage can irritate pain-sensitive structures such as blood vessels and meninges, through a cascade of inflammatory responses. Finally, hemorrhagic strokes cause inflammation in the brain tissue itself with inflammatory mediators sensitizing pain receptors. In hemorrhagic stroke, disruption of cerebral blood vessels and the inflammatory response can also contribute to vasospasm or vasodilation, further aggravating headaches.

Hemorrhagic strokes are particularly relevant in cardiovascular patients, as many are on anticoagulation or antiplatelet therapies. Initiating these therapies on a cardiovascular patient comes only after a thorough assessment of the risks and benefits. Moderately performing risk scores have been developed to facilitate this evaluation including the HAS-BLED, ATRIA, and DAPT, HEMORR2HAGES, and ORBIT (139) scores. Clinicians should maintain a high index of suspicion for hemorrhagic stroke especially in a patient on anticoagulation with a new-onset or changing headache, and have a low threshold for CT scan of the head to rule out this highly morbid condition.

Non-hemorrhagic Stroke

The cardiovascular patient is also at risk for cardioembolic (non-hemorrhagic) stroke due to atrial fibrillation, valvular disease, bioprosthetic or mechanical heart valves, dilated cardiomyopathy, or recent myocardial infarction (140). Ischemic stroke accounts for about 87% of strokes in the United States (141). Although the presence of headache at onset of ischemic stroke is often overshadowed by the presence of neurologic deficits, the prevalence of headache can range 7.4% to 34% (142, 143). Although severe headache is more commonly thought of at the onset of hemorrhagic stroke, headache can occur at onset of non-hemorrhagic stroke or TIA and is positively associated with younger age, female sex, history of migraine and posterior circulation or cerebellar strokes (144).

In addition to the aforementioned causes of headache in hemorrhagic stroke, the pathophysiology of headache associated with ischemic stroke/TIA is in part hypothesized to be related to triggering of cortical spreading depression as a result of ischemia. Trigeminovascular innervation has been found to be denser in the posterior circulation and this is thought to possibly contribute to higher prevalence of headache with ischemic stroke in this territory. Additionally, prothrombotic and inflammatory substances along with serotonin and prostaglandins released from platelet aggregation in the acute phase of the stroke may also play a role in the generation of headache. Headache occurs more frequently in larger sized ischemic strokes and strokes of the vertebrobasilar system or with cortical involvement. Small-vessel lacunar infarcts are associated with a lower incidence of headache (143).

Patients with a primary headache disorder who present with "the worst headache of my life" may simply be experiencing a severe episode of their typical headache rather than an acute stroke. Headaches associated with cerebrovascular accidents more commonly present as sudden onset, severe, and rapidly reaching maximum intensity (145) (Table 5.4). In a study on headache at the onset of ischemic stroke,

TABLE 5.4 Features of different stroke types and prevalence of associated headache

STROKE TYPE	HEADACHE PREVALENCE	FEATURES
Subarachnoid hemorrhage	78%	• "Worst headache of my life" • Traumatic vs nontraumatic (aneurysmal) • Increased intracranial pressure • Inflammatory mediators -> sensitization of pain structures • Vascular dysfunction -> vasospasm • Blood irritation of pain-sensitive meninges and vessels
Subdural hemorrhage	Up to 80% (chronic)	• More subacute onset • Less distinct headache presentation • Headache often progressive/worsening • See mechanisms above
Ischemic stroke	7.4–34% (headache at onset of stroke) (142, 143)	• New headache or headache with altered characteristics. Triggered CSD from ischemia • Associated with migraine with aura, younger adults, females, posterior circulation stroke • Cardio-embolic stroke sources (mechanical valve, potential intracardiac thrombus, atrial fibrillation/persistent flutter, mechanical heart valve, paradoxical emboli from a PFO)
Cervical artery dissection	65–95% (153)	• Unilateral sudden headaches ipsilateral to side of dissection • Often in young adults, associated with migraine headaches • Associated with FMD
Endocarditis	2–4% (headache as the sole neurologic complaint) (154, 155)	• Often in younger patients • Ischemic stroke from septic emboli • New or changing cardiac murmur • Fever, sequelae of septic emboli (Janeway lesions, Oslers nodes, splinter hemorrhages) • Risk factors: valvular or congenital heart disease, recent dental procedure, IV drug use

more than half of the patients who experienced headache at stroke onset had a headache that was either new or had altered characteristics. Additionally, headache at stroke onset was associated with a low prevalence of atherosclerosis and a significantly increased prevalence of cardioembolic stroke (146). In a large review (144) on headache at onset of stroke or TIA, vascular risk factors such as hypertension and smoking did not show a significant association. In a study to evaluate the presence of sentinel headache and its characteristics in the context of ischemic stroke (147), a new headache or headache with altered characteristics one week prior to stroke was found to be significantly more prevalent in ischemic stroke patients than controls. History of atrial fibrillation and attacks of arrhythmia during the 7 days prior to stroke was significantly associated with a sentinel headache.

Migraine with aura is associated with increased risk of stroke in young adults, women, and headache at onset of stroke and independent of vascular risk factors (144, 148–151). The risk of stroke may be in part related to the increased prevalence of PFO and paradoxical embolism. To determine if the PFO is incidental or related to the etiology of the stroke, the ROPE (Risk of Paradoxical Embolism) score (152) is used to estimate the likelihood that a PFO is causally related to a stroke and to furthermore guide management in the consideration of PFO closure to prevent stroke recurrence. In addition to paradoxical embolism from PFO, migraine with aura has also been shown to be strongly associated with atrial fibrillation (148). In a study on young adults with migraine with aura and history of ischemic stroke, atrial fibrillation and cervical artery dissection were the second leading cause of stroke behind a PFO (150).

Cervical artery dissection is a major cause of stroke in young adults and can cause sudden unilateral, ipsilateral headaches that may precede neurologic deficits (153). Ischemia from embolism from carotid dissection or cardioembolism can trigger cortical spreading depression and produce visual or sensory symptoms identical to migraine aura (143). Additionally, when thinking about embolic stroke, endocarditis is an important consideration, especially in young patients with unexplained fevers. Although headache as the sole neurologic complaint in endocarditis is rare, multiple case reports describe presentation of severe headache and late discovery of ischemic stroke from septic emboli and mycotic aneurysms from endocarditis (154, 155).

Ms. C underwent stat CT head imaging which demonstrated a large hemorrhagic stroke with subarachnoid hemorrhage, mass effect, and hydrocephalus. Further work up demonstrated a posterior fossa aneurysm within an AV malformation which was thought to be the cause of her stroke, conceivably secondary to hypertension.

SUMMARY

- Of prevalent types of cerebrovascular accidents, hemorrhagic strokes are most associated with headaches. However, ischemic strokes that are large, cortical, or involve the posterior circulation may also cause headache.
- Stroke is the one of the most morbid and feared outcomes of an acute headache and may be a catastrophic representation of failure of the blood vessel integrity.

CONCLUSIONS

Many questions regarding potential vascular mechanisms arise when confronted by a cardiovascular patient with a headache. First, is the headache acute and catastrophic, such as seen in intracranial hemorrhage or malignant hypertension? Or is the headache an inflammatory emergency, such as a patient with giant cell arteritis or growing mycotic aneurysm? In chronic headache, is the headache migrainous, or perhaps triggered by elevated blood pressure? Is it related to a patent foramen ovale or a new vasodilating medication? Critical vasomotor and pain mechanisms are yet to be elucidated. As noted by the case discussions, the interaction of cardiovascular disease and headache is an evolving story which includes the blood vessel and a thoughtful diagnostician.

REFERENCES

1. Ferrari A, Spaccapelo L, Gallesi D, Sternieri E. Focus on headache as an adverse reaction to drugs. *J Headache Pain.* 2009 Aug;*10*(4):235–9.
2. Ferrari A. Headache: one of the most common and troublesome adverse reactions to drugs. *Curr Drug Saf.* 2006 Jan;*1*(1):43–58.
3. White TJ, Arakelian A, Rho JP. Counting the costs of drug-related adverse events. *Pharmacoeconomics.* 1999 May;*15*(5):445–58.
4. Thadani U, Rodgers T. Side effects of using nitrates to treat angina. *Expert Opin Drug Saf.* 2006 Sep;*5*(5):667–74.
5. Tfelt-Hansen PC, Tfelt-Hansen J. Nitroglycerin headache and nitroglycerin-induced primary headaches from 1846 and onwards: a historical overview and an update. *Headache.* 2009 Mar;*49*(3):445–56.
6. Gupta S, Nahas SJ, Peterlin BL. Chemical mediators of migraine: preclinical and clinical observations. *Headache.* 2011 Jun;*51*(6):1029–45.
7. Bagdy G, Riba P, Kecskeméti V, Chase D, Juhász G. Headache-type adverse effects of NO donors: vasodilation and beyond. *Br J Pharmacol.* 2010 May;*160*(1):20–35.
8. Ashina M, Bendtsen L, Jensen R, Olesen J. Nitric oxide-induced headache in patients with chronic tension-type headache. *Brain.* 2000 Sep;*123* (Pt 9):1830–7.
9. Karsan N, Bose PR, Thompson C, Newman J, Goadsby PJ. Headache and non-headache symptoms provoked by nitroglycerin in migraineurs: A human pharmacological triggering study. *Cephalalgia.* 2020 Jul;*40*(8):828–841.
10. Young WB. Drug-induced headache. *Neurol Clin.* 2004 Feb;*22*(1):173–84.
11. The International Classification of Headache Disorders - ICHD-3. ICHD. (2023, February 24).
12. Hsi DH, Roshandel A, Singh N, Szombathy T, Meszaros ZS. Headache response to glyceryl trinitrate in patients with and without obstructive coronary artery disease. *Heart.* 2005 Sep;*91*(9):1164–6.
13. Askmark H, Lundberg PO, Olsson S. Drug-related headache. *Headache.* 1989 Jul;*29*(7):441–4.
14. Cohn JN, McInnes GT, Shepherd AM. Direct-acting vasodilators. *J Clin Hypertens (Greenwich).* 2011 Sep;*13*(9):690–2.
15. Jamieson DG. The safety of triptans in the treatment of patients with migraine. *Am J Med.* 2002 Feb 1;*112*(2):135–40.
16. Kalkman DN, Couturier EGM, El Bouziani A, Dahdal J, Neefs J, Woudstra J, Vogel B, Trabattoni D, MaassenVanDenBrink A, Mehran R, de Winter RJ, Appelman Y. Migraine and cardiovascular disease: what cardiologists should know. *Eur Heart J.* 2023 Aug 7;*44*(30):2815–2828.
17. Schoonman GG, van der Grond J, Kortmann C, van der Geest RJ, Terwindt GM, Ferrari MD. Migraine headache is not associated with cerebral or meningeal vasodilatation–a 3T magnetic resonance angiography study. *Brain.* 2008 Aug;*131*(Pt 8):2192–200.
18. Cleophas TJ, Niemeyer MG, van Der Wall EE. Nitrate-Induced Headache in Patients with Stable Angina Pectoris: Beneficial Effect of Starting on a Low Dosage. *Am J Ther.* 1996 Dec;*3*(12):802–806.
19. Abrams BM. Medication overuse headaches. *Med Clin North Am.* 2013 Mar;*97*(2):337–52. doi: 10.1016/j.mcna.2012.12.007. Epub 2013 Jan 5.
20. Diener HC, Limmroth V. Medication-overuse headache: a worldwide problem. *Lancet Neurol.* 2004 Aug;*3*(8):475–83.
21. Lopez JI, Holdridge A, Chalela J. Headache and vasculitis. *Curr Pain Headache Rep.* 2013;*17*:1–6.
22. Nahas SJ. Headache and temporal arteritis: when to suspect and how to manage. *Curr Pain Headache Rep.* 2012;*16*:371–378.
23. Wurmann P, Karsulovic C, Sabugo F, Hernandez C, Zamorano Soto P, Mac-Namara M. Cranial versus Extracranial Involvement in Giant Cell Arteritis: 15 Years Retrospective Cohort Analysis. *Open Access Rheumatol Res Rev.* Published online 2022:97–101.

24. Lensen KD, Voskuyl AE, Comans EF, Van Der Laken CJ, Smulders YM. Extracranial giant cell arteritis: a narrative review. *Neth J Med.* 2016;*74*(5):182–192.
25. Ling ML, Yosar J, Lee BW, et al. The diagnosis and management of temporal arteritis. *Clin Exp Optom.* 2020;*103*(5):572–582.
26. Saldanha G, Hongo J, Plant G, Acheson J, Levy I, Anand P. Decreased CGRP, but preserved Trk A immunoreactivity in nerve fibres in inflamed human superficial temporal arteries. *J Neurol Neurosurg Psychiatry.* 1999;*66*(3):390–392. doi:10.1136/jnnp.66.3.390
27. Tokushige S ichi, Matsuura H, Hideyama T, Tamura K, Maekawa R, Shiio Y. Hypertrophic pachymeningitis as a potential cause of headache associated with temporal arteritis. *Intern Med.* 2016;*55*(5):523–526.
28. Younger DS. Headaches and vasculitis. *Neurol Clin.* 2014;*32*(2):321–362.
29. Kutty RK, Maekawa M, Kawase T, Fujii N, Kato Y. Temporal arteritis with focal pachymeningitis: a deceptive association. *Nagoya J Med Sci.* 2020;*82*(1):143.
30. Karthik SN, Bhanu K, Velayutham S, Jawahar M. Hypertrophic pachymeningitis. *Ann Indian Acad Neurol.* 2011;*14*(3):203.
31. Karassa FB, Matsagas MI, Schmidt WA, Ioannidis JP. Meta-analysis: test performance of ultrasonography for giant-cell arteritis. *Ann Intern Med.* 2005;*142*(5):359–369.
32. Arida A, Kyprianou M, Kanakis M, Sfikakis PP. The diagnostic value of ultrasonography-derived edema of the temporal artery wall in giant cell arteritis: a second meta-analysis. *BMC Musculoskelet Disord.* 2010;*11*:1–8.
33. Duftner C, Dejaco C, Sepriano A, Falzon L, Schmidt WA, Ramiro S. Imaging in diagnosis, outcome prediction and monitoring of large vessel vasculitis: a systematic literature review and meta-analysis informing the EULAR recommendations. *RMD Open.* 2018;*4*(1):e000612.
34. Winkler A, True D. Giant cell arteritis: 2018 review. *Mo Med.* 2018;*115*(5):468.
35. Rubenstein E, Maldini C, Gonzalez-Chiappe S, Chevret S, Mahr A. Sensitivity of temporal artery biopsy in the diagnosis of giant cell arteritis: a systematic literature review and meta-analysis. *Rheumatology.* 2020;*59*(5):1011–1020.
36. Finelli PF. Biopsy negative giant cell arteritis–Revised diagnostic criteria: Giant cell arteritis diagnostic criteria. *J Stroke Cerebrovasc Dis.* 2022;*31*(10):106660.
37. Stone JH, Tuckwell K, Dimonaco S, et al. Trial of tocilizumab in giant-cell arteritis. *N Engl J Med.* 2017;*377*(4):317–328.
38. Mahr AD, Jover JA, Spiera RF, et al. Adjunctive methotrexate for treatment of giant cell arteritis: an individual patient data meta-analysis. *Arthritis Rheum.* 2007;*56*(8):2789–2797.
39. Proven A, Gabriel SE, Orces C, O'Fallon WM, Hunder GG. Glucocorticoid therapy in giant cell arteritis: duration and adverse outcomes. *Arthritis Care Res Off J Am Coll Rheumatol.* 2003;*49*(5):703–708.
40. Touzé E, Southerland AM, Boulanger M, et al. Fibromuscular dysplasia and its neurologic manifestations: a systematic review. *JAMA Neurol.* 2019;*76*(2):217–226.
41. Kesav P, Manesh Raj D, John S. Cerebrovascular Fibromuscular Dysplasia–A Practical Review. *Vasc Health Risk Manag.* Published online 2023:543–556.
42. Sarti C, Picchioni A, Telese R, et al. "When should primary angiitis of the central nervous system (PACNS) be suspected?": literature review and proposal of a preliminary screening algorithm. *Neurol Sci.* 2020;*41*:3135–3148.
43. Byram K, Hajj-Ali RA, Calabrese L. CNS vasculitis: an approach to differential diagnosis and management. *Curr Rheumatol Rep.* 2018;*20*:1–7.
44. Kraemer M, Berlit P. Primary central nervous system vasculitis–An update on diagnosis, differential diagnosis and treatment. *J Neurol Sci.* 2021;*424*:117422.
45. Burton TM, Bushnell CD. Reversible cerebral vasoconstriction syndrome: A diagnostic imaging review. *Stroke.* 2019;*50*(8):2253–2258.
46. Perillo T, Paolella C, Perrotta G, Serino A, Caranci F, Manto A. Reversible cerebral vasoconstriction syndrome: Review of neuroimaging findings. *Radiol Med (Torino).* 2022;*127*(9):981–990.
47. Ducros A. Reversible cerebral vasoconstriction syndrome. *Lancet Neurol.* 2012;*11*(10):906–917.
48. Cappelen-Smith C, Calic Z, Cordato D. Reversible cerebral vasoconstriction syndrome: recognition and treatment. *Curr Treat Options Neurol.* 2017;*19*:1–15.
49. Chen SP, Wang SJ. Pathophysiology of reversible cerebral vasoconstriction syndrome. *J Biomed Sci.* 2022;*29*(1):1–13.
50. Song TJ, Lee KH, Li H, et al. Reversible cerebral vasoconstriction syndrome: a comprehensive systematic review. Published online 2021.

51. Ashina M, Katsarava Z, Do TP, Buse DC, Pozo-Rosich P, Özge A, Krymchantowski AV, Lebedeva ER, Ravishankar K, Yu S, Sacco S, Ashina S, Younis S, Steiner TJ, Lipton RB. Migraine: epidemiology and systems of care. *Lancet*. 2021 Apr 17;*397*(10283):1485–1495.

52. Elgendy IY, Nadeau SE, Bairey Merz CN, Pepine CJ; American College of Cardiology Cardiovascular Disease in Women Committee; American College of Cardiology Cardiovascular Disease in Women Committee. Migraine Headache: An Under-Appreciated Risk Factor for Cardiovascular Disease in Women. *J Am Heart Assoc*. 2019 Nov 19;*8*(22):e014546.

53. VanderPluym J, Hoffman-Snyder C, Khoury J, Goodman, B. Migraine in Postural Orthostatic Tachycardia Syndrome (POTS). *Neurology Apr* 2018, *90* (15 Supplement) P3.126.

54. Bigal ME, Kurth T, Santanello N, Buse D, Golden W, Robbins M, Lipton RB. Migraine and cardiovascular disease: a population-based study. *Neurology*. 2010 Feb 23;*74*(8):628–35. doi: 10.1212/WNL.0b013e3181d0cc8b. Epub 2010 Feb 10.

55. Kalkman DN, Couturier EGM, El Bouziani A, Dahdal J, Neefs J, Woudstra J, Vogel B, Trabattoni D, MaassenVanDenBrink A, Mehran R, de Winter RJ, Appelman Y. Migraine and cardiovascular disease: what cardiologists should know. *Eur Heart J*. 2023 Aug 7;*44*(30):2815–2828.

56. Vargas BB, Dodick DW, Wingerchuk DM, Demaerschalk BM. Migraine with and without aura and risk for cardiovascular disease. *Curr Atheroscler Rep*. 2008 Oct;*10*(5):427–33.

57. Goadsby PJ, Edvinsson L, Ekman R. Release of vasoactive peptides in the extracerebral circulation of humans and the cat during activation of the trigeminovascular system. *Ann Neurol*. 1988 Feb;*23*(2):193–6.

58. Charles A, Pozo-Rosich P. Targeting calcitonin gene-related peptide: a new era in migraine therapy. *Lancet*. 2019 Nov 9;*394*(10210):1765–1774.

59. Mueller BR, Robinson-Papp J. Postural orthostatic tachycardia syndrome and migraine: A narrative review. *Headache*. 2022 Jul;*62*(7):792–800.

60. Jamieson DG. The safety of triptans in the treatment of patients with migraine. *Am J Med*. 2002 Feb 1;*112*(2):135–40.

61. Buettner C, Nir RR, Bertisch SM, Bernstein C, Schain A, Mittleman MA, Burstein R. Simvastatin and vitamin D for migraine prevention: A randomized, controlled trial. *Ann Neurol*. 2015 Dec;*78*(6):970–81.

62. MaassenVanDenBrink A, Meijer J, Villalón CM, Ferrari MD. Wiping Out CGRP: Potential Cardiovascular Risks. *Trends Pharmacol Sci*. 2016 Sep;*37*(9):779–788.

63. Favoni, V, Giani, L, Al-Hassany, L et al. CGRP and migraine from a cardiovascular point of view: what do we expect from blocking CGRP?. *J Headache Pain* 2019:*20*:27.

64. Anzola GP, Magoni M, Guindani M, Rozzini L, Dalla Volta G. Potential source of cerebral embolism in migraine with aura: a transcranial Doppler study. *Neurology*. 1999 May 12;*52*(8):1622–5.

65. Del Sette M, Angeli S, Leandri M, Ferriero G, Bruzzone GL, Finocchi C, Gandolfo C. Migraine with aura and right-to-left shunt on transcranial Doppler: a case-control study. *Cerebrovasc Dis*. 1998 Nov-Dec;*8*(6):327–30

66. Koppen H, Palm-Meinders IH, Mess WH, Keunen RW, Terwindt GM, Launer LJ, van Buchem MA, Kruit MC, Ferrari MD. Systemic right-to-left shunts, ischemic brain lesions, and persistent migraine activity. *Neurology*. 2016 May 3;*86*(18):1668–75.

67. Wilmshurst P, Nightingale S. Relationship between migraine and cardiac and pulmonary right-to-left shunts. *Clin Sci (Lond)*. 2001 Feb;*100*(2):215–20.

68. Kumar, Preetham, Kijima, Yasufumi, West, Brian H., Tobis, Jonathan M., The Connection Between Patent Foramen Ovale and Migraine, *Neuroimaging Clinics of North America*, 2019:*29*(2):261–270.

69. Tobis MJ, Azarbal B. Does patent foramen ovale promote cryptogenic stroke and migraine headache? *Tex Heart Inst J*. 2005;*32*(3):362–5.

70. Carroll, JD, Saver, JL, Thaler, DE, Smalling, R.W., Berry, S, MacDonald, LA, Marks, DS, & Tirschwell, DL. Closure of Patent Foramen Ovale versus Medical Therapy after Cryptogenic Stroke. *New England Journal of Medicine*, 2013:*368*(12):1092–1100.

71. Langholz D, Louie EK, Konstadt SN, Rao TL, Scanlon PJ. Transesophageal echocardiographic demonstration of distinct mechanisms for right to left shunting across a patent foramen ovale in the absence of pulmonary hypertension. *J Am Coll Cardiol*. 1991 Oct;*18*(4):1112–7.

72. Katsanos AH, Psaltopoulou T, Sergentanis TN, Frogoudaki A, Vrettou AR, Ikonomidis I, Paraskevaidis I, Parissis J, Bogiatzi C, Zompola C, Ellul J, Triantafyllou N, Voumvourakis K, Kyritsis AP, Giannopoulos S, Alexandrov AW, Alexandrov AV, Tsivgoulis G. Transcranial Doppler versus transthoracic echocardiography for the detection of patent foramen ovale in patients with cryptogenic cerebral ischemia: A systematic review and diagnostic test accuracy meta-analysis. *Ann Neurol*. 2016 Apr;*79*(4):625–35.

73. Mayerhofer E, Kanz D, Guschlbauer B, Anderson CD, Asmussen A, Grundmann S, Strecker C, Harloff A. Bubble Test and Carotid Ultrasound to Guide Indication of Transesophageal Echocardiography in Young Patients With Stroke. *Front Neurol.* 2022 Mar 4;*13*:836609.

74. Daniëls C, Weytjens C, Cosyns B, Schoors D, De Sutter J, Paelinck B, Muyldermans L, Van Camp G. Second harmonic transthoracic echocardiography: the new reference screening method for the detection of patent foramen ovale. *Eur J Echocardiogr.* 2004 Dec;*5*(6):449–52.

75. Pinto FJ. When and how to diagnose patent foramen ovale. *Heart.* 2005 Apr;*91*(4):438–40.

76. Sloan MA, Alexandrov AV, Tegeler CH, Spencer MP, Caplan LR, Feldmann E, Wechsler LR, Newell DW, Gomez CR, Babikian VL, Lefkowitz D, Goldman RS, Armon C, Hsu CY, Goodin DS; Therapeutics and Technology Assessment Subcommittee of the American Academy of Neurology. Assessment: transcranial Doppler ultrasonography: report of the Therapeutics and Technology Assessment Subcommittee of the American Academy of Neurology. *Neurology.* 2004 May 11;*62*(9):1468–81.

77. Truong, T, Slavin, L, Kashani, R, Higgins, J, Puri, A, Chowdhry, M, Cheung, P, Tanious, A, Child, JS, Perloff, JK, & Tobis, JM Prevalence of Migraine Headaches in Patients With Congenital Heart Disease. *The American Journal of Cardiology.* 2008; *101*(3), 396–400.

78. Volman, M, Mojadidi, MK, Gevorgyan, R, Kaing, A, Agrawal, H, & Tobis, J. Incidence of patent foramen ovale and migraine headache in adults with congenital heart disease with no known cardiac shunts. *Catheterization and Cardiovascular Interventions.* 2021; *81*(4), 643–647.

79. Post MC, van Gent MW, Plokker HW, Westermann CJ, Kelder JC, Mager JJ, Overtoom TT, Schonewille WJ, Thijs V, Snijder RJ. Pulmonary arteriovenous malformations associated with migraine with aura. *Eur Respir J.* 2009 Oct;*34*(4):882–7.

80. van Gent MW, Mager JJ, Snijder RJ, Westermann CJ, Plokker HW, Schonewille WJ, Thijs V, Post MC. Relation between migraine and size of echocardiographic intrapulmonary right-to-left shunt. *Am J Cardiol.* 2011 May 1;*107*(9):1399–404.

81. Post MC, Thijs V, Schonewille WJ, Budts W, Snijder RJ, Plokker HW, Westermann CJ. Embolization of pulmonary arteriovenous malformations and decrease in prevalence of migraine. *Neurology.* 2006 Jan 24;*66*(2):202–5

82. Deen M, Christensen CE, Hougaard A, Hansen HD, Knudsen GM, Ashina M. Serotonergic mechanisms in the migraine brain - a systematic review. *Cephalalgia.* 2017 Mar;*37*(3):251–264.

83. Gupta, S, Nahas, SJ, & B Matija Peterlin. Chemical Mediators of Migraine: Preclinical and Clinical Observations. *Headache.* 2011; *51*(6), 1029–1045.

84. Hanington E. Migraine: the platelet hypothesis after 10 years. Biomed Pharmacother. 1989;*43*(10):719–26.

85. Supornsilpchai W, Sanguanrangsirikul S, Maneesri S, Srikiatkhachorn A. Serotonin depletion, cortical spreading depression, and trigeminal nociception. *Headache.* 2006 Jan;*46*(1):34–9.

86. Borgdorff P, Tangelder GJ. Migraine: possible role of shear-induced platelet aggregation with serotonin release. *Headache.* 2012 Sep;*52*(8):1298–318.

87. Trabattoni D, Brambilla M, Canzano P, Becchetti A, Teruzzi G, Porro B, Fiorelli S, Muratori M, Tedesco CC, Veglia F, Montorsi P, Bartorelli AL, Tremoli E, Camera M. Migraine in Patients Undergoing PFO Closure: Characterization of a Platelet-Associated Pathophysiological Mechanism: The LEARNER Study. *JACC Basic Transl Sci.* 2022 Apr 13;*7*(6):525–540.

88. Bianca Biglione, Alexander Gitin, Philip B. Gorelick, Charles Hennekens. Aspirin in the Treatment and Prevention of Migraine Headaches: Possible Additional Clinical Options for Primary Healthcare Providers. *The American Journal of Medicine.* 2020;*133*(4):412–416.

89. Sommer, RJ, Nazif, T, Privitera, L, & Robbins, BT. Retrospective review of thienopyridine therapy in migraineurs with patent foramen ovale. *Neurology.* 2018; *91*(22), 1002–1009.

90. Rodés-Cabau J, Horlick E, Ibrahim R, Cheema AN, Labinaz M, Nadeem N, Osten M, Côté M, Marsal JR, Rivest D, Marrero A, Houde C. Effect of Clopidogrel and Aspirin vs Aspirin Alone on Migraine Headaches After Transcatheter Atrial Septal Defect Closure: The CANOA Randomized Clinical Trial. *JAMA.* 2015 Nov 24;*314*(20):2147–54.

91. Caputi, L, Usai, S, Maria Vincenza Carriero, Licia Grazzi, Domenico D'Amico, Falcone, C, Gian Paolo Anzola, Massimo Del Sette, Parati, E, & Bussone, G. Microembolic Air Load During Contrast-Transcranial Doppler: A Trigger for Migraine With Aura? *Headache.* 2010; *50*(8), 1320–1327.

92. Nozari, A, Dilekoz, E, Sukhotinsky, I, Stein, T, Eikermann-Haerter, K, Liu, C, Wang, Y, Frosch, MP, Waeber, C, Ayata, C, & Moskowitz, MA. Microemboli may link spreading depression, migraine aura, and patent foramen ovale. *Annals of Neurology.* 2010; *67*(2), 221–229.

93. Jesurum, JT, Fuller, CJ, Kim, CJ, Krabill, KA, Spencer, MP, Olsen, JV, Likosky, W, & Reisman, M. Frequency of Migraine Headache Relief Following Patent Foramen Ovale "Closure" Despite Residual Right-to-Left Shunt. *American Journal of Cardiology.* 2008; *102*(7), 916–920.

94. Mojadidi, MK, Kumar, P, Mahmoud, AN, Elgendy, IY, Shapiro, H, West, B, Charles, A, Mattle, H, Sorensen, SG, Meier, B, Silberstein, SD, & Tobis, JM. Pooled Analysis of PFO Occluder Device Trials in Patients With PFO and Migraine. *Journal of the American College of Cardiology.* 2021; *77*(6), 667–676.

95. Mojadidi MK, Khessali H, Gevorgyan R, Levinson RD, Tobis JM. Visual migraine aura with or without headache: association with right to left shunt and assessment following transcutaneous closure. *Clin Ophthalmol.* 2012; 6:1099–105.

96. Dowson, A, Mullen, MJ, Peatfield, R, Muir, K, Khan, AA, Wells, C, Lipscombe, SL, Rees, T, De Giovanni, JV, Morrison, WL, Hildick-Smith, D, Elrington, G, Hillis, WS, Malik, IS, & Rickards, A. Migraine Intervention With STARFlex Technology (MIST) trial: a prospective, multicenter, double-blind, sham-controlled trial to evaluate the effectiveness of patent foramen ovale closure with STARFlex septal repair implant to resolve refractory migraine headache. *Circulation.* 2008; *117*(11), 1397–1404.

97. Mattle HP, Evers S, Hildick-Smith D, Becker WJ, Baumgartner H, Chataway J, Gawel M, Göbel H, Heinze A, Horlick E, Malik I, Ray S, Zermansky A, Findling O, Windecker S, Meier B. Percutaneous closure of patent foramen ovale in migraine with aura, a randomized controlled trial. *Eur Heart J.* 2016 Jul 7;*37*(26):2029–36.

98. Tobis JM, Charles A, Silberstein SD, Sorensen S, Maini B, Horwitz PA, Gurley JC. Percutaneous Closure of Patent Foramen Ovale in Patients With Migraine: The PREMIUM Trial. *J Am Coll Cardiol.* 2017 Dec 5;*70*(22):2766–2774.

99. Wang YF, Wang SJ. Hypertension and migraine: Time to revisit the evidence. *Curr Pain Headache Rep.* 2021;*25*:1–9.

100. Zhang J, Mao Y, Li Y, et al. Association between migraine or severe headache and hypertension among US adults: A cross-sectional study. *Nutr Metab Cardiovasc Dis.* 2023;*33*(2):350–358.

101. Finocchi C, Sassos D. Headache and arterial hypertension. *Neurol Sci.* 2017;*38*:67–72.

102. Taylor DA. Hypertensive Crisis: A Review of Pathophysiology and Treatment. *Crit Care Nurs Clin North Am.* 2015;*27*(4):439–447.

103. Donnelly J, Aries MJ, Czosnyka M. Further understanding of cerebral autoregulation at the bedside: possible implications for future therapy. *Expert Rev Neurother.* 2015;*15*(2):169–185.

104. González-Quintanilla V, Madera J, Pascual J. Update on headaches associated with physical exertion. *Cephalalgia.* 2023 Mar;*43*(3):3331024221146989.

105. Muiesan ML, Padovani A, Salvetti M, et al. Headache: Prevalence and relationship with office or ambulatory blood pressure in a general population sample (the Vobarno Study). *Blood Press.* 2006;*15*(1):14–19.

106. Fuchs FD, Gus M, Moreira LB, Moreira WD, Goncalves SC, Nunes G. Headache is not more frequent among patients with moderate to severe hypertension. *J Hum Hypertens.* 2003;*17*(11):787–790.

107. Manandhar K, Risal A, Koju R, Linde M, Steiner TJ. If headache has any association with hypertension, it is negative. Evidence from a population-based study in Nepal. *Cephalalgia.* 2021;*41*(13):1310–1317.

108. Tronvik E, Stovner LJ, Hagen K, Holmen J, Zwart JA. High pulse pressure protects against headache: prospective and cross-sectional data (HUNT study). *Neurology.* 2008;*70*(16):1329–1336.

109. Hagen K, Zwart JA, Holmen J, Svebak S, Bovim G, Stovner LJ. Does hypertension protect against chronic musculoskeletal complaints?: The nord-trøndelag health study. *Arch Intern Med.* 2005;*165*(8):916–922.

110. Fagernaes CF, Heuch I, Zwart JA, Winsvold BS, Linde M, Hagen K. Blood pressure as a risk factor for headache and migraine: A prospective population-based study. *Eur J Neurol.* 2015;*22*(1):156–e11.

111. Virtanen R, Jula A, Huikuri H, et al. Increased pulse pressure is associated with reduced baroreflex sensitivity. *J Hum Hypertens.* 2004;*18*(4):247–252.

112. Cotta Ramusino M, Perini G, Capelli M, et al. Potential Contribution of Hypertension to Evolution of Chronic Migraine and Related Mechanisms. *J Oral Facial Pain Headache.* 2022;*36*.

113. Prudenzano MP, Monetti C, Merico L, et al. The comorbidity of migraine and hypertension. A study in a tertiary care headache centre. *J Headache Pain.* 2005;*6*:220–222.

114. Gudmundsson LS, Thorgeirsson G, Sigfússon N, Sigvaldason H, Jóhannsson M. Migraine patients have lower systolic but higher diastolic blood pressure compared with controls in a population-based study of 21 537 subjects. The Reykjavik Study. *Cephalalgia.* 2006;*26*(4):436–444.

115. Agostoni E, Aliprandi A. Migraine and hypertension. *Neurol Sci.* 2008;*29*:37–39.

116. Cirillo M, Stellato D, Lombardi C, De Santo NG, Covelli V. Headache and cardiovascular risk factors: positive association with hypertension. *Headache J Head Face Pain.* 1999;*39*(6):409–416.

117. Diener HC. The risks or lack thereof of migraine treatments in vascular disease. *Headache J Head Face Pain.* 2020;*60*(3):649–653.

118. Mancia G, Rosei EA, Ambrosioni E, et al. Hypertension and migraine comorbidity: prevalence and risk of cerebrovascular events: evidence from a large, multicenter, cross-sectional survey in Italy (MIRACLES study). *J Hypertens.* 2011;*29*(2):309–318.

119. Bigal ME, Kurth T, Santanello N, et al. Migraine and cardiovascular disease: a population-based study. *Neurology.* 2010;*74*(8):628–635.

120. Entonen AH, Suominen SB, Korkeila K, et al. Migraine predicts hypertension—a cohort study of the Finnish working-age population. *Eur J Public Health.* 2014;*24*(2):244–248.

121. Olesen J. The role of nitric oxide (NO) in migraine, tension-type headache and cluster headache. *Pharmacol Ther.* 2008;*120*(2):157–171.

122. Hermann M, Flammer A, Lüscher TF. Nitric oxide in hypertension. *J Clin Hypertens.* 2006;*8*:17–29.

123. Gevirtz R. The Role of the Autonomic Nervous System in Headache: Biomarkers and Treatment. *Curr Pain Headache Rep.* 2022;*26*(10):767–774.

124. Rauschel V, Straube A, Süß F, Ruscheweyh R. Responsiveness of the autonomic nervous system during paced breathing and mental stress in migraine patients. *J Headache Pain.* 2015;*16*:1–10.

125. Schrader H, Stovner LJ, Helde G, Sand T, Bovim G. Prophylactic treatment of migraine with angiotensin converting enzyme inhibitor (lisinopril): randomised, placebo controlled, crossover study. *BMJ.* 2001;*322*(7277):19.

126. Disco C, Maggioni F, Zanchin G. Angiotensin II receptor blockers: a new possible treatment for chronic migraine? *Neurol Sci.* 2015;*36*:1483–1485.

127. Paterna S, Di Pasquale P, D'Angelo A, et al. Angiotensin-converting enzyme gene deletion polymorphism determines an increase in frequency of migraine attacks in patients suffering from migraine without aura. *Eur Neurol.* 2000;*43*(3):133–136.

128. Wiehe M, Fuchs SC, Moreira LB, Moraes RS, Fuchs FD. Migraine is more frequent in individuals with optimal and normal blood pressure: a population-based study. *J Hypertens.* 2002;*20*(7):1303–1306.

129. Tzourio C, Gagniere B, El Amrani M, Alperovitch A, Bousser MG. Relationship between migraine, blood pressure and carotid thickness. A population-based study in the elderly. *Cephalalgia.* 2003;*23*(9):914–920.

130. GBD 2016 Neurology Collaborators. Global, regional, and national burden of neurological disorders, 1990–2016: a systematic analysis for the Global Burden of Disease Study 2016. *Lancet Neurol.* 2019 May;*18*(5):459–480.

131. Gorelick PB, Hier DB, Caplan LR, Langenberg P. Headache in acute cerebrovascular disease. *Neurology.* 1986;*36*(11):1445–1450. doi:10.1212/wnl.36.11.1445

132. Petridis AK, Kamp MA, Cornelius JF, et al. Aneurysmal subarachnoid hemorrhage: diagnosis and treatment. *Dtsch Ärztebl Int.* 2017;*114*(13):226.

133. Xu L, Wang W, Lai N, Tong J, Wang G, Tang D. Association between pro-inflammatory cytokines in cerebrospinal fluid and headache in patients with aneurysmal subarachnoid hemorrhage. *J Neuroimmunol.* 2022;*366*:577841.

134. Muroi C, Bellut D, Coluccia D, Mink S, Fujioka M, Keller E. Systemic interleukin-6 concentrations in patients with perimesencephalic non-aneurysmal subarachnoid hemorrhage. *J Clin Neurosci.* 2011 Dec; *18*(12):1626–9.

135. Yamada SM, Tomita Y, Murakami H, et al. Headache in patients with chronic subdural hematoma: analysis in 1080 patients. *Neurosurg Rev.* 2018;*41*(2):549–556. doi:10.1007/s10143-017-0889-x

136. Gao X, Cai X, Yang Y, Zhou Y, Zhu W. Diagnostic Accuracy of the HAS-BLED Bleeding Score in VKA- or DOAC-Treated Patients With Atrial Fibrillation: A Systematic Review and Meta-Analysis. *Front Cardiovasc Med.* 2021;*8*:757087. Published 2021 Nov 22.

137. Apostolakis S, Lane DA, Guo Y, Buller H, Lip GY. Performance of the HEMORR(2)HAGES, ATRIA, and HAS-BLED bleeding risk-prediction scores in patients with atrial fibrillation undergoing anticoagulation: the AMADEUS (evaluating the use of SR34006 compared to warfarin or acenocoumarol in patients with atrial fibrillation) study. *J Am Coll Cardiol.* 2012;*60*(9):861–867.

138. Montalto C, Ferlini M, Casula M, et al. DAPT Score to Stratify Ischemic and Bleeding Risk after Percutaneous Coronary Intervention: An Updated Systematic Review, Meta-Analysis, and Meta-Regression of 100,211 Patients. *Thromb Haemost.* 2021;*121*(5):687–689.

139. Wang C, Yu Y, Zhu W, Yu J, Lip GYH, Hong K. Comparing the ORBIT and HAS-BLED bleeding risk scores in anticoagulated atrial fibrillation patients: a systematic review and meta-analysis. *Oncotarget.* 2017;*8*(65):109703–109711. Published 2017 Aug 3.

140. Doufekias E, Segal AZ, Kizer JR. Cardiogenic and aortogenic brain embolism. J Am Coll Cardiol. 2008 Mar 18;*51*(11):1049–59.

141. Tsao CW, Aday AW, Almarzooq ZI, Alonso A, Beaton AZ, Bittencourt MS, Boehme AK, Buxton AE, Carson AP, Commodore-Mensah Y, Elkind MSV, Evenson KR, Eze-Nliam C, Ferguson JF, Generoso G, Ho JE, Kalani R, Khan SS, Kissela BM, Knutson KL, Levine DA, Lewis TT, Liu J, Loop MS, Ma J, Mussolino ME, Navaneethan SD, Perak AM, Poudel R, Rezk-Hanna M, Roth GA, Schroeder EB, Shah SH, Thacker EL, VanWagner LB, Virani SS, Voecks JH, Wang NY, Yaffe K, Martin SS. Heart Disease and Stroke Statistics-2022 Update: A Report From the American Heart Association. *Circulation.* 2022 Feb 22;*145*(8):e153–e639.

142. Lu J, Liu W, Zhao H. Headache in cerebrovascular diseases. *Stroke Vasc Neurol.* 2020 Jun;*5*(2):205–210.

143. Oliveira FAA, Sampaio Rocha-Filho PA. Headaches Attributed to Ischemic Stroke and Transient Ischemic Attack. *Headache.* 2019 Mar;*59*(3):469–476.

144. Tentschert S, Wimmer R, Greisenegger S, Lang W, Lalouschek W. Headache at stroke onset in 2196 patients with ischemic stroke or transient ischemic attack. *Stroke.* 2005 Feb;*36*(2):e1–3.

145. Rothrock JF, Diener HC. Headache secondary to cerebrovascular disease. *Cephalalgia.* 2021 Apr;*41*(4):479–492.

146. Lebedeva ER, Ushenin AV, Gurary NM, Tsypushkina TS, Gilev DV, Kislyak NV, Olesen J. Headache at onset of first-ever ischemic stroke: Clinical characteristics and predictors. *Eur J Neurol.* 2021 Mar;*28*(3):852–860.

147. Lebedeva ER, Ushenin AV, Gurary NM, Gilev DV, Olesen J. Sentinel headache as a warning symptom of ischemic stroke. *J Headache Pain.* 2020 Jun 10;*21*(1):70.

148. Gollion C, Gazagnes J, Fabry V, Barbieux-Guillot M, Lerebours F, Larrue V. Atrial fibrillation and migraine with aura in young adults with ischemic stroke. *Cephalalgia.* 2021 Mar;*41*(3):375–382.

149. Martinez-Majander N, Artto V, Ylikotila P, von Sarnowski B, Waje-Andreassen U, Yesilot N, Zedde M, Huhtakangas J, Numminen H, Jäkälä P, Fonseca AC, Redfors P, Wermer MJH, Pezzini A, Putaala J; SECRETO Study Group. Association between Migraine and Cryptogenic Ischemic Stroke in Young Adults. *Ann Neurol.* 2021 Feb;*89*(2):242–253.

150. Spector JT, Kahn SR, Jones MR, Jayakumar M, Dalal D, Nazarian S. Migraine headache and ischemic stroke risk: an updated meta-analysis. *Am J Med.* 2010 Jul;*123*(7):612–24.

151. Tietjen GE, Maly EF. Migraine and Ischemic Stroke in Women. *A Narrative Review. Headache.* 2020 May;*60*(5):843–863.

152. Kent DM, Ruthazer R, Weimar C, Mas JL, Serena J, Homma S, Di Angelantonio E, Di Tullio MR, Lutz JS, Elkind MS, Griffith J, Jaigobin C, Mattle HP, Michel P, Mono ML, Nedeltchev K, Papetti F, Thaler DE. An index to identify stroke-related vs incidental patent foramen ovale in cryptogenic stroke. *Neurology.* 2013 Aug 13;*81*(7):619–25.

153. Keser Z, Chiang CC, Benson JC, Pezzini A, Lanzino G. Cervical Artery Dissections: Etiopathogenesis and Management. *Vasc Health Risk Manag.* 2022 Sep 2;*18*:685–700.

154. Pruitt AA, Rubin RH, Karchmer AW, Duncan GW. Neurologic complications of bacterial endocarditis. *Medicine (Baltimore).* 1978 Jul;*57*(4):329–43.

155. Cahill TJ, Prendergast BD. Infective endocarditis. *Lancet.* 2016 Feb 27;*387*(10021):882–93. doi: 10.1016/S0140-6736(15)00067-7. Epub 2015 Sep 1.

Headache and Dermatologic Conditions

6

Twan Sia and Anne Lynn S. Chang

LEARNING OBJECTIVES

1. Explore links between headache and links to inflammatory skin disease
2. Describe links between headache and neurocutaneous conditions
3. Identify headache and viral skin infections

INTRODUCTION

The relationship between headache and skin disorders, as two seemingly unrelated entities, is often under-appreciated, even though the nervous system and skin share ectodermal lineage during development. In reality, several conditions present with headache (and, more broadly, neurologic disease) and dermatologic manifestations. Considering the full constellation of signs and symptoms can better inform treatment for the patient.

This chapter covers several conditions that commonly present with headache and dermatologic signs, such as inflammatory conditions, neurocutaneous disorders, and viral infections. In these conditions, the appearance and characteristics of the dermatologic signs can aid in narrowing the differential diagnosis, as well as inform treatment options and possible systemic sequelae. We also review emerging evidence that links headache with common dermatologic conditions that were previously considered unrelated. Understanding the molecular underpinnings of these relationships can highlight therapeutics that may be beneficial in the treatment of headache and dermatologic conditions.

INFLAMMATORY SKIN DISEASES AND HEADACHE

Atopic Dermatitis

Atopic dermatitis is a common chronic inflammatory condition of the skin characterized by pruritus and rash. There are many notable similarities in the pathophysiology of migraine and atopy, such as a strong genetic element, involvement of vasoactive mediators, and certain exacerbating factors like stress or environmental elements. In several observational studies, atopic dermatitis and childhood migraine, as well as migraine in adults (Shreberk-Hassidim et al., 2017; Han et al., 2023; Fan et al., 2023; Medina and Diamond, 1976; Muñoz-Jareño et al., 2011; Aupiais et al., 2017) and headache in general were associated (Silverberg, 2016). Given the association of atopic dermatitis and migraine, it is unsurprising that other groups have also reported a positive relationship between migraine and asthma, as well as allergic rhinitis (Wei et al., 2018; Wang et al., 2017; Graif et al., 2018). As such, atopy in a pediatric patient presenting with paroxysmal headaches can support the diagnosis of migraine (Mortimer et al., 1993).

There is preliminary evidence suggesting that the presence of atopy may influence the phenotype of migraine. Atopy was more common in patients with migraine with aura than migraine without aura and tension-type headache. The atopy and migraine association was strongest in patients aged 11–14 years old (Özge et al., 2014). Less severe atopy in patients was associated with less frequent and less severe migraine in patients under age 45, while more severe atopy was associated with more frequent migraine (Martin et al., 2011).

Beyond observational studies, investigations into the link between atopy and migraine are sparse. A preliminary multicenter, double-blind, randomized, controlled trial of montelukast, a leukotriene receptor antagonist used in the treatment of asthma, has been investigated for migraine prevention. Though montelukast was well tolerated, it was not effective at reducing migraine frequency (Brandes et al., 2004). The precise molecular linkage between migraine and atopy/allergy remains elusive but may serve as a future target for migraine prevention in atopic patients. As a possible example, the histamine receptors have been noted to play roles in both atopy and migraine (Ohsawa and Hirasawa, 2014; Worm et al., 2019). Subcutaneous histamine has been investigated by one group in Mexico, finding promising migraine prevention activity. However, their results are not known to have been attempted to be replicated elsewhere (Millán-Guerrero et al., 2007; Millán-Guerrero et al., 2008; Millán-Guerrero et al., 2009). Cyproheptadine, a serotonin and histamine antagonist, was also found to be effective at preventing migraine by several groups (Okuma et al., 2013; Lewis et al., 2004; Eiland et al., 2007).

Rosacea

Rosacea is a chronic inflammatory disease of the face that presents with facial erythema, papules, pustules, flushing, telangiectasia, and ocular symptoms. Rosacea and migraine have been observed to be associated with each other since 1976, with recent analyses finding the co-occurrence of rosacea and migraine to be over 50% (Christensen et al., 2018; Weinholtz et al., 2022). The precise mechanism underlying this association is likely multifactorial, leading to several possible hypotheses. The leading hypothesis focuses on the vascular abnormalities in both conditions. Of note, several vasoactive neuropeptides (calcitonin gene-related peptide, CGRP; pituitary adenylate cyclase-activating peptide, PACAP; vasoactive intestinal peptide, VIP) and the transient receptor potential vanilloid-1 (TRPV1) receptor have been observed to be elevated in patients with rosacea and patients with migraine, suggesting that they may play a role in the shared pathogenesis (Pérez-Pereda et al., 2020; Meentz et al., 2010; Lonne-Rahm et al., 2004; Helfrich et al., 2015; Sulk et al., 2012). Other similarities in both diseases include that they are recurrent and have similar triggers, such as stress and alcohol (Alia and Feng, 2022; Marmura, 2018). Both diseases also show evidence of heritability (Anttila et al., 2018; Aldrich et al., 2015). These similarities may play a role in the co-occurrence of rosacea and migraine. Rosacea has been noted to co-occur with other neurological diseases, as reviewed by Holmes et al., 2018.

CGRP is a vasoactive neuropeptide that has been successfully targeted for both the preventive and acute treatment of migraine (Dodick, 2019). CGRP monoclonal antibodies have been shown to improve rosacea signs and symptoms in patients with rosacea and migraine in an exploratory, retrospective cohort study (Sia et al., in press). A CGRP monoclonal antibody is currently being investigated in a prospective open-label trial (NCT04419259). If found to be safe and effective, CGRP monoclonal antibodies may be a therapeutic choice for patients with rosacea and migraine. VIP, PACAP, and TRPV1 have also been hypothesized to be potential pharmacologic targets in the treatment of migraine but have yet to show efficacy (Al-Hassany et al., 2023).

Psoriasis

Psoriasis is a chronic immune-mediated skin disease that is characterized by erythematous patches with silver-white scales, primarily involving extensor surfaces. Psoriasis is associated with several conditions, with the most notable being psoriatic arthritis in approximately one-third of psoriasis patients. Other comorbidities include cardiometabolic, psychiatric, and inflammatory bowel diseases (Armstrong and Read, 2020).

Based on the observation that psoriasis and migraine share cardiovascular comorbidities, several groups investigated the possible correlation between psoriasis and migraine. Egeberg et al. reported the adjusted incidence rate ratio of new-onset migraine to be 1.37 (95% CI, 1.30–1.45) in mild psoriasis, 1.55 (95% CI, 1.29–1.86) in severe psoriasis, and 1.92 (95% CI, 1.65–2.22) in psoriatic arthritis (Egeberg et al., 2015). The observation that more severe psoriasis and psoriatic arthritis were strongly associated with migraine was later corroborated by Sarkhani et al. (2023). Galili et al. found an association between overall chronic headaches, intermediate-frequency migraine, low-frequency migraine, and nonmigraine headaches in patients with moderate-to-severe psoriasis (Galili et al., 2018). Taheri et al. also reported relatively high prevalence of migraine (20.8%) in psoriasis vulgaris patients (Taheri et al., 2021). Conversely, Capo et al. found a higher prevalence of migraine with aura and a higher average number of monthly migraine attacks in psoriasis patients versus healthy controls, suggesting more severe migraine in psoriasis patients (Capo et al., 2018). In contrast, Yang et al. investigated a variety of possible comorbidities in psoriasis patients, finding no significantly increased risk of migraine (Yang et al., 2011).

Besides the aforementioned work, there currently exists no literature studying the mechanism underlying the association of psoriasis and migraine. Neuroinflammatory mediators such as nerve growth factor, substance P (SP), and CGRP have been hypothesized to be possible culprits (Galili et al., 2018). Of note, SP and CGRP-positive nerve afferents were more abundant in psoriatic epidermis (Jiang et al., 1998). Future research may consider investigating whether anti-psoriatic agents may be beneficial in the treatment of migraine or vice versa. These investigations may also provide more insight into possibly implicated molecular pathways.

It should be noted that some treatments for psoriasis are associated with headaches as a common adverse effect, including efalizumab (Gaylor and Duvic, 2004) and secukinumab (Abrouk et al., 2017). In the case of aprelimast, headaches were associated with the discontinuation of apremilast (Ighani et al., 2018).

Other Inflammatory Skin Conditions and Migraine

Hidradenitis suppurativa (HS) is a chronic scarring condition of the intertriginous skin, commonly presenting with painful, inflamed nodules, abscesses, and sinus tracts. Inflammation in HS is not limited to the skin but is considered systemic, affecting several other organs. Patients with HS are at higher risk for metabolic syndrome, type 2 diabetes mellitus, and inflammatory bowel disease, among other conditions (Sabat et al., 2020). A preliminary study found that the prevalence of migraine was 12.6% in patients with HS. Though the authors did not compare to controls, the prevalence was similar to the prevalence of migraine in the general population, suggesting that HS and migraine may not be associated. However, interestingly, they also found that HS patients with migraine were more likely to have psoriasis than HS patients without migraine (Kluger et al., 2019). It is unclear if this association between migraine and psoriasis was strengthened in patients with HS or not. Given that migraine, psoriasis, and HS have similar cardiometabolic risk factors, there may be a possible association between the three conditions.

Sarcoidosis is a multisystemic disorder characterized by granulomatous inflammation, most commonly in the lungs, skin, eye, liver, and lymph nodes. Headache in patients with sarcoidosis is a common clinical manifestation of neurosarcoidosis, but in a preliminary study using a validated migraine instrument, migraine was found in 29% of patients with sarcoidosis versus 13% of healthy controls. Patients with neurosarcoidosis were not more likely to have migraine than patients without neurosarcoidosis (Gelfland et al., 2018).

NEUROCUTANEOUS SYNDROMES

Neurocutaneous syndromes are a group of rare congenital disorders impacting ectodermal and mesodermal development, resulting in various skin and nervous system manifestations. Given that neurocutaneous disorders are heterogenous, we seek to summarize the inheritance, pathology, and dermatologic and neurologic clinical manifestations (with particular attention to headache) for each disorder, bearing in mind that space limitations mean that some syndromes may not be discussed here.

Parry–Romberg Syndrome

Parry–Romberg syndrome (PRS) is characterized by progressive atrophy of the skin, subcutaneous, and fat tissues of the face. Though PRS commonly affects dermatomes of one or more branches of the trigeminal nerve, the characteristic atrophy has been reported to also sometimes progress to the arms, trunk, and legs. Atrophy in PRS usually begins in the first decade of life, progresses over 2 to 20 years, and then stabilizes. PRS is typically unilateral, while bilateral progressive atrophies have been suggested to be reclassified as Barraquer–Simons syndrome instead.

Common cutaneous manifestations of PRS include alopecia (band-like hair loss that may also involve the eyes and eyebrows), ipsilateral pigmentation changes on the face and neck, and thin, soft skin without sclerosis. Neurologic symptoms manifest in approximately 15%–20% of PRS patients. Neurologic symptoms can include pain (headache, facial pain, trigeminal neuralgia), epilepsy, cerebrovascular events, speech abnormalities, and movement disorders (muscle spasms, synkinesia, dystonia). Neuro-ophthalmologic (oculomotor and trochlear nerve palsy, Horner's syndrome, and optic neuropathy) and neuropsychiatric (hallucinations, cognitive disturbances) manifestations are also reported. Other extracutaneous symptoms of PRS include hypoplasia of facial bones, hypertrophic cardiomyopathy, and metabolic disorders.

A commonly associated condition with PRS is linear scleroderma *en coup de sabre*, which is a subtype of localized scleroderma to the face and skull with extracutaneous manifestations such as epilepsy, dementia, and other neurologic deficits. It is debated if the two are distinct entities or clinical subtypes of each other.

PRS is believed to be sporadic, but familial cases have been reported without a clear pattern of inheritance. To date, no specific genes have been linked to PRS. On the population level, PRS appears to be more common in females than males (3:1).

The precise etiology of PRS remains elusive and debated. One of the most accepted theories is that PRS is an autoimmune condition, given its overlap with linear scleroderma and its possible association with other autoimmune diseases, such as rheumatoid arthritis, inflammatory bowel disease, and vitiligo, among others. Other theories generally fall into the category of either neurologic or induced causes. Suggested neurologic causes of PRS include sympathetic dysfunction, dysregulation of neural crest cell migration in development, dysfunction of the trophic fibers of trigeminal nerves, and interstitial neurovasculitis. Theories of induced PRS suggest that physical trauma/head injury or certain viral infections (varicella zoster, herpes simplex virus, *Borrelia burgdorferi*) may be risk factors for PRS (Shah and Chhabra, 2023; El-Kehdy et al., 2012).

Sturge–Weber Syndrome

Sturge–Weber syndrome (SWS) is regarded as the third most common neurocutaneous syndrome, with an estimated incidence of 1 in every 20,000 to 50,000 live births. SWS typically presents with an abnormal vasculature in the face, resulting in a port-wine stain. Abnormal vasculature in the eyes and brain may also be observed, resulting in glaucoma and leptomeningeal angiomatosis.

The port-wine stain initially appears at birth as flat, red-pink patches, traditionally noted in the ophthalmic division of the trigeminal nerve. The port-wine stain progresses to hypertrophic red-purple lesions and eventually becomes papular or nodular overgrowths, causing dysmorphism, asymmetry, and occasional bleeding. The port-wine stain occurs in approximately 0.3% of live births. They are generally not considered pathognomonic, as brain involvement is frequently used to make the diagnosis of SWS. However, the causative somatic mutation underlying SWS and port-wine stains were found to be the same, so some authors suggest that SWS and port-wine stains not be considered distinct entities. Besides, the phenotypes of SWS exist on a spectrum: some patients with isolated brain involvement, some with isolated eye involvement, and most with port-wine stains and brain and eye involvement. Port-wine stains with exclusive involvement of the maxillary or mandibular branches of the trigeminal nerve are associated with leptomeningeal angiomatosis but not glaucoma. However, it should be noted that more recent work on PWS deviates from using the traditional dermatomal distributions of the trigeminal nerve branches to describe the involved area. Rather, more recent literature focuses on the frontal placode as a predictor of neurologic/ophthalmic symptoms. The frontal placode is the triangular area from the forehead midline, outer edge of the eye, to the top of the ear. This area develops vasculature derived from the prosencephalon and anterior mesencephalon. Regardless, any patient with a port-wine stain should be worked up with neuroimaging (typically T1-weighted magnetic resonance imaging with gadolinium contrast and susceptibility-weighted imaging) to identify intracranial involvement.

The most common neurologic manifestations of SWS include epilepsy, cognitive impairment, and headaches. Most patients with SWS develop seizures within the first two years of life (over 75%). There appears to be an increased susceptibility for fever-induced seizures as the onset of seizures is noted in approximately 30% of cases. Patients typically suffer from focal motor seizures, though a variety of different seizures have been reported, including generalized tonic-clonic seizures, partial seizures, infantile spasms, gelastic seizures, and status epilepticus. Indicators of poor prognoses are early onset of seizures, refractory to medication, bilateral intracranial involvement, and severe unilateral lesions.

Cognitive impairment is reported in over 50% of patients with SWS. Early onset and treatment of refractory epilepsy were associated with more severe intellectual disability. Besides intellectual disability, mental disorders are also common, including depressed mood, attention deficit/hyperactivity disorder, oppositional-defiant disorder, and conduct disorder. Of note, depression in patients with SWS has been associated with the presence and size of the port-wine stain. Thus, treatment of the port-wine stain in early infancy may be critical to improving SWS patient outcomes.

Though headache was thought to be a less common symptom in SWS than epilepsy and cognitive impairment, a self-reported questionnaire found that 81% of respondents with SWS reported suffering from both headaches and seizures, with almost half noting that their headaches were more bothersome than their seizures. Only a third of patients noted taking prophylactic medication for their headaches, suggesting that headaches may be undertreated in patients with SWS. Headache characteristics in patients with SWS appear to vary from migraine with aura to hemiplegic migraine with contralateral involvement. Migraine onset occurs at a young age, with a prevalence in children with SWS of 31%.

SWS appears to be sporadic and noninherited. The primary causative somatic mutation is noted to be a single nucleotide variant in *GNAQ*, which results in a single amino acid substitution in the guanine nucleotide-binding protein G(q) subunit alpha (c.548G→A, p.Arg183Gln). The mutation is an activating mutation upstream of the mitogen-activated protein kinase (MAPK) pathway, which is involved in cell proliferation. Thus, dysregulation of the MAPK pathway may result in the capillary malformations observed in patients with SWS and port-wine stains. This mutation was identified in 88% of patients with SWS and 92% of patients with nonsyndromic port-wine stains. The *GNAQ* mutation was found to be absent in unaffected tissues, explaining the mosaic phenotype observed in port-wine stains and SWS.

RASA1 is another gene that has been studied in the pathogenesis of SWS. *RASA1* encodes for p120-RasGTPase-activating protein, which is a negative regulator of the MAPK pathway. Mutations in *RASA1* have been observed in capillary and arteriovenous malformations. In SWS, *RASA1* mutations are much less frequent than GNAQ mutations, though *RASA1* mutations have been suggested to lead to familial inheritance patterns of SWS or port-wine stains (Comi, 2015; Sudarsanam and Ardern-Holmes, 2014; Higueros et al., 2017).

Neurofibromatoses

Neurofibromatosis is a group of three neurocutaneous syndromes that are characterized by neoplasms of neural origin: neurofibromatosis type 1 (NF1), neurofibromatosis type 2 or NF2-related schwannomatosis (NF2), and schwannomatosis. The three neurofibromatoses are clinically and genetically distinct from each other.

NF1 is the most common of the three, with an approximate global prevalence of 1 case in 3,000 individuals. Approximately half of NF1 cases are autosomal dominantly inherited, and the other half are secondary to *de novo* mutations. NF1 is caused by a germline mutation in the appropriately named *NF1* gene, which encodes for neurofibromin. Neurofibromin is a protein that is expected to act as a GTPase-activating protein that functions to inactivate RAS. Therefore, the loss of neurofibromin, as in NF1 patients, results in dysregulation of the MAPK pathway due to overactive RAS and subsequent increased cell proliferation. Postzygotic mutations in *NF1* result in mosaic or segmental variations of NF1.

In NF1, neurofibromas typically form in close association with cranial, spinal, or peripheral nerves. Over 80% of patients with NF1 develop neurofibromas by puberty, and the majority continue to develop neurofibromas over time. Other neoplasms are less common, but include malignant peripheral nerve sheath tumors, pilocytic astrocytomas, and other gliomas. Besides neoplasms, skin manifestations and headaches are common.

The most common skin manifestations are café au lait macules, which are flat patches of hyperpigmentation that appear in early infancy. Though the general population may have café au lait macules, the presence of six or more café au lait macules creates clinical suspicion for NF1. Other cutaneous manifestations include skinfold freckling (Crowe sign), intracutaneous tumors, and Lisch nodules, which are raised, tan hamartomas of the iris. Other signs and symptoms include skeletal abnormalities, behavioral deficits, and vasculopathies. Patients with NF1 have a reduced life expectancy of approximately 8–21 years, with the most common cause of death being due to malignant neoplasms (Gutmann et al., 2017; Plotkin and Wick, 2018).

The prevalence of headaches in patients with NF1 is widely variable, from 30% to 78%, depending on the study. Regardless, the prevalence appears to be greatly increased compared to the general population. Some authors report cases of NF1 where headache is the only neurologic symptom (Gao et al., 2022). The characteristics of the headache also seem to vary greatly, as some note a majority as migraine, while others report a majority as tension-type headaches (Afridi et al., 2015; Clementi et al., 1996; DiMario and Langshur, 2000; Pinho et al., 2014). Secondary headaches in NF1 patients may be attributed to neoplasms or vasculopathies. The mechanism underlying headaches in NF1 has been hypothesized to be related to the decreased level of neurofibromin, resulting in increased collapsing response mediator protein 2 (CRMP2) expression intracellularly, thus increasing the release of CGRP (White et al., 2014). Therefore, CGRP inhibitors have been hypothesized as possibly effective therapeutics in the prevention of primary headaches and migraine in patients with NF1; however, no systematic studies have been done on this topic to date.

Primary headaches are less common in NF 2 and schwannomatosis but are discussed next.

With a frequency of 1 case in 25,000 live births, NF2 is less common than NF1. NF2 is characterized by an increased predisposition to develop several tumors, particularly bilateral vestibular schwannomas, cranial and spinal meningiomas, and intraspinal indolent ependymomas. Headaches in NF2 are noted to be more likely to be secondary to intracranial tumors than in NF1 (Nandyala and Dougherty, 2022; Evans, 2015). The skin is a helpful tool to distinguish NF1 and NF2. Patients with NF2 will have more café au lait macules than the general population, but approximately 99% will have less than six, which is the threshold for suspicion of NF1. Approximately 70% of NF2 patients will have cutaneous tumors, and 10% will have more than ten cutaneous tumors (Evans et al., 1992). These tumors have the following characteristics: (1) plaque-like, raised, hyperpigmented lesion, often with excess hair; (2) subcutaneous nodular tumors, sometimes distributed along major peripheral nerves; or (3) intracutaneous tumors, similar to those in NF1. These tumors are mostly schwannomas, though neurofibromas have been reported (Evans, 2015). Though NF2 is autosomal dominant, approximately 50%–60% of cases are due to *de novo* mutations. The causative mutation is in the *NF2* gene, which encodes merlin, a protein with tumor suppressor function upstream of the MAPK and phosphatidylinositol-3-kinase (PI3K) pathways. The specific mutation appears to influence the phenotype.

Schwannomatosis is differentiated from NF2 by the presence of nonintradermal schwannomas and absence of vestibular schwannomas. Patients typically present with pain and/or a mass. Headaches are not a commonly reported condition in schwannomatosis. Schwannomatosis is a genetically distinct condition from NF1 and NF2, as mutations are typically noted in *SMARCB1* and *LZTR1* (Plotkin and Wick, 2018).

Tuberous Sclerosis Complex

Tuberous sclerosis complex (TSC) is a multisystemic disorder and is one of the most common neurocutaneous syndromes, affecting approximately 1 in every 6,000 to 10,000 live births. TSC has a heterogeneous clinical phenotype with varying degrees of severity. TSC is typically characterized by hamartoma formation in various organs, especially the brain (notably, malformations of the cerebral cortex are called tubers), skin, eyes, kidneys, lungs, and heart. Cutaneous manifestations include hypomelanocytic macules (90% of patients with TSC), facial angiofibromas (75%), ungual fibromas (20%–80%), shagreen patches (>50%), and fibrous cephalic plaques (25%; Teng et al., 2014). Neurologic manifestations of TSC include epilepsy, subependymal giant cell astrocytoma, and various neuropsychiatric disorders. Notably, headaches in TSC happen to be secondary in nature (Wan et al., 2019; Konakondla et al., 2016). To our knowledge, there currently do not exist any systemic studies on primary headaches in TSC, though the literature on headache in TSC remains limited. Other manifestations of tuberous sclerosis include pulmonary lymphangioleiomyomatosis, renal angiomyolipomas, and cardiac rhabdomyomas.

TSC is autosomal dominant, though only a third of cases are inherited. The causative mutations are in *TSC1*, which encodes for hamartin, and *TSC2*, which encodes for tuberin. Both proteins are negative regulators in the mammalian target of rapamycin (mTOR) signaling pathway. Mutations leading to TSC allow for overactivation of the mTOR signaling pathway, resulting in cell proliferation and thus hamartomas and neoplasms (Henske et al., 2016).

PHACE Syndrome

PHACE (Posterior fossa malformation, Hemangioma, Arterial anomalies, Coarctation of the aorta/Cardiac defects, and Eye abnormalities) syndrome is a relatively rare neurocutaneous disorder with poorly understood pathophysiology. There is currently no evidence of a genetic basis for PHACE syndrome. The estimated prevalence in European countries ranges from 0.59–6.5 per million (Disse et al., 2020). It also disproportionately affects female patients (9:1).

The most obvious sign that creates clinical suspicion for PHACE syndrome is infantile hemangiomas of the head and neck. PHACE syndrome occurs in 2%–3% of infantile hemangiomas. The presence of segmental or large infantile facial hemangiomas increases the likelihood by 20%–31% (Rotter et al., 2018). As implied by the name of the syndrome, the clinical manifestation of PHACE syndrome is multisystemic; however, abnormalities of the brain, aorta, and other arteries are most likely to cause long-term morbidity in PHACE syndrome patients (Garzon et al., 2016; Rotter et al., 2018; Winter et al., 2016).

Given the vascular and structural changes in the brain, it is unsurprising that PHACE patients frequently experience headaches (62%–89%). In addition, headache develops at an early age (48.8 months) with migrainous features, including nausea (62.5%), vomiting (37.5%), photophobia (75%), and phonophobia (75%; Stefanko et al., 2019; Yu et al., 2016). In patients with PHACE syndrome who develop new onset of headaches, evaluation for secondary headache causes such as vasculopathies or cerebral ischemia are indicated according to consensus guidelines, regardless of the findings on initial MRI (Garzon et al., 2016). Of note, given that PHACE syndrome patients suffer from arterial abnormalities, vasoconstrictive headache pharmacologic agents such as triptans, dihydroergotamine, and ergotamine tartrate should be considered contraindicated. Other neurologic issues in patients with PHACE syndrome include epilepsy, neurodevelopmental abnormalities, and hearing impairments. The pattern of cutaneous manifestations of PHACE syndrome may help predict the extracutaneous sequelae, including neurologic issues. Large facial infantile hemangiomas in the frontotemporal, maxillary, mandibular, and frontonasal distribution (S1-4 distribution) were associated with cerebral and vascular disorders. While those only affecting the frontotemporal distribution (S1) were associated with ocular disorders, those only affecting the mandibular distribution (S3) were associated with airway or ventral/cardiac disorders (Oza et al., 2008).

VIRAL INFECTIONS

Viral infections often manifest with skin findings and, therefore, may be a critical sign in the evaluation of a patient presenting with a headache. For example, herpes zoster (commonly referred to as shingles) is caused by the reactivation of the varicella-zoster virus, the virus that causes chicken pox. Herpes zoster can commonly present with headache, fever, malaise, and skin itching, burning, or pain, which is then followed by the appearance of a characteristic exanthematous rash. The maculopapular rash typically has a single unilateral dermatomal distribution, with new lesions appearing proximally to distally. The lesions typically crust over seven to ten days and heal within two to four weeks; however, scarring and pigmentation changes are common (Cohen, 2019). Postherpetic neuralgia is another common complication of herpes zoster, which is defined by pain in a dermatomal distribution for at least 90 days following the resolution of the rash. The pain in postherpetic neuralgia can be characterized as three types: (1) spontaneous and ongoing pain, (2) paroxysmal shooting pain or electric shock-like pain, or (3) evoked sensations such as allodynia/hyperalgesia.

Herpes zoster and the subsequent postherpetic neuralgia are not uncommon. In the United States alone, there are over 1 million cases of herpes zoster annually, with a rate of 3–4 cases per 1,000 persons. Postherpetic neuralgia is reported in 20% of herpes zoster patients three months after the onset of symptoms and in 15% of patients two years after the onset of symptoms. Major risk factors for herpes zoster and postherpetic neuralgia include increasing age, unvaccinated status, and impaired cell-mediated immunities. Other risk factors for herpes zoster include female sex, white race/ethnicity, previous family history, and comorbidities such as autoimmune conditions (Kawai and Yawn, 2017). Though many risk factors of herpes zoster and postherpetic neuralgia are similar, the evidence regarding the association of sex and postherpetic neuralgia remains conflicting (Forbes et al., 2016).

Prevention is a mainstay in the management of herpes zoster, primarily with infection control and vaccination. In patients with active herpes zoster, oral guanosine analogues (acyclovir, famciclovir, or valacyclovir) should be initiated within 72 hours of onset of the rash or after 72 hours if complications are still present. Patients should be advised that common adverse effects of these antivirals are mild to moderate headaches that generally resolve without intervention (Mubareka et al., 2010). Glucocorticoids, acetaminophen, or nonsteroidal anti-inflammatory agents may be considered as an adjunct therapy for the management of acute pain in herpes zoster (Saguil et al., 2017). Management of postherpetic neuralgia management primarily focuses on symptom control with topical treatment (capsaicin or lidocaine) or oral agents (gabapentin, pregabalin, opioids, or tricyclic antidepressants) (Johnson and Rice, 2014).

Besides postherpetic neuralgia, other neurologic complications of herpes zoster include cranial and peripheral palsies, myelitis, and vasculopathies. Of note, cranial and peripheral nerve palsies are the second most common complication of herpes zoster, after postherpetic neuralgia, occurring in 0.5% to 5% of patients with herpes zoster (Yaszay et al., 2000; Amlie-Lefond and Jubelt, 2009). Some neurologic complications of herpes zoster may be life-threatening and require emergent treatment. For example, a patient presenting with a severe headache and a unilateral dermatomal rash may have herpes zoster ophthalmicus (Catron and Hern, 2008) or autonomic dysreflexia secondary to herpes zoster (Wells, 2021).

Other neurotropic viral infections can clinically present with a constellation, including headaches and rashes. In patients with clinical suspicion of neurotropic viral infections, the differential may be narrowed by the appearance of the rash, exposure history, risk factors, and epidemiology. However, to be sure, the rash's appearance in the context of a headache is not pathognomonic, and the diagnosis should still be confirmed. Characteristics of common viruses or viruses of emerging interest that may present with a rash and headache are summarized in Table 6.1.

TABLE 6.1   Summary of neurologic and dermatologic conditions that co-occur and overlapping treatments, if any

CATEGORY	EXAMPLE DERMATOLOGIC CONDITION	EXAMPLE NEUROLOGIC CONDITION
Inflammatory conditions	Atopic dermatitis	Headache/migraine, epilepsy, autism spectrum disorder, attention deficit hyperactivity disorder, depression
	Rosacea	Migraine, depression, anxiety, Parkinson's disease, glioma, Alzheimer's disease, dementia, multiple sclerosis
	Seborrheic dermatitis	Parkinson's disease/parkinsonism, brachycephaly, spinal cord injury, nerve lesions, stroke, tardive dyskinesia, epilepsy
	Psoriasis	Migraine, multiple sclerosis, epilepsy, restless leg syndrome, Guillain-Barré syndrome, myasthenia gravis, depression, bipolar mood disorder, anxiety, psychosis, cognitive impairment, personality change, sexual disorders, sleep disturbance, eating disorders
Neurocutaneous syndromes	PRS • Atrophy of the skin • Alopecia (in band-like distribution, may also involve the eyes and eyebrows) • Ipsilateral pigmentation changes on face and neck	Headache, facial pain, trigeminal neuralgia, epilepsy, cerebrovascular events, speech abnormalities, muscle spasms, synkinesia, dystonia, oculomotor and trochlear nerve palsy, Horner's syndrome, optic neuropathy, hallucinations, cognitive disturbances
	SWS • Port-wine stain	Headache, epilepsy, cognitive impairment, hemiparesis, delayed neuropsychological development, visual field defects, glaucoma
	Neurofibromatosis type 1 • Café au lait macules (typically more than 6) • Skinfold freckling (Crowe sign) • Intracutaneous tumors • Lisch nodules	Headache, neoplastic manifestations (such as neurofibromas), macrocephaly, epilepsy, hydrocephalus, aqueductal stenosis, Moyamoya disease, attention deficit hyperactivity disorder, autism spectrum disorder
	TSC • Hypomelanocytic macules • Facial angiofibromas • Ungual fibromas • Shagreen patches • Fibrous cephalic plaques	Secondary headache, epilepsy, subependymal giant cell astrocytoma, retinal hamartomas, optic nerve hamartomas, elevated intracranial pressure, cerebral nerve palsies, visual field defects, anxiety, mood disorder, adjustment disorder, attention deficit hyperactivity disorder
	PHACE syndrome • Segmental or large infantile hemangiomas of the head and neck	Headache, posterior fossa brain abnormality, Dandy-Walker complex, optic nerve hypoplasia, seizures, developmental delays, hypotonia, dysphagia, opisthotonus, hearing loss

(Continued)

TABLE 6.1   (Continued) Summary of neurologic and dermatologic conditions that co-occur and overlapping treatments, if any

CATEGORY	EXAMPLE DERMATOLOGIC CONDITION	EXAMPLE NEUROLOGIC CONDITION
Viral Infections	Herpes zoster • Exanthematous, maculopapular rash with a single unilateral dermatomal distribution. New papules appear proximal to distal, crust over in seven to ten days and heal in two to four weeks	Headache, postherpetic neuralgia, cranial and peripheral nerve palsies, herpes zoster ophthalmicus, autonomic dysreflexia
	Measles (rubeola): • Exanthem (erythematous maculopapular rash that first appears on the face and spreads to the neck, trunk, and extremities) • Koplik spots	Acute encephalitis, subacute sclerosing panencephalitis, measles inclusion body encephalitis (Patterson, 2020)
	Rubella: • Exanthem (generalized erythematous maculopapular rash)	Encephalitis, progressive rubella panencephalitis, microcephaly, developmental delay (Winter and Moss, 2022)
	Human immunodeficiency virus (HIV) • Acute HIV exanthem (maculopapular rash on face, trunk, and arms) • Other rashes can include herpes simplex virus, herpes zoster, dermatophytosis (Khambaty and Hsu, 2010)	HIV-associated neurocognitive disorder, HIV-associated vacuolar myelopathy, distal symmetric polyneuropathy (Bilgrami and O'Keefe, 2014)
	Monkeypox (2022 outbreak) • Lesions appear primarily in anogenital, arms and legs, trunk, and face. Lesions progress through macular, papular, vesicular, then pustular stages	Myalgia, headache, encephalitis, seizure, confusion (Mitjà et al., 2023)

A COMMON THERAPEUTIC IN NEUROLOGY AND DERMATOLOGY: BOTULINUM A TOXIN

Botulinum A toxin (BoNT-A) is a neurotoxin synthesized by *Clostridium botulinum* that was frequently used as a neuromuscular blocking agent to control wrinkles. Following observations that migraine appeared to improve in patients receiving BoNT-A for cosmetic purposes, BoNT-A injects were extensively studied in the context of migraine, ultimately showing that BoNT-A was an effective migraine preventive agent (Herd et al., 2018).

Later mechanistic research showed that BoNT-A inhibited the release of neurotransmitters by cleaving SNAP-25 in motor and sensory nerve terminals. By blocking the release of acetylcholine and neurotransmitters that mediate pain, BoNT-A caused muscle relaxation and reduction of pain signaling. Further, BoNT-A reduces cell surface expression of presynaptic ion channels and sensory receptors by preventing exocytic fusion to the membrane (Martinelli et al., 2020).

BoNT-A injections are also used in the treatment of hyperhidrosis, which is an idiopathic, chronic condition characterized by excessive sweating, particularly on the hands, feet, or axillae. BoNT-A injections are safe and effective in treating hyperhidrosis when injected into the axillary, palmar, or plantar surfaces (Doft et al., 2012). BoNT-A injections have also been studied for the off-label treatment of clinically related diseases: chromhidrosis and bromhidrosis (Wu et al., 2005; Tato et al., 2012; He et al., 2012).

BoNT-A has also been investigated as a treatment for several other dermatologic conditions that have a prominent neurologic component.

Pachyonychia congenita (PC) is a genodermatosis characterized by hypertrophic nails, painful palmar and plantar keratoma and hyperhidrosis, pilosebaceous cysts, and follicular keratosis. PC is autosomally inherited. Causative mutations for PC encode for various keratin. Given the antihidrotic effect of BoNT-A observed in patients with hyperhidrosis, coupled with its analgesic effect in migraine, BoNT-A was investigated in the treatment of PC. Early research suggested that BoNT-A was able to effectively ameliorate hyperhidrosis, blistering, and pain in PC patients (Swartling and Vahlquist, 2006; Swartling et al., 2010; González-Ramos et al., 2016; Koren et al., 2020).

Cephalgia alopecia (CA) is a recurrent headache disorder with burning and stabbing pain, which is then followed by hair loss at the same location of the headache. Headaches in CA are thought to cause overstimulation of trigeminal and upper cervical nerves that innervate hair cells, which leads to depletion of SP and CGRP. These neuropeptides play a role in mediating hair growth. Thus, the loss of SP and CGRP results in hair loss. CA has been shown to be refractory to traditional headache therapeutic options, such as nonsteroidal anti-inflammatory agents, tricyclic antidepressants, propranolol, topiramate, and gabapentin (Bedrin and Dougherty, 2020). BoNT-A has been suggested to block the release of SP and CGRP by primary sensory neurons in the skin (Aoki, 2005). Outcomes of BoNT-A in patients with CA were positive, and BoNT-A is one of the mainstays of treatment for CA to date, though treatment is not remittive (Bedrin and Dougherty, 2020). Scalp biopsies in patients with CA following treatment with BoNT-A showed elevated levels of SP and CGRP-positive fibers (Cutrer et al., 2010).

A similar condition, alopecia areata (AA), is a common dermatologic condition with patches of non-scarring hair loss, often on the scalp. The pathophysiology of AA is not fully elucidated, though it is likely multifactorial in nature. Nevertheless, it is likely that neuropeptides like CGRP and SP play a similar role in AA as they do in CA. Scalp biopsies from patients with AA showed decreased levels of CGRP and SP (Rossi et al., 1997). Thus, BoNT-A was investigated as a possible therapeutic. In 2010, an open-label trial of BoNT-A in seven patients with AA showed no effect on hair growth (Cho et al., 2010). It is currently not clear what is responsible for the differences in results of BoNT-A on CA versus AA.

Given the role that SP and CGRP may also play in the pathophysiology of psoriasis (Jiang et al., 1998), BoNT-A may be of interest in psoriasis as well due to the hypothesis that it may block neuropeptide release. Scant observational reports of patients with plaque psoriasis and inverse psoriasis show that BoNT-A may be effective (Zanchi et al., 2008; Gilbert et al., 2014), though further research is needed.

Other dermatologic diseases in which BoNT-A injections have been investigated include keloids/hypertrophic scars, Hailey-Hailey disease, linear IgA bullous dermatosis, epidermolysis bullosa simplex Weber-Cockayne subtype, Darier disease, HS, aquagenic keratoderma, AA, androgenetic alopecia, notalgia paresthetica, facial erythema/flushing, Raynaud phenomenon, and postherpetic neuralgia, which are reviewed by other works (Campanati et al., 2017; Kim et al., 2017; Guida et al., 2018).

SUMMARY

- Neurocutaneous disorders are rare genetic conditions that often have characteristic dermatologic signs, as well as extracutaneous manifestations. Headaches are especially implicated in PRS, SWS, NF1, TSC, and PHACE syndrome.
- Viral infections that present with a headache can frequently also have cutaneous manifestations, with herpes zoster being a notable example.

- Emerging evidence supports an association between headaches and several common dermatologic conditions, such as rosacea, atopic dermatitis, and psoriasis. Future research is focused on identifying mechanistic linkages and using them as possible drug targets.
- BoNT-A is a safe and effective treatment for migraine presentation and hyperhidrosis by inhibiting neurotransmitter release, thus modulating nociceptive and hidrotic pathways. BoNT-A has been investigated for the treatment of several other dermatologic diseases, such as PC, alopecia, and psoriasis.

REFERENCES

Abrouk M, Gandy J, Nakamura M, et al. Secukinumab in the treatment of psoriasis and psoriatic arthritis: A review of the literature. *Skin Therapy Letter* 2017;*22*(4):1–6.

Afridi SK, Leschziner GD, Ferner RE. Prevalence and clinical presentation of headache in a National Neurofibromatosis 1 Service and impact on quality of life. *American Journal of Medical Genetics Part A.* 2015;*167*(10):2282–2285. Doi:10.1002/ajmg.a.37186

Aldrich N, Gerstenblith M, Fu P, et al. Genetic vs environmental factors that correlate with Rosacea: A cohort-based survey of twins. *JAMA Dermatology* 2015;*151*(11):1213–1219. Doi:10.1001/jamadermatol.2015.2230

Al-Hassany L, Boucherie DM, Creeney H, et al. Future targets for migraine treatment beyond CGRP. *The Journal of Headache and Pain* 2023;*24*(1):76. Doi:10.1186/s10194-023-01567-4

Alia E, Feng H. Rosacea pathogenesis, common triggers, and dietary role: The cause, the trigger, and the positive effects of different foods. *Clinics in Dermatology* 2022;*40*(2):122–127. Doi:10.1016/j.clindermatol.2021.10.004

Amlie-Lefond C, Jubelt B. Neurologic manifestations of varicella zoster virus infections. *Current Neurology and Neuroscience Reports* 2009;*9*(6):430–434. Doi:10.1007/s11910-009-0064-z

Anttila V, Wessman M, Kallela M, Palotie A. Chapter 31 – Genetics of migraine. In: Geschwind DH, Paulson HL, Klein C, eds. *Handbook of Clinical Neurology.* Vol *148.* Neurogenetics, Part II. Elsevier; 2018:493–503. Doi:10.1016/B978-0-444-64076-5.00031-4

Aoki KR. Review of a proposed mechanism for the antinociceptive action of botulinum toxin type A. *Neurotoxicology* 2005;*26*(5):785–793. Doi:10.1016/j.neuro.2005.01.017

Armstrong AW, Read C. Pathophysiology, clinical presentation, and treatment of psoriasis: A review. *Journal of the American Medical Association* 2020;*323*(19):1945–1960. Doi:10.1001/jama.2020.4006

Aupiais C, Wanin S, Romanello S, et al. Association between migraine and atopic diseases in childhood: A potential protective role of anti-allergic drugs. *Headache: The Journal of Head and Face Pain.* 2017;*57*(4):612–624. Doi:10.1111/head.13032

Bedrin KO, Dougherty C. Cephalgia alopecia. *Current Pain and Headache Reports* 2020;*24*(9):46. Doi:10.1007/s11916-020-00880-w

Bettley FR, Marten RH. Unilateral Seborrheic Dermatitis Following a Nerve Lesion. *AMA Archives of Dermatology.* 1956;*73*(2):110–115. Doi:10.1001/archderm.1956.01550020010002

Bilgrami M, O'Keefe P. Chapter 90 - Neurologic diseases in HIV-infected patients. In: Biller J, Ferro JM, eds. *Handbook of Clinical Neurology.* Vol *121.* Neurologic Aspects of Systemic Disease Part III. Elsevier; 2014:1321–1344. Doi:10.1016/B978-0-7020-4088-7.00090-0

Brandes JL, Visser WH, Farmer MV, et al. Montelukast for Migraine Prophylaxis: A Randomized, Double-Blind, Placebo-Controlled Study. *Headache: The Journal of Head and Face Pain.* 2004;*44*(6):581–586. Doi:10.1111/j.1526-4610.2004.446006.x

Burton JL, Pye RJ. Seborrhoea is not a feature of seborrheic dermatitis. *British Medical Journal (Clinical Research Ed.)* 1983;*286*(6372):1169–1170. Doi:10.1136/bmj.286.6372.1169

Campanati A, Martina E, Giuliodori K, Consales V, Bobyr I, Offidani A. Botulinum toxin off-label use in dermatology: A review. *Skin Appendage Disorders.* 2017;*3*(1):39–56. Doi:10.1159/000452341

Capo A, Affaitati G, Giamberardino MA, Amerio P. Psoriasis and migraine. *Journal of the European Academy of Dermatology and Venereology* 2018;*32*(1):57–61. Doi:10.1111/jdv.14472

Catron T, Hern HG. Herpes zoster ophthalmicus. *The Western Journal of Emergency Medicine* 2008;*9*(3):174–176.

Cho HR, Lew BL, Lew H, Sim WY. Treatment effects of intradermal botulinum toxin type A injection on alopecia areata. *Dermatologic Surgery* 2010;*36*(s4):2175–2181. Doi:10.1111/j.1524-4725.2010.01709.x

Christensen CE, Andersen FS, Wienholtz N, Egeberg A, Thyssen JP, Ashina M. The relationship between migraine and rosacea: Systematic review and meta-analysis. *Cephalalgia* 2018;*38*(7):1387–1398. Doi:10.1177/0333102417731777

Clementi M, Battistella PA, Rizzi L, Boni S, Tenconi R. Headache in patients with neurofibromatosis type 1. *Headache: The Journal of Head and Face Pain.* 1996;*36*(1):10–13. Doi:10.1046/j.1526-4610.1996.3601010.x

Cohen D, Shpitalni G, Lifshitz Y, Anani S, Eyal A, Segal G. A Stroke in the Young with Surprising Recovery. *Eur J Case Rep Intern Med.* 2019;*6*(5):000200. Doi:10.12890/2019_000200

Comi AM. Chapter 11 – Sturge–Weber syndrome. In: Islam MP, Roach ES, eds. *Handbook of Clinical Neurology.* Vol *132.* Neurocutaneous Syndromes. Elsevier; 2015:157–168. Doi:10.1016/B978-0-444-62702-5.00011-1

Cowley NC, Farr PM, Shuster S. The permissive effect of sebum in seborrheic dermatitis: an explanation of the rash in neurological disorders. *The British Journal of Dermatology* 1990;*122*(1):71–76. Doi:10.1111/j.1365-2133.1990.tb08241.x

Cutrer F, Sandroni P, Wendelschafer-Crabb G. Botulinum toxin treatment of cephalalgia alopecia increases substance P and calcitonin gene-related peptide-containing cutaneous nerves in scalp. *Cephalalgia* 2010;*30*(8):1000–1006. Doi:10.1111/j.1468-2982.2009.01987.x

Dall'Oglio F, Nasca MR, Gerbino C, Micali G. An overview of the diagnosis and management of seborrheic dermatitis. *Clinical, Cosmetic and Investigational Dermatology* 2022;*15*:1537–1548. Doi:10.2147/CCID.S284671

Dessinioti C, Katsambas A. Seborrheic dermatitis: Etiology, risk factors, and treatments: Facts and controversies. *Clinics in Dermatology* 2013;*31*(4):343–351. Doi:10.1016/j.clindermatol.2013.01.001

DiMario FJ, Langshur S. Headaches in patients with neurofibromatosis-1. *Journal of Child Neurology* 2000;*15*(4):235–238. Doi:10.1177/088307380001500406

Disse SC, Toelle SP, Schroeder S, et al. Epidemiology, clinical features, and use of early supportive measures in PHACE syndrome: A European multinational observational study. *Neuroepidemiology* 2020;*54*(5):383–391. Doi:10.1159/000508187

Dodick DW. CGRP ligand and receptor monoclonal antibodies for migraine prevention: Evidence review and clinical implications. *Cephalalgia* 2019;*39*(3):445–458. Doi:10.1177/0333102418821662

Doft MA, Hardy KL, Ascherman JA. Treatment of hyperhidrosis with botulinum toxin. *Aesthetic Surgery Journal* 2012;*32*(2):238–244. Doi:10.1177/1090820X11434506

Egeberg A, Mallbris L, Hilmar Gislason G, Skov L, Riis Hansen P. Increased risk of migraine in patients with psoriasis: A Danish nationwide cohort study. *Journal of the American Academy of Dermatology* 2015;*73*(5):829–835. Doi:10.1016/j.jaad.2015.08.039

Eiland LS, Jenkins LS, Durham SH. Pediatric Migraine: Pharmacologic Agents for Prophylaxis. *The Annals of Pharmacotherapy* 2007;*41*(7-8):1181–1190. Doi:10.1345/aph.1K049

El-Kehdy J, Abbas O, Rubeiz N. A review of parry-romberg syndrome. *Journal of the American Academy of Dermatology* 2012;*67*(4):769–784. Doi:10.1016/j.jaad.2012.01.019

Evans D, Huson S, Donnai D, et al. A clinical study of type 2 neurofibromatosis. *QJM: An International Journal of Medicine.* 1992;*84*(1):603–618. Doi:10.1093/oxfordjournals.qjmed.a068699

Evans DGR. Chapter 5 – neurofibromatosis type 2. In: Islam MP, Roach ES, eds. *Handbook of Clinical Neurology.* Vol *132.* Neurocutaneous Syndromes. Elsevier; 2015:87–96. Doi:10.1016/B978-0-444-62702-5.00005-6

Fan R, Leasure AC, Damsky W, Cohen JM. Migraine among adults with atopic dermatitis: A cross-sectional study in the All of Us research programme. *Clinical and Experimental Dermatology* 2023;*48*(1):24–26. Doi:10.1093/ced/llac004

Forbes HJ, Thomas SL, Smeeth L, et al. A systematic review and meta-analysis of risk factors for postherpetic neuralgia. *Pain* 2016;*157*(1):30–54. Doi:10.1097/j.pain.0000000000000307

Galili E, Barzilai A, Shreberk-Hassidim R, Merdler I, Caspi T, Astman N. Neuropsychiatric comorbidity among adolescents with psoriasis. *The British Journal of Dermatology* 2018;*178*(4):910–916. Doi:10.1111/bjd.16031

Gao M, Liu H, Sun Q, Yang G. The gene diagnosis of neurofibromatosis type I with headache as the main symptom: A case report and review of the literature. *Frontiers in Neurology* 2022;*13*:874613. Doi:10.3389/fneur.2022.874613

Garzon MC, Epstein LG, Heyer GL, et al. PHACE Syndrome: Consensus-Derived Diagnosis and Care Recommendations. The Journal of Pediatrics. 2016;*178*:24–33. Doi:10.1016/j.jpeds.2016.07.054

Gaylor MLN, Duvic M. Generalized pustular psoriasis following withdrawal of efalizumab. *Journal of Drugs in Dermatology* 2004;*3*(1):77–79.

Gelfand JM, Gelfand AA, Goadsby PJ, Benn BS, Koth LL. Migraine is common in patients with sarcoidosis. *Cephalalgia* 2018;*38*(14):2079–2082. Doi:10.1177/0333102418768037

Gilbert E, Ward NL. Efficacy of botulinum neurotoxin type A for treating recalcitrant plaque psoriasis. *Journal Drugs Dermatology* 2014;*13*(11):1407–1408.

González-Ramos J, Sendagorta-Cudós E, González-López G, Mayor-Ibarguren A, Feltes-Ochoa R, Herranz-Pinto P. Efficacy of botulinum toxin in pachyonychia congenita type 1: Report of two new cases. *Dermatologic Therapy* 2016;*29*(1):32–36. Doi:10.1111/dth.12297

Graif Y, Shohat T, Machluf Y, Farkash R, Chaiter Y. Association between asthma and migraine: A cross-sectional study of over 110 000 adolescents. *The Clinical Respiratory Journal*. 2018;*12*(10):2491–2496. Doi:10.1111/crj.12939

Guida S, Farnetani F, Nisticò SP, et al. New trends in botulinum toxin use in dermatology. *Dermatol Pract Concept*. 2018;*8*(4):277–282. Doi:10.5826/dpc.0804a05

Gutmann DH, Ferner RE, Listernick RH, Korf BR, Wolters PL, Johnson KJ. Neurofibromatosis type 1. *Nature Reviews. Disease Primers* 2017;*3*(1):1–17. Doi:10.1038/nrdp.2017.4

Han JH, Lee HJ, Yook HJ, Han K, Lee JH, Park YM. Atopic disorders and their risks of migraine: A nationwide population-based cohort study. *Allergy, Asthma & Immunology Research* 2022;*15*(1):55–66. Doi:10.4168/aair.2023.15.1.55

Han ZA, Choi JY, Ko YJ. Dermatological problems following spinal cord injury in Korean patients. *The Journal of Spinal Cord Medicine*. 2015;*38*(1):63–67. Doi:10.1179/2045772313Y.0000000154

He J, Wang T, Dong J. A close positive correlation between malodor and sweating as a marker for the treatment of axillary bromhidrosis with Botulinum toxin A. *The Journal of Dermatological Treatment* 2012;*23*(6):461–464. Doi:10.3109/09546634.2011.594869

Helfrich YR, Maier LE, Cui Y, et al. Clinical, histologic, and molecular analysis of differences between erythematotelangiectatic rosacea and telangiectatic photoaging. *JAMA Dermatology* 2015;*151*(8):825–836. Doi:10.1001/jamadermatol.2014.4728

Henske EP, Jóźwiak S, Kingswood JC, Sampson JR, Thiele EA. Tuberous sclerosis complex. *Nature Reviews. Disease Primers* 2016;*2*(1):1–18. Doi:10.1038/nrdp.2016.35

Herd CP, Tomlinson CL, Rick C, et al. Botulinum toxins for the prevention of migraine in adults. *Cochrane Database of Systematic Reviews* 2018;(6). Doi:10.1002/14651858.CD011616.pub2

Higueros E, Roe E, Granell E, Baselga E. Sturge-Weber Syndrome: A Review. *Actas Dermo-Sifiliográficas (English Edition)*. 2017;*108*(5):407–417. Doi:10.1016/j.adengl.2017.03.034

Holmes AD, Spoendlin J, Chien AL, Baldwin H, Chang AS. Evidence-based update on rosacea comorbidities and their common physiologic pathways. *Journal of the American Academy of Dermatology* 2018;*78*(1):156–166. Doi:10.1016/j.jaad.2017.07.055

Ighani A, Georgakopoulos JR, Shear NH, Walsh S, Yeung J. Short-term reasons for withdrawal and adverse events associated with apremilast therapy for psoriasis in real-world practice compared with in clinical trials: A multicenter retrospective study. *Journal of the American Academy of Dermatology* 2018;*78*(4):801–803. Doi:10.1016/j.jaad.2017.09.067

Jiang WY, Raychaudhuri SP, Farber EM. Double-labeled immunofluorescence study of cutaneous nerves in psoriasis. *International Journal of Dermatology* 1998;*37*(8):572–574. Doi:10.1046/j.1365-4362.1998.00533.x

Johnson RW, Rice ASC. Postherpetic Neuralgia. *New England Journal of Medicine* 2014;*371*(16):1526–1533. Doi:10.1056/NEJMcp1403062

Kawai K, Yawn BP. Risk factors for herpes zoster: A systematic review and meta-analysis. *Mayo Clinic Proceedings* 2017;*92*(12):1806–1821. Doi:10.1016/j.mayocp.2017.10.009

Khambaty MM, Hsu SS. Dermatology of the patient with HIV. *Emergency Medicine Clinics of North America* 2010;*28*(2):355–368. Doi:10.1016/j.emc.2010.01.001

Kim YS, Hong ES, Kim HS. Botulinum Toxin in the Field of Dermatology: Novel Indications. *Toxins*. 2017;*9*(12):403. Doi:10.3390/toxins9120403

Kluger N, Nuutinen P, Lybeck E, Ruohoalho T, Salava A. Migraine is not the most common comorbidity in hidradenitis suppurativa patients. *Journal of the European Academy of Dermatology and Venereology* 2019;*33*(9):e330–e331. Doi:10.1111/jdv.15625

Konakondla S, Jayarao M, Skrade J, Giannini C, Workman MJ, Morgan CJ. Subependymal giant cell astrocytoma in a genetically negative tuberous sclerosis complex adult: Case report. *Clinical Neurology and Neurosurgery* 2016;*150*:177–180. Doi:10.1016/j.clineuro.2016.09.015

Koren A, Sprecher E, Reider E, Artzi O. A treatment protocol for botulinum toxin injections in the treatment of pachyonychia congenita-associated keratoderma. *The British Journal of Dermatology* 2020;*182*(3):671–677. Doi:10.1111/bjd.18169

Lewis DW, Diamond S, Scott D, Jones V. Prophylactic Treatment of Pediatric Migraine. *Headache: The Journal of Head and Face Pain*. 2004;*44*(3):230–237. Doi:10.1111/j.1526-4610.2004.04052.x

Lonne-Rahm S, Nordlind K, Edström DW, Ros AM, Berg M. Laser treatment of Rosacea: A Pathoetiological Study. *Archives of Dermatology* 2004;*140*(11):1345–1349. Doi:10.1001/archderm.140.11.1345

Marmura MJ. Triggers, Protectors, and Predictors in Episodic Migraine. *Current Pain and Headache Reports* 2018;*22*(12):81. Doi:10.1007/s11916-018-0734-0

Martin VT, Taylor F, Gebhardt B, et al. Allergy and Immunotherapy: Are They Related to Migraine Headache? *Headache: The Journal of Head and Face Pain.* 2011;*51*(1):8–20. Doi:10.1111/j.1526-4610.2010.01792.x

Martinelli D, Arceri S, Tronconi L, Tassorelli C. Chronic migraine and Botulinum Toxin Type A: Where do paths cross? *Toxicon* 2020;*178*:69–76. Doi:10.1016/j.toxicon.2020.02.017

Mastrolonardo M, Diaferio A, Logroscino G. Seborrheic dermatitis, increased sebum excretion, and Parkinson's disease: a survey of (im)possible links. *Medical Hypotheses* 2003;*60*(6):907–911. Doi:10.1016/S0306-9877(03)00094-X

Medina JL, Diamond S. Migraine and Atopy. *Headache: The Journal of Head and Face Pain.* 1976;*15*(4):271–274. Doi:10.1111/j.1526-4610.1976.hed1504271.x

Meents JE, Neeb L, Reuter U. TRPV1 in migraine pathophysiology. *Trends in Molecular Medicine* 2010;*16*(4):153–159. Doi:10.1016/j.molmed.2010.02.004

Millán-Guerrero RO, Isais-Millán R, Barreto-Vizcaíno S, et al. Subcutaneous histamine versus sodium valproate in migraine prophylaxis: A randomized, controlled, double-blind study. *European Journal of Neurology* 2007;*14*(10):1079–1084. Doi:10.1111/j.1468-1331.2007.01744.x

Millán-Guerrero RO, Isais-Millán R, Barreto-Vizcaíno S, et al. Subcutaneous histamine versus topiramate in migraine prophylaxis: A double-blind study. *European Neurology* 2008;*59*(5):237–242. Doi:10.1159/000115637

Millán-Guerrero RO, Isais-Millán S, Barreto-Vizcaíno S, Rivera-Castaño L, Rios-Madariaga C. Subcutaneous histamine versus botulinum toxin type A in migraine prophylaxis: A randomized, double-blind study. *European Journal of Neurology* 2009;*16*(1):88–94. Doi:10.1111/j.1468-1331.2008.02352.x

Mitjà O, Ogoina D, Titanji BK, et al. Monkeypox. *Lancet* 2023;*401*(10370):60–74. Doi:10.1016/S0140-6736(22)02075-X

Morís G, Ribacoba R, Solar D, Vidal J. SUNCT syndrome and seborrheic dermatitis associated with craneosynostosis. *Cephalalgia* 2001;*21*(2):157–159. Doi:10.1046/j.1468-2982.2001.00183.x

Mortimer MJ, Kay J, Gawkrodger DJ, Jaron A, Barker DC. The prevalence of headache and migraine in atopic children: an epidemiological study in general practice. *Headache* 1993;*33*(8):427–431. Doi:10.1111/j.1526-4610.1993.hed3308427.x

Mubareka S, Leung V, Aoki FY, Vinh DC. Famciclovir: A focus on efficacy and safety. *Expert Opinion on Drug Safety* 2010;*9*(4):643–658. Doi:10.1517/14740338.2010.485189

Muñoz-Jareño N, Fernández-Mayoralas DM, Martínez-Cervell C, Campos-Castelló J. [Relationship between migraine and atopy in childhood: a retrospective case-control study]. *Revista de Neurologia* 2011;*53*(12):713–720.

Nandyala A, Dougherty C. Dermatologic symptoms and syndromes associated with headache. *Current Pain and Headache Reports* 2022;*26*(10):719–723. Doi:10.1007/s11916-022-01080-4

Ohsawa Y, Hirasawa N. The role of histamine H1 and H4 receptors in atopic dermatitis: from basic research to clinical study. *Allergology International* 2014;*63*(4):533–542. Doi:10.2332/allergolint.13-RA-0675

Okuma H, Iijima K, Yasuda T, Tokuoka K, Kitagawa Y. Preventive effect of cyproheptadine hydrochloride in refractory patients with frequent migraine. *Springerplus* 2013;*2*(1):573. Doi:10.1186/2193-1801-2-573

O'Neill CJA, Richardson MD, Charlett A, et al. Could seborrheic dermatitis be implicated in the pathogenesis of parkinsonism? *Acta Neurologica Scandinavica* 1994;*89*(4):252–257. Doi:10.1111/j.1600-0404.1994.tb01675.x

Oza VS, Wang E, Berenstein A, et al. PHACES association: A neuroradiologic review of 17 patients. *American Journal of Neuroradiology* 2008;*29*(4):807–813. Doi:10.3174/ajnr.A0937

Özge A, Öksüz N, Ayta S, et al. Atopic disorders are more common in childhood migraine and correlated headache phenotype. *Pediatrics International* 2014;*56*(6):868–872. Doi:10.1111/ped.12381

Patterson MC. Neurological Complications of Measles (Rubeola). *Current Neurology and Neuroscience Reports* 2020;*20*(2):2. Doi:10.1007/s11910-020-1023-y

Pérez-Pereda S, Toriello-Suárez M, Ocejo-Vinyals G, et al. Serum CGRP, VIP, and PACAP usefulness in migraine: a case–control study in chronic migraine patients in real clinical practice. *Molecular Biology Reports* 2020;*47*(9):7125–7138. Doi:10.1007/s11033-020-05781-0

Pérez Tato B, Zamora Martínez E, Sánchez Albisua B, et al. Facial and axillary apocrine chromhidrosis. *Dermatology Online Journal* 2012;*18*(3):13.

Pinho RS, Fusão EF, Paschoal JKSF, et al. Migraine is frequent in children and adolescents with neurofibromatosis type 1. *Pediatrics International* 2014;*56*(6):865–867. Doi:10.1111/ped.12375

Plotkin SR, Wick A. Neurofibromatosis and Schwannomatosis. *Seminars in Neurology* 2018;*38*(1):73–85. Doi:10.1055/s-0038-1627471

Rossi R, Del Bianco E, Isolani D, Baccari MC, Cappugi P. Possible involvement of neuropeptidergic sensory nerves in alopecia areata. *Neuroreport* 1997;*8*(5):1135–1138. Doi:10.1097/00001756-199703240-00015

Rotter A, Samorano LP, Rivitti-Machado MC, Oliveira ZNP, Gontijo B. PHACE syndrome: clinical manifestations, diagnostic criteria, and management. *Anais Brasileiros de Dermatologia* 2018;*93*:405–411. Doi:10.1590/abd1806-4841.20187693

Rubin-Asher D, Zeilig G, Klieger M, Adunsky A, Weingarden H. Dermatological findings following acute traumatic spinal cord injury. *Spinal Cord* 2005;*43*(3):175–178. Doi:10.1038/sj.sc.3101697

Sabat R, Jemec GBE, Matusiak Ł, Kimball AB, Prens E, Wolk K. Hidradenitis suppurativa. *Nature Reviews. Disease Primers* 2020;*6*(1):1–20. Doi:10.1038/s41572-020-0149-1

Saguil A, Kane S, Mercado M, Lauters R. Herpes zoster and postherpetic neuralgia: Prevention and management. *American Family Physician* 2017;*96*(10):656–663.

Sandyk R. Seborrhea and Persistent Tardive Dyskinesia. *International Journal of Neuroscience* 1990;*50*(3–4):223–226. Doi:10.3109/00207459008987175

Sarkhani M, Rostami Mogaddam M, Fattahzadeh-Ardalani G, Fouladi N. Evaluation of the relationship between migraine and psoriasis: a case-control study. *Anais Brasileiros de Dermatologia* 2023;*98*:316–323. Doi:10.1016/j.abd.2022.04.009

Shah SS, Chhabra M. Parry-Romberg Syndrome. In: *StatPearls*. StatPearls Publishing; 2023. Accessed July 31, 2023. http://www.ncbi.nlm.nih.gov/books/NBK574506/

Shreberk-Hassidim R, Hassidim A, Gronovich Y, Dalal A, Molho-Pessach V, Zlotogorski A. Atopic Dermatitis in Israeli Adolescents from 1998 to 2013: Trends in Time and Association with Migraine. *Pediatric Dermatology* 2017;*34*(3):247–252. Doi:10.1111/pde.13084

Sia T, Webb T, Li S, Moskatel LS, Chang AS. An exploratory, comparative case series of calcitonin gene-related peptide monoclonal antibodies in migraine patients with rosacea. *The British Journal of Dermatology* In press.

Silverberg JI. Association between childhood eczema and headaches: An analysis of 19 US population-based studies. *The Journal of Allergy and Clinical Immunology.* 2016;*137*(2):492–499. Doi:10.1016/j.jaci.2015.07.020

Stefanko NS, Cossio ML, Powell J, et al. Natural history of PHACE syndrome: A survey of adults with PHACE. *Pediatric Dermatology* 2019;*36*(5):618–622. Doi:10.1111/pde.13871

Sudarsanam A, Ardern-Holmes SL. Sturge–Weber syndrome: From the past to the present. *European Journal of Paediatric Neurology* 2014;*18*(3):257–266. Doi:10.1016/j.ejpn.2013.10.003

Sulk M, Seeliger S, Aubert J, et al. Distribution and Expression of Non-Neuronal Transient Receptor Potential (TRPV) Ion Channels in Rosacea. *Journal of Investigative Dermatology* 2012;*132*(4):1253–1262. Doi:10.1038/jid.2011.424

Swartling C, Karlqvist M, Hymnelius K, Weis J, Vahlquist A. Botulinum toxin in the treatment of sweat-worsened foot problems in patients with epidermolysis bullosa simplex and pachyonychia congenita. *The British Journal of Dermatology* 2010;*163*(5):1072–1076. Doi:10.1111/j.1365-2133.2010.09927.x

Swartling C, Vahlquist A. Treatment of pachyonychia congenita with plantar injections of botulinum toxin. *The British Journal of Dermatology* 2006;*154*(4):763–765. Doi:10.1111/j.1365-2133.2005.07115.x

Taheri R, Nekuvaght Tak A, Masoudian N. Prevalence of migraine headache in patients with psoriasis vulgaris referred to dermatologists in Semnan, Iran: a crosssectional study. *Iranian Journal of Dermatology.* 2021;*24*(3):166–171. Doi:10.22034/ijd.2020.222747.1040

Tato BP, Martínez EZ, Albisua BS, et al. Facial and axillary apocrine chromhidrosis. *Dermatology Online Journal.* 2012;*18*(3). doi:10.5070/D34md22376

Teng JMC, Cowen EW, Wataya-Kaneda M, et al. Dermatologic and dental aspects of the 2012 international tuberous sclerosis complex consensus statements. *JAMA Dermatology* 2014;*150*(10):1095–1101. Doi:10.1001/jamadermatol.2014.938

Vadgama N, Lamont D, Hardy J, Nasir J, Lovering RC. Distinct proteomic profiles in monozygotic twins discordant for ischaemic stroke. *Molecular and Cellular Biochemistry* 2019;*456*(1):157–165. Doi:10.1007/s11010-019-03501-2

Wan MJ, Chan KL, Jastrzembski BG, Ali A. Neuro-ophthalmological manifestations of tuberous sclerosis: current perspectives. *Eye and Brain.* 2019;*11*:13–23. Doi:10.2147/EB.S186306

Wang IC, Tsai JD, Shen TC, Lin CL, Li TC, Wei CC. Allergic conjunctivitis and the associated risk of migraine among children: A nationwide population-based cohort study. *Ocular Immunology and Inflammation* 2017;*25*(6):802–810. Doi:10.1080/09273948.2016.1178303

Wei CC, Lin CL, Shen TC, Chen AC. Children with allergic diseases have an increased subsequent risk of migraine upon reaching school age. *Journal of Investigative Medicine* 2018;*66*(7):1064–1068. Doi:10.1136/jim-2018-000715

Wells T. Medical emergency: rash, headache and spinal cord injury. *BML Case Reports* 2021;*14*(4):e238285. Doi:10.1136/bcr-2020-238285

White S, Prado BM de, Russo AF, Hammond DL. Heat hyperalgesia and mechanical hypersensitivity induced by calcitonin gene-related peptide in a mouse model of neurofibromatosis. *PLoS One* 2014;*9*(9):e106767. Doi:10.1371/journal.pone.0106767

Wienholtz NKF, Christensen CE, Zhang DG, et al. Clinical characteristics of combined rosacea and migraine. *Front Med (Lausanne)*. 2022;*9*:1026447. Doi:10.3389/fmed.2022.1026447

Winter AK, Moss WJ. Rubella. *Lancet* 2022;*399*(10332):1336–1346. Doi:10.1016/S0140-6736(21)02691-X

Winter PR, Itinteang T, Leadbitter P, Tan ST. PHACE syndrome – clinical features, aetiology and management. *Acta Paediatrica* 2016;*105*(2):145–153. Doi:10.1111/apa.13242

Worm J, Falkenberg K, Olesen J. Histamine and migraine revisited: mechanisms and possible drug targets. *The Journal of Headache and Pain* 2019;*20*(1):30. Doi:10.1186/s10194-019-0984-1

Wu JM, Mamelak AJ, Nussbaum R, McElgunn PSJ. Botulinum toxin a in the treatment of chromhidrosis. *Dermatologic Surgery* 2005;*31*(8 Pt 1):963–965. Doi:10.1097/00042728-200508000-00014

Yang YW, Keller JJ, Lin HC. Medical comorbidity associated with psoriasis in adults: A population-based study. *The British Journal of Dermatology* 2011;*165*(5):1037–1043. Doi:10.1111/j.1365-2133.2011.10494.x

Yaszay B, Jablecki CK, Safran MR. Zoster paresis of the shoulder. Case report and review of the literature. *Clinical Orthopaedics and Related Research* 2000;(*377*):112–118.

Yell JA, Marren PM. Skin changes in epilepsy. *Journal of the European Academy of Dermatology and Venereology* 1993;2(3):217–224. Doi:10.1111/j.1468-3083.1993.tb00039.x

Yu J, Siegel DH, Drolet BA, et al. Prevalence and clinical characteristics of headaches in PHACE syndrome. *Journal of Child Neurology* 2016;*31*(4):468–473. Doi:10.1177/0883073815599261

Zanchi M, Favot F, Bizzarini M, Piai M, Donini M, Sedona P. Botulinum toxin type-A for the treatment of inverse psoriasis. *Journal of the European Academy of Dermatology and Venereology* 2008;*22*(4):431–436. Doi:10.1111/j.1468-3083.2007.02457.x

Endocrine Causes of Headache

7

Susan M. Seav and Marina Basina

LEARNING OBJECTIVES

1. Identify endocrine conditions that can cause or exacerbate headaches
2. Review initial evaluation for suspicious endocrine conditions
3. Review general principles for treatment of endocrine conditions that may lead to headache resolution

Case 1

Ms. F is a 54-year-old female who presents with the recent onset of a nonspecific headache for the past three months. She denies any previous history of headache, as well as any family history of headache. The headaches can be severe and can be associated with some nausea but without photophobia or phonophobia. During this time, she has also noticed some visual disturbances. She reports going through menopause five years earlier. She is given a diagnosis of migraine with aura and started on nortriptyline. After a three-month trial, she reports that her headaches are worse, and she has noticed that her vision continues to worsen.

PITUITARY

Nonfunctional Pituitary Adenomas

Clinically, nonfunctional pituitary adenomas (NFPA) are pituitary adenomas that are not hormonally active and therefore not associated with any clinical syndromes, such as Cushing's disease or acromegaly. They are often discovered incidentally or through signs and symptoms related to mass effect, including headache and visual field defects.

The prevalence of NFPA is 7–22 per 100,000 population, with an incidence rate of 1.02 per 100,000 per year.[1] They are usually diagnosed in the fifth decade of life and have an equal sex distribution. Although they are not the most common type of pituitary adenoma in general (falling second to prolactinomas), they are the most frequent cause of large pituitary macroadenomas, defined as pituitary lesions > 1 cm. Approximately 50% of nonfunctioning macroadenomas will increase at five years, and among these, 50% will lead to symptoms related to mass effect. On the other hand, nonfunctioning microadenomas (< 1 cm) tend not to increase in size.[2]

Most NFPAs present with headache, visual field defects, and/or hypopituitarism as a result of local pressure produced by the tumor on surrounding structures. Approximately 30%–70% of patients with pituitary adenomas report headache symptoms.[3, 4] The cause for headaches is thought to be dural stretch and invasion into the cavernous sinus.[3] Notably, there are mixed data regarding the association between tumor size and headache intensity or frequency.[4, 5] There is also conflicting data on an association with a family history of headache. Levy et al. reported on clinical headache scores for 63 patients initially seen for pituitary tumor and found a strong association between pituitary-associated headache and a family history of headache.[5] However, Gondim et al. conducted a similarly sized, prospective study and did not demonstrate any association with family history.[4]

Headache associated with NFPA tends to be nonspecific. They do not occur in any particular location, although bifrontal or retro-orbital locations are reported often. A prospective study in 2005 attempted to classify clinical headache phenotypes according to the International Headache Society (IHS) diagnostic criteria.[6] In this study, a total of 84 patients with pituitary tumors and troublesome headache were investigated, 24% of which had NFPA. Chronic migraine (46%) was the most common presentation, followed by episodic migraine (30%), primary stabbing headache (27%), short-lasting unilateral neuralgiform headache attacks with conjunctival injection and tearing (SUNCT; 5%), cluster headache (4%), and hemicrania continua (1%). Six headache presentations (7%) could not be classified according to the IHS criteria. Most other studies characterizing pituitary-associated headaches did not use the IHS criteria.

Surgery is the initial treatment for NFPA, especially if there is evidence of mass effect, such as persistent headache or optic nerve compression. However, there are no clear guidelines on patient selection or optimal timing of surgery. A study in Norway showed that patients with NFPA who underwent surgical treatment had better resolution of headache symptoms (85%) than patients who did not undergo surgery.[7] Surgical resection of nonfunctional microadenomas that do not cause any symptoms or biochemical hormonal derangements is generally not indicated since tumor growth is fairly rare (3%–13%), and less than 5% will grow more than 1 cm during long-term follow-up.[7] These microadenomas can be monitored with routine magnetic resonance imaging (MRI).

When to suspect NFPA

Patients with recent-onset, persistent headache or a change in characteristic from prior headaches associated with visual disturbances, exacerbated by increased intracranial pressure, and/or signs and symptoms of hypopituitarism.

Workup to consider

- Detailed history and physical examination to assess for hypopituitarism and bitemporal hemianopsia, as well as any clinical signs of acromegaly, Cushing's disease, or prolactinoma
- MRI of the sella
- Prolactin (PRL), thyroid-stimulating hormone (TSH), free thyroxine (FT4), morning cortisol, adrenocorticotropic hormone (ACTH), insulin-like growth factor 1 (IGF-1), luteinizing hormone (LH), follicle-stimulating hormone (FSH), testosterone (in men), estradiol (in women)

Case 2

Mr. T is a 58-year-old male with no previous history of headache who presents for headache after being referred from neurology. He reports that six months ago, he had the onset of a throbbing headache in the occiput that has been associated with nausea and sensitivities to light and sound. The neurologist diagnosed him with chronic migraine and elected to start him on metoprolol given his blood pressure of 146/84. After a three-month course of metoprolol, his headaches did not improve, and his blood pressure is unchanged. Physical exam demonstrated more coarse facial features and possible spacing of his teeth and initial labs showed a fasting glucose of 164.

Functional Pituitary Adenomas

Acromegaly

Acromegaly is a rare clinical syndrome of growth hormone (GH) excess. The annual incidence rate is 6–8 per million people. It is most often caused by a functional pituitary tumor arising from somatotroph cells secreting excessive GH. It can rarely be caused by ectopic secretion of GH or occur in the setting of other clinical syndromes, such as McCune Albright or Carney syndrome. Excessive GH leads to overproduction of IGF-1 by the liver. Both of these hormones cause the somatic overgrowth distinct to acromegaly. The clinical manifestations of acromegaly include gigantism (if disease onset is prior to long bone fusion), skin thickening, acral and soft tissue overgrowth, and visceral organ enlargement, as well as diabetes and hypertension.[8]

Headache is also a common feature of acromegaly. As discussed in the prior section, large pituitary masses (either functional or nonfunctional) can cause headache by mass effect. Although only 8% of patients with acromegaly may present with headache, approximately 60% will eventually develop headache as elevated serum GH may directly lead to headache, regardless of tumor size.[9] Chronic migraine is a common headache type in patients with acromegaly.[10] Additionally, treatment with somatostatin analogues has been shown to rapidly ameliorate headache symptoms by biochemical normalization of acromegaly, again independent of tumor size. Further supporting the notion that GH directly contributes to headache pathogenesis is the significant proportion of patients reporting headaches as a side effect of GH replacement therapy when used to treat GH deficiency. This side effect is more commonly seen in children.

The primary treatment for acromegaly is surgical resection, even with microadenomas. However, the recurrence rate is about 10% with microadenomas and up to 50% with macroadenomas, and often, these patients will have nonresectable residual tumors.[11] In these cases, medical therapy with somatostatin analogues (octreotide, lanreotide, pasireotide) can be used. Somatostatin analogues have been shown to have impressive analgesic properties, improving acromegaly associated headache in 64% of cases in one report.[6] Other therapies include GH receptor antagonist (pegvisomant), which can quickly lower IGF-1 levels; however, due to its mechanism of action, pegvisomant does not decrease GH levels, nor does it cause tumor shrinkage. It is unclear how effective pegvisomant is in improving headaches in patients with acromegaly. However, in the ACROSTUDY where 1288 patients on pegvisomant for a mean of 3.7 years were followed for adverse events, only 26 (2%) reported headaches, which is certainly a much smaller headache prevalence compared to untreated patients with acromegaly.[12]

Dopamine agonists like cabergoline have also been used off-label to treat acromegaly, especially in prolactin/GH dual-secreting tumors, although headache has been reported as an adverse effect with cabergoline therapy.[11] In a 2011 meta-analysis including ten studies reviewing cabergoline monotherapy in the management of acromegaly, Sandret et al. found that only 2.5% of patients noted persistent headache during treatment.[13]

When to suspect acromegaly

Patients with new-onset, unremitting headaches (especially migraine-like headaches) associated with a change in hat/ring/shoe size, change in bite size or facial appearance, recent-onset diabetes/arthralgias/obstructive sleep apnea, and/or visual disturbances.

Workup to consider

- Detailed history and exam to assess for large prominent facial features such as frontal bossing, prognathism, spacing of teeth, swelling/puffiness of soft tissue in hands and feet, skin tags, coarse skin, signs of carpal tunnel syndrome, bitemporal hemianopsia
- MRI of the sella
- Morning, fasting IGF-1, PRL, TSH, FT4, morning cortisol, LH, FSH, testosterone (in men), estradiol (in women)

Prolactinoma

Prolactinomas are the most common type of pituitary adenoma, accounting for over 50% of all pituitary adenomas. They arise from lactotroph cells and secrete prolactin. Women are ten times more likely to develop these tumors, with a mean age of diagnosis of about 30–37 years in women and 38–47 years in men.[14] Although hypogonadal symptoms and galactorrhea are the two most common clinical manifestations (experienced by 93% and 85% of women with prolactinoma, respectively), one study showed that a substantial proportion (46%) of patients also presented with headache.[15]

Headaches caused by prolactinomas have been described to be similar to migraines and trigeminal autonomic cephalalgias (TACs). In a small, retrospective study characterizing headache quality of 12 patients with prolactinoma, all patients treated with dopamine agonist endorsed an improvement in their headaches, with one patient endorsing the immediate return of headache after temporarily pausing treatment.[16] Similar findings have been shown in other studies.[17] However, there are some reported cases of worsening headache with dopamine agonist treatment.[6]

Unlike with other functional, hormone-secreting pituitary tumors, medical therapy with dopamine agonists (cabergoline, bromocriptine) can be used as the first-line therapy for prolactinomas as long as there is no significant mass effect such as optic nerve compression. Cases of severe headaches that do not improve with medical therapy should also be considered for surgery.

When to suspect prolactinoma

Patients (especially women) with recent-onset, persistent headache, or a change in characteristics from prior headaches associated with galactorrhea, amenorrhea, decrease in libido, and/or visual disturbances.

Workup to consider

- Detailed history and physical examination to assess for expressible galactorrhea, irregular menses, bitemporal hemianopsia
- MRI of the sella
- PRL, TSH, FT4, morning cortisol, morning fasting IGF-1, LH, FSH, testosterone (in men), estradiol (in women)

Pituitary Apoplexy

Pituitary apoplexy is a rare clinical syndrome caused by the abrupt hemorrhage and/or infarction of the pituitary gland. It is a complication of approximately 2%–12% of pituitary tumors, especially nonfunctioning adenomas, and has a prevalence rate of about 6.2 cases per 100,000 people.[18] It occurs more commonly in men and most frequently in the fifth and sixth decades of life.

Headaches associated with pituitary apoplexy are very specific and often the main presenting symptom. These headaches are described as severe and of a sudden onset. In numerous case reports and retrospective studies, apoplexy presented with sudden onset headache in 92%–100% of the cases.[19] Other presenting features may include visual disturbances if the optic nerve is physically perturbed. During apoplexy, corticotropic deficiency leading to adrenal insufficiency may cause life-threatening hemodynamic instability if left untreated. Head imaging with computed tomography (CT) or MRI is the primary method of confirming the diagnosis.[18]

Although pituitary apoplexy has the potential to be lethal, the outcomes from acute apoplexy are extremely variable and difficult to predict. Some patients suffer from intracranial bleeding secondary to the hemorrhaging pituitary or cerebral ischemia secondary to reactive cerebral vasospasm, as well as pituitary hormone deficiencies and visual loss. Others, however, suffer very little permanent sequelae and can be managed conservatively without the need for any surgical intervention. Because of this, treatment of apoplexy is evolving to a more watch-and-wait approach as opposed to emergent neurosurgical intervention.[20]

When to suspect pituitary apoplexy

Patients with acute onset, severe headache associated with profound fatigue, hemodynamic instability, hyponatremia or hypoglycemia, nausea/vomiting, and/or visual disturbances.

Workup to consider

- Detailed history and physical examination to assess for adrenal insufficiency, hypothyroidism, panhypopituitarism, and/or bitemporal hemianopsia
- MRI of the sella (can also perform CT head if more accessible given urgency)
- Random stat cortisol, TSH, FT4, sodium, glucose, and morning cortisol on the next day, morning fasting IGF-1, LH, FSH, testosterone (in men), estradiol (in women)

Hypophysitis

Hypophysitis occurs when there is a lymphocytic infiltration of the pituitary gland. This can be further characterized as primary or secondary. Primary pituitary hypophysitis is an organ-specific autoimmune infiltration that can be further divided into five categories based on the histopathologic features: lymphocytic hypophysitis (LHP), granulomatous hypophysitis (GHP), IgG-4 hypophysitis (IgG4HP), xanthomatous hypophysitis (XH), and necrotizing hypophysitis (NHP). Secondary hypophysitis is the sequela of a more systemic autoimmune disorder (such as sarcoidosis and Chron's disease; see Table 7.1) and is becoming a more frequently occurring entity in the setting of immune checkpoint inhibitor use for cancer treatment.

Autoimmune hypophysitis presents similarly to nonfunctional pituitary tumors, where headache and visual disturbances are the most commonly presenting symptoms. Anterior pituitary hormone deficiencies and arginine vasopressin deficiency (previously known as central diabetes insipidus) may also occur if the autoimmune infiltration disrupts normal cellular function and hormone secretion. Sometimes, hyperprolactinemia can be seen due to stalk effect, whereby the large sellar mass disrupts the negative feedback from dopamine traveling from the hypothalamus to lactotroph cells in the pituitary gland. In one literature review of 36 cases of XH, headache and irregular menses were the two most common clinical manifestations, both occurring in about 70% of the cases.[21]

A challenge in managing hypophysitis is establishing the diagnosis and etiology. A combination of imaging findings, inflammatory markers, antibody testing, and the presence or absence of other comorbid diseases can assist in diagnosing primary versus secondary hypophysitis. Of note, primary hypophysitis is a diagnosis of exclusion. A literature review by Caturegli et al. analyzed 379 patients with LHP and noted that MRI findings in LHP tended to have more homogeneous enhancement, intact sellar floor, stalk thickening, and loss of posterior hyperintensity compared to MRI findings of a pituitary macroadenoma. In LHP, stalk displacement and asymmetric mass were less commonly seen compared to the macroadenomas.

The treatment of hypophysitis is primarily symptomatic. This includes reducing the size of the pituitary mass if there is mass affect and/or replacing hormone deficiencies. Mass effect reduction can be achieved by pituitary surgery, lympholytic drugs (glucocorticoids, azathioprine, or methotrexate), or radiotherapy. If hypophysitis is secondary to a systemic autoimmune disorder or iatrogenically induced, such as with immune checkpoint inhibitors, then treatment of the underlying condition or discontinuation of the offending agent is recommended.

When to suspect hypophysitis

Patients (especially those with pre-existing autoimmune disorders or under immunotherapy treatment) presenting with recent-onset, persistent headache, or a change in characteristic from prior headaches associated with visual disturbances and/or signs and symptoms of hypopituitarism.

Workup to consider

- Detailed history and physical examination to assess for signs of systemic autoimmune disease, medications/treatments that augment the immune system, hypopituitarism, or bitemporal hemianopsia
- MRI of the sella
- PRL, TSH, FT4, morning cortisol, morning fasting IGF-1, LH, FSH, testosterone (in men), estradiol (in women)

Nonpituitary Sellar Masses

There are several other structures located in the sella that can present with headache if abnormal. Rathke's cleft cysts are benign cysts that arise from the embryologic remnant of the Rathke pouch, a dorsal invagination of the stomodeal ectoderm. In addition to mass effect, some hypothesize that headaches associated with Rathke's cleft cysts can be due to slow secretion of the cystic content, leading to an inflammatory response in the brain.[22] In a meta-analysis of surgical outcomes following Rathke's cleft cyst removal, Altuwaijri et al. found that 70% of patients experienced headache resolution.[23]

Craniopharyngiomas are malformational tumors arising along the craniopharyngeal duct. Although they have low histological malignancy, they can behave rather aggressively with complex and expansive invasion into nearby structures and are known to recur. In a retrospective study of 39 children and 150 adults diagnosed with craniopharyngiomas, acute visual symptoms, headache, and nausea/vomiting were the most frequently reported. Acute symptoms were more frequent among children (28%) than among adults (9%) (P < 0.01).[23]

Other less commonly found sellar masses that can present with headache include chordoma, epidermoid tumors, meningioma, metastatic tumors, lymphoma, vascular malformations, mucoceles, and abscesses.[24]

When to suspect nonpituitary sellar masses

Patients presenting with recent-onset, persistent headache, or a change in characteristic from prior headaches associated with visual disturbances, nausea/vomiting, and/or signs and symptoms of hypopituitarism.

TABLE 7.1 Systemic conditions that can affect the pituitary gland

SYSTEMIC INFLAMMATORY CONDITIONS	INFECTIONS	VASCULITIDES
Sarcoidosis disease	Tuberculosis	Wegener's granulomatosis
Langerhans cell histiocytosis	Syphilis	Takaysu's arteritis
	Fungal	Polyarteritis nodosa
		Churg-Strauss syndrome
		Kawasaki disease

Workup to consider

- Detailed history and physical examination to assess for hypopituitarism, malignancy, infection, and/or bitemporal hemianopsia
- MRI of the sella
- PRL, TSH, FT4, morning cortisol, morning fasting IGF-1, LH, FSH, testosterone (in men), estradiol (in women)

Systemic Conditions Affecting the Pituitary Gland

There are several systemic conditions that can directly affect or infiltrate the pituitary gland and cause headache. When patients present with multi-organ symptoms and new-onset or worsening headaches, head imaging should be considered to determine any intracranial involvement (Table 7.1).

THYROID

Hypothyroidism

Hypothyroidism is a common condition of thyroid hormone deficiency. It is seen in up to 3.7% of the population in the US and up to 5.3% in Europe.[25] It occurs more frequently in women over 65 years of age and more commonly in people with other autoimmune disorders such as type 1 diabetes and celiac disease. The clinical manifestations include fatigue, unintentional weight gain, cold intolerance, depressed mood, and constipation. In addition, up to one-third of patients with hypothyroidism will endorse headaches.[26] Interestingly, the prevalence of hypothyroidism has been found to occur more often in patients with tension-type headache (3.9%), migraine (3.2%), trigeminal neuralgia (6.1%), and occipital neuralgia (6.3%).[27]

According to the *International Classification of Headache Disorders, 3rd Edition* (*ICHD-3*; beta version), headache attributed to hypothyroidism (HAH) tend to be bilateral, nonpulsatile, and resolve after normalization of thyroid hormone levels.[26] A prospective cross-sectional study followed 73 patients with HAH for 12 months and noted that 78% reported alleviation in symptoms after treatment with levothyroxine. Even among patients with subclinical hypothyroidism (defined as elevated TSH but normal thyroxine hormone levels), there was improvement in headache symptoms with treatment.[28] The pathophysiology of HAH is unknown. Some speculate that the high TSH seen in primary hypothyroidism leads to pituitary gland growth, which causes increased intrasellar pressure.[29] Others attribute this disorder to a lower pain threshold in patients with hypothyroidism.[30]

A literature review conducted by Spanou et al. tried to identify any association between primary headaches (migraine and tension-type headache) and hypothyroidism.[31] The results of this review showed a possible bidirectional relationship between the aforementioned conditions; however, the data reviewed were considered to be of poor quality and too heterogenous to perform a meta-analysis. The authors nevertheless believe that headache, particularly migraines, may increase the risk of developing hypothyroidism. To explain this, there are also several unverified proposed mechanisms, such as alterations in the immune system leading to thyroid autoimmunity, a decrease in sympathetic function during interictal periods leading to hypothyroidism, and shared genetic/environmental disturbances that would lead to the development of both conditions.

Diagnostic criteria for headache attributed to hypothyroidism[26]

A. Headache fulfilling criterion C (evidence of causation)
B. Hypothyroidism has been demonstrated
C. Evidence of causation demonstrated by at least two of the following:
    1. Headache has developed in temporal relation to the onset of hypothyroidism or led to its discovery
    2. Either or both of the following:
        a. Headache has significantly worsened in parallel with worsening of the hypothyroidism
        b. Headache has significantly improved or resolved in parallel with improvement in or resolution of the hypothyroidism
    3. Headache has at least one of the following three characteristics:
        a. Bilateral location
        b. Nonpulsatile quality
        c. Constant over time
D. Not better accounted for by another *ICHD-3* diagnosis.

When to suspect hypothyroidism

Patients presenting with headaches in the setting of unintentional weight gain, hair loss, dry skin, constipation, and/or new-onset or worsening depressed mood.

Workup to consider

*   Detailed history and physical examination for signs and symptoms of hypothyroidism
*   TSH and FT4

Hyperthyroidism

Hyperthyroidism is a condition of thyroid hormone excess. In the United States, the prevalence of hyperthyroidism is approximately 1.2% (0.5% overt and 0.7% subclinical). The most common causes of hyperthyroidism are Graves' disease, toxic multinodular goiter, and autonomously functioning adenoma (also known as a hot or toxic nodule).[32] Hyperthyroidism typically occurs between the ages of 20 and 40 years and is much more common in women. The clinical manifestations include chest palpitations, heat intolerance, unintentional weight loss, hand tremors, increased frequency of bowel movements, and shortness of breath. In older patients, hyperthyroidism can present more atypically with apathy instead of hyperactivity.

Unlike with hypothyroidism, there is less association between primary hyperthyroidism and headache. Nevertheless, there are several case reports describing headache as the primary or initial presenting symptom in patients eventually diagnosed with thyrotoxicosis in whom symptoms resolved when thyroid hormones normalized.[33–35]

When to suspect hyperthyroidism

Patients (especially women) with headaches in the setting of unintentional weight loss, diarrhea, hand tremors, restlessness, new or worsening anxiety, and/or chest palpitations.

Workup to consider

- Detailed history and physical examination to assess for hyperthyroidism
- TSH, FT4, and total triiodothyronine (TT3)

ADRENAL

Pheochromocytoma and Paraganglioma (PPGL)

A pheochromocytoma is a neuroendocrine tumor that arises from catecholamine-secreting chromaffin cells in the adrenal medulla. A paraganglioma is a tumor that arises from extra-adrenal chromaffin cells found in the sympathetic paravertebral ganglia located in the thorax, abdomen, and pelvis; these can also secrete catecholamines. Paragangliomas can also arise from the parasympathetic ganglia located along the glossopharyngeal and vagal nerves in the neck and at the base of the skull. However, unlike the aforementioned tumors, these neck and skull base paragangliomas do not secrete catecholamines. About 80%–85% of chromaffin-cell tumors are pheochromocytomas, and 10%–15% are paragangliomas.[36] Together, they will be referred to as PPGL.

PPGL are very rare, with a prevalence rate of about 0.2%–0.6% in patients with hypertension. Mean age of diagnosis is 40–50 years, and in approximately one-third of cases, pheochromocytoma occurs in the context of familial syndromes such as multiple endocrine neoplasia syndromes (MEN 2A, MEN 2B), type I neurofibromatosis, von Hippel Lindau disease, and Sturge-Weber syndrome.[37]

One of the hallmark features of PPGL is headache. The classic triad associated with PPGL is paroxysmal headache, excessive sweating, and heart palpitations. Nevertheless, less than 25% of patients actually present with all three symptoms.[38] The headache characteristic associated with PPGL can be described as paroxysmal and migraine-like. However, there is significant variability in quality and intensity among patients. In a retrospective study of 27 patients with pheochromocytoma, 20 experienced headaches, and there was no association between headache quality and the amount of catecholamine produced. Furthermore, the authors noted that the lability of headaches was more linked to the rate of change of blood pressure than the absolute blood pressure values.[39] It is thought that the variable duration and intensity of headaches in patients with PPGL is due to the extent of intracranial vasoconstriction caused by the secreted catecholamines.

Treatment of PPGL is surgical resection. Pre-operative alpha-adrenergic receptor blockade is recommended to prevent pheochromocytoma crisis and its cardiovascular complications perioperatively.

When to suspect PPGL

Patients with paroxysmal headaches associated with episodes of diaphoresis, chest palpitations, elevated blood pressure, or panic attack–like symptoms.

Workup to consider

- Detailed history and physical examination to assess for PPGL
- CT or MRI of chest and abdomen/adrenal glands
- Plasma-fractionated metanephrines and/or 24-hour urine-fractionated metanephrines/catecholamines

GONADAL

Menstrual Migraine

Menstrual migraine (MM) is migraine that is mainly associated with menstruation. Pure MM attacks only occur with menstruation and have a prevalence rate of about 1%. In some female patients with migraine, the MM can attack during the time of menses and at other times during the menstrual cycle as well. These are called menstrually related migraines and have a higher prevalence rate of about 6%–7%. Compared to more typical migraines, MM are usually without aura, more intense, longer lasting, and more resistant to standard treatment. MM attacks can start two to three days prior to actual menstrual bleeding.[40]

MM is attributed to the dramatic changes in estrogen levels.[41] During the menstrual cycle, estrogen levels peak during the mid-follicular phase, just prior to ovulation, and decline soon afterward with a significant drop just a few days prior to menses. One of the first studies to support this theory was conducted in 1972 by Somerville et al., where they showed that intramuscular injections of estradiol a few days prior to menses delayed the onset of headache attacks in female migraineurs.[42] A similar trial done in 1986 by De Lignieres et al. with estrogen gel showed a decrease in duration and intensity of MM attacks in the treatment group compared to placebo.[43] Several additional studies have continued to show similar conclusions; however, the minimal estrogen threshold to trigger a migraine attack remains unclear.

Treatment options for MM are divided into three categories: acute, short-term prophylaxis, and daily preventative therapy. In a 2017 literature review by Maasumi et al., the authors found that for acute treatment, among the triptans, rizatriptan had the strongest efficacy data for pain relief within the first 24 hours of symptom onset. In short-term prophylaxis treatment, women are advised to start treatment a few days prior to menses for about a week every month, and zolmitriptan has a Food and Drug Administration indication for this use. Chronic daily preventative therapy can include antiepileptics. However, these must be used with caution, as some may have interactions with estrogen metabolism and oral contraceptive efficacy, especially with topiramate.[40]

When to consider MM

Women with monthly headaches that tend to occur just before or during menses and resolve before the next menstrual cycle.

Workup to consider

- Detailed history to assess any correlation between timing/severity of headache with menstrual cycle

Polycystic ovarian syndrome

Polycystic ovarian syndrome (PCOS) is the most common endocrine/metabolic disorder among women of reproductive age, with a prevalence rate of about 6%–10%.[44] The hallmark features of PCOS include androgen excess, ovulatory dysfunction, and/or polycystic ovaries. Although PCOS can lead to several sex hormone imbalances and infertility, it can also lead to significant cardiometabolic consequences, such as diabetes, obesity, dyslipidemia, and sleep apnea. Studies have shown that there is a high proportion of metabolic syndrome in patients with migraine. One report found that up to 32% of people with migraine also have metabolic syndrome, and 11% of patients with migraine have insulin resistance (IR).[45] However, this entity is controversial, with mixed data in the literature.

Alpha-lipoic acid (ALA), a cofactor of pyruvate dehydrogenase and alpha-ketoglutarate dehydrogenase, has been shown to have potent anti-inflammatory effects that improve IR in patients with PCOS.[46] In 2018, Cavestro et al. administered oral ALA to 32 patients with migraines and assessed IR as determined by the quantitative insulin-sensitivity check index. The authors found almost a 50% decrease in migraine attack rates at six months of treatment compared to baseline.[47] The authors concluded that ALA has the potential to be a treatment option for patients with migraine and IR. Some of the authors even postulated that a low-carbohydrate coupled with metformin could be used as well. However, there were many limitations to this study, including a small sample size, lack of a control arm, and exclusion of patients with PCOS. Based on reported glucose values, none of the patients had diabetes, and a significant portion (41%) were of normal weight; 9% were even underweight. In 2009, Pourabolghasm et al. conducted headache interviews with 133 women with PCOS and 107 women without PCOS and noted no significant difference in the prevalence of headaches in general or of migraine headaches.[48] Two other studies also did not show an increased prevalence of migraines in patients with IR.[49, 50]

Obstructive sleep apnea (OSA) is also common in PCOS as part of the metabolic syndrome, as well as with hyperandrogenism. OSA is certainly a risk factor for daytime headaches too. Obesity in itself has also been reported as a risk factor for higher migraine burden.[51] Although still unclear, the systemic inflammatory state associated with obesity is hypothesized to be the link with migraines.

The treatment of PCOS is very symptom-based.[52] As this condition has a very wide spectrum of clinical manifestations, treatment is aimed toward the most bothersome or concerning features. If patients have signs of metabolic syndrome or are overweight, then weight loss is advised. If hyperandrogenism or irregular menses is present, then oral combined contraceptive pills can be prescribed. Mineralocorticoid receptor antagonists can also be used to treat unwanted male-pattern hair growth in women with PCOS but do not necessarily lower serum testosterone levels.

When to consider PCOS

Female patients with headaches in the setting of elevated body mass index, irregular periods, unwanted or male-pattern hair growth, IR, and/or other signs of metabolic syndrome.

Workup to consider

- Detailed history and physical examination assessing for hirsutism, oligomenorrhea, acanthosis nigricans (evidence of diabetes)
- Testing for associated conditions: fatty liver disease, hypertension, dyslipidemia, OSA
- Pelvic ultrasound
- LH, FSH, testosterone, A1c, lipid panel, liver panel

DYSGLYCEMIA

In an observational study conducted in 1997 by Split and Szydlowska, the authors found a much higher prevalence of headache in patients with noninsulin-dependent diabetes compared to controls. In a total of 154 patients with diabetes, 82% endorsed headaches (nearly double that of the control group). Of these patients, 75% had migraine, a rate that is astonishingly much higher than the general population.[53] However, it is unclear if headaches in patients with diabetes are due to hyperglycemia or intermittent episodes of hypoglycemia.

For instance, fasting is a commonly known trigger for headaches in both patients with or without a chronic headache condition. In a similar observational study done by Blau and Pyke, who reviewed 36 patients with both diabetes and migraine diagnoses, they found that patients with nocturnal hypoglycemia had headache symptoms upon arousal. However, notably over 50% of the patients reviewed reported that diabetes in no way influenced their migraines.[54] Other studies have also reported mixed findings, and some argue that it is not the absolute glucose value that triggers headache but rather the rate of glucose decline. Nevertheless, the pathophysiology of how hypoglycemia triggers headaches is unclear. It is important to note that although peripheral venous hypoglycemia may occur, patients with diabetes, to a certain degree, are able to preserve normal brain glucose due to adapted regional differences in their cerebral blood flow and glucose utilization. There are theories that hypoglycemia leads to other metabolic processes that change the amount of free fatty acids, ketones, and other hormonal regulators such as dopamine and serotonin that can make certain patients more susceptible to pain and headache attacks.[55]

Besides uncontrolled diabetes, pancreatic neuroendocrine tumors (PNETs) can also cause significant dysglycemia. PNETs are neoplasms that arise from endocrine tissues in the pancreas. They are extremely rare, occurring at about four cases per one million patients per year. Although an estimated 50%–70% of these tumors are nonfunctional, they have the potential to secrete various hormones, including insulin, glucagon, gastrin, and vasoactive intestinal peptide. Of those, insulinomas are the most common and can lead to profound recurrent hypoglycemia. However, the most common symptoms associated with insulinomas are neuroglycopenic symptoms, such as confusion and lightheadedness. There was one case abstract that described a patient with five years of chronic headaches that were alleviated by eating or consuming sugary drinks. She was eventually diagnosed with an insulinoma with improvement in symptoms after tumor resection.[56]

When to consider dysglycemia

Patients with headaches in the context of diabetes associated with episodes of hypoglycemia or patients with no known history of diabetes but presenting with signs and symptoms of recurrent hypoglycemia.

Workup to consider

- Detailed history and physical examination to assess if headache episodes occur during periods of hypoglycemia or rapid changes in blood glucose levels
- Placement of a continuous glucose monitoring system
- Seventy-two-hour fasting test for suspected insulinoma

Figure 7.1 provides a comprehensive overview of determining an endocrine cause for headaches.

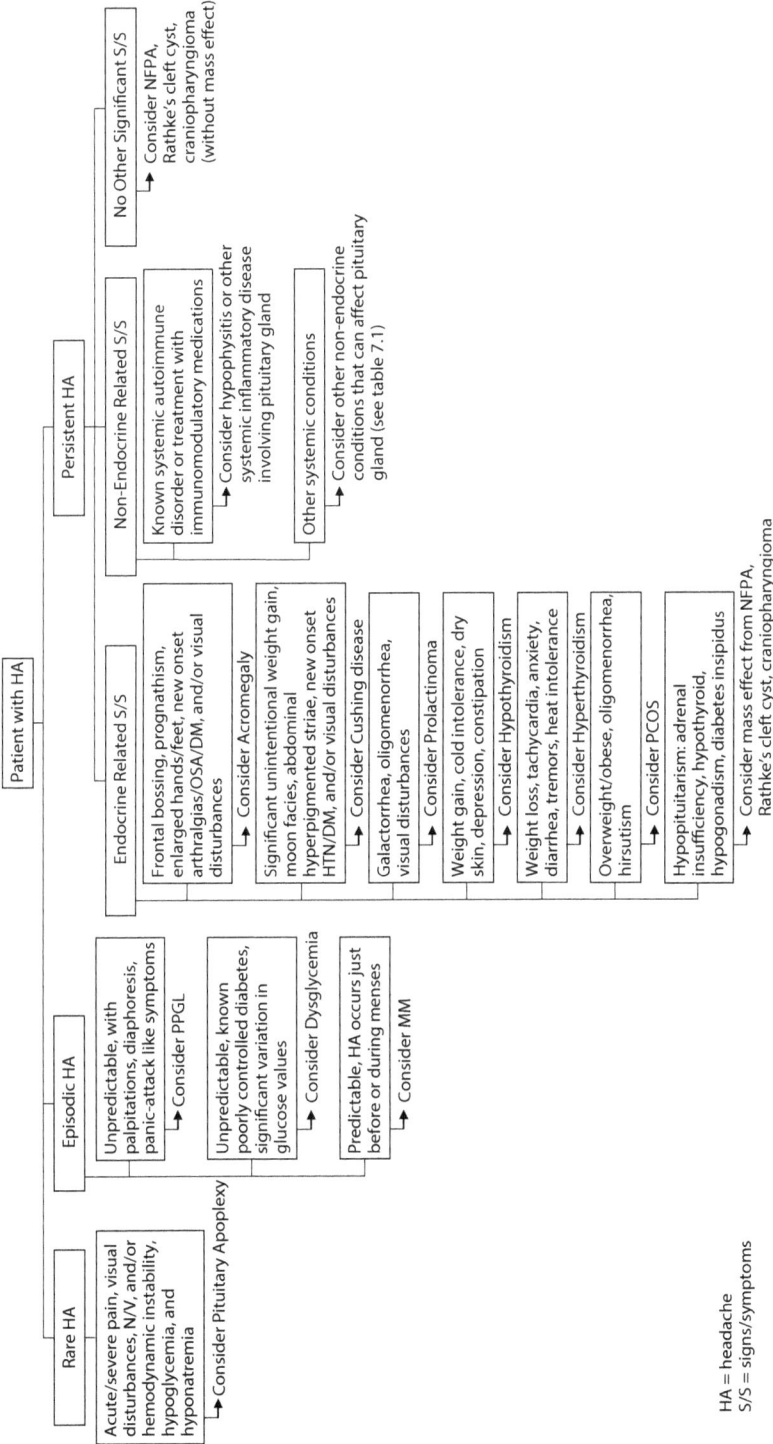

FIGURE 7.1   Algorithm for determining an endocrine cause for headaches.

REFERENCES

1. Fernandez A, Karavitaki N, Wass J. Prevalence of pituitary adenomas: a community-based, cross-sectional study in Banbury (Oxfordshire, UK). *Clin Endocrinol.* 2010;*72*(3):377–382.

2. Karavitaki N, Collison K, Halliday J, et al. What is the natural history of nonoperated nonfunctioning pituitary adenomas? *Clin Endocrinol (Oxf).* 2007;*67*(6):938–943. doi:10.1111/j.1365-2265.2007.02990.x

3. Kreitschmann-Andermahr I, Siegel S, Weber Carneiro R, Maubach JM, Harbeck B, Brabant G. Headache and pituitary disease: a systematic review. *Clin Endocrinol (Oxf).* 2013;*79*(6):760–769. doi:10.1111/cen.12314

4. Gondim JA, De Almeida JPC, De Albuquerque LAF, Schops M, Gomes É, Ferraz T. Headache associated with pituitary tumors. *J Headache Pain.* 2009;*10*(1):15–20. doi:10.1007/s10194-008-0084-0

5. Levy MJ, Jäger HR, Powell M, Matharu MS, Meeran K, Goadsby PJ. Pituitary volume and headache: Size is not everything. *Arch Neurol.* 2004;*61*(5):721. doi:10.1001/archneur.61.5.721

6. Levy MJ, Matharu MS, Meeran K, Powell M, Goadsby PJ. The clinical characteristics of headache in patients with pituitary tumours. *Brain.* 2005;*128*(8):1921–1930. doi:10.1093/brain/awh525

7. Esposito D, Olsson DS, Ragnarsson O, Buchfelder M, Skoglund T, Johannsson G. Nofunctioning pituitary adenomas: indications for pituitary surgery and post-surgical management. *Pituitary.* 2019;*22*(4):422–434. doi:10.1007/s11102-019-00960-0

8. nejmra062453.pdf.

9. Slagboom TNA, Van Bunderen CC, De Vries R, Bisschop PH, Drent ML. Prevalence of clinical signs, symptoms and comorbidities at diagnosis of acromegaly: a systematic review in accordance with PRISMA guidelines. *Pituitary.* 2023;*26*(4):319–332. doi:10.1007/s11102-023-01322-7

10. Kaniuka-Jakubowska S, Levy M, Pal A, et al. A study of acromegaly-associated headache with somatostatin analgesia. *Endocr Relat Cancer.* 2023;*30*(3):e220138.

11. Ershadinia N, Tritos NA. Diagnosis and treatment of acromegaly: An update. *Mayo Clin Proc.* 2022;*97*(2): 333–346. doi:10.1016/j.mayocp.2021.11.007

12. Van Der Lely AJ, Biller BMK, Brue T, et al. Long-term safety of pegvisomant in patients with acromegaly: Comprehensive review of 1288 subjects in ACROSTUDY. *J Clin Endocrinol Metab.* 2012;*97*(5):1589–1597. doi:10.1210/jc.2011-2508

13. Sandret L, Maison P, Chanson P. Place of cabergoline in acromegaly: A meta-analysis. *J Clin Endocrinol Metab.* 2011;*96*(5):1327–1335. doi:10.1210/jc.2010-2443

14. Tritos NA, Miller KK. Diagnosis and management of pituitary adenomas: A review. *JAMA.* 2023;*329*(16):1386. doi:10.1001/jama.2023.5444

15. Drange MR, Fram NR, Herman-Bonert V, Melmed S. Pituitary Tumor Registry: A Novel Clinical Resource. *J. Clin. Endocrinol. Metab.* 2000;*85*(1): 168–174.

16. Kallestrup MM, Kasch H, Østerby T, Nielsen E, Jensen TS, Jørgensen JO. Prolactinoma-associated headache and dopamine agonist treatment. *Cephalalgia.* 2014;*34*(7):493–502. doi:10.1177/0333102413515343

17. Al-Karagholi MAM, Kalatharan V, Ghanizada H, Gram C, Dussor G, Ashina M. Prolactin in headache and migraine: A systematic review of clinical studies. *Cephalalgia.* 2023;*43*(2):033310242211362. doi:10.1177/03331024221136286

18. Briet C, Salenave S, Bonneville JF, Laws ER, Chanson P. Pituitary Apoplexy. *Endocr Rev.* 2015;*36*(6): 622–645. doi:10.1210/er.2015-1042

19. Kreitschmann-Andermahr I, Siegel S, Weber Carneiro R, Maubach JM, Harbeck B, Brabant G. Headache and pituitary disease: a systematic review. *Clin Endocrinol (Oxf).* 2013;*79*(6):760–769. doi:10.1111/cen.12314

20. Barkhoudarina G, Kelly D. Pituitary Apolexy. *Neurosurgery Clinics of North America.* 2019;*30*(4):457–463.

21. Zhu J, Wang Z, Wang W, et al. Xanthomatous Hypophysitis: A Case Report and Comprehensive Literature Review. *Front Endocrinol.* 2021;*12*:735655. doi:10.3389/fendo.2021.735655

22. Altuwaijri N, Cote DJ, Lamba N, et al. Headache Resolution After Rathke Cleft Cyst Resection: A Meta-Analysis. *World Neurosurg.* 2018;*111*:e764–e772. doi:10.1016/j.wneu.2017.12.170

23. Nielsen EH, Jørgensen JO, Bjerre P, et al. Acute presentation of craniopharyngioma in children and adults in a Danish national cohort. *Pituitary.* 2013;*16*(4):528–535. doi:10.1007/s11102-012-0451-3

24. Freda P, Post K. Differential Diagnosis of Sellar Masses. *Endocrinol. Metab. Clin. North Am.* 1999;*28*(1):81–117.

25. Chaker L, Antonio B, Jacqueline J, Robin P. Hypothyroidism. *The Lancet.* 2017;*390*(10101):1550–1562.

26. Headache Classification Committee of the International Headache Society (IHS). The International Classification of Headache Disorders, 3rd edition (beta version). *Cephalalgia*. 2013;*33*(9):629–808. doi:10.1177/0333102413485658

27. Fernández-Garza LE, Marfil A. Comorbidity between hypothyroidism and headache disorders in a Mexican population. *Rev Neurol*. 2022;*75*(1):13–16.

28. Lima Carvalho MDF, De Medeiros JS, Valença MM. Headache in recent onset hypothyroidism: Prevalence, characteristics and outcome after treatment with levothyroxine. *Cephalalgia*. 2017;*37*(10):938–946. doi:10.1177/0333102416658714

29. Arafah BM, Prunty D, Ybarra J, Hlavin ML, Selman WR. The Dominant Role of Increased Intrasellar Pressure in the Pathogenesis of Hypopituitarism, Hyperprolactinemia, and Headaches in Patients with Pituitary Adenomas. *J. Clin. Endocrinol. Metab*. 2000;*85*(5): 1789–93.

30. Guieu R, Harley J, Blin O, Pouget G, Serratrice G. Nociceptive Threshold in Hypothyroid Patients. *Acta Neurol (Napoli)*. 1993;*15*(3):183–188.

31. Spanou I, Bougea A, Liakakis G, et al. Relationship of Migraine and Tension-Type Headache With Hypothyroidism: A Literature Review. *Headache J Head Face Pain*. 2019;*59*(8):1174–1186. doi:10.1111/head.13600

32. Ross DS, Burch HB, Cooper DS, et al. 2016 American Thyroid Association Guidelines for Diagnosis and Management of Hyperthyroidism and Other Causes of Thyrotoxicosis. *Thyroid*. 2016;*26*(10):1343–1421. doi:10.1089/thy.2016.0229

33. Takizawa T, Kurihara I, Suzuki N, Nakahara J, Shibata M. Painless Thyroiditis Presenting with Headache. *Intern Med*. 2021;*60*(16):2693–2696. doi:10.2169/internalmedicine.6975-20

34. Ashawesh K, Abdulqawi R, Ahmad S. Hyperthyroidism presenting with persistent vomiting, headache and deranged liver function tests. *Eur J Intern Med*. 2008;*19*(1):72. doi:10.1016/j.ejim.2007.06.002

35. Huang C, Shen S, Yao J. Subacute thyroiditis presenting as simple acute headache was misdiagnosed as meningitis: case report and literature review. *BMC Endocr Disord*. 2023;*23*(1):53. doi:10.1186/s12902-023-01313-6

36. Lenders JWM, Duh QY, Eisenhofer G, et al. Pheochromocytoma and Paraganglioma: An Endocrine Society Clinical Practice Guideline. *J Clin Endocrinol Metab*. 2014;*99*(6):1915–1942. doi:10.1210/jc.2014-1498

37. Anyfanti P, Mastrogiannis K, Lazaridis A, et al. Clinical presentation and diagnostic evaluation of pheochromocytoma: case series and literature review. *Clin Exp Hypertens*. 2023;*45*(1):2132012. doi:10.1080/10641963.2022.2132012

38. Westover C, Conran RM. Educational Case: Pheochromocytoma. *Acad Pathol*. 2018;*5*:2374289518780500. doi:10.1177/2374289518780500

39. Lance J, Hinterberger H. The headaches of phaeochromocytoma. *Proc Aust Assoc Neurol*. 1975;*12*:49–53.

40. Maasumi K, Tepper SJ, Kriegler JS. Menstrual Migraine and Treatment Options: Review. *Headache J Head Face Pain*. 2017;*57*(2):194–208. doi:10.1111/head.12978

41. Nappi R, Tiranini L, Sacco S, De Matteis E, De Icco R, Tassorelli C. Role of Estrogens in Menstrual Migraine. *Cells*. 2022;*11*(8):1355. doi:10.3390/cells11081355

42. Somerville BW. The role of estradiol withdrawal in the etiology of menstrual migraine. *Neurology*. 1972;*22*(4):355–355. doi:10.1212/WNL.22.4.355

43. de Lignieres B, Vincens M, Mauvais-Jarvis P, Mas J, Touboul P, Bouser M. Prevention of menstrual migraine by percutaneous oestradiol. *Br MEd J (Clin Res Ed)*. 1986;*293*(6561):1540.

44. Bozdag G, Mumusoglu S, Zengin D, Karabulut E, Yildiz BO. The prevalence and phenotypic features of polycystic ovary syndrome: a systematic review and meta-analysis. *Hum Reprod*. 2016;*31*(12):2841–2855. doi:10.1093/humrep/dew218

45. Bhoi SK, Kalita J, Misra UK. Metabolic syndrome and insulin resistance in migraine. *J Headache Pain*. 2012;*13*(4):321–326. doi:10.1007/s10194-012-0416-y

46. Masharani U, Gjerde C, Evans JL, Youngren JF, Goldfine ID. Effects of Controlled-Release Alpha Lipoic Acid in Lean, Nondiabetic Patients with Polycystic Ovary Syndrome. *J Diabetes Sci Technol*. 2010;*4*(2):359–364. doi:10.1177/193229681000400218

47. Cavestro C, Bedogni G, Molinari F, Mandrino S, Rota E, Frigeri MC. Alpha-Lipoic Acid Shows Promise to Improve Migraine in Patients with Insulin Resistance: A 6-Month Exploratory Study. *J Med Food*. 2018;*21*(3):269–273. doi:10.1089/jmf.2017.0068

48. Pourabolghasem S, Najmi S, Arami MA. Polycystic Ovary Syndrome and Migraine Headache, Is There Any Correlation? *Eur Neurol*. 2009;*61*(1):42–45. doi:10.1159/000165349

49. Sacco S, Altobelli E, Ornello R, Ripa P, Pistoia F, Carolei A. Insulin resistance in migraineurs: Results from a case-control study. *Cephalalgia*. 2014;*34*(5):349–356. doi:10.1177/0333102413511155

50. Ozcan R, Ozmen S. The Association Between Migraine, Metabolic Syndrome, Insulin Resistance, and Obesity in Women: A Case-Control Study. *Sisli Etfal Hastan Tip Bul actions Search in PubMed Search in NLM Catalog Add to Search.* 2019;*53*(4):395–402.

51. Cervoni C, Bond D, Keng E. Behavioral Weight Loss Treatments for Individuals with Migraine and Obesity. *Curr Pain Headache Rep.* 2016;*20*(2):13.

52. Legro RS, Arslanian SA, Ehrmann DA, et al. Diagnosis and Treatment of Polycystic Ovary Syndrome: An Endocrine Society Clinical Practice Guideline. *J Clin Endocrinol Metab.* 2013;*98*(12):4565–4592. doi:10.1210/jc.2013-2350

53. Split W, Szydlowska M. Headaches in non insulin-dependent diabetes mellitus. *Funct Neurol.* 1997;*12*(6):327–332.

54. Blau JN, Pyke DA. Effect Of Diabetes on Migraine. *The Lancet.* 1970;*296*(7666):241–243. doi:10.1016/S0140-6736(70)92588-2

55. Jacome DE. Hypoglycemia Rebound Migraine. *Headache J Head Face Pain.* 2001;*41*(9):895–898. doi:10.1111/j.1526-4610.2001.01163.x

56. Demaj E, Kermaj M. A case report of insulinoma in a patient with chronic headache. *Endocrine Abstracts.* 2017;*49*:EP634.

Gastrointestinal Symptoms and Comorbid Conditions in Migraine

8

Brandon K. Chu, Elisa Karhu, B.U.K. Li, and Irene Sonu

LEARNING OBJECTIVES

1. Review the similarities and differences between migraine, abdominal migraine, and cyclic vomiting syndrome
2. Learn the pathophysiology of migraine and comorbid gastrointestinal conditions
3. Identify the treatment of acute gastrointestinal symptoms during migraine attacks
4. Understand the key clinical features and management of cyclic vomiting syndrome and cannabinoid hyperemesis syndrome
5. Understand the key clinical features and management of abdominal migraine
6. Recognize the clinical features and management of acute and chronic nausea
7. List the chronic, comorbid conditions associated with migraine headaches and how to diagnose and manage them

---

INTRODUCTION

Patients with headache disorders commonly present with multiple gastrointestinal (GI) complaints. A survey of nearly 30,000 participants in the United States reports that 73% of patients with migraine experience nausea, and 29% experience vomiting [1]. Nausea is the most common GI symptom seen in patients with migraine but other GI symptoms include vomiting, diarrhea, reflux, and constipation [1, 2]. GI conditions such as cyclic vomiting syndrome (CVS) and abdominal migraines (AM) are considered migraine-equivalent conditions. Other chronic GI conditions ranging from irritable bowel syndrome (IBS) to celiac disease have also been associated with migraine. Recognizing, managing, and appropriately referring these comorbid GI conditions in patients with migraine is key to ensuring high care for these patients.

DOI: 10.1201/b23330-8

TABLE 8.1 Symptom overlap among patients with migraine headaches, CVS and AM

	MIGRAINE HEADACHE[a] (%)	CVS[a] (%)	ABDOMINAL MIGRAINE[a] (%)
Core Symptoms			
Vomiting	40–73	100	39–72
Abdominal Pain	10–55	3–81	100
Headache	100	38–59	31–50
Associated Symptoms			
Pallor	23–88	87	90–100
Lethargy		91	
Anorexia	13–93	74	91–98
Nausea	29–100	72	73–91
Photophobia	27–81	32	1–42

Note:
[a] Data from Reference [1, 2, 26]

Migraine, AM, and CVS each have different diagnostic criteria; however, there is significant phenotypic overlap among these disorders (Table 8.1). In the absence of diagnostic biomarkers, differentiating each disorder relies on a thorough history to ascertain the most troublesome symptom, as well as the timing and duration of symptoms, to ensure an accurate diagnosis. Severe episodes characterized by pulsating headaches predominate for migraine, whereas debilitating, periodic bouts of abdominal pain lasting 1–72 hours highlight AM. Recurring episodes of relentless nausea and vomiting are the hallmark features of CVS. Accompanying symptoms, such as pallor, flushing, photophobia, phonophobia, and nausea, can be observed in all three disorders. All conditions share similar precipitating events, including stress, travel, fatigue, and alleviating factors such as rest and sleep [3]. All three respond to antimigraine therapies. These conditions were historically considered periodic syndromes with severe, debilitating symptoms during acute exacerbations followed by symptom resolution. In each, patients may report a prodromal phase lasting minutes to hours as well as a recovery phase following an acute episode, with eventual return to baseline health. The interepisodic phase may last weeks to months at a time, with minimal or no symptoms [4, 5].

Although considered separate conditions, migraine, AM, and CVS may represent a continuum of a single disorder in which patients progress from one to the other [6, 7]. Pediatric school-based surveys have shown that the peak age of children with CVS is 5 years, AM is 9 years, and migraine is 11 years. Children with CVS begin to outgrow it at age 9 and may then develop AM but more typically develop migraine, and it is predicted that 75% of children will develop migraine by age 18 [7]. This progression of symptoms is not always linear. For instance, in the adult population, patients who develop adult-onset CVS may report a previous history of AM or migraine as a child. For clinicians, eliciting whether a patient exhibited any childhood symptoms of these related episodic disorders can be a useful clue to diagnosis.

PATHOPHYSIOLOGY

The pathophysiology of migraine and GI comorbidities is complex, with several potential shared pathways of overlap having been identified (Figure 8.1) [8]. These include a complex interplay of neurotransmitters, neuropeptides, inflammatory mediators, and changes in the microbiome [9]. The autonomic nervous system (ANS) is thought to play an important role in the overlap of migraine and GI dysfunction given shared symptoms of nausea, vomiting, dyspepsia, and motility disturbances and documented ANS abnormalities in migraine and various GI disorders [8, 10]. The nucleus tractus solitarius (NTS) in the brainstem is also involved in regulating vomiting and GI motility and may contribute to the nausea, vomiting, and reduced gastric motility that has been documented in migraine [8].

Gut–Brain Axis

GI tract functions:
➤ Digestion/absorption
➤ Sensory
➤ Secretion
➤ Motility
➤ Gut microbiota

Bi-directional communication
mediated by:
➤ CNS
➤ ENS
➤ Vagal nerve
➤ Microbiota-derived
  neurotransmitters and
  metabolites
➤ Inflammatory cytokines
➤ Hormones
➤ Alterations in intestinal
  permeability

Brain functions:
➤ Cognition
➤ Behavior
➤ Nociception
➤ Salience

Pathology:
➤ CVS
➤ Abdominal migraine
➤ IBS
➤ IBD
➤ GERD/PUD
➤ FD/Gastroparesis
➤ Celiac Disease

Pathology:
➤ Migraine
➤ CVS
➤ Abdominal migraine
➤ Depression
➤ Anxiety
➤ Neurodegenerative
  disorders

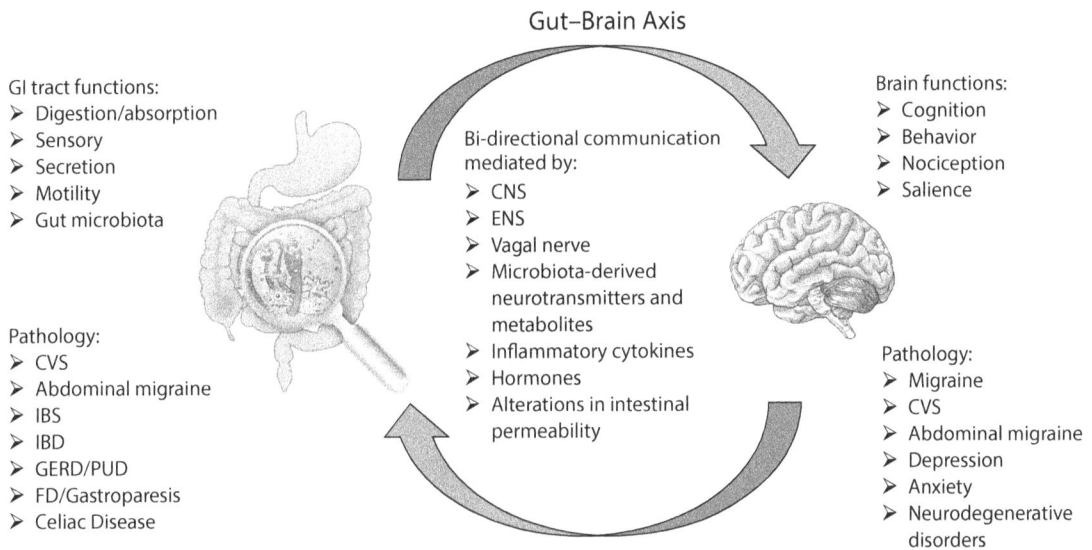

FIGURE 8.1 CNS, Central nervous system; ENS, Enteric nervous system; GI, Gastrointestinal; CVS, Cyclic vomiting syndrome; IBS, Irritable bowel syndrome; IBD, Inflammatory bowel disease; GERD, Gastroesophageal reflux disease; PUD, Peptic ulcer disease; FD, Functional dyspepsia.

Neurotransmitters

The neurotransmitter serotonin has been implicated in the pathophysiology of migraine and GI disorders [8]. Serotonin can act as both a vasodilator and vasoconstrictor, modulating nociceptive pain. Decreased activity of $5\text{-HT}_{1B/1D}$ receptors has also been thought to activate the trigeminovascular (TGV) system involved in the initiation of a migraine attack and through subsequent neuronal activation in the NTS [8]. Further, over 95% of the body's total serotonin is housed in the GI tract within the enteric nervous system, where it regulates GI motility and secretion, thus resulting in GI symptoms [11–14]. Serotonin activation is a key mechanism in the modulation of chronic abdominal pain in disorders of gut-brain interaction (DGBIs), such as IBS, which commonly are seen in patients with migraine [15]. Serotonin receptors are also found on immune cells, including monocytes, macrophages, lymphocytes, and dendritic cells, supporting their role in immune modulation [16]. Given its immunomodulatory effects, serotonin has a role in increasing the susceptibility to inflammatory GI diseases, such as inflammatory bowel disease (IBD), celiac disease, and diverticulitis [16].

Glutamate, another neurotransmitter, acts in an excitatory fashion and contributes to migraine through central sensitization, cortical spreading depression, and stimulation of the TGV system. Studies have found increased levels of glutamate in the plasma and cerebrospinal fluid of patients with migraines [9, 17]. Disturbances in glutamate pathways are thought to be involved in the pathogenesis of numerous GI disorders, including IBD, IBS, and gastroesophageal reflux disease (GERD) [9]. In the GI tract, glutamate has been implicated in inflammation and oxidative stress, motility, and modulation of visceral hypersensitivity [18].

Neuropeptides

Neuropeptides are thought to play a role in the development of both migraine and GI disorders. The neuropeptide calcitonin gene-related peptide (CGRP) is widely distributed in the central and peripheral nervous system and is predominantly expressed in sensory and enteric neurons, innervating a variety of areas within the digestive system [19]. CGRP has been shown to inhibit gastric acid secretion and may suppress food intake, potentially leading to alterations in the microbiome as well as the digestion and absorption of food [20]. Neuropeptides, including CGRP, are hypothesized to exert an antimicrobial impact on the gut microbiota and influence the gut-brain axis [9]. CGRP is also released from trigeminal nerves in migraine, and monoclonal antibodies and small molecule inhibitors targeting CGRP have gained widespread clinical use for the acute and preventive treatment of migraine [19, 21–23].

Inflammatory Mediators and Microbiota

Various inflammatory mediators, including IL-1β, IL-6, IL-8, and TNF-α, can influence the development of migraine as well as GI symptoms. In migraine, these inflammatory mediators can affect nociceptive responses in the trigeminal pathway, triggering migraine attacks, while GI symptoms may be mediated by the bidirectional association between inflammation and intestinal permeability. Proinflammatory cytokines can increase intestinal permeability, which can in turn stimulate inflammation through lipopolysaccharide (LPS) leakage [9].

The gut microbiome can become disrupted through stress, including diet, infections, inactivity, psychological stress, and sleep disturbances. The microbiome is an important mediator of pain and GI symptoms through indirect signaling of microbiota-derived neurotransmitters, inflammatory molecules, and hormones, as well as direct stimulation of end terminals of the vagus nerve [9]. Short-chain fatty acids, including butyrate, propionate, and acetoacetate, produced by intestinal bacteria through fermentation of indigestible carbohydrates are not only important for the maintenance of intestinal epithelial lining but have also been shown to exert neuroprotective and anti-inflammatory effects [24]. Neuroprotective effects in the brain include promoting cell proliferation and differentiation in the dentate gyrus, increasing the expression of brain-derived neurotrophic factor and glia-derived neurotrophic factor, and improving memory performance [24]. In turn, anti-inflammatory effects in the gut and brain are mediated through the prevention of TNF-α induction by the endotoxin LPS via the suppression of nuclear factor κB [24]. The gram-negative bacteria-derived LPS in the setting of a compromised intestinal barrier can gain entry into circulation, promoting endotoxemia and systemic inflammation. One study showed that antibiotic disruption of the microbiome prolonged migraine-like pain in mice, while administration of probiotics inhibited the antibiotic-mediated pain prolongation [25].

In summary, several shared pathophysiological pathways, including serotonin, neuropeptides, inflammatory mediators, and microbiome effects, have been proposed to explain the relationship between migraine and GI disorders.

GASTROINTESTINAL SYMPTOMS AND MANAGEMENT IN ACUTE MIGRAINE

Patients with migraine may experience a variety of GI symptoms during acute migraine episodes or due to chronic comorbid GI conditions. Nausea, vomiting, retching, abdominal pain, and inability to tolerate food are frequently reported during an acute episode and can be as debilitating as the headache itself. In fact, nausea and vomiting are the most common GI manifestations of migraine and are part of the *International Classification of Headache Disorders, 3rd Edition* (*ICHD-3*) diagnostic criteria for it. Approximately 90% of patients with migraine experience nausea, and 70% experience vomiting [26]. Nausea, vomiting, and retching may appear at the same time as pain but typically develop an hour after the onset of a headache. Severe nausea and vomiting may necessitate hospitalization for dehydration, electrolyte imbalance, and symptom management with intravenous (IV) medications. Nausea and vomiting also hinder migraine management, as nearly 30% of patients who experience nausea report that they interfer with their ability to take their oral migraine medications [27].

Abdominal pain and dyspepsia are symptoms that can be associated with migraine. Dyspepsia is defined as having one or more symptoms of bothersome epigastric pain, burning, postprandial fullness, or early satiety. Associated symptoms may include belching, nausea, vomiting, or heartburn. Examples of organic causes of dyspepsia include peptic ulcer disease (PUD), GERD, and gastric cancer [28]. Functional dyspepsia is a DGBI where there is no structural disease to explain symptoms. Several theories have been proposed to explain the association between migraine and dyspepsia. Gastric dysmotility (gastroparesis) has been observed both during migraine attacks and interictal periods, which may result in dyspeptic symptoms [29].

Treatment of Key GI Symptoms during Acute Migraines

The main goal of migraine management is to initiate acute treatment as soon as possible once an attack has begun. Acute therapies include acetaminophen, nonsteroidal anti-inflammatory drugs (NSAIDs), triptans, dihydroergotamine (DHE), and CGRP antagonists. Oral medications are usually well tolerated; however, they become less effective in patients who have concomitant nausea and vomiting, presumably due to delayed gastric emptying and drug bioavailability [27]. For patients who have a high frequency of nausea and vomiting during migraine attacks, several other treatment options are available (Table 8.2).

Dopamine$_2$ receptor antagonists such as prochlorperazine and metoclopramide have been extensively studied and are effective agents for nausea and vomiting in migraineurs. These agents, when administered via IV, can also serve as monotherapy for acute migraine attacks. The most common side effects are sedation and drowsiness, and they may also cause extrapyramidal side effects. IV diphenhydramine can be

TABLE 8.2   Treatment of gastrointestinal symptoms in acute migraine headaches

	Nausea and Vomiting
Initial management	➤ Abortive therapies for migraine headaches (e.g., triptans, DHE, CRGP antagonists) ➤ Volume assessment and hydration, electrolyte replacement if necessary ➤ Simple analgesics (NSAIDs and acetaminophen)
First-line therapies	➤ Prochlorperazine or metoclopramide ➤ Consider the addition of diphenhydramine to reduce the risk of akathisia and acute dystonic reactions ➤ Consider addition of NSAIDs with metoclopramide
Second-line or adjunctive therapies	➤ Droperidol or haloperidol for refractory nausea and vomiting ➤ Promethazine as an adjunctive therapy. Avoid in patients younger than 2 years ➤ Consider ondansetron; monitor for constipation and QTc prolongation ➤ Consider aprepitant and fosaprepitant
	Dyspepsia/Abdominal Pain
Initial management	➤ Rule out pathologic causes of abdominal pain
First-line therapies	➤ Trial course of proton pump inhibitor
Second-line or adjunctive therapies	➤ Tricyclic antidepressants such as amitriptyline or nortriptyline ➤ Metoclopramide or other prokinetic agents for refractory symptoms ➤ Consider antinociceptive agents such as gabapentin ➤ Limit opiates and NSAIDs; acetaminophen is acceptable

given as a premedicating agent to reduce the risk of akathisia and acute dystonic reactions [30]. IV/intramuscular (IM) administration of metoclopramide is the preferred route of administration. However, oral administration in the absence of vomiting is acceptable. A combination of oral metoclopramide and NSAIDs has been found to be as effective as oral sumatriptan in managing headache symptoms and more effective in the treatment of nausea [31]. IV/IM prochlorperazine is also the preferred route of administration for migraine, but a recent randomized control trial found a buccally absorbed form of prochlorperazine to be equally efficacious with lower rates of extrapyramidal side effects [32]. Droperidol and haloperidol are first-generation dopamine agonists that have been used for nausea, vomiting, and migraine attacks, but due to increased risks of extrapyramidal side effects, some societies have recommended against their use as first-line agents [33]; they can be used as second-line agents if patients continue to have ongoing nausea and vomiting despite initial medical treatment.

Ondansetron and granisetron are 5-HT_3 antagonists that act centrally in the chemoreceptor trigger zone of the area postrema and peripherally on afferent vagus nerves [34]. There are limited studies evaluating their efficacy in patients with migraine, and several case series have noted increased frequency of headaches following administration of ondansetron [35, 36]. These agents can also result in constipation and cardiac effects, including QTc prolongation. In light of the limited efficacy data and side effect profile, several guidelines recommend against the use of granisetron during migraine attacks [33, 37].

Promethazine is a phenothiazine derivative with antidopaminergic, antihistamine, and anticholinergic properties. It has not been independently studied for efficacy in migraine, but it has been used as an adjunctive therapy due to its sedative and antiemetic properties [38]. The preferred route of administration is IM due to the risk of severe tissue injury, including tissue necrosis from IV extravasation. Promethazine should not be used in pediatric patients younger than two years because of the risk of fatal respiratory depression [39].

Benzodiazepines have anxiolytic, sedative, and mild antiemetic properties. When taken chronically, benzodiazepines are associated with serious side effects such as addiction and sedation, as well as worsening headaches. There are limited studies specifically evaluating benzodiazepines for acute migraine. A randomized controlled trial involving 90 patients found that compared to ibuprofen monotherapy, the combination of ibuprofen 200 mg and 1 mg of lorazepam was as effective in treating headache symptoms and more effective in resolving nausea and vomiting [40]. While these results seem promising, larger studies are needed. Although benzodiazepines have been used sparingly as an adjunct for acute migraines in select cases, current guidelines do not recommend the routine use of benzodiazepines for migraine attacks [41].

Aprepitant and fosaprepitant are neurokinin-1 (NK1) receptor antagonists that have an excellent safety profile and, unlike other antiemetics, do not prolong QTc and lack sedative effects [42]. Despite the efficacy of these medications in treating nausea and vomiting in CVS, there are limited data evaluating their role in migraine. A retrospective chart review (74 patients) found aprepitant was effective in treating DHE-induced nausea and emesis when dopamine receptor antagonists, 5-HT_3 receptor antagonists, and antihistamines failed. The study also found that aprepitant was effective in migraine patients with marked nausea even before DHE administration [43]. Further studies are needed to support the role of NK1 receptor antagonists in migraine, but given their excellent safety profile, they should be considered as an adjunctive antiemetic when first-line agents are unsuccessful.

Those who develop chronic dyspepsia with migraine have several options to help alleviate their symptoms. After ruling out alternative pathologic causes (e.g., H. pylori), a trial of antisecretory agents such as proton pump inhibitors (PPIs) has been effective in relieving overall dyspepsia symptoms. Patients with ongoing symptoms of dyspepsia despite a trial of PPIs may benefit from the initiation of a tricyclic antidepressant such as amitriptyline or nortriptyline [44]. Prokinetic agents such as metoclopramide may also be used for those who have exhausted other therapies [45]. Although NSAIDs are effective in migraine, they may worsen dyspeptic symptoms and should therefore be limited if possible. Likewise, opiates should be limited as well due to their adverse side effect profile, especially the risk of dependency. Analgesics such as acetaminophen are safe and permissible to use in moderation. There is growing evidence that antinociceptive agents such as gabapentin may be effective in improving symptoms of dyspepsia, though further studies are needed [46, 47].

CYCLIC VOMITING SYNDROME

CVS is characterized by recurrent, stereotypical bouts of nausea and vomiting with intervening periods of normalcy between episodes [48]. It has been considered a migraine-equivalent disorder with predominantly GI manifestations. CVS affects both adults and children with a significant impact on the quality of life for patients due to recurrent disruptive episodes, emergency department visits and hospitalizations, and comorbid symptoms that persist in between attacks. The prevalence of CVS is estimated to be 2% in both children and adults [49, 50]. In children, the average age of symptom onset is around 5 years, with around a two-year delay in formal diagnosis. There is a slight female predominance (55:45) in children. The majority of pediatric patients experience resolution at a median age of 9.9 years but often then develop migraine [51, 52]. In adults, the mean age of onset for CVS is believed to be around the age of 35 [50]. In adults, there is presently no clearly defined sex predominance.

CVS is considered a DGBI and is included in both the Rome IV and ICHD-3 classifications (Table 8.3) [53, 54]. The characteristic features of CVS include recurrent episodes of vomiting that occur in a stereotypical pattern within individuals. The vomiting is typically projectile, occurring multiple times per hour, and significantly debilitating for patients. Interestingly, once the stomach is emptied, retching may continue at the same pace, suggesting a central rather than gastric driver. Nausea, for many, is the most distressing symptom and is often difficult to treat, but it may improve with sleeping or sedation. Midline abdominal pain during episodes is a common physical complaint. Migraine features, including headache, photophobia, and phonophobia, have been frequently reported as well, although in less than half of affected children. Other associated signs and symptoms include pallor, diaphoresis, anxiety, profound fatigue, and lethargy [50].

Episodes occur at regular or varying intervals in half of patients each. Some patients also identify antecedent triggers such as emotional stress or physical stressors, such as infection or lack of sleep. Following an episode, patients typically return to normal or baseline health, though up to 36% of adults will have continued symptoms, usually persistent daily nausea, during the interictal phase. It is noteworthy that approximately one-half of adults with CVS reported a history of physical or sexual abuse as a child [55].

The treatment of CVS in adults is divided into the acute management of emetic episodes and prophylactic treatment to prevent future episodes. Those during the prodromal phase may respond to abortive nasal or subcutaneous sumatriptan, similar to those with migraine [18]. Once the patient is in a well-established episode, no treatment will stop it, and care becomes supportive and symptom-directed. For patients who present to the hospital, the 2019 adult guidelines recommend a supportive regimen of antiemetics, analgesics, and sedation [48]. Recommended antiemetics include IV ondansetron, followed by IV prochlorperazine or fosaprepitant. Managing pain is also indicated, and ketorolac is preferred over opioids. Sedation with IV diphenhydramine, lorazepam, or droperidol is an important adjunct in the acute treatment of CVS and potentially the only means to attenuate symptoms. Patients may benefit from staying in a dark, quiet room with limited sensory stimulation, as many are hyperaesthetic to sound, light, and even touch, similar to some patients with migraine.

For patients who experience frequent (e.g., monthly) and debilitating episodes of CVS, prophylactic therapy should be considered. Lifestyle modification, including sleep hygiene, regular meals, hydration, exercise, and stress reduction (e.g., meditation) are recommended. Tricyclic antidepressants (TCAs), such as amitriptyline up to doses of 75 to 100 mg per day, are the first-line choice for pharmacologic prophylaxis. Second-line prophylactic agents include aprepitant or anticonvulsants, such as topiramate, zonisamide and levetiracetam. Mitochondrial supplements such as coenzyme Q10 and riboflavin have been used successfully as adjunctive therapy in conjunction with other prophylactic agents.

Cannabinoid hyperemesis syndrome (CHS), a newer entity that overlaps with CVS, is fast-rising in states with legalized recreational cannabis. The first and still best characterized series of nine patients was described by Allen et al. in South Australia [56]. The largest review of 376 patients revealed that 69%–72% with CHS were male, mean age 29 years, the duration of cannabis use before onset was 6.6–8.0 years, and hot

TABLE 8.3   Diagnostic criteria for CVS and AM

		DIAGNOSTIC CRITERIA
CVS[a]	ROME IV	*Must include **all** of the following*:*

*Must include **all** of the following*:*

1. Stereotypical episodes of vomiting regarding onset (*acute*) and duration (*less than one week*)
2. At least three discrete episodes in the prior year and two episodes in the past six months, occurring at least one week apart
3. Absence of vomiting between episodes, but other milder symptoms can be present between cycles

*Criteria fulfilled for the last three months with symptom onset at least six months prior to diagnosis

ICHD-3

A. At least five attacks of intense nausea and vomiting, fulfilling criteria B and C
B. Stereotypical in the individual patient and recurring with predictable periodicity
C. All of the following:
   1. Nausea and vomiting occur at least four times per hour
   2. Attacks last for ≥ 1 hour, up to 10 days
   3. Attacks occur ≥ 1 week apart
D. Complete freedom from symptoms between attacks
E. Not attributed to another disorder

Abdominal migraine[b]   ROME IV   *Must include **all** of the following occurring at least twice*:*

1. Paroxysmal episodes of intense, acute periumbilical, midline, or diffuse abdominal pain lasting one hour or more (should be the most severe and distressing symptom)
2. Episodes are separated by weeks to months
3. The pain is incapacitating and interferes with normal activities
4. Stereotypical pattern and symptoms in the individual patient
5. The pain is associated with ***two or more*** of the following: anorexia, nausea, vomiting, headache, photophobia, or pallor
6. After appropriate evaluation, the symptoms cannot be fully explained by another medical condition

*Criteria fulfilled for at least six months prior to diagnosis

ICHD-3

A. At least five attacks of abdominal pain, fulfilling criteria B–D
B. Pain has at least two of the following three characteristics:
   1. Midline location, periumbilical or poorly localized
   2. Dull or "just sore" quality
   3. Moderate or severe intensity
C. At least two of the following four associated symptoms or signs:
   1. Anorexia
   2. Nausea
   3. Vomiting
   4. Pallor
D. Attacks last 2–72 hours when untreated or unsuccessfully treated
E. Complete freedom from symptoms between attacks
F. Not attributed to another disorder

Note:
[a] Sourced from [53, 54].
[b] Sourced from [54, 68, 103].

water bathing was used therapeutically in 75%–86% [48]. Other key clinical features included the recurrence of episodes every one to four months and resolution of symptoms after cessation of cannabis. CHS also occurs in adolescents with a mean age of 16, 62%–64% girls, daily usage for 3.5 years, but with similarly high rates of response to hot water hydrotherapy 71%–91% [57]. Response to hot water bathing, once thought to be pathognomonic for CHS, also occurs in 48% of CVS without cannabis use [58]. In Colorado, the first state to legalize recreational cannabis in 2012, the rates of emergency department visits for CHS doubled in an eight-year span, and hospitalizations increased 46% over five years [59, 60]. After a careful review of these, the task force concluded that CHS is a subset of CVS triggered by chronic high-dose recreational usage [48].

The endocannabinoid system helps attenuate the stress response. Cannabis sativa, the main marijuana species grown commercially, consists of > 450 constituents. The two main medicinal components are Δ^9-tetrahydrocannabinol (THC), the psychoactive component, which acts on CB1 receptors, and cannabidiol (CBD), which is not psychoactive and acts upon $5HT_{1A}$ [61]. The advent of CHS appears to be related both to the 20-fold increase in potency in addition to legalization. Chronic usage is known to reduce the number of CB1Rs both in animals and humans. As THC is a weak CB1R agonist and hence a weak antiemetic, it has been postulated that THC displaces stronger endocannabinoids on fewer remaining receptors, resulting in the antiemetic effect falling below a critical threshold [62].

Based on limited anecdotal data, agents used to treat CVS, such as ondansetron and metoclopramide, do not appear effective in CHS [63]. Two unique modalities appear more effective in CHS. First, hot water hydrotherapy is used in the majority of CHS patients and half of those with CVS [64]. Patients respond within 5–10 minutes, and the therapeutic effect dissipates within 10–30 minutes after stopping. Hot water at 43°C is known to activate TRPV-1 receptors that can act as a central antiemetic [65]. Second, topical capsaicin from chili peppers applied topically to the abdomen also stimulates TRPV-1 receptors and appears effective [66]. Interestingly, central CB1Rs are part of the endogenous thermoregulatory response. As CB1Rs and TRPV-1 receptors are co-localized on the same neurons, both may be actively involved in the therapeutic antiemetic effect during acute attacks. At present, whether standard prophylactic therapy (TCAs, anticonvulsants, or aprepitant) used to treat CVS is effective in the prevention of recurring CHS attacks is unknown [67]. If the key therapeutic principle is the restoration of the normal density of CB1Rs, then the definitive treatment is either complete cannabis cessation or at least below a critical threshold.

ABDOMINAL MIGRAINE

AM is a disorder characterized by recurring severe episodes of poorly localized abdominal pain that interferes with normal activities in an otherwise healthy individual. AM is considered a migraine equivalent. This condition is primarily recognized in children but has been reported occasionally in adults. The prevalence of AM in the pediatric population ranges from 0.4%–4% [3]. It affects more girls, with most being between 3–10 years of age. Children who have AM have a propensity to subsequently develop migraine headaches (MH) and recurrent abdominal pain as adults. Epidemiologic data on adults is limited, likely because it is often underdiagnosed given the significant overlap with other causes of recurrent abdominal pain in adults, such as IBS.

AM should be considered an etiology when an adult presents with recurrent, discrete bouts of abdominal pain rather than daily pain and a completely negative GI evaluation. AM is included in both Rome IV and ICHD-3 to facilitate a consistent diagnosis (Table 8.3) [54, 68, 69]. Patients typically present with recurrent, severe attacks of abdominal pain and, similar to migraines, become largely asymptomatic between attacks separated by weeks to months at a time [7]. Symptoms are reported to range between 2–72 hours in duration, with average episodes lasting 17 hours [70]. The attacks can be associated with nausea, vomiting, headache, anorexia, photophobia, and pallor. Prodromal symptoms may precede an attack and may include flushing, diarrhea, visual auras, slurred speech, and numbness [5]. Patients with

AM may report a history of migraine or a family history of migraine [71]. Common triggers of AM are similar to those of migraine, such as stress, sleep deprivation, and dehydration.

There is limited evidence-based treatment for AM, especially in the adult population. Most treatment approaches are derived from the treatment of migraine and from the pediatric population. In the acute setting, analgesics such as ibuprofen and acetaminophen are helpful if taken soon after the onset of pain. Intranasal sumatriptan has also been reported as effective in aborting an attack [72, 73]. In children, refractory to abortive care, IV sodium valproate, and DHE have been reported to resolve episodes of AM [74, 75]. Nonpharmacologic therapies include stress reduction, adequate hydration, adequate sleep hygiene, limiting external stimulation, and resting in a dark and quiet room. A few studies have shown symptom improvement in response to an oligoantigenic diet if a food allergen is suspected. Prophylactic treatment with reported efficacy in children includes pizotifen (in Canada and United Kingdom), propranolol, cyproheptadine, and flunarizine [72]. In adult-onset AM, case reports have reported successful prophylactic treatment with propranolol, pizotifen, topiramate, valproate, and verapamil [73]. Although CGRP monoclonal antagonists have been shown to be effective in the treatment of migraine, there is no data on their efficacy in AM.

ACUTE NAUSEA AND CHRONIC FUNCTIONAL NAUSEA IN MIGRAINE HEADACHE

Nausea, with its queasy subjective epigastric sensation, is typically associated with vomiting as both an antecedent and accompanying symptom. However, vomiting may occur in the absence of nausea and may occur by itself in DGBIs as chronic or functional nausea. It is a prominent symptom of migraine, AM, and CVS, and many describe it as more distressing than the primary symptoms of headache, pain, or vomiting. There is also increasing recognition of disabling chronic nausea and vomiting in adults and functional nausea without vomiting [53, 76, 77]. Chronic nausea could also be due to undiagnosed autonomic dysfunction. Recently, Gosalvez-Tejada et al. found that 40% of adolescents with episodic CVS at 14 years of age developed autonomic dysautonomia (e.g., postural orthostatic tachycardia), resulting in chronic daily nausea [78]. Despite its 7% prevalence in adults and its troublesome and disabling impact, relatively little is known about the pathophysiology, and there are no efficacious medications to treat it [79].

The accompanying symptoms of nausea include pallor, mydriasis, hypersalivation, diaphoresis, and tachycardia mediated through the ANS. Afferent inputs that lead to nausea and vomiting may arise from the GI tract, vestibular, and central nervous system and arrive at the nucleus tractus solitarus in the brainstem [79]. These are integrated to produce vagal efferent output that results in the autonomic expression of nausea and the coordinated motor response of vomiting. It has been proposed that mild stimulation produces nausea, whereas more intense input leads to vomiting. Many transmitters are involved, including histamine, dopamine, serotonin, norepinephrine, acetylcholine, substance P, cortisol, ß-endorphin, and vasopressin.

Although an array of testing is available to evaluate the anatomy (upper GI radiographs), the mucosa (endoscopy), and the functioning of the stomach (gastric emptying study), if nausea and vomiting are limited to the migraine or CVS episode, no further evaluation is warranted. In one series of 45 adolescents with functional nausea, endoscopy results were negative for a cause [80]. The exception is if, in association with vomiting, there is concomitant iCVS, in which we typically discover prolapse gastropathy or Mallory-Weiss tear, or if the nausea and vomiting persist between episodes, then other chronic conditions should be considered. Specific conditions that should be considered include medical use of opiates or long-term cannabis use (CHS). In long-term insulin-dependent diabetic or postviral state, gastroparesis should be considered. In an adolescent or younger woman, bulimia and hyperemesis gravidarum from pregnancy should be considered. Beyond those are the host of GI disorders commonly found in the general population, such as PUD.

There is no effective medication for nausea by itself, whereas there are very effective antiemetics even for the highly emetogenic chemotherapy regimens. Most agents discussed next have not been studied in chronic functional nausea alone but have been evaluated in postoperative, chemotherapy-induced, and pregnancy nausea and vomiting [81]. Even in CVS and migraine, there is minimal data on the specific efficacy of agents in the acute management of emesis. The first line of management in migraine, AM, and CVS is to attempt to abort the attack early on, which in turn may resolve the nausea and vomiting. In migraine, this may include nasal or subcutaneous triptans, nasal DHE, or oral gepants if administered before the onset of emesis [82]. In CVS, intravenous ondansetron or oral aprepitant have both been used as abortive agents, with greater success with the latter [48]. Among adolescents who developed chronic daily nausea, 27% of whom had antecedent CVS and 71% had familial migraine, 40% had a ≥50% response to amitriptyline, a higher rate compared to that with a proton pump inhibitor or ondansetron [80]. Treatment options have been extensively covered in the migraine, AM, and CVS sections.

CHRONIC GASTROINTESTINAL COMORBIDITIES

Several chronic GI comorbidities have been associated with migraine. Recognizing, managing, and appropriately referring patients with these conditions is essential in providing comprehensive care for these patients. These conditions are detailed as follows and summarized in Table 8.4.

Gastroesophageal Reflux Disease and Peptic Ulcer Disease

GERD develops when stomach acid flows retrograde into the esophagus, provoking symptoms such as heartburn and regurgitation, and in severe cases, causing damage to the esophageal mucosa, such as erosive esophagitis and peptic strictures [83]. Diagnosis is based on a combination of symptom presentation, endoscopic evaluation of esophageal mucosa, reflux monitoring, or response to therapeutic intervention—namely, the administration of PPIs [84]. There is now a growing body of literature demonstrating the association of migraine with reflux symptoms [85]. A significant correlation between MH and GERD symptoms has been reported in the literature [86]. One study noted that almost half of the surveyed patients with migraine reported GERD [87]. Conversely, MH has also been found to be more prevalent

TABLE 8.4 Management of common migraine comorbidities

MIGRAINE COMORBIDITY	MANAGEMENT
GERD	NSAID avoidance, lifestyle and dietary change, PPI and H2 antagonist
PUD	NSAID avoidance, H. pylori testing and treatment
IBD	Referral to GI for therapy, NSAID avoidance
IBS	Lifestyle and dietary change, antidiarrheals or laxatives, behavioral therapy, neuromodulators
Chronic diarrhea	Removal of dietary triggers, determine if related to medication side effects and switch to different agent if needed, antidiarrheals
Chronic constipation	Lifestyle and dietary change, determine if related to medication side effects and switch to different agent if needed, laxatives
Gastroparesis/FD	Dietary change, determine if related to medication side effects, prokinetics, neuromodulators
Celiac disease	Gluten-free diet, referral to GI and dietician

Note: IBS, irritable bowel syndrome; IBD, inflammatory bowel disease; GERD, gastroesophageal reflux disease; PUD, peptic ulcer disease; FD, functional dyspepsia among those with reflux symptoms [2]. The exact cause of this association is unclear, but the frequent treatment of migraine with NSAIDs may offer one explanation. NSAIDs are known to cause PUD and exacerbate erosive esophageal disease, with one study finding prescription NSAIDs nearly doubled the risk of developing GERD [87, 88]. Use of NSAIDs for migraine has been found to be common among diagnosed GERD patients and even more so in those with undiagnosed GERD symptoms [87]. This highlights the need for caution in the use of NSAIDs for migraine treatment. If NSAIDs are needed, the smallest dose necessary should be used to prevent GI toxicity. Additionally, concomitant prophylactic therapy with PPIs may be considered, especially in patients who have additional risk factors for GI bleeding [83]. One small case series has reported the resolution of headache with PPI treatment in patients with headaches associated with reflux [89]. However, more studies are needed to establish a causal relationship between reflux with headaches.

In addition to NSAID-induced GERD and PUD, H. pylori has also been implicated as a potential contributor to migraine. A meta-analysis of five case-control studies found H. pylori in approximately 45% of patients with migraine, while the prevalence among healthy controls was approximately 33% [90]. In addition, treatment of H. pylori has been shown to resolve or reduce migraine symptoms in a portion of patients. A review study reported that at 6 and 12 months, H. pylori eradication in migraine patients was associated with resolution of symptoms in 23% and 28% of cases, respectively, and a significant decrease in intensity, frequency, and duration of attacks in the remaining patients [91]. The mechanism for the association between migraine and H. pylori is not well understood; however, it has been proposed that the infection may induce immune, inflammatory, and vascular responses with subsequent release of immune cells and inflammatory and vasoactive agents into the gastric mucosa that leads to hypersensitivity to pain [90]. Inflammatory mediators such as IL-12 and IL-10 have been found at increased levels in patients with H. pylori, and interestingly, higher IL-10 plasma levels have been observed during migraine attacks [85]. The chronic inflammation caused by H. pylori infection may also trigger neuroendocrine cell release of other migraine mediators, such as serotonin, substance P, and vasoactive intestinal polypeptide [90]. Additionally, CGRP levels, which may play a potential role in both migraine physiology and GI symptoms as described earlier in this chapter, have been found to be elevated in duodenal ulcers in H. pylori–positive individuals [85]. Thus, in patients with migraine and comorbid reflux or PUD, eradication of H. pylori and avoidance of NSAIDs is advisable.

Clinical Case 1

The patient is a 45-year-old male with a history of ulcerative colitis who is referred to headache clinic for treatment options. His ulcerative colitis (UC) has been previously well controlled on mesalamine; however, he had a recent flare of symptoms after requiring multiple days of ibuprofen due to a prolonged migraine attack. While his UC has now improved, his gastroenterologist has referred him to clinic for evaluation of better acute treatment options for acute migraine attacks that will not exacerbate his UC.

Discussion with the patient reveals that he typically has two migraine days per month, which he typically does not treat with medication but instead will lay down in a quiet, dark room with an ice pack until symptoms improve; the recent migraine episodes have been more severe than his previous episodes, prompting him to try the ibuprofen. Since NSAIDs are relatively contraindicated in patients with IBD, starting a triptan is discussed, and the patient elects to try zolmitriptan nasal spray initially to bypass gut absorption. He also raises concerns about being on "too many medications," and so remote electrical neuromodulation (REN) is also presented to the patient. Two months later, the patient returns to clinic and reports that he has had two migraine attacks since seeing you in clinic. He states that while the zolmitriptan nasal spray significantly improved the severity of his head pain, he found the medication's taste repulsive. Consequently, with his second episode, he instead tried REN and found it effective and well tolerated – he decided to use this as the sole treatment going forward. He also reports that he has not had additional flares of his UC.

Inflammatory Bowel Disease

IBD is a chronic relapsing-remitting inflammatory condition affecting the gastrointestinal tract that is comprised of Crohn's disease and UC [92]. Multiple studies have suggested increased migraine prevalence in patients with IBD compared to the general population, although the mechanism for the reported overlap has not been fully elucidated [9]. Autoimmune-inflammatory responses, malabsorption, and endothelial dysfunction found in patients with IBD have been hypothesized to contribute to the pathophysiology relating to IBD and migraine [9]. Additionally, the immunosuppressive treatments commonly prescribed for IBD may play a role, as migraine has been found to be more prevalent among those on anti-TNF-α agents [9]. A study investigating the overlap of migraine and IBD concluded that migraine is unrelated to IBD clinical activity, and thus migraine could be considered an extraintestinal manifestation of IBD [93]. The authors hypothesized that slight inflammatory activity could maintain migraine activity in the absence of major intestinal manifestations; however, this should be further investigated given the poor correlation between clinical and endoscopic activity in IBD [93]. Given that migraine prevalence was found to be twice as high as that in the general population of equivalent age, screening for migraine in patients with IBD may be warranted. Currently, migraine is not considered an extraintestinal manifestation of IBD, and thus systematic screening is not part of the recommended guidelines. However, comorbid migraine occurs more frequently than joint involvement, which is considered to be the most frequent extraintestinal manifestation [93]. As in multiple other comorbid GI conditions, NSAIDs should be avoided in the treatment of migraine, as they can precipitate an IBD flare. In IBD, triptans should be used as first-line migraine treatment [93, 94]. Close collaboration with the patient's gastroenterologist is needed if immunosuppressive treatments are suspected to play a role in migraine symptoms. In most cases, the benefit gained in IBD treatment and remission with immunosuppressive agents may outweigh the potential association with increased migraine prevalence.

Clinical Case 2

The patient is a 28-year-old female who presents to your clinic for recurrent headache episodes. On discussion, her headaches are consistent with high-frequency episodic migraine, including 12 headache days per month. Additional questioning finds that the patient also has recurrent episodes of abdominal pain and diarrhea, consistent with the Rome IV criteria for IBS. The patient is interested in starting both acute and preventive treatments for migraine. She elects to try as-needed rizatriptan and daily nortriptyline. You also provide her with handouts about a diet low in fermentable oligo-, di-, and monosaccharides and polyols (FODMAP).

Four months later, the patient returns and happily expresses that she is feeling much better. Her headaches have been reduced to five headache days per month, and they respond well to rizatriptan. In addition, she has significantly fewer episodes of abdominal pain and diarrhea after starting the nortriptyline and switching to the FODMAP diet.

Irritable Bowel Syndrome, Chronic Diarrhea, and Chronic Constipation

A common association between migraine and IBS has been established in the literature. The Rome IV criteria used to diagnose IBS requires recurrent abdominal pain, on average, at least one day per week in the last three months, associated with two or more of the following criteria: related to defecation, associated with a change in frequency of stool, or associated with a change in form (appearance) of stool. These criteria should be fulfilled for the last three months, with symptom onset at least six months before diagnosis [95]. IBS has been found to be common among those with migraine with

2.5-fold increased prevalence over those without migraine [96]. Likewise, chronic headache has been reported in 34%–50% of patients with IBS, reflecting considerable overlap in these conditions [10]. Both disorders are also frequently associated with multiple other comorbidities, including interstitial cystitis, fibromyalgia, chronic fatigue, sleep disturbances, and anxiety [97]. As with most noted instances of overlap of GI disease and migraine, the precise pathophysiological mechanism is poorly understood. Central, visceral, and cutaneous hypersensitization are common among both disorders and may contribute to the comorbidity [97]. Likewise, gut dysbiosis has been reported in both migraine and IBS and may lead to alterations in the gut-brain axis and inflammatory responses [9]. Furthermore, food allergies and intolerances can trigger both migraine attacks as well as IBS flares. It has been suggested that IgG-based elimination diets may improve symptoms of both IBS and migraine [98]. Serotonin may also play a role in the association between the disorders given that agents modulating serotonin receptors are effective in both groups of patients [9]. Besides the aforementioned overlapping treatments, other therapies that may address both conditions include neuromodulators, such as TCAs, which improve visceral hypersensitivity and act as migraine prophylaxis; behavioral therapies; and complementary therapies, such as acupuncture [97]. The treatment of IBS should be multifaceted and comanaged with a primary care provider or gastroenterologist. A general approach to treatment involves lifestyle and dietary modification, such as soluble fiber and diets low in FODMAP, which have been helpful in improving global IBS symptoms. Behavioral therapies such as cognitive-behavioral therapy and gut-directed hypnotherapy have also been shown to improve global IBS symptoms. Patients who have persistent symptoms may benefit from pharmacologic therapies such as TCAs, which may also be effective in the management of migraine. Although antispasmodic agents such as dicyclomine and hyoscyamine are commonly prescribed in IBS patients, the American College of Gastroenterology has found limited evidence to support their use and recommends against using these agents. Peppermint oil is an effective alternative due to its antispasmodic properties. Patients with recent onset diarrhea-predominant IBS may benefit from a course of rifaximin. Patients with constipation-predominant IBS may benefit from guanylate cyclase-C agonists, such as linaclotide, or Cl–channel activators, such as lubiprostone [99].

Isolated chronic idiopathic diarrhea in the absence of associated abdominal pain may also co-exist in patients with migraine. In the absence of other causes, chronic diarrhea may reflect the altered autonomic function in migraine and can be a premonitory symptom [83]. Conversely, diarrhea is also often associated with specific therapeutic agents in migraine, such as magnesium or the anti-seizure medication topiramate [83]. If caused by altered autonomic function, migraine treatment may improve this form of diarrhea. Diarrhea caused by migraine medications would be expected to continue or worsen, and switching to an alternative medication not associated with diarrhea may resolve the issue.

Chronic idiopathic constipation is also a common symptom in migraine patients. It is more prevalent in patients with migraine, but again, the mechanism underlying this association is unclear [83]. Similar to diarrhea, it may reflect altered autonomic function in migraine or be caused by medications used to treat headaches. Medications used for migraine associated with constipation side effects include tricyclic antidepressants (TCAs), certain anti-seizure medications such as valproate, Ca^{2+}-channel blockers (CCBs), and ß-blockers. Atenolol and metoprolol are ß-blockers more frequently associated with GI side effects, including constipation, while these are less commonly observed with propranolol and nadolol [83]. A case report suggests treating constipation may reduce headache frequency [10]. If a constipating medication is otherwise felt to be effective in the treatment of migraine, alternatives to switching to a different prophylactic migraine medication include encouraging behavioral changes such as adequate fluid and fiber intake effective defecatory positioning, and, if necessary, the addition of laxatives. Over-the-counter and prescription laxatives can be effective. Osmotic laxatives such as polyethylene glycol form a good starting point to which stimulant laxatives such as senna or bisacodyl may be added.

GASTROPARESIS

Gastroparesis is a disorder of delayed gastric emptying that can be idiopathic or caused by another condition, such as viral infection, diabetes, or surgery, which can result in vagal nerve injury and autonomic dysfunction. Patients most commonly present with symptoms of nausea and vomiting, but abdominal pain, bloating, weight loss, postprandial fullness, and early satiety are also common. A diagnosis of gastroparesis is confirmed with a four-hour gastric scintigraphy, wireless capsule motility test, or C^{13}-*Spirulina* breath test and exclusion of other etiologies. Gastroparesis is another GI disorder that may be comorbid with migraine. In patients with idiopathic gastroparesis and abdominal pain, those with severe abdominal pain were more likely to have overlapping migraine than those with milder symptoms [8]. Interestingly, individuals with migraine have also been noted to experience reduced gastric motility both during and outside of migraine attacks [8]. Gastroparesis is typically treated with dietary changes and prokinetic medications such as metoclopramide or macrolide antibiotics.

Gastric emptying can be affected by medications. Opiates can slow motility throughout the gastrointestinal tract and cause opioid-induced bowel dysfunction, including gastroparesis [83]. Given the already documented alterations in gastric emptying among migraine patients, avoidance of opioids as acute or chronic treatment of migraine is important. Gastric emptying can also be enhanced by certain medications, lending an opportunity to simultaneously treat both GI and migraine symptoms. The Ca^{2+}-channel blocker flunarizine, which has demonstrated efficacy in the prophylactic treatment of migraine, was shown to result in significant improvement of both headache and GI symptoms in patients with overlapping migraine and delayed gastric emptying but is not available in the United States [100].

Clinical Case 3

The patient is a 21-year-old female who presents to your clinic for evaluation. She reports eight days per month of severe headaches associated with nausea, photophobia, and phonophobia, which no longer respond to acetaminophen. Further questioning also reveals that she has had increasing diarrhea and fatigue over the past few years. On physical examination, the patient is thin and has grouped excoriated papules and vesicles on her knees. A diagnosis of episodic migraine is made, and a broad workup for malabsorption disease is sent. Her tissue transglutaminase (tTG)-IgA antibody returns positive, and she establishes with gastroenterology where an upper endoscopy with biopsy shows atrophic mucosa. A diagnosis of celiac disease is made. The patient is started on sumatriptan for acute treatment of migraine and counseled by a nutritionist on starting a gluten-free diet.

The patient returns three months later to clinic. She reports that she now has only three headache days per month that are responsive to sumatriptan. She also notes that she has successfully gained ten pounds.

Celiac Disease

Celiac disease is an immune-mediated disorder that occurs in patients following gluten exposure. The immune response causes intraepithelial lymphocytic infiltration, villous atrophy, and crypt hyperplasia in small intestinal mucosa. Patients can be asymptomatic or experience a range of intestinal and extraintestinal symptoms such as diarrhea, bloating, weight loss, fatigue, anemia, rash (dermatitis herpetiformis), macro- and micronutrient malabsorption, and neurological manifestations [101]. The diagnosis is made through serological testing (anti-tissue transglutaminase IgA antibody) and confirmed by duodenal biopsies via upper endoscopy. Up to 30% of patients with celiac disease suffer from migraine, but the reason for this association is unclear. Conversely, patients with migraine were more likely to have celiac disease, with a 2.4% prevalence of celiac disease in children with MH compared to 1.0%–1.4% of the general population [9, 102]. Treatment is with a gluten-free diet.

CONCLUSION

Patients with migraine experience both significant acute GI morbidity during headache episodes and chronic GI comorbid conditions between attacks. These headache and GI manifestations may share common pathophysiological mechanisms through the action of neurotransmitters, neuropeptides, inflammatory mediators, and changes in the microbiome. Given the high prevalence of GI symptoms such as nausea and vomiting in patients with MH and the effect these symptoms may have on medication tolerance and efficacy, it is important that neurologists and primary care physicians are equipped with effective treatment strategies. In many instances, GI comorbidity and symptoms may guide the selection of medication for the treatment of migraine, either through avoidance of exacerbating medications such as PPI in patients with PUD or through selection of treatment that is effective for both GI symptoms and migraine, such as the use of TCAs in patients with IBS. Similarly, recognizing, managing, and appropriately referring patients with migraine and common comorbid GI conditions is vital for the optimal care of these patients.

SUMMARY

- Patients with headache disorders may present with multiple GI complaints ranging from acute symptoms such as nausea, vomiting, and abdominal pain to chronic, comorbid conditions.
- The underlying pathophysiology for headaches and GI manifestations include a complex interplay of the gut-brain axis with neurotransmitters, neuropeptides, inflammatory mediators, and changes in the microbiome.
- Acute therapies for migraine can help reduce the severity of both migraine and GI symptoms. For patients with a high frequency of nausea and vomiting during migraine, antiemetics such as metoclopramide and prochlorperazine are first-line agents. Patients who develop dyspepsia should trial a course of PPIs once alternative pathologic causes have been excluded.
- CVS is characterized by recurrent episodes of nausea and vomiting with intervening periods of normalcy between episodes. Acute management involves abortive therapies during the prodromal phase and antiemetics/supportive care during the emetic phase. Prophylactic therapies include TCAs, anti-seizure medications, or aprepitant.
- CHS is fast-rising in states with legalized recreational cannabis use. There is significant symptom overlap with CVS. Response to hot water bathing can be observed in both CHS and CVS patients. Agents used for CVS treatment have not been found to be effective for CHS. Treatment involves cessation of cannabis.
- AM is a migraine equivalent that is characterized by recurrent severe episodes of poorly localized abdominal pain. The condition is primarily recognized in children and should be considered in adults with recurrent, discrete bouts of abdominal pain. There is limited evidence-based treatment for AM, but most treatment approaches are derived from the treatment of migraine.
- Several chronic GI conditions have been associated with migraine, including GERD, IBD, IBS, gastroparesis, and celiac disease.

REFERENCES

1. Lipton RB, Stewart WF, Diamond S, Diamond ML, Reed M (2001) Prevalence and burden of migraine in the United States: data from the American Migraine Study II. *Headache 41*:646–657.
2. Aamodt AH, Stovner LJ, Hagen K, Zwart JA (2008) Comorbidity of headache and gastrointestinal complaints. *Head-HUNT Study Cephalalgia 28*:144–151.
3. Napthali K, Koloski N, Talley NJ (2015) Abdominal migraine. *Cephalalgia 36*:980–986.
4. Raucci U, Borrelli O, Di Nardo G, Tambucci R, Pavone P, Salvatore S, Baldassarre ME, Cordelli DM, Falsaperla R, Felici E, Ferilli MAN, Grosso S, Mallardo S, Martinelli D, Quitadamo P, Pensabene L, Romano C, Savasta S, Spalice A, Strisciuglio C, Suppiej A, Valeriani M, Zenzeri L, Verrotti A, Staiano A, Villa MP, Ruggieri M, Striano P, Parisi P (2020) Cyclic vomiting syndrome in children. *Front Neurol 11*:583425.
5. Winner P (2016) Abdominal migraine. *Semin Pediatr Neurol 23*:11–13.
6. Russell G, Abu-Arafeh I, Symon DN (2002) Abdominal migraine: Evidence for existence and treatment options. *Paediatr Drugs 4*:1–8.
7. Azmy DJ, Qualia CM (2020) Review of abdominal migraine in children. *Gastroenterol Hepatol 16*:632–639.
8. Aurora SK, Shrewsbury SB, Ray S, Hindiyeh N, Nguyen L (2021) A link between gastrointestinal disorders and migraine: Insights into the gut-brain connection. *Headache 61*:576–589.
9. Arzani M, Jahromi SR, Ghorbani Z, Vahabizad F, Martelletti P, Ghaemi A, Sacco S, Togha M (2020) Gut-brain Axis and migraine headache: a comprehensive review. *J Headache Pain 21*:15.
10. Cámara-Lemarroy CR, Rodriguez-Gutierrez R, Monreal-Robles R, Marfil-Rivera A (2016) Gastrointestinal disorders associated with migraine: A comprehensive review. *World J Gastroenterol 22*:8149–8160.
11. Coleman NS, Marciani L, Blackshaw E, Wright J, Parker M, Yano T, Yamazaki S, Chan PQ, Wilde K, Gowland PA, Perkins AC, Spiller RC (2003) Effect of a novel 5-HT3 receptor agonist MKC-733 on upper gastrointestinal motility in humans. *Aliment Pharmacol Ther 18*:1039–1048.
12. Degen L, Matzinger D, Merz M, Appel-Dingemanse S, Osborne S, Lüchinger S, Bertold R, Maecke H, Beglinger C (2001) Tegaserod, a 5-HT4 receptor partial agonist, accelerates gastric emptying and gastrointestinal transit in healthy male subjects. *Aliment Pharmacol Ther 15*:1745–1751.
13. Gershon MD (2004) Review article: serotonin receptors and transporters -- roles in normal and abnormal gastrointestinal motility. *Aliment Pharmacol Ther 20* Suppl 7:3–14.
14. Talley NJ, Van Zanten SV, Saez LR, Dukes G, Perschy T, Heath M, Kleoudis C, Mangel AW (2001) A dose-ranging, placebo-controlled, randomized trial of alosetron in patients with functional dyspepsia. *Aliment Pharmacol Ther 15*:525–537.
15. Törnblom H, Drossman DA (2021) Psychopharmacologic therapies for irritable bowel syndrome. *Gastroenterol Clin North Am 50*:655–669.
16. Mittal R, Debs LH, Patel AP, Nguyen D, Patel K, O'Connor G, Grati M, Mittal J, Yan D, Eshraghi AA, Deo SK, Daunert S, Liu XZ (2017) Neurotransmitters: The critical modulators regulating gut-brain axis. *J Cell Physiol 232*:2359–2372.
17. Noseda R, Borsook D, Burstein R (2017) Neuropeptides and neurotransmitters that modulate thalamo-cortical pathways relevant to migraine headache. *Headache 57* Suppl 2:97–111.
18. Filpa V, Moro E, Protasoni M, Crema F, Frigo G, Giaroni C (2016) Role of glutamatergic neurotransmission in the enteric nervous system and brain-gut axis in health and disease. *Neuropharmacology 111*:14–33.
19. Edvinsson L, Ho TW (2010) CGRP receptor antagonism and migraine. *Neurotherapeutics 7*:164–175.
20. Fischer JA, Born W (1985) Novel peptides from the calcitonin gene: expression, receptors and biological function. *Peptides 6* Suppl 3:265–271.
21. Dodick DW, Lipton RB, Ailani J, Lu K, Finnegan M, Trugman JM, Szegedi A (2019) Ubrogepant for the Treatment of Migraine. *N Engl J Med 381*:2230–2241.
22. Lipton RB, Croop R, Stock EG, Stock DA, Morris BA, Frost M, Dubowchik GM, Conway CM, Coric V, Goadsby PJ (2019) Rimegepant, an Oral Calcitonin Gene-Related Peptide Receptor Antagonist, for Migraine. *N Engl J Med 381*:142–149.
23. Ho TW, Edvinsson L, Goadsby PJ (2010) CGRP and its receptors provide new insights into migraine pathophysiology. *Nat Rev Neurol 6*:573–582.
24. Noble EE, Hsu TM, Kanoski SE (2017) Gut to Brain Dysbiosis: Mechanisms Linking Western Diet Consumption, the Microbiome, and Cognitive Impairment. *Front Behav Neurosci 11*:9.

25. Tang Y, Liu S, Shu H, Yanagisawa L, Tao F (2020) Gut Microbiota Dysbiosis Enhances Migraine-Like Pain Via TNFα Upregulation. *Mol Neurobiol 57*:461–468.
26. Min YW, Lee JH, Min BH, Lee JH, Kim JJ, Chung CS, Rhee PL (2013) Clinical Predictors for Migraine in Patients Presenting With Nausea and/or Vomiting. *J Neurogastroenterol Motil 19*:516–520.
27. Láinez MJ, García-Casado A, Gascón F (2013) Optimal management of severe nausea and vomiting in migraine: improving patient outcomes. *Patient Relat Outcome Meas 4*:61–73.
28. Oustamanolakis P, Tack J (2012) Dyspepsia: Organic Versus Functional. *J Clin Gastroenterol 46*:175–190.
29. Di Stefano M, Pucci E, Miceli E, Pagani E, Brondino N, Nappi G, Corazza GR, Di Sabatino A (2019) Prevalence and pathophysiology of postprandial migraine in patients with functional dyspepsia. *Cephalalgia 39*:1560–1568.
30. Kelley NE, Tepper DE (2012) Rescue therapy for acute migraine, part 2: neuroleptics, antihistamines, and others. *Headache 52*:292–306.
31. Tfelt-Hansen P, Henry P, Mulder LJ, Scheldewaert RG, Schoenen J, Chazot G (1995) The effectiveness of combined oral lysine acetylsalicylate and metoclopramide compared with oral sumatriptan for migraine. *Lancet (London, England) 346*:923–926.
32. Fernando T, Lumanauw DD, Youn S, Shimada M, Yadav K, Chappell B, Horeczko T, Tanen DA (2019) Buccally absorbed vs intravenous prochlorperazine for treatment of migraines headaches. *Acta Neurol Scand 140*:72–77.
33. Orr SL, Aubé M, Becker WJ, Davenport WJ, Dilli E, Dodick D, Giammarco R, Gladstone J, Leroux E, Pim H, Dickinson G, Christie SN (2015) Canadian Headache Society systematic review and recommendations on the treatment of migraine pain in emergency settings. *Cephalalgia 35*:271–284.
34. Naylor RJ, Rudd JA (1992) Pharmacology of ondansetron. *Eur J Anaesthesiol Suppl 6*:3–10.
35. Veneziano M, Framarino Dei Malatesta M, Bandiera AF, Fiorelli C, Galati M, Paolucci A (1995) Ondansetron-induced headache. *Eur J Gynaecol Oncol 16*:203–207.
36. Singh V, Sinha A, Prakash N (2010) Ondansetron-induced migraine-type headache. *Can J Anaesth 57*:872–873.
37. Silberstein SD (2000) Practice parameter: evidence-based guidelines for migraine headache (an evidence-based review): Report of the Quality Standards Subcommittee of the American Academy of Neurology. *Neurology 55*:754–762.
38. Gelfand AA, Goadsby PJ (2012) A neurologist's guide to acute migraine therapy in the emergency room. *Neurohospitalist 2*:51–59.
39. Starke PR, Weaver J, Chowdhury BA (2005) Boxed warning added to promethazine labeling for pediatric use. *N Engl J Med 352*:2653.
40. Rad RE, Ghaffari F, Fotokian Z, Ramezani A (2017) The effectiveness of ibuprofen and lorazepam combination therapy in treating the symptoms of acute migraine: A randomized clinical trial. *Electron Physician 9*:3912–3917.
41. Backonja M, Beinlich B, Dulli D, Schutta HS (1989) Haloperidol and lorazepam for the treatment of nausea and vomiting associated with the treatment of intractable migraine headaches. *Arch Neurol 46*:724–724.
42. Marbury TC, Jin B, Panebianco D, Murphy MG, Sun H, Evans JK, Han TH, Constanzer ML, Dru J, Shadle CR (2009) Lack of effect of aprepitant or its prodrug fosaprepitant on QTc intervals in healthy subjects. *Anesth Analg 109*:418–425.
43. Chou DE, Tso AR, Goadsby PJ (2016) Aprepitant for the management of nausea with inpatient IV dihydroergotamine. *Neurology 87*:1613–1616.
44. Jackson JL, O'Malley PG, Tomkins G, Balden E, Santoro J, Kroenke K (2000) Treatment of functional gastrointestinal disorders with antidepressant medications: a meta-analysis. *Am J Med 108*:65–72.
45. Pittayanon R, Yuan Y, Bollegala NP, Khanna R, Lacy BE, Andrews CN, Leontiadis GI, Moayyedi P (2019) Prokinetics for functional dyspepsia: A systematic review and meta-analysis of randomized control trials. *Am J Gastroenterol 114*:233–243.
46. Shafigh-Ardestani MH, Karami-Horestani M, Emami B, Arjmandpour A (2019) Evaluating the effect of oral gabapentin on the improvement of gastrointestinal symptoms in patients with functional dyspepsia resistant to conventional treatments. *Adv Biomed Res 8*:53.
47. Staller K, Thurler AH, Reynolds JS, Dimisko LR, McGovern R, Skarbinski KF, Kuo B (2019) Gabapentin improves symptoms of functional dyspepsia in a retrospective, open-label cohort study. *J Clin Gastroenterol 53*:379–384.
48. Venkatesan T, Levinthal DJ, Tarbell SE, Jaradeh SS, Hasler WL, Issenman RM, Adams KA, Sarosiek I, Stave CD, Sharaf RN, Sultan S, Li BUK (2019) Guidelines on management of cyclic vomiting syndrome in adults by the American neurogastroenterology and motility society and the cyclic vomiting syndrome association. *Neurogastroenterol Motil 31* Suppl 2:e13604.

49. Sperber AD, Bangdiwala SI, Drossman DA, Ghoshal UC, Simren M, Tack J, Whitehead WE, Dumitrascu DL, Fang X, Fukudo S, Kellow J, Okeke E, Quigley EMM, Schmulson M, Whorwell P, Archampong T, Adibi P, Andresen V, Benninga MA, Bonaz B, Bor S, Fernandez LB, Choi SC, Corazziari ES, Francisconi C, Hani A, Lazebnik L, Lee YY, Mulak A, Rahman MM, Santos J, Setshedi M, Syam AF, Vanner S, Wong RK, Lopez-Colombo A, Costa V, Dickman R, Kanazawa M, Keshteli AH, Khatun R, Maleki I, Poitras P, Pratap N, Stefanyuk O, Thomson S, Zeevenhooven J, Palsson OS (2021) Worldwide prevalence and burden of functional gastrointestinal disorders, results of rome foundation global study. *Gastroenterology* 160:99–114.

50. Sunku B (2009) Cyclic vomiting syndrome: A disorder of all ages. *Gastroenterol Hepatol* 5:507–515.

51. Guandalini S (2004) *Textbook of pediatric gastroenterology and nutrition*, CRC Press

52. Li BU (1995) Cyclic vomiting: The pattern and syndrome paradigm. *J Pediatr Gastroenterol Nutr 21* Suppl 1:S6–10.

53. Stanghellini V, Chan FK, Hasler WL, Malagelada JR, Suzuki H, Tack J, Talley NJ (2016) Gastroduodenal disorders. *Gastroenterology* 150:1380–1392.

54. (2018) Headache classification committee of the international headache society (IHS) the international classification of headache disorders, 3rd edition. *Cephalalgia* 38:1–211.

55. Fleisher DR, Gornowicz B, Adams K, Burch R, Feldman EJ (2005) Cyclic Vomiting Syndrome in 41 adults: the illness, the patients, and problems of management. *BMC Med 3*:20.

56. Allen JH, de Moore GM, Heddle R, Twartz JC (2004) Cannabinoid hyperemesis: cyclical hyperemesis in association with chronic cannabis abuse. *Gut 53*:1566–1570.

57. Zhu JW, Gonsalves CL, Issenman RM, Kam AJ (2021) Diagnosis and acute management of adolescent cannabinoid hyperemesis syndrome: A systematic review. *J Adolesc Health* 68:246–254.

58. Venkatesan T, Sengupta J, Lodhi A, Schroeder A, Adams K, Hogan WJ, Wang Y, Andrews C, Storr M (2014) An Internet survey of marijuana and hot shower use in adults with cyclic vomiting syndrome (CVS). *Exp Brain Res* 232:2563–2570.

59. Kim HS, Anderson JD, Saghafi O, Heard KJ, Monte AA (2015) Cyclic vomiting presentations following marijuana liberalization in Colorado. *Acad Emerg Med* 22:694–699.

60. Bhandari S, Jha P, Lisdahl KM, Hillard CJ, Venkatesan T (2019) Recent trends in cyclic vomiting syndrome-associated hospitalisations with liberalisation of cannabis use in the state of Colorado. *Intern Med J* 49:649–655.

61. Legare CA, Raup-Konsavage WM, Vrana KE (2022) Therapeutic potential of cannabis, cannabidiol, and cannabinoid-based pharmaceuticals. *Pharmacology* 107:131–149.

62. Hillard CJ (2023) Personal Communication.

63. Simonetto DA, Oxentenko AS, Herman ML, Szostek JH (2012) Cannabinoid hyperemesis: a case series of 98 patients. *Mayo Clin Proc* 87:114–119.

64. Rosen S, Diaz R, Garacci Z, Kumar VCS, Thyarala SR, Hillard CJ, Venkatesan T (2021) Hot-water bathing improves symptoms in patients with cyclic vomiting syndrome and is modulated by chronic cannabis use. *Dig Dis Sci* 66:1153–1161.

65. Louis-Gray K, Tupal S, Premkumar LS (2022) TRPV1: A common denominator mediating antinociceptive and antiemetic effects of cannabinoids. *Int J Mol Sci* 23 (17): 10016.

66. Pourmand A, Esmailian G, Mazer-Amirshahi M, Lee-Park O, Tran QK (2021) Topical capsaicin for the treatment of cannabinoid hyperemesis syndrome, a systematic review and meta-analysis. *Am J Emerg Med* 43:35–40.

67. Patel M, Partovi O, Mooers H, Kovacic K, Garacchi Z, Venkatesan T (2023) Efficacy of aprepitant as a prophylactic medication in adults with cyclic vomiting syndrome. *Neurogastroenterol Motil* 35:e14530.

68. Napthali K, Koloski N, Talley NJ (2016) Abdominal migraine. *Cephalalgia* 36:980–986.

69. Lenglar TL, Caula C, Moulding T, Lyles A, Wohrer D, Titomanlio L (2021) Brain to belly: Abdominal variants of migraine and functional abdominal pain disorders associated with migraine. *J Neurogastroenterol Motil* 27:482–494.

70. Evans RW, Whyte C (2013) Cyclic vomiting syndrome and abdominal migraine in adults and children. *Headache* 53:984–993.

71. Al-Twaijri WA, Shevell MI (2002) Pediatric migraine equivalents: occurrence and clinical features in practice. *Pediatr Neurol* 26:365–368.

72. Angus-Leppan H, Saatci D, Sutcliffe A, Guiloff RJ (2018) Abdominal migraine. *BMJ (Clinical research ed)* 360:k179.

73. Kunishi Y, Iwata Y, Ota M, Kurakami Y, Matsubayashi M, Kanno M, Kuboi Y, Yoshie K, Kato Y (2016) Abdominal migraine in a middle-aged woman. *Int Med* 55:2793–2798.

74. Raina M, Chelimsky G, Chelimsky T (2013) Intravenous dihydroergotamine therapy for pediatric abdominal migraines. *Clin Pediatr* 52:918–921.

75. Tan V, Sahami AR, Peebles R, Shaw RJ (2006) Abdominal migraine and treatment with intravenous valproic Acid. *Psychosomatics 47*:353–355.
76. Hyams JS, Di Lorenzo C, Saps M, Shulman RJ, Staiano A, van Tilburg M (2016) Functional disorders: Children and Adolescents. *Gastroenterology 150*:1456–1468.
77. Drossman DA, Hasler WL (2016) Rome IV-functional GI disorders: Disorders of gut-brain interaction. *Gastroenterology 150*:1257–1261.
78. Gosalvez-Tejada A, Li BUK, Simpson P, Zhang L, Kovacic K (2023) Natural history of pediatric cyclic vomiting syndrome: Progression to dysautonomia. *J Pediatr Gastroenterol Nutr 76*:737–742.
79. Lacy BE, Parkman HP, Camilleri M (2018) Chronic nausea and vomiting: evaluation and treatment. *Am J Gastroenterol 113*:647–659.
80. Kovacic K, Miranda A, Chelimsky G, Williams S, Simpson P, Li BU (2014) Chronic idiopathic nausea of childhood. *J Pediatr 164*:1104–1109.
81. Heckroth M, Luckett RT, Moser C, Parajuli D, Abell TL (2021) Nausea and vomiting in 2021: A comprehensive update. *J Clin Gastroenterol 55*:279–299.
82. Ailani J, Burch RC, Robbins MS (2021) The American headache society consensus statement: Update on integrating new migraine treatments into clinical practice. *Headache 61*:1021–1039.
83. Ailani J, Kaiser EA, Mathew PG, McAllister P, Russo AF, Vélez C, Ramajo AP, Abdrabboh A, Xu C, Rasmussen S, Tepper SJ (2022) Role of calcitonin gene-related peptide on the gastrointestinal symptoms of migraine-clinical considerations: A narrative review. *Neurology 99*:841–853.
84. Katz PO, Dunbar KB, Schnoll-Sussman FH, Greer KB, Yadlapati R, Spechler SJ (2022) ACG clinical guideline for the diagnosis and management of gastroesophageal reflux disease. *Am J Gastroenterol 117*:27–56.
85. Mönnikes H, van der Voort IR, Wollenberg B, Heymann-Monnikes I, Tebbe JJ, Alt W, Arnold R, Klapp BF, Wiedenmann B, McGregor GP (2005) Gastric perception thresholds are low and sensory neuropeptide levels high in helicobacter pylori-positive functional dyspepsia. *Digestion 71*:111–123.
86. Saberi-Firoozi M, Yazdanbakhsh MA, Heidari ST, Khademolhosseini F, Mehrabani D (2007) Correlation of gastroesophageal reflux disease with positive family history and headache in Shiraz city, southern Iran. *Saudi J Gastroenterol 13*:176–179.
87. Katić BJ, Golden W, Cady RK, Hu XH (2009) GERD prevalence in migraine patients and the implication for acute migraine treatment. *J Headache Pain 10*:35–43.
88. Kotzan J, Wade W, Yu HH (2001) Assessing NSAID prescription use as a predisposing factor for gastroesophageal reflux disease in a Medicaid population. *Pharm Res 18*:1367–1372.
89. Spierings EL (2002) Reflux-triggered migraine headache originating from the upper gum/teeth. *Cephalalgia 22*:555–556.
90. Su J, Zhou XY, Zhang GX (2014) Association between Helicobacter pylori infection and migraine: a meta-analysis. *World J Gastroenterol 20*:14965–14972.
91. Savi L, Ribaldone DG, Fagoonee S, Pellicano R (2013) Is Helicobacter pylori the infectious trigger for headache?: A review. *Infect Disord Drug Targets 13*:313–317.
92. Cai Z, Wang S, Li J (2021) Treatment of Inflammatory Bowel Disease: A Comprehensive Review. *Front Med (Lausanne) 8*:765474.
93. Moisset X, Bommelaer G, Boube M, Ouchchane L, Goutte M, Dapoigny M, Dallel R, Guttmann A, Clavelou P, Buisson A (2017) Migraine prevalence in inflammatory bowel disease patients: A tertiary-care centre cross-sectional study. *Eur J Pain 21*:1550–1560.
94. Singh S, Graff LA, Bernstein CN (2009) Do NSAIDs, antibiotics, infections, or stress trigger flares in IBD? *Am J Gastroenterol 104*:1298–1313.
95. Mearin F, Lacy BE, Chang L, Chey WD, Lembo AJ, Simren M, Spiller R (2016) Bowel disorders. *Gastroenterology 150*:1393–1470.
96. Wongtrakul W, Charoenngam N, Ungprasert P (2022) Increased prevalence of irritable bowel syndrome in migraine patients: a systematic review and meta-analysis. *Eur J Gastroenterol Hepatol 34*:56–63.
97. Chang FY, Lu CL (2013) Irritable bowel syndrome and migraine: bystanders or partners? *J Neurogastroenterol Motil 19*:301–311.
98. Aydinlar EI, Dikmen PY, Tiftikci A, Saruc M, Aksu M, Gunsoy HG, Tozun N (2013) IgG-based elimination diet in migraine plus irritable bowel syndrome. *Headache 53*:514–525.
99. Lacy BE, Pimentel M, Brenner DM, Chey WD, Keefer LA, Long MD, Moshiree B (2021) ACG clinical guideline: Management of irritable bowel syndrome. *Am J Gastroenterol 116*:17–44.
100. Boccia G, Del Giudice E, Crisanti AF, Strisciuglio C, Romano A, Staiano A (2006) Functional gastrointestinal disorders in migrainous children: efficacy of flunarizine. *Cephalalgia 26*:1214–1219.

101. Fanaeian MM, Alibeik N, Ganji A, Fakheri H, Ekhlasi G, Shahbazkhani B (2021) Prevalence of migraine in adults with celiac disease: A case control cross-sectional study. *PLoS One 16*:e0259502.

102. Zis P, Julian T, Hadjivassiliou M (2018) Headache associated with coeliac disease: A systematic review and meta-analysis. *Nutrients 10*:1445.

103. Lenglar TL, Caula C, Moulding T, Lyles A, Wohrer D, Titomanlio L (2021) Brain to belly: Abdominal variants of migraine and functional abdominal pain disorders associated with migraine. *J Neurogastroenterol Motil 27*:482–494.

General Internal Medicine for the Headache Specialist

9

Sloane Heller

LEARNING OBJECTIVES

1. Define the primary care approach to diagnosing and managing headache
2. Discuss diagnosis and management of common headache comorbidities
3. Address concerns in treating primary headache in medically complex patients

---

PRIMARY CARE APPROACH TO HEADACHE

Primary care physicians are often the first health-care professionals to address headache. The first task for a primary care physician is to determine if there are any red flag symptoms present. The SNOOP^{4}E criteria (systemic symptoms, neurologic symptoms, onset with maximal intensity, older age at onset, progression, precipitated by Valsalva, postural, papilledema, exertional) is recommended by the American Academy of Family Physicians for use in primary care [1]. If any of these conditions are met, patients are referred for further workup, which can include outpatient imaging or evaluation in an emergency room.

Second, it must be determined if headaches are occurring in isolation or as part of a symptom complex, which can include a comorbid headache disorder. The differential for headache includes primary headache disorders, as well as chronic pain syndromes, such as fibromyalgia, brittle diabetes with episodes of hypo or hyperglycemia, acute hypertensive urgency or emergency, insomnia, obstructive sleep apnea, mood disorders (including depression, anxiety, adjustment disorder, or complex grief processes), and underlying trauma, including intimate partner violence. When headaches are felt to represent a more systemic process, treatment is usually directed at the underlying process rather than at the headache. Serotonin and norepinephrine reuptake inhibitors such as duloxetine and/or neuropathic pain agents such as gabapentin or pregabalin are often used to treat chronic or systemic pain and mood disorders in patients with concomitant headaches. NSAIDs and acetaminophen are also frequently employed [2]. When headaches are felt to represent primarily a mood disorder, therapy may be targeted to management of the mood disorder primarily with the use of selective serotonin reuptake inhibitors and/or counseling. If the headaches do not respond to these therapies but the other aspects of the underlying disorder do

DOI: 10.1201/b23330-9

improve, the question of whether the headaches are a distinct issue from the underlying issue should be readdressed.

Headaches that do not appear to be part of another syndrome or symptom complex are most often viewed through the framework of migraine, tension, or cluster headaches, as these primary headache disorders are the ones discussed in primary care guidelines and education materials [1]. Many primary care physicians will initiate treatment for chronic headaches using oral therapies, and there are more and more resources dedicated to educating primary care providers about the anti-calcitonin gene-related peptide (CGRP) agents. Patients who fail oral agents or who exhibit atypical headache symptoms are likely to be referred to neurology.

Headache and Preventative Vaccines

Headache is a frequently reported complaint following preventative vaccines. According to the Vaccine Adverse Events Reporting System (VAERS), headache was the fifth most common reported adverse effect, with the most common culprit vaccines being those for influenza and herpes zoster. Post-vaccine headache appears to affect women more commonly than men, with the highest prevalence among elderly women. The vast majority of these were mild, with fewer than 30% characterized as serious adverse events. Headache phenotype types reported include tension-type and migraine.

Headache is also one of the most common symptoms reported after receiving one of the mRNA-based vaccines for Sars-CoV2 (COVID-19). Again, the vast majority of these events were classified as mild, most commonly tension-type or migraine. There have been reports of headache associated with cerebral venous sinus thrombosis; however, this has been seen rarely with the administration of the adenovirus-based vaccine (produced by Johnson and Johnson) and has not been reported to be associated with the mRNA-based vaccines [3–5].

A Note on Hypertension in Headache

While hypertension can be associated with headache, primary chronic hypertension is largely asymptomatic and should not explain the development of headache. Headache can be caused by hypertensive urgency or emergency though, both of which are defined as blood pressure $\geq$ 180/110 mm Hg. Hypertensive emergency is distinguished from hypertensive urgency by the presence of new or acutely worsening end-organ damage (Table 9.1) and requires immediate inpatient management. Headache without an acute stroke does not constitute end-organ damage and can therefore be seen in both conditions. Hypertensive urgency does not require referral to an emergency room necessarily, although referral might be required for diagnostic testing to differentiate between urgency and emergency [6].

Pheochromocytomas and pituitary adenomas, both of which are causes of secondary hypertension, can cause headaches, although not due to hypertension without urgency or emergency.

TABLE 9.1 End-organ damage associated with hypertension [6, 10]

ORGAN SYSTEM	EFFECT
Brain	Strokes, posterior reversible encephalopathy syndrome (PRES), vascular dementia
Eye	Retinopathy, hemorrhage
Heart	Left ventricular hypertrophy, obstructive cardiomyopathy, heart failure, accelerated CAD, myocardial infarction
Vasculature	Atherosclerotic disease with organ or limb ischemia, aortic aneurysm, arterial dissection (including aortic)
Kidneys	Albuminuria, CKD, end-stage renal disease (kidney failure)

CLINICAL CASE 1: HEADACHE DUE TO OBSTRUCTIVE SLEEP APNEA

The patient is a 48-year-old male who presents for evaluation of morning headaches. He reports that over the past four years, he has gained substantial weight, and his body mass index (BMI) is now 32, increased from 27. He reports that over the past year, he wakes up most mornings with a pounding headache that will slowly improve over the course of the morning. He also notes that he is often very tired throughout the day and has been told that he snores very loudly. On physical examination, his blood pressure is 144/86. HemoglobinA1c returns at 6.7%.

A comprehensive management plan for obstructive sleep apnea, hypertension, and diabetes was discussed with the patient. He declines a referral for polysomnography but is interested in trying an oral appliance. He is also amenable to starting a scheduled aerobic exercise program, as well as daily metformin.

The patient returns four months later and notes that he has greatly enjoyed the exercise and has lost 15 pounds through exercise and diet. He notes that the oral appliance was initially a bit difficult to tolerate, but he became used to it and his headaches have been greatly improved, although still present. He initially had some diarrhea associated with the metformin, but that has improved as well.

Common Comorbidities and Risk of Headache Progression

Obstructive sleep apnea (OSA) and metabolic syndrome complex disorders are common and are also often comorbid with headache. There is evidence that these disorders are also risk factors for the progression of migraine. It is important for headache specialists to determine if their patients have been appropriately diagnosed and managed from this perspective. We will discuss evidence-based diagnosis and management of these disorders from the primary care perspective.

OSA

Background

OSA is a disorder that causes episodic narrowing and/or collapse of the upper airway during sleep. It is defined by reduced airflow, referred to as hypopnea, or completely absent airflow, referred to as apnea, that lasts for at least 10 seconds during sleep and is associated with cortical arousal and/or decreased blood oxygen saturation. It is estimated to affect approximately 25% of adults in the United States, with a higher prevalence in men and those over 60 years of age. OSA is associated with increased morbidity and mortality in general, with an especially close correlation to cardiovascular conditions, including atrial fibrillation and heart failure. Symptoms of OSA include excessive daytime sleepiness, snoring, gasping, or choking while asleep, in addition to headaches (classically morning headaches) and sometimes cognitive changes. Current guidelines do not recommend screening of asymptomatic adults in primary care; however, those who report signs and symptoms of OSA are recommended to undergo evaluation [7, 8].

Diagnosis

Patients who report symptoms of sleep-disordered breathing as described earlier or for whom there is clinical concern for OSA should undergo a risk assessment for this disorder. The STOP-BANG questionnaire is quick and easy to administer and has a 90% sensitivity for the detection of OSA. Although it was initially developed as a preoperative risk score, it is recommended for use in the primary care setting. A score of ≥ 3 indicates a moderate-high risk of OSA and should trigger a referral for polysomnography.

Polysomnography (PSG), or a sleep study, is the definitive diagnostic test for OSA. These are performed in dedicated laboratories and involve measurement of both sleep and respiratory metrics. These metrics include airflow through the nose and mouth, respiratory effort, peripheral oxygen saturation, presence of snoring, and body and leg position. Electroencephalogram and electrocardiogram are also performed to monitor the stage of sleep, cortical arousal, and cardiac rhythm. Home sleep studies, which are significantly less expensive to perform and more convenient for patients, include measures of airflow, respiratory effort, and oxygen saturation but do not measure the other parameters included in PSGs. Home sleep studies have been proven to show acceptable sensitivity and specificity for OSA; however, in patients with a high pretest probability of disease, the rates of false negatives are up to 50%. Therefore, patients with a negative home sleep study but a high clinical suspicion of OSA should undergo a full laboratory PSG.

OSA is diagnosed and quantified by the apnea-hypopnea index (AHI), which is defined as the number of apneic events plus the number of hypopnic events per hour of sleep (or hour of recording on home tests). An AHI of 4–14.9 indicates mild OSA, an AHI of 15–29.9 indicates moderate OSA, and an AHI of ≥ 30 corresponds to severe OSA.

Treatment

Positive airway pressure (PAP) is the mainstay of treatment for symptomatic OSA. These devices deliver pressurized air through a mask worn over the nose and mouth, preventing airway collapse. This can be administered as a continuous amount of pressure (CPAP) or as different amounts of pressure for inhalation and exhalation, referred to as bilevel positive pressure. Bilevel PAP may be helpful for patients who need higher levels of pressure, who have difficulty exhaling against a fixed pressure (such as patients with chronic obstructive pulmonary disease), or when there is a hypoventilation component (such as obesity hypoventilation syndrome). Nasal masks, in which pressurized air is delivered via a device over the nose only, are preferred by patients in terms of comfort but can only deliver continuous pressure and have limited efficacy for severe OSA. When the device is fitted correctly and worn as prescribed, it reduces AHI in 90% of patients.

In patients with mild OSA, oral devices can be considered prior to the initiation of PAP therapy. Oral devices consist of plates fitted to the teeth that temporarily realign the maxilla relative to the mandible to help open the upper airway and prevent collapse. Weight loss can also be considered an initial treatment in mild OSA, although it has been shown to improve both the AHI and the associated morbidity and mortality risks of OSA at all levels of disease severity.

CLINICAL CASE 2

The patient is a 45-year-old female who presents for evaluation of headache. The patient reports that on 11 days of the month, she will have unilateral headaches associated with nausea that last for 6 hours and require her to go home from work early. She has not previously tried any medications for the prevention of migraine, and physical examination reveals a blood pressure of 142/82, consistent with what she has measured on her home machine. In discussion with the patient, she states that she is eager to be on as few medications as possible and asks about a medication to treat her episodic migraine and presumed hypertension. In addition to starting lisinopril, daily aerobic exercise is discussed as a helpful treatment for both of these conditions. She is also eager to start the Dietary Approaches to Stop Hypertension (DASH) diet.

Three weeks after this visit, the patient sends a message that she has taken up daily jogging but also notes that she has developed a chronic cough. Lisinopril is discontinued and candesartan started instead. Two months later, the patient is seen in follow-up and notes that her headache frequency has decreased to five days per month and her blood pressure is now 134/78.

Metabolic Syndrome

Background

The term metabolic syndrome is used to describe the co-occurrence of insulin resistance, hypertension, dyslipidemia, and increased adiposity. Metabolic syndrome is a useful construct to understand the way that these seemingly disparate disease processes interact to produce a pro-inflammatory and pro-thrombotic state, increasing the risk of atherosclerotic cardiovascular disease (ASCVD) and progression of headache disorders. Diabetes, hyperlipidemia, and obesity are processes within this spectrum of disease, although all patients with metabolic syndrome will not meet full criteria for those illnesses. Given that management of metabolic syndrome consists of managing the component pathologies, we will discuss diagnosis and management of diabetes, hypertension, hyperlipidemia, and obesity in addition to metabolic syndrome as a whole [9–17].

Diagnosis

Metabolic syndrome is defined as the presence of at least three out of the following five metrics: elevated waist circumference ($\geq$ 40 inches for men, $\geq$ 35 inches for women), triglyceride level $\geq$150 mg/dL or on triglyceride lowering treatment, HDL < 40 mg/dL for men or <50 mg/dL for women, systolic blood pressure >130 mm Hg or diastolic blood pressure >80 mm Hg (or on antihypertensive treatment), fasting glucose $\geq$ 100 mg/dL, or on glucose-lowering treatment.

Diabetes

Diabetes can be broken down into four categories: type 1 (autoimmune mediated), type 2 (insulin resistance mediated), gestational, or diabetes due to other causes (disease process that target the pancreas or use of medications such as glucocorticoids). In this text, diabetes refers to type 2, although all syndromes are diagnosed using the same serum metrics, and management is largely similar. Diabetes may be diagnosed using any of the following criteria: a fasting plasma glucose of $\geq$ 126 mg/dL, plasma glucose of $\geq$ 200 mg/dL two hours after ingestion of glucose solution during an oral glucose tolerance test, a random plasma glucose of $\geq$ 200 mg/dL in a patient with symptoms of hyperglycemia, or a hemoglobin A1c of $\geq$ 6.5%. Hemoglobin A1c is the easiest test to perform and is the metric used to diagnose diabetes most often in primary care settings. Prediabetes is defined as a hemoglobin A1c of 5.7%–6.4%.

Obesity

Obesity is defined as a BMI of $\geq$ 30. A BMI of 30–34.9 is considered class I obesity, a BMI of 35–39.9 is considered class II obesity, and a BMI of $\geq$ 40 is considered class III or severe obesity.

CLINICAL CASE 3

The patient is a 65-year-old male who presents for transition of care after moving to the area. His episodic migraine is currently well controlled on nightly nortriptyline and rizatriptan as needed. His last migraine episode was more than a year ago, and he has not used his rizatriptan since. It has been a similar time since he's seen a doctor. He is having some numbness in his feet and is urinating frequently and with hesitation. Hemoglobin A1C is found to be 9.5%. Nortriptyline is discontinued given his low headache frequency and urinary hesitation.

On follow-up six months later, he reports that his headaches have reappeared but remain infrequent, occurring up to once per month and are responsive to his rizatriptan. He was able to establish with primary care, where he was started on metformin, but it was discontinued due to gastrointestinal side effects, and he was then started on empagliflozin. He has also lost weight after stopping night snacks. His repeat hemoglobin A1c is 6.9%, and he reports that his urinary frequency and hesitation have improved.

Hypertension

Hypertension is defined as a systolic blood pressure of ≥ 130 mm Hg or a diastolic blood pressure of ≥ 80 mm Hg made on at least two occasions, with proper technique and an appropriate-sized cuff. Stage I hypertension is defined as systolic blood pressure of 130–139 mm Hg or diastolic blood pressure of 80–89 mm Hg, with Stage 2 hypertension including systolic blood pressure ≥ 140 or diastolic blood pressure ≥ 90. This definition was adopted in 2017 by the American College of Cardiology–American Heart Association Hypertension Guidelines and was supported by data from the SPRINT trial. With this change, the prevalence of hypertension in the United States increased from approximately 30% to approximately 45%.

Once diagnosed, the patient's medical and family history, comorbidities, and lifestyle should be assessed for anything to suggest secondary hypertension. The development of hypertension before age 30, or sudden onset, severe, or refractory hypertension should prompt an evaluation for secondary causes of hypertension. However, a gradual onset that coincides with increasing age and weight, especially in those with a family history of hypertension, is consistent with primary hypertension. If there is concern for "white-coat hypertension" in which patients have hypertension in the clinic but not at home, ambulatory blood pressure monitoring can be performed with home blood pressure cuffs. Masked hypertension, which occurs when patients have normal blood pressure in clinic but hypertension outside of it, should be suspected when there is evidence of end-organ damage from hypertension out of proportion to the blood pressures that are measured in clinic (Table 9.1).

Hyperlipidemia

Hyperlipidemia refers to elevated serum lipid levels. Lipids commonly measured are total cholesterol, high-density lipoprotein (HDL), low-density lipoprotein (LDL), and triglycerides. The term "dyslipidemia" refers to disorders of lipid metabolism and can include low levels of HDL. There is an inverse relationship between HDL and ASCVD risk, although this is complex and not clearly causal. LDL is the most atherogenic of the lipids commonly measured, and management of hyperlipidemia is generally geared toward lowering LDL to a specific target. Severe hypertriglyceridemia (fasting triglycerides ≥500 mg/dL) is the exception, in which case therapy should be targeted toward lowering the triglyceride level primarily.

Serum LDL levels should be kept at ≤190 mg/dL for all individuals regardless of medical history or ASCVD risk. Depending on age and medical history, different LDL goals should be adopted, which are discussed in the treatment section. Although hypertriglyceridemia is defined as serum triglyceride level ≥150 mg/dL, treatment is not required until levels reach ≥500 mg/dL.

Treatment

Management of metabolic syndrome boils down to treatment of the individual disease processes that make up the syndrome. The overall goal is to reduce the risk of ASCVD; therefore, patients are risk stratified based on their ten-year risk of ASCVD events. Clinical ASCVD includes acute coronary syndrome, unstable angina or stable angina with revascularization, coronary artery disease with or without revascularization, ischemic stroke or TIA, and symptomatic peripheral artery disease, including aortic aneurysm. Acute coronary syndrome, ischemic strokes, and symptomatic peripheral artery disease are considered major ASCVD events. Risk is calculated using the ASCVD score, which is a composite risk score calculated based on the patient's age, gender, and presence of atherosclerotic risk factors, including blood pressure, cholesterol levels, and presence or absence of diabetes and tobacco use. High-risk patients are those with an ASCVD score of >20%, intermediate risk are those with a score of between 7.5% and 20%, borderline risk are those with a score of 5%–7.5%, and low-risk patients have a score of <5%. This score can only be calculated for those

TABLE 9.2   Management of metabolic syndrome [9–17]

DISEASE PROCESS	TARGET	TREATMENT
Obesity/increased adiposity	BMI ≤ 25 Waist circumference <40 inches for men, < 35 for women	Lifestyle modifications – 30–60 minutes of aerobic exercise at least 5 days/week – reduced calorie intake, diets low in simple sugars and saturated fats Medications (oral vs. injectable) Bariatric surgery
Hypertension	BP <130/80	Lifestyle modifications, antihypertensive medications (see section on treatment of hypertension)
Dyslipidemia/hyperlipidemia	LDL ≤ 70 for very high risk, LDL ≤100 intermediate-high risk, LDL ≤ 160 low risk	Statins – High-intensity statins for high-risk category – Moderate-high intensity for intermediate risk category – Moderate-intensity statin for those with diabetes regardless of score, high intensity for those with diabetes + ASCVD >7.5% – Low-moderate intensity for low risk
Impaired glucose tolerance	For nondiabetics: hemoglobin A1c < 6.5% For diabetics: hemoglobin A1c <7%	Oral antihyperglycemics Injectable antihyperglycemics Insulin
Pro-thrombotic state		High risk: initiate low-dose aspirin Moderate risk: consider low-dose aspirin

between the ages of 40–75 years old without known ASCVD and whose LDL levels are less than 190 mg/dL. Patients with a history of ASCVD or LDL >190 mg/dL are automatically considered at least high risk. Very high-risk patients are those with a history of multiple major ASCVD events or a single major ASCVD event and multiple high-risk conditions (older age, diabetes, hypertension, coronary artery disease, chronic kidney disease, congestive heart failure, active tobacco use, LDL ≥ 100 mg/dL despite maximal medical therapy).

Lifestyle modifications, including adoption of a heart-healthy diet and aerobic exercise, are recommended for all patients. In addition, pharmacologic therapies are used to target specific goal metrics for each disease process that makes up metabolic syndrome (Table 9.2). We will discuss the therapies for each disease process separately in the following sections.

Diabetes

The first step in management of diabetes is to set a treatment goal. Hemoglobin A1c (HbA1c) is the target metric used in diabetes diagnosis and management. The standard target is HbA1c <7.0%. However, this should be modified as needed on an individualized basis as the risks of side effects, including hypoglycemia, are not insignificant. Elderly patients, those with long-standing, resistant disease, those who have already developed significant vascular complications, and those with other life-limiting comorbidities might all benefit from a more liberal goal.

The tools available to manage diabetes include lifestyle modifications (low glycemic index diet, aerobic exercise), oral and injectable anti-hyperglycemic medications, and insulin. Lifestyle modifications are recommended for all patients and can be used as monotherapy in those with prediabetes. Most patients with diabetes require medication for optimal management, although occasionally, patients can meet their goal HbA1c with lifestyle modifications alone. Metformin is the first-line therapy in patients without chronic kidney disease; if target HbA1c is not met with metformin monotherapy, other antihyperglycemics are added. Categories of antihyperglycemic medications include SGLT2 inhibitors, GLP1-receptor antagonists, DDP-4 inhibitors, sulfonylureas, and thiazolidinediones. Each of these has a different benefit and side effect profile and decisions on which class of medication to initiate in which order should be individualized (Table 9.3). Generally, once patients are on three agents without optimal control, basal insulin is started. If HbA1c is still not at goal, then mealtime insulin boluses are added. Once patients are on a basal/bolus regimen of insulin, other agents are discontinued, and insulin can be titrated up as needed to reach goals.

In recent years, the benefits of bariatric surgery for management of type 2 diabetes have been established. A consensus document from several international diabetes medical societies was published in 2016, which recommended bariatric surgery for all patients with diabetes and class III obesity, for those with class II obesity and inadequately controlled blood sugar despite maximal medical therapy, and those with class I obesity and inadequately controlled blood sugar despite medical therapy, including insulin.

TABLE 9.3 Oral medications for diabetes [13–14, 18]

DRUG CLASS (EXAMPLES)	METHOD OF ADMINISTRATION	ADVANTAGES	DISADVANTAGES
Biguanides (metformin)	Oral	Inexpensive, no hypoglycemia, weight neutral – mild weight loss	Cannot be used in CKD, can cause lactic acidosis and B12 deficiency, can have GI side effects
SGLT2 inhibitors (dapagliflozin, empagliflozin)	Oral	Mild weight loss, reduction in BP and cardiovascular events, can be used to treat heart failure, no risk of hypoglycemia	Increased risk of lower urinary tract infections, Fournier's gangrene, risk of hypovolemia, risk of euglycemic diabetic ketoacidosis (DKA), need to adjust for renal insufficiency
GLP-1 receptor agonists (liraglutide, semaglutide)	Subcutaneous (semaglutide only) Oral	Significant weight loss, decrease in cardiovascular events, no hypoglycemia	Nausea/vomiting, increased risk of thyroid C cell carcinoma, theoretical risk of pancreatitis, no dose adjustments available for renal insufficiency
GIP/GLP-1 receptor agonist (tirzepatide)	Subcutaneous	Very significant weight loss	Not well studied in renal disease, nausea/vomiting, risk of thyroid C cell carcinoma, theoretical risk of pancreatitis
DPP-4 inhibitors (sitagliptin, linagliptin, saxagliptin)	Oral	No hypoglycemia, side effects are rare	Hypersensitivity reactions, risk of acute pancreatitis, bullous pemphigoid
Second-generation sulfonylureas (glipizide, glyburide, glimepiride)	Oral	Cheaper, proven to decrease microvascular complications	Risk of hypoglycemia, glyburide not recommended in CKD, weight gain, cardiovascular risk with first generation only
Thiazoledindiones (pioglitazone, rosiglitazone)	Oral	No hypoglycemia, pioglitazone associated with decreased cardiovascular events	Weight gain, edema, associated with bone fractures, rosiglitazone possibly associated with increased risk of MI

Note: SGLT2 = sodium-glucose cotransporter 2, GLP1 = glucagon-like peptide 1, GIP = gastric inhibitory peptide, DPP-4 = dipeptidyl peptidase 4, CKD = chronic kidney disease, MI = myocardial infarction

All diabetics should receive yearly eye and foot exams and urinalysis to screen for diabetic retinopathy, neuropathy, and nephropathy, respectively.

Obesity

The field of obesity medicine has had tremendous development in recent years. The latest guidelines from the American Heart Association/American College of Cardiology/The Obesity Medicine Society for management of obesity were published in 2014. These guidelines are focused on comprehensive lifestyle management with diet and exercise, as well as reduction of atherosclerotic and cardiovascular risk. All adults should have annual screenings with BMI measurement, and those with a BMI ≥ 25 and an obesity-related condition or a BMI ≥ 30 should be counseled on weight loss. Although the most reduction of ASCVD risk occurs with weight loss that normalizes BMI, there is robust evidence to suggest that a reduction in body weight of 3%–5% can reduce the cardiovascular risk profile to some degree. Initial treatment strategies include a calorie-restricted diet and participation in a comprehensive lifestyle management program that includes instruction on diet and exercise participation. It can be very difficult to find available and affordable comprehensive lifestyle management programs, and if there are no in-person programs available, there is evidence to support telephone or electronic-based programs that involve trained health professionals. Pharmacotherapy should be initiated for those with a BMI ≥30 or BMI ≥27 with obesity-related conditions who do not achieve or sustain 5% body weight reduction with lifestyle modifications.

Options for pharmacotherapy to manage obesity include appetite suppressants, bupropion/naltrexone, and, more recently, GLP1-receptor agonists. Appetite suppressants include phentermine (with or without topiramate) and diethylproprion; these are the oldest medications and the least efficacious. Appetite suppressants generally cause a modest weight loss of 3–6 kg. These medications can also worsen hypertension and are contraindicated in moderate-severe hypertension, cardiovascular disease, and hyperthyroidism. Bupropion and naltrexone in combination have a slightly higher efficacy with weight loss of 5–7 kg; however, this combination has shown to cause significant constipation, nausea, dizziness, and headaches. In the premarketing studies, 20% of subjects were not able to tolerate it. Lorcaserin, a serotonin agonist, was a medication initially approved for weight loss but was removed from the market in 2020 due to the discovery of an increased risk of cancer.

The GLP-1 receptor agonists that have been approved by the Food and Drug Administration for weight loss are liraglutide and semaglutide, with semaglutide additionally approved for the treatment of diabetes. Liraglutide is modestly effective, with an expected weight loss of 5–10 kg. Semaglutide has shown to be the most effective agent, with over half of all subjects experiencing at least a 10% reduction in body weight in multiple clinical trials. This translates to an approximately 10–20 kg weight loss on average. However, there was a significant amount of nausea and gastrointestinal distress. Tirzepatide, which is a combined GIP/GLP-1 receptor agonist, has been shown to be the most effective, with half of all subjects in the premarket trial losing at least 20% of body weight. This is the newest agent, and therefore it has the least amount of data behind it, although what is there is promising. None of the pharmacologic agents have demonstrated sustained weight loss once the medication is stopped.

For patients with a BMI of ≥40 or a BMI of ≥35 with an obesity-related condition (i.e., diabetes or metabolic syndrome) who have not had success with lifestyle modification, bariatric surgery is recommended. This requires referral to a bariatric surgery center.

Hypertension

Pharmacologic treatment of hypertension to goal BP < 130/80 is recommended for all individuals with Stage 2 hypertension, as well as those with Stage 1 hypertension who are over 65 years of age, those with comorbid diabetes or chronic kidney disease, or an ASCVD score of ≥ 10%. Note that this recommendation applies to those over 65 years of age who are in a community dwelling and ambulatory; for frail older adults, an individualized approach to lowering blood pressure is recommended.

First-line agents include thiazide diuretics, angiotensin-converting-enzyme (ACE) inhibitors, angiotensin-receptor blockers (ARBs), and calcium channel blockers. In African American individuals, thiazides and calcium channel blockers have been shown to be more effective than ACE inhibitors as first-line therapy. Patients with chronic kidney disease with albuminuria should be started on an ACE inhibitor or an ARB. Thiazides should be used with caution in the elderly and those with chronic hyponatremia.

Beta-blockers and loop diuretics are considered second-line agents and are only used when there is another comorbid condition requiring their use (i.e., chronic kidney disease, heart failure, or cirrhosis). Spironolactone is considered an adjunct for refractory hypertension. These drugs are further discussed in the considerations for prescribing section.

Lifestyle modification is recommended for all individuals with Stage 1 or 2 hypertension and can be used as an initial treatment prior to initiating medication for those with Stage 1 hypertension without other comorbidities or an ASCVD score of $\leq 10\%$. These modifications include weight loss, restricting sodium intake to less than 1,500 mg daily, limiting alcohol use (fewer than two drinks daily for men and fewer than one drink daily for women), and performing aerobic exercise for 90 to 150 minutes per week. The DASH diet, which encourages increased consumption of whole grains, fresh produce, and low-fat dairy, as well as limited sodium, has been proven equally effective at lowering blood pressure as some of the first-line medications.

Hyperlipidemia

The mainstay of treatment for hyperlipidemia is statin therapy. Statins are divided into high-intensity agents (high-dose atorvastatin and rosuvastatin), moderate intensity (low-dose atorvastatin and rosuvastatin; high-dose simvastatin, pravastatin, lovastatin, fluvastatin, pitavastatin), and low intensity (low-dose simvastatin, pravastatin, lovastatin, fluvastatin). High-intensity statins lower LDL levels by $\geq 50\%$, moderate-intensity agents lower LDL levels by 30–49%, and low-intensity agents lower LDL levels by $\leq 30\%$.

Nonstatin therapies include ezetimibe and bile acid sequestrants, which have modest LDL-lowering effects. Niacin and fibrates primarily lower triglyceride levels but may have some small LDL-lowering effect in patients with normal triglycerides. These drugs can be used for monotherapy or as add-ons to statins. PCSK9 inhibitors, which are a newer class of agents, have powerful LDL-lowering effects. These agents are mainly indicated in the very high-risk group of patients who cannot tolerate statin therapy or who have ASCVD events despite maximal statin therapy.

Treatment of hyperlipidemia begins with the selection of the appropriate intensity statin and a target LDL level if appropriate. A goal LDL of ≤ 70 mg/dL should be used for very high-risk patients and individuals between the ages of 40 and 75 years old with diabetes. All very high-risk patients should be prescribed a high-intensity statin, while all diabetics between the ages of 40 and 75 years old should be prescribed at least a moderate-intensity statin, with consideration of initiating a high-intensity statin if their lipids are not at goal or they have other high-risk comorbidities. High-risk patients should target an LDL of ≤ 100 mg/dL and should be treated with a high-intensity statin. Patients between the ages of 40 and 75 years old without diabetes who fall into the intermediate or borderline risk categories should begin treatment with a moderate-intensity statin if there are other risk factors present, such as chronic kidney disease, or if they meet full criteria for metabolic syndrome. If metabolic syndrome is present, these patients should target an LD of ≤ 130 mg/dL. Low-risk patients should be counseled on diet and exercise with a view toward maintaining their low-risk status, and a target LDL of ≤ 160 mg/dL should be established. If LDL goals are not met with initial statin therapy, doses or intensities should be increased, and if this is not effective nonstatin agents may be added.

Note that the most recent guidelines from the American College of Cardiology/American Heart Association recommend initiation of therapy with moderate-intensity statins rather than low-intensity statins. However, low-intensity statin therapy remains an option for patients who experience side effects (mainly myalgias) with moderate-intensity therapy or who are able to maintain their target LDLs with low-intensity agents.

In patients over 75 years old, the decision to initiate treatment for hyperlipidemia should be individualized based on other chronic conditions and life expectancy.

SPECIAL POPULATIONS: CONSIDERATIONS FOR PRESCRIBING HEADACHE TREATMENTS

In this section, we will discuss considerations for prescribing headache medications in special medical populations [18, 19]. This information, summarized in Table 9.4, is meant as a general guide, not to replace case-by-case risk and benefit assessments made by physicians for individual patients.

TABLE 9.4   Special populations and considerations for prescribing headache medications [18, 19]

PATIENT POPULATION	DISEASE TARGETED TREATMENT	PREFERRED HEADACHE MEDICATIONS	USE WITH CAUTION	HEADACHE MEDICATIONS TO AVOID
Elderly	None, although often have comorbid conditions listed below	Triptans CGRP antagonists/ inhibitors Gabapentin ACE inhibitors/ ARBs	DHE Beta-blockers Topiramate	NSAIDs (occasional use is acceptable) TCAs Lasmitidan
CHF	Beta-blockers (metoprolol, carvedilol, atenolol) ACE/ARB vs. ARNI SGLT2-inhibitor (dapagliflozin) Mineralcorticoid antagonist (spironolactone, eplenerone) Diuretics as needed	CGRP antagonists/ inhibitors Valproic acid TCAs Topiramate Metoclopramide	Lasmitidan	Calcium channel blockers NSAIDs Propranolol DHE Triptans
CAD	Antiplatelet therapy (aspirin, clopidogrel vs. ticagrelor, dual antiplatelet therapy if recent intervention) Statin	CGRP antagonists/ inhibitors Metoclopramide Valproic acid Topiramate TCAs Beta-blockers Calcium channel blockers Lasmitidan	Triptans (stable, mild disease, no recent intervention)	Triptans (recent intervention) DHE
Atrial fibrillation	Anticoagulation Rate-control agent (beta-blocker, calcium channel blocker) Maybe rhythm control agent (amiodarone, digoxin)	Triptans CGRP antagonists/ inhibition Metoclopramide Topiramate ACE inhibitor/ ARBs	Lasmitidan Valproic acid (adverse interactions with some anti-coagulants)	DHE Propranolol NSAIDs (if on anticoagulation) TCAs

(Continued)

TABLE 9.4 (Continued) Special populations and considerations for prescribing headache medications [18, 19]

PATIENT POPULATION	DISEASE TARGETED TREATMENT	PREFERRED HEADACHE MEDICATIONS	USE WITH CAUTION	HEADACHE MEDICATIONS TO AVOID

CKD	ACE inhibitor/ARB
	Diuretic as needed
		Metoclopramide
		CGRP antagonists/
		  inhibitors
		Valproic acid
		Topiramate
		TCAs
		Beta-blockers
		Calcium channel
		  blockers
		Lasmitidan
			Triptans
			(reduced dose)
				NSAIDs

ESRD	Sodium bicarbonate if
	  needed for acidemia
	Diuretics if not anuric
	Iron supplement/
	  erythropoietin stimulating
	  agent
	Phosphate binder
	Calcium supplement
		CGRP antagonists/
		  inhibitors
		Beta-blockers
		Calcium channel
		  blockers
			Triptans
			(reduced doses)
			TCAs
			Lasmitidan
			Valproic acid
				NSAIDs
				ACE inhibitors/
				  ARBs
				Topiramate
				DHE

Cirrhosis	Lactulose/rifaximin
	Propranolol/nadolol
	  Pantoprazole
	Diuretics as needed
		Metoclopramide
		Topiramate
		TCAs
		ACE inhibitor/
		  ARBs
		Acetaminophen
		(2 gm/24 hr
		maximum)
			Calcium channel
			  blockers
			Triptans
			(reduced doses)
			CGRP
			antagonists/
			inhibitors
				NSAIDs
				Lasmitidan
				Valproic acid
				DHE
				Acetaminophen
				(more than 2
				mg/24 hrs)

HIV	HAART, often combination
	pill (classes include
	nucleoside and nucleotide
	reverse transcriptase
	inhibitors (NRTIs), non-
	nucleoside reverse
	transcriptase inhibitors
	(NNRTIs), protease inhibitors,
	fusion inhibitors, integrase
	strand transfer inhibitors
	(INSTIs), less commonly
	capsid inhibitor, attachment
	or post-attachment inhibitor,
	CCR5 antagonist)
	Prophylactic antimicrobials
	depending on CD4
	count (most commonly
	sulfamethoxazole-
	trimethoprim, azithromycin
	if CD4 count <50 cells/
	microL, antifungals and/
	or tuberculosis regimen
	depending on location)
		Triptans
		CGRP antagonists/
		  inhibitors
		Valproic acid
		Topiramate (except
		  with protease
		  inhibitor use)
		TCAs
		Beta-blockers
		Calcium channel
		  blockers
			ACE inhibitor/
			  ARB
			NSAIDs
			Metoclopramide	

(Continued)

TABLE 9.4   (Continued) Special populations and considerations for prescribing headache medications [18, 19]

PATIENT POPULATION	DISEASE TARGETED TREATMENT	PREFERRED HEADACHE MEDICATIONS	USE WITH CAUTION	HEADACHE MEDICATIONS TO AVOID
Asthma, COPD	Inhaled anticholinergics (short or long acting) Inhaled beta agonists (short or long acting) Possibly inhaled or oral corticosteroids	Triptans CGRP antagonists/ inhibitors Metoclopramide Valproic acid TCAs Topiramate ACE inhibitor/ARB	Lasmitidan	Beta-blockers
Inflammatory Bowel Disease	Possibilities include mesalamine /sulfasalazine (ulcerative colitis only), azathioprine, methotrexate, anti-TNF α agents (infliximab, adalimumab, certolizumab pegol, golimumab), anti-integrin agents (natalizumab, vedolizumab), anti-cytokine agents (ustekinumab, tofacitinib), steroids	Triptans DHE TCAs Lasmitidan ACE inhibitor/ ARBs	Topiramate Metoclopramide Valproic acid NSAIDs CGRP antagonists/ inhibitors	
Inflammatory disorders: SLE, rheumatoid arthritis, Sjogren's disease, scleroderma, sarcoidosis, vasculitis	Possibilities include steroids Cyclophosphamide Methotrexate Mycofenolate mofetil Azathioprine Hydroxychloroquine Anti-TNF α agents Anakinra Abatacept Rituximab	Triptans DHE TCAs Lasmitidan Topiramate Metoclopramide ACE inhibitors/ARBs (in scleroderma, ACE inhibitors should be used to manage renal manifestations, avoid ARB)	Valproic acid NSAIDs CGRP small-molecule inhibitors	ARB (in scleroderma) CGRP monoclonal antibodies

Note: This information is meant as a general guide, not to replace case-by-case risk and benefit and medication safety assessments made by physicians for individual patients.CHF = congestive heart failure, CKD = chronic kidney disease, ESRD = end-stage renal disease, COPD = chronic obstructive pulmonary disease, HIV = human immunodeficiency virus, SLE= systemic lupus erythematosus, ARNI = angiotensin-receptor/neprilisyn inhibitor, NSAIDs = nonsteroidal anti-inflammatory drugs, TCA = tricyclic antidepressents, DHE = dihydroergotamine

Lisinopril, Candesartan (ACE Inhibitor/ARB)

ACE inhibitors and ARBs are a part of management of congestive heart failure and chronic kidney disease. ACE inhibitors in particular are also recommended for use to prevent neurohormonal remodeling in the heart after a myocardial infarction and in diabetics with albuminuria to prevent the development of diabetic nephropathy. When used as neurohormonal agents only, ACE inhibitors are dosed at less than 10 mg daily.

Populations who should not be on ACE inhibitors or ARBs include patients with end-stage renal disease or chronic hyperkalemia and pregnant women. Additionally, caution should be exercised in utilizing these agents in populations who are predisposed to acute kidney injury and renal insufficiency. The rise in creatinine seen with the initiation of ACE inhibitors and ARBs is normally transient; however, some patients with very vulnerable renal function may not be able to recover. These populations include decompensated cirrhosis and patients with HIV on highly active antiretroviral therapy (HAART), as some very common HAART agents predispose to kidney injury.

Propranolol (Beta-Blockers)

Beta-blockers are similarly a key part of management of congestive heart failure and are also a mainstay of prevention of variceal bleeding in decompensated cirrhosis, as well as rhythm control in atrial fibrillation and other tachyarrhythmias. Selective beta-blockers are used for heart failure and heart rate control; examples include metoprolol, bisoprolol, carvedilol, and esmolol. Nonselective beta-blockers are used in cirrhosis and include propranolol and nadolol. Beta-blockers are generally well tolerated, with the exception of patients with asthma or (to a lesser degree) chronic obstructive pulmonary disease and those with orthostatic hypotension.

Propranolol is the primary beta-blocker used for headache management. However, it is not effective for management of heart failure and less effective for rhythm control in atrial fibrillation. Patients with these conditions should be on a selective beta-blocker only, and propranolol should not be initiated, as these patients should not take more than one beta-blocker simultaneously.

Lastly, beta-blockers can cause orthostatic hypotension and falls. This is a special concern in the elderly, and these agents should be used with significant caution in this population.

Verapamil (Calcium Channel Blockers)

Calcium channel blockers can exacerbate heart failure and should be avoided in patients with severe heart failure. Note that calcium channel blockers are effective rate-control agents in atrial fibrillation and can be combined with beta-blockers for optimal rate control if needed. However, caution should be exercised in prescribing calcium channel blockers to patients who are also taking beta-blockers in the absence of elevated heart rates, as the combination can produce bradycardia and possibly hypotension.

Topiramate

Topiramate can provoke nephrolithiasis and therefore should be avoided in patients already predisposed to this condition—namely, patients with Crohn's disease and patients with HIV on protease inhibitors, as protease inhibitors can also cause this problem. Similarly, topiramate can provoke acute angle closure glaucoma, and should be avoided in patients with underlying narrow angle glaucoma. Topiramate is primarily renally cleared and doses can fluctuate significantly with hemodialysis. Lastly, topiramate can suppress appetite and cause weight loss and should therefore be used with caution in patients with inflammatory bowel disease who are already struggling to maintain a healthy body weight.

Tricyclic Antidepressants (TCAs)

TCAs have anticholinergic effects and can provoke cognitive symptoms in the elderly. TCAs are primarily renally metabolized; while not contraindicated in those with chronic kidney disease (CKD) or end stage renal disease (ESRD), patients with decreased renal function are more vulnerable to side effects and should be initiated on low doses and titrated up slowly. TCAs should not be prescribed to patients who are also taking an SSRI or SNRI due to the risk of serotonin syndrome.

Valproic Acid

Valproic acid is primarily hepatically metabolized and can cause hyperammonemia, and should therefore be avoided in those with cirrhosis or severe hepatic dysfunction. Many immune suppressive agents, including methotrexate and anti-TNF α agents, can cause hepatotoxicity, so caution should be exercised when prescribing valproic acid to a patient already taking one of these medications. Care should be taken to avoid using valproic acid in women of childbearing potential, as it is teratogenic. Additionally, valproic acid can cause thrombocytopenia and platelet dysfunction and should be used with caution in patients with preexisting platelet dysfunction, including ESRD and cirrhosis.

Nonsteroidal Anti-Inflammatories (NSAIDs)

NSAIDs can cause bleeding diathesis, acute kidney injury, and gastritis with gastrointestinal bleeding. The elderly are especially vulnerable to these complications, and chronic NSAID use should be avoided in that population. Occasional or time-limited use is acceptable; however, the decision about whether to use NSAIDs in the elderly should be made based on the frequency of headaches, the planned duration of use, and the individual patient risk factors for the aforementioned. Note that concomitant use of NSAIDs and anticoagulation is not recommended given the increased risk for bleeding complications. The risk of both bleeding diathesis and gastritis is higher when NSAIDs are combined with steroids, so care should be taken when prescribing NSAIDs to patients on chronic steroid therapy (autoimmune disease, chronic obstructive pulmonary disease).

NSAIDs should also be avoided in those at significant risk of kidney injury, namely those with CKD or ESRD. Patients with heart failure are at a higher risk of NSAID-induced kidney injury due to lower effective circulating blood volume in this condition. Those with decompensated cirrhosis have two reasons to avoid NSAIDs: an acute kidney injury in a patient with decompensated cirrhosis can precipitate hepatorenal syndrome and renal failure, and these patients are at risk for bleeding complications due to coagulopathy and thrombocytopenia. Caution should be used in using NSAIDs in patients with HIV on HAART, as many medications used in HAART predispose to kidney injury. NSAIDs can worsen hypertension and should not be used in patients with resistant hypertension.

Metoclopramide

The primary concern in using metoclopramide is QTc prolongation. Therefore, metoclopramide should be used with caution in HIV patients on HAART, as some of the most common HAART agents can also prolong the QTc. Metoclopramide can also increase gut motility and should be avoided in patients with inflammatory bowel disease, as it can worsen diarrhea and abdominal pain.

Triptans

Triptans are vasoconstrictive agents and therefore cannot be used in those with significant coronary artery disease (CAD), unstable angina, or ischemic heart disease. These agents are cleared both renally and hepatically, and therefore have prolonged clearance in patients with cirrhosis or renal insufficiency. In patients with chronic renal or liver disease, triptans should be used in lower doses and titrated slowly.

CGRP Antagonists/Inhibitors

These agents have very few side effects and are generally well tolerated. One thing to note is that the only notable side effect seems to be constipation, which should be watched for closely in patients with cirrhosis, as constipation may trigger or worsen hepatic encephalopathy.

Dihydroergotamine (DHE)

DHE can provoke cardiac arrythmias and should be avoided in those with preexisting atrial fibrillation or other risk factors for arrythmias, including CAD and heart failure. It cannot be used in those with ESRD or cirrhosis due to issues with clearance. Lastly, the IV formulation requires inpatient monitoring, which can cause significant morbidity in certain populations, namely the elderly.

Lasmitidan

Lasmitidan can cause significant sedation and should therefore be avoided in the elderly. Caution should also be exercised in those with COPD and chronic respiratory failure, as any sedating medications can cause respiratory depression. It is hepatically cleared and is contraindicated in cirrhosis due to significantly prolonged clearance, but it can be used in renal disease. Lasmitidan can also cause bradycardia and should be used with caution in those already on beta-blockers or calcium channel blockers—i.e., those with heart failure and atrial fibrillation.

SUMMARY

- The primary care approach to headache management involves first ruling out red flag symptoms, then assessing for secondary headache/headaches as part of other disease syndromes, and, lastly, attempting treatment
- Mild, temporary headaches and/or transient worsening of primary headache syndromes are common side effects of routine vaccinations
- OSA and metabolic syndrome are incredibly common, and when mismanaged, they can worsen headache control; understanding appropriate management of these comorbidities is essential to ensure optimal control of primary headaches
- Familiarity with the medications used in diseases commonly comorbid with headache, as well as in specific systemic conditions, is necessary for optimal medication management in headache

REFERENCES

1. Ford B, Dore M, Harris E. Outpatient Primary Care Management of Headaches: Guidelines from the VA/DoD. *Am Fam Physician.* 2021 Sep 1;*104*(3):316–320. PMID: 34523900.
2. Crenshaw B et al. "AAFP Chronic Pain Toolkit" HOP20012003 2021
3. Cocores AN, Goadsby PJ, Monteith TS. Post-vaccination Headache Reporting: Trends According to the Vaccine Adverse Events Reporting System. *Headache.* 2023 Feb;*63*(2):275–282. doi: 10.1111/head.14458. Epub 2023 Jan 18. PMID: 36651626.
4. Ekizoglu E, Gezegen H, Yalınay Dikmen P, Orhan EK, Ertaş M, Baykan B. The Characteristics of COVID-19 Vaccine-related Headache: Clues Gathered from the Healthcare Personnel in the Pandemic. *Cephalalgia.* 2022 Apr;*42*(4–5):366–375. doi: 10.1177/03331024211042390. Epub 2021 Sep 12. PMID: 34510919; PMCID: PMC8988457.
5. Mouliou DS, Dardiotis E. Current Evidence in SARS-CoV-2 mRNA Vaccines and Post-Vaccination Adverse Reports: Knowns and Unknowns. *Diagnostics (Basel).* 2022 Jun 26;*12*(7):1555. doi: 10.3390/diagnostics12071555. PMID: 35885461; PMCID: PMC9316835.
6. Varon J. The Diagnosis and Treatment of Hypertensive Crises. *Postgrad Med.* 2009 Jan;*121*(1):5–13. doi: 10.3810/pgm.2009.01.1950. PMID: 19179809.

7. Semelka M, Wilson J, Floyd R. Diagnosis and Treatment of Obstructive Sleep Apnea in Adults. *Am Fam Physician*. 2016 Sep 1;*94*(5):355–60. PMID: 27583421.

8. US Preventive Services Task Force; Mangione CM, Barry MJ, Nicholson WK, Cabana M, Chelmow D, Rucker Coker T, Davidson KW, Davis EM, Donahue KE, Jaén CR, Kubik M, Li L, Ogedegbe G, Pbert L, Ruiz JM, Stevermer J, Wong JB. Screening for Obstructive Sleep Apnea in Adults: US Preventive Services Task Force Recommendation Statement. JAMA. 2022 Nov 15;*328*(19):1945–1950. doi: 10.1001/jama.2022.20304. PMID: 36378202.

9. Taler SJ. Initial Treatment of Hypertension. *N Engl J Med*. 2018 Feb 15;*378*(7):636–644. doi: 10.1056/NEJMcp1613481. PMID: 29443671.

10. Whelton PK, Carey RM, Aronow WS, Casey DE Jr, Collins KJ, Dennison Himmelfarb C, DePalma SM, Gidding S, Jamerson KA, Jones DW, MacLaughlin EJ, Muntner P, Ovbiagele B, Smith SC Jr, Spencer CC, Stafford RS, Taler SJ, Thomas RJ, Williams KA Sr, Williamson JD, Wright JT Jr. 2017 ACC/AHA/AAPA/ABC/ACPM/AGS/APhA/ASH/ASPC/NMA/PCNA Guideline for the Prevention, Detection, Evaluation, and Management of High Blood Pressure in Adults: A Report of the American College of Cardiology/American Heart Association Task Force on Clinical Practice Guidelines. *Hypertension*. 2018 Jun;*71*(6):e13–e115. doi: 10.1161/HYP.0000000000000065 Epub 2017 Nov 13. Erratum in: Hypertension. 2018 Jun;71(6):e140–e144. PMID: 29133356.

11. Grundy SM, Cleeman JI, Daniels SR, Donato KA, Eckel RH, Franklin BA, Gordon DJ, Krauss RM, Savage PJ, Smith SC Jr, Spertus JA, Costa F; American Heart Association; National Heart, Lung, and Blood Institute. Diagnosis and Management of the Metabolic Syndrome: An American Heart Association/National Heart, Lung, and Blood Institute Scientific Statement. *Circulation*. 2005 Oct 25;*112*(17):2735–52. doi: 10.1161/CIRCULATIONAHA.105.169404. Epub 2005 Sep 12. Erratum in: Circulation. 2005 Oct 25;112(17):e297. Erratum in: Circulation. 2005 Oct 25;112(17):e298. PMID: 16157765.

12. Brito JP, Montori VM, Davis AM. Metabolic Surgery in the Treatment Algorithm for Type 2 Diabetes: A Joint Statement by International Diabetes Organizations. *JAMA*. 2017 Feb 14;*317*(6):635–636. doi: 10.1001/jama.2016.20563. PMID: 28196240; PMCID: PMC5557277.

13. Inzucchi SE, Bergenstal RM, Buse JB, Diamant M, Ferrannini E, Nauck M, Peters AL, Tsapas A, Wender R, Matthews DR. Management of Hyperglycemia in Type 2 Diabetes, 2015: A Patient-centered Approach: Update to a Position Statement of the American Diabetes Association and the European Association for the Study of Diabetes. *Diabetes Care*. 2015 Jan;*38*(1):140–9. doi: 10.2337/dc14-2441. PMID: 25538310.

14. American Diabetes Association. Standards of Care in Diabetes-2023 Abridged for Primary Care Providers. *Clin Diabetes*. 2022 Winter;*41*(1):4–31. doi: 10.2337/cd23-as01. Epub 2022 Dec 12. Erratum in: Clin Diabetes. 2023 Spring;41(2):328. PMID: 36714254; PMCID: PMC9845083.

15. Arnett DK, Blumenthal RS, Albert MA, Buroker AB, Goldberger ZD, Hahn EJ, Himmelfarb CD, Khera A, Lloyd-Jones D, McEvoy JW, Michos ED, Miedema MD, Muñoz D, Smith SC Jr, Virani SS, Williams KA Sr, Yeboah J, Ziaeian B. 2019 ACC/AHA Guideline on the Primary Prevention of Cardiovascular Disease: A Report of the American College of Cardiology/American Heart Association Task Force on Clinical Practice Guidelines. *J Am Coll Cardiol*. 2019 Sep 10;*74*(10):e177–e232. doi: 10.1016/j.jacc.2019.03.010. Epub 2019 Mar 17. Erratum in: J Am Coll Cardiol. 2019 Sep 10;74(10):1429–1430. Erratum in: J Am Coll Cardiol. 2020 Feb 25;75(7):840. PMID: 30894318; PMCID: PMC7685565.

16. Jastreboff AM, Aronne LJ, Ahmad NN, Wharton S, Connery L, Alves B, Kiyosue A, Zhang S, Liu B, Bunck MC, Stefanski A; SURMOUNT-1 Investigators. Tirzepatide Once Weekly for the Treatment of Obesity. *N Engl J Med*. 2022 Jul 21;*387*(3):205–216. doi: 10.1056/NEJMoa2206038. Epub 2022 Jun 4. PMID: 35658024.

17. Grundy SM, Stone NJ, Bailey AL, Beam C, Birtcher KK, Blumenthal RS, Braun LT, de Ferranti S, Faiella-Tommasino J, Forman DE, Goldberg R, Heidenreich PA, Hlatky MA, Jones DW, Lloyd-Jones D, Lopez-Pajares N, Ndumele CE, Orringer CE, Peralta CA, Saseen JJ, Smith SC Jr, Sperling L, Virani SS, Yeboah J. 2018 AHA/ACC/AACVPR/AAPA/ABC/ACPM/ADA/AGS/APhA/ASPC/NLA/PCNA Guideline on the Management of Blood Cholesterol: A Report of the American College of Cardiology/American Heart Association Task Force on Clinical Practice Guidelines. *Circulation*. 2019 Jun 18;*139*(25):e1082–e1143. doi: 10.1161/CIR.0000000000000625. Epub 2018 Nov 10. Erratum in: Circulation. 2019 Jun 18;139(25):e1182–e1186. Erratum in: Circulation. 2023 Aug 15;148(7):e5. PMID: 30586774; PMCID: PMC7403606.

18. Lexicomp, Wolters Kluwar Health (2023) https://www.wolterskluwer.com/en/solutions/lexicomp/lexicomp

19. Kasper et al. *Harrison's Principles of Internal Medicine*. 19th ed. McGraw-Hill, 2015.

Hematologic/ Oncologic Causes of Headache

10

Diana V. Maslov, Shanley Banaag, Charisma Mylavarapu, Quinne Sember, John Garrett, and Carrie Costantini

---

LEARNING OBJECTIVES

1. Identify the hematologic and oncologic conditions and complications that can lead to headache, including sickle cell disease, leukemia, myeloproliferative neoplasms, and solid tumors that have metastasized to the brain
2. Describe mechanisms of anticancer medications that can be associated with headache
3. Describe mechanisms of supportive agents used in oncologic care that can be associated with headache
4. Understand that treatment plans for oncology patients may require modifications based on the development of medication side effects

---

Clinical Case #1

A 19-year-old female presents to the emergency room with headache, fatigue, and heavy vaginal bleeding. Workup is notable for a white blood cell count of 120,000, hemoglobin 6.3g/dL, and platelets 14,000. There are blasts identified on her peripheral smear. Bone marrow biopsy is consistent with acute lymphocytic leukemia (ALL).

ACUTE LEUKEMIAS

Diagnosis of acute leukemias is typically preceded by symptoms associated with cytopenias related to their replaced bone marrow, as well as constitutional symptoms such as fatigue, unintentional weight loss, night sweats, early satiety, or unexplained fevers. While central nervous system (CNS) involvement is not common with most initial diagnoses of acute leukemias, when present, it can be associated with significant morbidity and mortality.

There is a known association between ALL and CNS involvement, with 5%–15% of adults presenting with CNS disease at the time of diagnosis[1] and approximately 5% of relapses occurring in the CNS. As such, routine staging at the time of diagnosis includes assessment of CNS leukemic involvement and prophylaxis or treatment for CNS disease in ALL patients. Risk factors associated with CNS involvement in ALL include younger age, hyperleukocytosis (WBC>100k), KMT2 rearrangements, Philadelphia chromosome-positive ALL, mature B- or T-cell immunophenotypes, high proliferative index, and presence of extramedullary disease.[2]

Acute myeloid leukemia (AML) can also be associated with CNS disease, though less commonly than in ALL. Risk factors for AML CNS involvement in AML include young age, hyperleukocytosis, elevated Lactate Dehydrogenase, FLT3-ITD mutations, chromosomal 11q23 abnormalities, and monocytic M4 or M5 phenotype.[3]

Manifestations of CNS involvement in acute leukemias are highly variable and can include increased intracranial pressure associated with leptomeningeal involvement, cranial nerve palsy, cord compression from extramedullary blasts (chloroma), and bleeding as a result of thrombocytopenia or coagulopathy. As such, symptoms are dependent on the anatomic location and burden of disease. These may be nonspecific and can be misinterpreted as treatment-related side effects such as headache, nausea/vomiting, dizziness, mood changes, and irritability. Thus a high degree of suspicion is warranted in the evaluation of headache or any neurologic of the aforementioned symptoms.

Diagnosis of CNS disease requires CSF evaluation via lumbar puncture, as well as MRI of the brain and/or spinal cord if symptoms warrant. MRI is the preferred study, as it has demonstrated greater sensitivity than CT in detecting smaller lesions or leptomeningeal involvement.[4]

Treatment and prophylaxis of CNS leukemic infiltration are reliant on systemic therapies with the ability to penetrate the blood–brain barrier, such as high-dose methotrexate (HD-MTX) and high-dose cytarabine (HD-AraC). Intrathecal chemotherapy with methotrexate and cytarabine are essential components of management of CNS leukemia. More than half of ALL patients who do not receive intrathecal treatment may develop a CNS relapse in the future.[5]

Unfortunately, these therapies do not come without their own CNS toxicities. Through possible direct toxicity or disruption of CNS folate homeostasis, HD-MTX can be associated with headache, seizures, or stroke-like symptoms. HD-AraC has been associated with cerebellar toxicities like ataxia, delirium, and ocular toxicities.[6] Table 10.1 describes MTX, HD-AraC, as well as other medications later mentioned in this chapter that can cause headache (Table 10.1).

TABLE 10.1   Treatments for hematologic and oncologic conditions and headache

TREATMENT	MECHANISM OF ACTION	SIDE EFFECTS RELATED TO HEADACHE
Methotrexate	Blocks dihydrofolate reductase, inhibiting the conversion of dihydrofolate to tetrahydrofolate, preventing cell division[106]	Headache[106]
High-Dose Cytarabine	Pauses DNA replication in the S phase of the cell cycle[107]	Neurotoxicity, delirium, ataxia, headache, ocular toxicity[107]
Hydroxyurea	Increases Hemoglobin F; converts to free radical nitroxide in vivo and ultimately inhibits S phase of cell cycle, halting DNA synthesis[108]	Headache, dizziness, and seizures[109]
Anagrelide	Anticyclic AMP phosphodiesterase that inhibits platelet aggregation[110]	Headache[36]
Ruxolitinib	Janus kinase (JAK) inhibitor that inhibits the ATP-binding site on JAK1 and JAK2[111]	Headache, anemia[111]

(Continued)

TABLE 10.1   (Continued) Treatments for hematologic and oncologic conditions and headache

TREATMENT	MECHANISM OF ACTION	SIDE EFFECTS RELATED TO HEADACHE
Platinum agents (cisplatin, carboplatin)	Forms reactive platinum complexes inside cells that modify DNA structure and inhibits DNA synthesis[75]	Changes in vision, tinnitus, headache[75]
Paclitaxel	Stabilizes microtubules to prevent cell division and arrests cells in G2/M-phase of the cell cycle[112]	Hypertension, hypotension[112]
Docetaxel	Stabilizes microtubules to prevent cell division and arrests cells in G2/M–phase of the cell cycle, induces bcl-2 phosphorylation promoting apoptotic cell death[112]	Changes in vision, infusion reaction[112]
Methotrexate	Inhibits the conversion of dihydrofolate to tetrahydrofolate, inhibiting cell division[113]	Thrombosis, seizures[113]
Ifosfamide	Alkylation of DNA prevents DNA from dividing[114]	Hallucinations, CNS toxicity[114]
Etoposide	Inhibits DNA topoisomerase II, producing free radicals and causing DNA strand breaks and induction of apoptosis[115]	Dehydration[115]
Vinblastine	Binds to microtubular proteins in the mitotic spindle and inhibits cell division during metaphase[116]	Headache, convulsions, tinnitus[116]
VEGFi (bevacizumab, aflibercept, ranibizumab, sorafenib, dasatinib, sunitinib, nilotinib, pazopanib)	Inhibits growth of blood vessels (angiogenesis)[117]	Hemorrhage, arterial thrombosis, hypertension, reversible posterior leukoencephalopathy syndrome (PRES)[98]
Tamoxifen	Competes with 17Beta-estradiol (E2) at the receptor site to block the promotion of estrogen in breast cancer, as well as binds to DNA to initiate carcinogenesis[118]	Thrombosis, hot flashes, headache[118]
Aromatase inhibitors (anastrozole, letrozole, exemestane)	Inhibits the action of the aromatase enzyme, which converts androgens into estrogens[86]	Hot flashes, headache[87]
Gonadotropin-releasing hormone agonist (leuprolide)	Suppresses gonadotrope secretion of luteinizing hormone and follicle-stimulating hormone that suppresses gonadal sex steroid production[119]	Hot flashes, headache[95]
Gonadotropin-releasing hormone inhibitor (degarelix)	Competitively and reversibly binds luteinizing hormone-releasing hormone receptors in the pituitary gland, resulting in suppression of luteinizing hormone and follicular stimulating hormone[94]	Hot flashes, dizziness, headache[94]

Outside of leukemia involvement of the CNS, leukostasis can be related to acute and, less commonly, chronic leukemias. This can be a life-threatening condition caused by decreased tissue perfusion due to increased blood viscosity by large numbers of circulating immature leukemic blasts. These immature white blood cells are less malleable and can lead to congestion of the microvasculature.[7] Manifestations of leukostasis are commonly seen in the CNS (30% in AML and 15.3% in ALL), as well as with respiratory symptoms (38.5% in AML and 23% in ALL[8]). Neurologic findings include headache, visual changes, dizziness, tinnitus, ataxia, and altered mental status. Treatment of leukostasis involves therapies to rapidly reduce the leukocyte count and include hydroxyurea (a cytoreductive therapy), leukapheresis, and initiation of systemic chemotherapy for the underlying leukemia.

Answer to Clinical Case #1

This patient has been diagnosed with ALL. ALL has an association with CNS disease at the time of diagnosis and at the time of relapse, and may present with headache. Primary treatment and prophylaxis of CNS leukemic infiltration is through systemic and intrathecal chemotherapies. The treatments themselves may also lead to headache.

ANEMIA

In addition to the malignant hematologic etiologies for headache, iron deficiency anemia can also commonly present with headache and fatigue. A questionnaire-based study revealed those with iron deficiency anemia reported an incidence of headache at 80%, with over one-third demonstrating features consistent with migraine.[9] Treatment of iron deficiency involves either oral or parenteral iron supplementation.[10]

SICKLE CELL DISEASE

Sickle cell disease (SCD) is a genetic disorder resulting from mutations in the beta-globin gene. The most common genotype is hemoglobin SS, which is synonymous with sickle cell anemia. The disease is inherited in an autosomal recessive pattern, with hemoglobin S causing abnormal cell polymerization and a characteristic sickled appearance of red blood cells in a low-oxygen environment.[11] Due to the deformity of the hemoglobin structure, this predisposes patients with sickle cell anemia to complications such as vaso-occlusive events, vascular ischemia, oxidative stress, and hemolytic anemia. These can manifest as pain crises, acute chest syndrome, stroke, and organ dysfunction. Pain, especially vaso-occlusive crises, is a common cause of morbidity, requiring acute opioid therapy and medications like hydroxyurea to reduce pain episodes.[12] Hydroxyurea helps increase the level of Hemoglobin F[13], which helps increase the level of hemoglobin for the patient and decrease the sickling episodes.

Headache in sickle cell anemia patients can result from primary or secondary causes. The prevalence of recurrent headache in studies of children and adolescents with SCD is estimated between 17.8 and 43.9%,[14] with an increased rate of headache reported in SCD patients compared with age-matched controls.[15]

Primary headaches experienced in SCD patients are typically tension-type headache or migraines.[16] While primary headaches do not typically produce the severe morbidity associated with secondary causes of headache in this population, patients with frequent headache were more likely to experience vaso-occlusive crises.[17]

Secondary causes of headache in SCD patients are more concerning and can include acute stroke, intracranial hemorrhage, posterior reversible encephalopathy syndrome (PRES), moyamoya syndrome, and cerebral venous thrombosis. Stroke is a leading cause of morbidity and mortality in SCD.[18] In addition to supportive management of stroke patients, the treatment for acute ischemic stroke is red blood cell exchange transfusion. Patients should receive simple transfusion to increase the hemoglobin level until exchange transfusion can be performed as it is more effective at lowering hemoglobin S percentage.

PRES can manifest in SCD patients, especially those with acute chest syndrome or following transfusions. It is characterized as headache, vision changes, confusion, nausea, and seizures, classically in the setting of elevated blood pressure. Treatment is supportive to control hypertension, seizures, and address reversible causes.

Clinical Case #2

A 57-year-old male presents with new-onset headache, skin reddening, and itching after hot showers. His laboratory testing shows hemoglobin 18.6 g/dL and hematocrit 58%; the remainder of his complete blood count is within normal limits. He is tested for mutations in the JAK-STAT pathway and found to have a JAK2 V617F mutation.

MYELOPROLIFERATIVE NEOPLASMS

Polycythemia vera (PV) is a myeloproliferative neoplasm (MPN). MPNs arise from clonal proliferation of myeloid cells.[19] PV differs from other MPNs by its increased red blood cell mass, though this finding is not specific to PV, as it can also be observed in patients with chronic hypoxia or erythropoietin-stimulating tumors. A JAK2 mutation is identified in the vast majority of patients with PV and is known to be the driving mutation in the pathogenesis of the disorder.[19] While some patients are diagnosed with PV upon further investigation of an elevated hemoglobin or hematocrit performed on routine complete blood count, others are diagnosed based on clinical manifestations or sequelae of untreated disease. Common clinical features of PV include hypertension, splenomegaly, ruddy cyanosis, gout flare, along with vasomotor symptoms such as erythromelalgia, aquagenic pruritus, headache, dizziness, visual disturbances, and paresthesias. Venous and arterial thrombosis and, rarely, significant hemorrhage can also occur.[19]

The pathogenesis of headache in PV is thought to be related to increased blood viscosity, leading to interruption in capillary microcirculation. Subsequently, this can lead to headache and vision changes.[20] While migraine more commonly affects those with vasomotor-related headache, cluster headache can occasionally happen as well. Popescu[21] cited a case involving a patient with cluster-like headache, who was later found to have underlying PV and responded dramatically to treatment with phlebotomy, an essential component of treatment in PV. Pharmacologic therapies such as hydroxyurea, aspirin, and alternative agents such as interferon, busulfan, and ruxolitinib may also be considered in the treatment of PV. Treatment is typically geared toward disease control of the MPN.

Essential thrombocythemia/essential thrombocytosis (ET) is another disease within the MPN classification and often presents with an elevated platelet count. It is known to cause similar vasomotor symptoms to PV.[22] While the exact pathogenesis of ET is not fully understood, it is thought to be a clonal stem cell disorder leading to excess production of platelets through the upregulation of the JAK-STAT pathway,[23] also driven by somatic mutations in JAK2, as well as CALR, or MPL in 90% of cases.[24] As in PV, a large proportion of patients are found to have this disease incidentally when thrombocytosis is identified on routine laboratory testing. Others may present with symptoms including, but not limited to, headache, vision changes, or dizziness.

Headache can occur in ET, though the specific pathogenesis remains largely unknown. A prospective study was able to identify a relationship between onset of headache and hematologic relapse of ET.[25] Other theories regarding platelet dysfunction to headache include serotonin receptor hypersensitivity or increased levels of serotonin circulating in the plasma. Serotonin is known to be a significant neurotransmitter involved in the etiology of migraine, and platelets are known to release serotonin in response to collagen.[26, 27] Moreover, a study by Michiels cited transient neurologic symptoms, such as headache, preceding or following erythromelalgia, further supporting the relationship between platelet dysfunction and headache in ET.[28]

Increased nitric oxide levels have also been an area of inquiry with regard to the underlying mechanism of headache in ET. Nitric oxide plays an essential role in both intracranial and extracranial blood flow. While platelets are known to produce nitric oxide when activated, this activation serves as negative feedback to preclude further platelet recruitment. A study by Rejto et al. demonstrates that in patients with chronic myeloproliferative neoplasms involving thrombocytosis, the nitric oxide response is attenuated, which is thought to be secondary to platelet dysfunction. Furthermore, these findings suggest that the impaired nitric oxide response may lead to platelet proliferation and subsequent thrombotic complications.[29]

The generally accepted approach to treatment of ET-related headache, among other vasomotor symptoms of ET, is with low-dose aspirin as well as treatment of the underlying condition.[30] Aside from vasomotor-related headache, one should also take into consideration that headache in a patient with ET or PV could reflect a stroke or intracranial bleed.

Medications used in the treatment of myeloproliferative neoplasms may cause headaches. Hydroxyurea is a commonly used cytoreductive medication for treatment of high-risk PV and ET. Nitric oxide production has been shown to be increased in patients with ET after administration of hydroxyurea. It is thought that this higher level of nitric oxide may lead to vasodilation and headache symptoms (Table 10.1).

Myelofibrosis (MF) is both a primary and secondary MPN disorder. Primary myelofibrosis is caused by disruption of the JAK-STAT pathway and subsequent defects in hematopoietic stem cells, followed by downstream abnormalities in megakaryocytic and granulocytic proliferation. As a result, inflammatory cytokines are secreted, and myeloproliferation, bone marrow fibrosis, and extramedullary hematopoiesis take place.[31] Secondary myelofibrosis can evolve from ET or PV.[32] Clinically, patients experience significant fatigue, early satiety, or abdominal pain related to splenomegaly or constitutional symptoms.[33, 34] Most do not experience the same vasomotor symptoms as those with PV or ET. Therefore, clinicians should rule out dangerous pathologies such as a stroke when evaluating a patient with myelofibrosis presenting with a headache. If treatment of myelofibrosis is indicated, there are various medications used that are known to cause headache, including hydroxyurea, as mentioned earlier (Table 10.1). Ruxolitinib is a JAK2 inhibitor commonly used in the treatment of myelofibrosis. Headache is a reported side effect of this medication as well, though the mechanism is not well understood (Table 10.1).[35] Anagrelide is another medication utilized in the treatment of MPNs by inhibiting megakaryocyte differentiation in the bone marrow.[36, 37] In clinical trials, headache was the most common side effect, reported to have occurred in 52% of patients with an MPN taking anagrelide hydrochloride capsules (Table 10.1).[36] Headache from anagrelide was found to decrease over time while on the drug and was noted to be dose related.[37]

Answer to Clinical Case #2

The patient has PV with a JAK2 mutation. Myeloproliferative neoplasms, such as PV and ET, are associated with vasomotor symptoms such as headache. Headache may also be associated with pharmacologic agents used for treatment of the underlying disease. It is also important to consider that headache in patients with MPNs can be secondary to thrombosis.

THROMBOTIC THROMBOCYTOPENIC PURPURA

Thrombotic thrombocytopenic purpura (TTP) is a thrombotic microangiopathic disorder characterized by the formation of microthrombi within the vascular walls of arterioles and capillaries. The pathogenesis stems from a deficiency of a key protease, ADAMTS13, to a value of less than 10%.[38] ADAMTS13 is responsible for cleaving proteins such as large Von Willebrand Factor (VWF) molecules. If ADAMTS13 activity is reduced, the large VWF molecules accumulate, forming multimers on the endothelial surface where platelets aggregate, leading to clot formation.[38] This clot formation culminates in the consumption of platelets and microangiopathic hemolytic anemia evidenced by schistocytes on peripheral blood smear, among other findings.[39] While deficiency of ADAMTS13 remains the only causative factor identified thus far, there are other precipitating factors, such as inflammation, sepsis, and pregnancy, which can increase VWF levels and potentially lead to an acute episode.[39, 40] Clinically, it has long been thought that patients with TTP present with a classic pentad of symptoms: fevers, thrombocytopenia, neurologic symptoms, microangiopathic hemolytic anemia, and renal insufficiency. However, this presentation is rarely the case, and more often, patients present with severe thrombocytopenia, microangiopathic hemolytic anemia, and associated symptoms including, but not limited to, fatigue, generalized weakness, skin and/or mucosal bleeding, and dyspnea. Neurologic manifestations can be extensive, ranging from confusion and headache to stroke, seizures, and even coma.[39]

While headache may be the initial presentation of a patient suffering from an acute TTP episode, they are also, unfortunately, a common sequela following an acute episode. This was studied by Saultz et al. in their single-center cross-sectional survey study examining headache prevalence following recovery from TTP. Patients who had an acute episode of TTP over three months prior were surveyed. The results showed a statistically significant increase in the impact of headache on quality of life in patients with TTP compared to sex-matched controls. This study sheds light on a lesser-recognized symptom in patients recovering from TTP and adds to the differential when assessing the etiology of a TTP patient's chronic headache.[41]

HYPERCOAGULABLE STATES

Blood clots may also lead to headache, particularly those that form in the cerebral venous system. Patients who have thrombophilias such as factor V Leiden mutation, antiphospholipid antibody syndrome, protein C or S deficiency, prothrombin gene mutations, or antithrombin III deficiency may be more susceptible to these types of thromboses. Therefore, patients with a history of deep vein thrombosis or pulmonary embolism who develop a cerebral venous thrombosis should be evaluated for these thrombophilias with further testing. One type of cerebral venous clot is cerebral venous sinus thrombosis (CVST). The usage of hormonal therapies such as oral contraceptive pills is associated with the formation of these thromboses. These clots can cause sinus occlusion, which leads to a backflow of blood in the vascular system, which can cause cerebral edema. Eighty percent of patients with CVST will present with headache.[42] Patients may also present with seizures, vision changes, papilledema, or encephalopathy. Treatment involves anticoagulation including options of unfractionated heparin, low-molecular-weight heparin, warfarin, or direct oral anticoagulants. There are no large-scale randomized trials available to compare the efficacy of these therapies and the choice of treatment may depend on whether or not the patient has an underlying thrombophilia. Patients who fail to improve with anticoagulation may require thrombolysis.[42]

Clinical Case #3

A 40-year-old female with a history of Stage II triple-negative, right-sided breast cancer presents with worsening headache and difficulty with balance. A brain MRI with contrast notes multiple well-circumscribed contrast-enhancing lesions in the frontal lobe and cerebellum, concerning for metastatic disease.

BRAIN METASTASES

Patients with a history of malignancy or an active malignancy with new or worsening headache should be assessed for the possibility of metastatic disease involving the brain. Approximately only 50% of patients who have a brain tumor complain of headache. The brain parenchyma does not contain pain receptors. Therefore, headache caused by brain metastases or tumors are typically caused by traction on the dura, vasculature, subcutaneous tissue, or skin (which do contain these pain receptors). Brain metastases can also cause vasogenic cerebral edema.[43] This is due to leakage of plasma across the vessel wall and into the parenchyma because of disruption to the blood–brain barrier. If the edema is not controlled, this can increase the intracranial pressure and also present as headache.[44] The quality of headache pain caused by brain tumors may vary and can include migraine-type or tension-type.[45] Other symptoms associated with brain metastasis include vomiting (26%), nausea (23%), hemiparesis (22%), visual changes (13%), and seizures (12%).[46] Therefore, patients who present with headache in addition to blurred or double vision, nausea, vomiting, cognitive changes, focal neurologic changes on physical exam, or new seizures should immediately be evaluated for brain metastases.

The most common malignancies with a propensity for brain metastases are lung cancer, breast cancer, melanoma, and renal cell carcinoma. The pathogenesis of brain metastasis is due to hematogenous spread of malignant cells. Brain metastases are usually localized to the gray-white matter junction, specifically the cerebral hemispheres and cerebellum, and less commonly the brainstem.[47, 48] Imaging with a contrast-enhanced MRI remains the preferred modality in evaluating a patient with suspected brain metastasis.[49]

Breast cancer is a common malignancy with a risk of brain metastases. Approximately 15%–30% of patients with metastatic breast cancer will develop brain metastases.[50] There are notable differences in brain metastases incidence among different subtypes of breast cancer. Metastatic hormone-receptor-positive breast cancer carries a three-year cumulative incidence of brain metastasis of 20%, whereas the incidence in patients with triple-positive disease (hormone-receptor positive and HER2 positive) is 39%, hormone negative and HER2 positive 59%, and triple-negative breast cancer 55%.[51] The variability may be explained by the complex tumor microenvironment and gene expression profiles of the primary tumor with upregulation of genes involved in cell cycle control (Wnt, Notch, and epidermal growth factor receptors)[52]. As with other solid tumors, brain metastasis in breast cancer portends a poor prognosis. Based on a SEER database review between 2010 and 2014, the difference in median overall survival between metastatic breast cancer patients with or without brain metastases was 11 months and 30 months, respectively.[53]

Treatment of brain metastases requires a multidisciplinary approach, including surgery, radiation, and systemic therapy. Local aggressive treatment with surgical resection is typically limited to patients with good performance status and a single solitary brain lesion.[54] The benefits of surgery compared to radiation therapy (RT) are more rapid cerebral decompression, shorter duration of use of steroids, and additional tissue for diagnosis or additional analysis. RT with whole brain radiation (WBRT) or stereotactic radiosurgery (SRS) can be considered for patients with multiple lesions or lesions that are not surgically accessible. Both of these strategies can be complicated by both early and late neurotoxicity. While WBRT can provide timely relief of neurological symptoms and improved quality of life, neurocognitive dysfunction resulting from WBRT poses a significant challenge.

Systemic therapies are limited in brain metastasis in any type of cancer due to the inability of many cytotoxic medications to cross the blood–brain barrier. The tight junctions and lack of fenestrations of the blood–brain barrier limit the penetration of cytotoxic drugs into the CNS.[54] The brain tissue itself has a unique immune environment involving astrocytes and complex interactions with cytokines, which may play a role in immune evasion and brain metastasis development.[54]

Cancer can metastasize to the CNS as leptomeningeal disease, wherein cancer cells permeate the leptomeninges and subarachnoid space. The most common solid tumors giving rise to leptomeningeal disease are breast cancer (12%–35%), lung cancer (10%–26%), and melanoma (5%–25%).[55] Median overall survival of breast cancer patients with leptomeningeal disease has been reported at four to five months.[55] Leptomeningeal disease can manifest as cranial neuropathies, radiculopathy or cauda equina syndrome, confusion, cerebellar dysfunction, headache, or seizures.[56] There is no role for surgical intervention in leptomeningeal disease. Local therapy with radiation can target symptomatic lesions; however, the mainstay of treatment is systemic therapy.

Metastatic lung cancer to the brain has been reported to occur in 10%–36% of lung cancer cases, though this range has been felt to underestimate the true incidence. Overall survival for lung cancer patients who develop brain metastases has been cited at only 3.4 months, though this may improve with the development of new therapeutic agents.[57] Patients with non-small-cell lung cancer (NSCLC), those with epidermal growth factor receptor (EGFR), anaplastic lymphoma kinase rearrangement (ALK), or human epidermal growth factor receptor (HER2) mutations or alterations have an increased proclivity for brain metastasis.[58–60] Leptomeningeal disease may also occur in patients with lung cancer.

Up to 30%–40% of melanoma patients with advanced disease will have brain metastases at the time of diagnosis. For many years, melanoma patients were excluded from clinical trials evaluating the efficacy of systemic therapies. Recently, clinical trials have been developed that show that patients with brain metastases from melanoma can have responses in the brain to systemic therapies used for treatment of non-CNS disease. Immunotherapies targeting the PD-1/PD-L1/CTLA-4 pathway are commonly used in the treatment of melanoma. Several studies have now shown that patients with brain metastases treated with immunotherapy may have a reduction in their brain metastatic disease.[61] Melanoma patients are also tested for alterations in BRAF as therapies targeting both BRAF and MEK have shown to have activity in these patients. There are also now several trials showing intracranial responses in patients with brain metastases and BRAF mutations treated with combined BRAF/MEK inhibition.[61]

Renal cell carcinoma (RCC) has a low prevalence of brain metastases at the time of diagnosis (1.5%), but throughout the disease course, this incidence increases to 10%–15%.[62] As with other solid tumors, brain metastasis portends a poor prognosis in patients with RCC, with median overall survival being less than ten months.[63] Risk factors associated with brain metastasis development include Caucasian ethnicity, sarcomatoid differentiation, larger size of the primary tumor, and lymph node infiltration.[62] RCC brain metastases are unique in that they harbor an increased risk for hemorrhage due to increased tumor vascularity and development in intraventricular regions and in proximity to the choroid plexus.[64, 65]

Answer to Clinical Case #3

Patients with a history of malignancy who present with new-onset or worsening headache should be evaluated for brain metastases, especially in the setting of additional symptoms such as vision changes, nausea, vomiting, cognitive changes, focal neurologic changes on physical exam, or new seizures. Patients should undergo imaging with brain MRI with contrast. The treatment of brain metastases depends on the primary malignancy but may involve surgery, radiation, and/or systemic therapies, though only a subset of systemic therapies can cross the blood–brain barrier. The development of brain metastases is a poor prognostic factor.

Clinical Case #4

A 50-year-old male has been diagnosed with stage IV small-cell lung cancer. He has started chemotherapy with cisplatin and etoposide. During his first cycle, he experienced severe headache and mild nausea. He took ondansetron for his nausea, which reduced his nausea, but the headache remained. He returns to the clinic prior to cycle two. He states his skin and lips feel very dry. He reports that about five days after receiving chemotherapy, he developed a severe persistent frontal pressure headache that he rates an 8/10 on the pain scale. He feels weak and tired, as well as dizzy and short of breath with ambulation. He denies unilateral weakness or mental status changes. His vital signs show a temperature of 98.8 degrees Celsius, blood pressure of 90/50 mmHg, and heart rate of 110 beats/minute. He had a brain MRI prior to starting chemotherapy, which was normal. What is the most likely cause of his headache?

CHEMOTHERAPY-INDUCED HEADACHE

Chemotherapeutic medications can precipitate a headache. Etoposide is a topoisomerase II inhibitor that prevents DNA synthesis and induces breaks in double-stranded DNA.[66] This chemotherapy agent is commonly used for treating small-cell lung cancer and germ-cell tumors. Etoposide contains ethanol, polyethylene glycol, and benzyl alcohol as additives.[68] These alcohol products can dehydrate the patient and induce a headache.[69] These headaches can be refractory and may ultimately require treatment to be changed.[70] The pathophysiology of dehydration and headache is not fully understood.[71] The Monro-Kellie doctrine suggests that a water deficit in the body results in dural venous stretching, provoking a headache.[72]

Other chemotherapies are associated with headache. Vinblastine is a vinca alkaloid chemotherapeutic agent that binds to microtubular proteins in the mitotic spindle and inhibits cell division during metaphase. This chemotherapy can commonly cause neurotoxicities such as paresthesias, peripheral neuritis, depression, convulsions, and headache.[73] It can lead to both auditory and vestibular damage to the eighth cranial nerve with the potential of partial or total deafness, as well as difficulties with balance, dizziness, nystagmus, and vertigo. All of these symptoms may precipitate or be concurrent with headache.[74]

Carboplatin and cisplatin are both platinum-based chemotherapeutic agents. They work by forming reactive platinum complexes inside cells that modify DNA structure and inhibit DNA synthesis.[75] Platinum chemotherapies can cause ototoxic effects such as tinnitus, which can precipitate headache.[75] Caution must be used if administering platinum therapies in combination with vinca alkaloids discussed earlier, as the combined neurotoxic effects may produce more significant headache. These treatments are also described in Table 10.1.

ANTIEMETICS

Many chemotherapy agents are highly emetogenic. It is considered standard of care for patients to receive prophylactic antiemetics while receiving chemotherapy. 5-HT3 antagonists are common medications prescribed to cancer patients to help reduce nausea and emesis. These medications block serotonin both on the gastrointestinal (GI) vagal nerve terminals and the central chemoreceptors.[77] Ondansetron is a commonly used 5-HT3 antagonist. Its half-life is approximately 3.5 hours, and it is generally well tolerated. It can safely be taken every 4–6 hours as needed. However, headache is the most commonly reported side effect.[78] The exact mechanism of ondansetron-induced headache is unknown. It is known that 5-hydroxytryptamine (5-HT) is an endogenous serotonin. Normal levels of this prevent migraine.[79] One study evaluated the side effects of ondansetron in more than 2,500 cancer patients who received intravenous doses. Headache occurred in 14% of patients.[80] Higher doses of ondansetron not only increase its antiemetic effect but also magnify its side effect profile. In an early study examining the clinical safety of ondansetron, there was a higher incidence of headache with a 32 mg dose (25%) compared to an 8 mg dose (18%). In 2012, the 32 mg dose of ondansetron was removed from the market due to increased risk for irregular heart rhythms. The highest recommended dose is now 16 mg.[81]

Due to concerns about safety and toxicities with large doses of 5-HT3 antagonists, a multimodal approach for adequately preventing nausea and vomiting is used in oncologic treatments. Patients are often given antiemetics targeting alternative pathways in addition to 5-HT3 antagonists prior to the chemotherapeutic agent to prevent nausea.

One class of medication that may be used are the NK-1 receptor antagonists (aprepitant, rolapitant, fosaprepitant, and netupitant). These medications prevent both chemotherapy-induced nausea and vomiting by blocking NK-1 receptor activation of substance P in the CNS, which releases the emetogenic signal from chemotherapy.[82] The most common side effects of NK-1 receptor antagonists are fatigue, anorexia, constipation or diarrhea, and hiccups.[83] In studies of NK-1 receptor antagonists such as aprepitant, headache have been a listed adverse effect.

Other medications that are used to prevent chemotherapy-induced nausea and vomiting include benzodiazepines (such as lorazepam), D2 dopamine receptor antagonists (such as olanzapine, prochlorperazine, metoclopramide), and steroids (such as dexamethasone).[84] By utilizing a multimodal approach for emetic prophylaxis, a smaller dose of each medication can be given in combination with others with similar or even improved efficacy. This multimodal approach also allows for medications that may have caused headache to be completely eliminated from the prophylactic regimen while still maintaining appropriate symptom control.

The antiemetics mentioned earlier are described further in Table 10.2.

TABLE 10.2 Supportive agents and headache

SUPPORTIVE AGENT	MECHANISM OF ACTION	SIDE EFFECTS
5-HT3 antagonists (ondansetron, granisetron, and palonosetron)	Block serotonin both on the gastrointestinal (GI) vagal nerve terminals and the central chemoreceptors[77]	Serotonin syndrome, headache[79]
NK-1 receptor antagonists (aprepitant, rolapitant, fosaprepitant, and netupitant)	Block NK-1 receptor activation of substance P in the CNS, which releases the emetic signal from chemotherapy[121]	Possible headache (controversial)[121]
Bisphosphonates (risedronate, alendronate, ibandronate, zoledronic acid, pamidronate)	Inhibit osteoclastic bone resorption[122]	Mild headache[122]
Opiates (buprenorphine, codeine, fentanyl, hydrocodone, hydromorphone, methadone, morphine, oxycodone, tramadol)	Bind to MOP receptors in central and peripheral nervous system in an agonist manner to elicit analgesia[123]	Medication-overuse headache[103]

Answer to Clinical Case #4

The patient had significant headache during his first cycle of chemotherapy. His complaints and vital signs are also indicative of dehydration. His dehydration is likely due to the alcohol-based components of etoposide leading to hypovolemia. If not appropriately managed with fluid resuscitation, dehydration can lead to secondary headache that can be debilitating and impair the patient's ability to continue to receive cancer-directed therapies. He also took ondansetron to help manage his nausea. This could have contributed to his headache as well. It is recommended for patients to use a multimodal approval for antiemetics in order to lower the dose of each in hopes of preventing migraine. The use of intravenous fluids while receiving chemotherapy or in between cycles, as well as using lower doses of multiple antiemetics, may allow the patient to better tolerate his chemotherapy.

Clinical Case #5

A 65-year-old female with a history of migraines has been diagnosed with stage I left hormone-receptor-positive breast cancer. She is treated with lumpectomy and is subsequently started on anastrozole to reduce the risk of breast cancer recurrence. She has a bone density scan, which shows osteoporosis. She is started on zoledronic acid to prevent further thinning of her bones. She presents to the clinic the day after receiving her first infusion of zoledronic acid and states that she has experienced an increased frequency of her migraine since starting anastrozole and had a headache after zoledronic acid yesterday as well.

HORMONAL THERAPIES

Hormone-targeting agents such as tamoxifen and aromatase inhibitors are used in patients with hormone-receptor-positive breast cancer. Both medications modify or reduce the actions of estrogen in the body. Tamoxifen works by competing with 17beta-estradiol (E2) at the receptor site to block the promotion of estrogen in breast cancer, as well as binding to DNA to initiate carcinogenesis.[85] Aromatase inhibitors block the conversion of androgens to estrogen.[86]

Studies have shown that migraine may be linked to hormonal changes and fluctuations. The use of hormonal contraception or hormonal replacement therapy can modify migraines.[87] In 1972, Somerville demonstrated that injection of estradiol shortly before menstruation delayed the onset of migraine in females. A level of estradiol less than 45–50 pg/mL was likely to trigger headache in those with a history of menstrual migraines.[88] Another study confirmed this in postmenopausal women who had a decrease in migraines when taking hormone replacement therapy as well as intramuscular estrogen injections.[89]

Side effects of tamoxifen include hot flashes, increased risk of blood clots, increased risk of uterine cancer, fatigue, and headache (Table 10.1).[90] Aromatase inhibitor side effects include asthenia, hot flashes, joint pain, osteoporosis, and headache as well (Table 10.1).[91] These medications could intensify headache due to their effects on estrogen in the body, particularly in women with a history of low-estrogen-induced headache. One study found that patients who smoke tobacco had an increased amount of tamoxifen-related side effects, including migraine.[92] It is important for patients with a history of menstrual/postmenopausal migraines to be aware of the potential for exacerbation of migraines prior to starting anti-estrogen medications.

In men, androgens are targeted in the treatment of prostate cancer. Leuprolide acetate is a gonadotropin-releasing hormone (GnRH) agonist used to suppress testosterone.[93] Degarelix is a GnRH inhibitor that also decreases androgen production. Inhibiting androgens is an effective way to target prostate cancer, as it is understood that prostate cancer cell growth is stimulated by testosterone.[94]

Studies have identified a relationship between hypogonadism and refractory headache.[95] One study showed that among 14 males with a history of chronic migraines, the average testosterone level was 322 ng/dL (in the lower 5% of the reference range of 300–1080 ng/dL).[95] Another small study analyzed seven males and two females with treatment-resistant cluster headaches who had low serum testosterone levels.[96] The male patients were treated with testosterone, while female patients were treated with a combination of testosterone and estrogen therapy. The study found that all male patients with low testosterone achieved remission of headache. This data suggests that low testosterone may be correlated to headache in male patients.

Headache as a side effect of GnRH inhibition is not well documented. However, it should be discussed with prostate cancer patients before starting treatment based on the literature presented (Table 10.1).

VASCULAR ENDOTHELIAL GROWTH FACTOR INHIBITORS

Vascular endothelial growth factor inhibitors work by inhibiting VEGF, a protein involved in angiogenesis, which is closely linked to tumor growth. VEGF inhibitors are used in the treatment of cancer, degenerative eye conditions, and other inflammatory diseases. VEGF may be targeted by monoclonal antibodies, such as bevacizumab, or by tyrosine-kinase inhibitors, such as cabozantinib, pazopanib, sorafenib, regorafenib, and lenvatinib.[97] Side effects of VEGF inhibitors include hemorrhage, arterial thrombosis, hypertension, impaired wound healing, PRES, and proteinuria.[98] As discussed earlier in this chapter, PRES is a clinico-radiological syndrome characterized by headache, seizures, altered mental status, and vision loss. Imaging findings show white matter vasogenic edema affecting the posterior lobes of the brain. PRES itself requires a headache for its diagnosis.

BONE MODIFYING AGENTS

Bisphosphonates are commonly used in oncology. Hormonal therapies used in breast and prostate cancer can lead to bone thinning and osteoporosis, which can increase the risk of fractures.[99] To counteract this, oncologists often prescribe bisphosphonates, a class of drugs that help to strengthen bones and reduce the risk of bone-related complications. They are also used to prevent skeletal-related adverse events in patients with bone metastases. Bisphosphonates work by inhibiting osteoclastic bone resorption.[100] This helps to maintain bone strength in those with osteoporosis or with osseous metastatic lesions. Acute reactions to bisphosphonates may include flu-like symptoms such as fever, achiness, and headache (Table 10.2).[101] These symptoms typically respond to ibuprofen or acetaminophen and resolve within a few days. These side effects tend to occur more frequently with the use of intravenous bisphosphonate therapies such as zoledronic acid.

Answer to Clinical Case #5

This patient was started on an aromatase inhibitor, which alters the amount of estrogen in her body. She has a history of migraines, and changes in hormone levels in the body are known to have the potential to worsen migraines. She also received zoledronic acid for treatment of her osteoporosis, which can be associated with mild headache.

MEDICATION-OVERUSE HEADACHE

Another important tool used to manage symptoms associated with cancer is analgesics, including opiates. Approximately 65% of patients with advanced cancer have pain, and 30%–50% of those experiencing pain that negatively impacts their quality of life.[102] Opiates are commonly used to treat this pain.

Patients who take opiate medications may frequently develop medication-overuse headache (MOH) (Table 10.2).[103] Patients with headache may overuse medication for their acute pain and inadvertently increase the frequency and dose in which a cycle of further drug consumption can develop. This may ultimately lead to a treatment for headache becoming the cause. Diagnostic criteria for MOH are a headache occurring greater than or equal to 15 days per month for a patient with preexisting headache, a regular medication overuse for greater than 3 months or more, or a headache without another cause for diagnosis. Many cancer patients will need to take opiates for many months. Using opiates can cause previously episodic migraines to transition to chronic migraines.[104] This is because opiates may activate toll-like receptor-4 on glial cells, resulting in increased inflammation that may present as pain/headache.[105] Treatment is the cessation of the medication, which can be difficult when opiates are often necessary to treat cancer-related pain.

SUMMARY

- ALL has an association with CNS involvement at the time of diagnosis and at the time of relapse. This may present with headache.
- Primary treatment and prophylaxis of CNS leukemic infiltration is with systemic and intrathecal chemotherapies. These treatments may lead to headache.
- Headache can be a manifestation of iron deficiency anemia with patients having an 80% reported rate of headache.
- SCD can be associated with headache, including primary headache, as well as headache related to secondary causes such as acute stroke or PRES.
- Myeloproliferative neoplasms, such as PV and ET, are associated with vasomotor symptoms, such as headache, though headache can also occur secondary to thrombosis. Headache may be associated with pharmacologic agents used for treatment of the underlying disease.
- TTP is a disorder characterized by the formation of microthrombi and can present with a headache, though these patients may also experience chronic headache months after an acute episode.

- Blood clots involving the cerebral venous system, such as CVST, often present with headache.
- Patients with a history of malignancy with new or worsening headache need to be evaluated for the presence of metastatic disease to the brain, especially in the setting of other associated symptoms, such as vision changes, headache, nausea, vomiting, cognitive changes, seizures, or focal neurologic changes. Contrast-enhanced MRI is the initial imaging modality of choice in diagnosing brain metastasis.
- Chemotherapeutic agents can cause headache through direct mechanisms of action or through secondary causes such as dehydration.
- 5-HT3 antagonists, such as ondansetron, can directly cause headache. A multimodal approach may need to be considered when treating patients for chemotherapy side effects such as nausea in order to limit the dose of 5-HT3 antagonists and reduce the risk of headache.
- Hormonal therapies used in cancer therapies can induce headache and should be considered when treating patients with a history of migraines.
- Opiates, which are often used for pain control in those with malignancy, may cause MOH. Treatment is the withdrawal of the medication.

REFERENCES

1. Lazarus HM, Richards SM, Chopra R, et al. Medical Research Council (MRC)/National Cancer Research Institute (NCRI) Adult Leukaemia Working Party of the United Kingdom and the Eastern Cooperative Oncology Group. Central nervous system involvement in adult acute lymphoblastic leukemia at diagnosis: results from the international ALL trial MRC UKALL XII/ECOG E2993. *Blood.* 2006 Jul 15;*108*(2):465–72. doi: 10.1182/blood-2005-11-4666.
2. Kantarjian HM, Walters RS, Smith TL, et al. Identification of risk groups for development of central nervous system leukemia in adults with acute lymphocytic leukemia. *Blood.* 1988 Nov;*72*(5):1784–9. PMID: 3052630.
3. Johnston DL, Alonzo TA, Gerbing RB, et al. Risk factors and therapy for isolated central nervous system relapse of pediatric acute myeloid leukemia. *J Clin Oncol.* 2005;*23*:9172–8. doi: 10.1200/jco.2005.02.7482.
4. Shen H, Zhao Y, Shi Y, et al. The diagnostic and prognostic value of MRI in central nervous system involvement of acute myeloid leukemia: a retrospective cohort of 84 patients. *Hematology.* 2020 Dec;*25*(1):258–263. doi: 10.1080/16078454.2020.1781500. PMID: 32567523.
5. Cortes J, O'Brien SM, Pierce S, et al. The value of high-dose systemic chemotherapy and intrathecal therapy for central nervous system prophylaxis in different risk groups of adult acute lymphoblastic leukemia. *Blood.* 1995 Sep 15;*86*(6):2091–7. PMID: 7662956.
6. Neurotoxicity associated with high dose cytarabine. (2021). eviQ. Retrieved December 17, 2023, from https://www.eviq.org.au/clinical-resources/side-effect-and-toxicity-management/neurological-and-sensory/1742-neurotoxicity-associated-with-high-dose-cytar.
7. Röllig C, Ehninger G. How I treat hyperleukocytosis in acute myeloid leukemia. *Blood.* 2015;*125*:3246–52. doi: 10.1182/blood-2014-10-551507.
8. Porcu P, Cripe LD, Ng EW, Bhatia S, Danielson CM, Orazi A, McCarthy LJ. Hyperleukocytic leukemias and leukostasis: a review of pathophysiology, clinical presentation and management. *Leuk Lymphoma.* 2000 Sep;*39*(1–2):1–18. doi: 10.3109/10428190009053534. PMID: 10975379.
9. Pamuk GE, Top MS, Uyanik MS, et al. Is iron-deficiency anemia associated with migraine? Is there a role for anxiety and depression? *Wien Klin Wochenschr.* 2016;*128*(Suppl 8):576–80. 10.1007/s00508-015-0740-8.
10. Macher S, Herster C, Holter M, et al. The effect of parenteral or oral iron supplementation on fatigue, sleep, quality of life and restless legs syndrome in iron-deficient blood donors: a secondary analysis of the IronWoMan RCT. *Nutrients.* 2020;*12*(5). doi: 10.3390/nu12051313.
11. Rees DC, Williams TN, Gladwin MT. Sickle-cell disease. *Lancet.* 2010 Dec 11;*376*(9757):2018–31. doi: 10.1016/S0140-6736(10)61029-X. Epub 2010 Dec 3. PMID: 21131035.
12. Charache S, Terrin ML, Moore RD, et al. Effect of hydroxyurea on the frequency of painful crises in sickle cell anemia. Investigators of the Multicenter Study of Hydroxyurea in Sickle Cell Anemia. *N Engl J Med.* 1995 May 18;*332*(20):1317–22. doi: 10.1056/NEJM199505183322001. PMID: 7715639.

13. Agrawal RK, Patel RK, Shah V, et al. Hydroxyurea in sickle cell disease: drug review. *Indian J Hematol Blood Transfus.* 2014 Jun;*30*(2):91–6. doi: 10.1007/s12288-013-0261-4.

14. Vgontzas A, Charleston L, Robbins MS. Headache and facial pain in sickle cell disease. *Curr Pain Headache Rep.* 2016 Mar;*20*(3):20. doi: 10.1007/s11916-016-0546-z. PMID: 26879878.

15. Kehinde MO, Temiye EO, Danesi MA. Neurological complications of sickle cell anemia in Nigerian Africans–a case-control study. *J Natl Med Assoc.* 2008 Apr;*100*(4):394–9. doi: 10.1016/s0027-9684(15)31271-2. PMID: 18481477.

16. Palermo TM, Platt-Houston C, Kiska RE, et al. Headache symptoms in pediatric sickle cell patients. *J Pediatr Hematol Oncol.* 2005;*27*(8):420–4.

17. Niebanck AE, Pollock AN, Smith-Whitley K, et al. Headache in children with sickle cell disease: prevalence and associated factors. *J Pediatr.* 2007 Jul;*151*(1):67–72. doi: 10.1016/j.jpeds.2007.02.015.

18. Alkan O, Kizilkilic E, Kizilkilic O, et al. Cranial involvement in sickle cell disease. *Eur J Radiol.* 2010;*76*:151–6.

19. Tefferi A, Barbui T. Polycythemia vera and essential thrombocythemia: 2021 update on diagnosis, risk-stratification and management. *Am J Hematol.* 2020 Dec;*95*(12):1599–613. doi: 10.1002/ajh.26008. Epub 2020 Oct 23. PMID: 32974939.

20. Ickenstein GW, Klotz JM, Langohr HD. Kopfschmerz bei Polycythaemia vera. Klassifikation eines Kopfschmerzes bei Stoffwechselstörungen [Headache caused by polycythemia vera. Classification of a headache under the heading of metabolic disturbances]. *Schmerz.* 1999 Aug 19;*13*(4):279–82. German. doi: 10.1007/s004829900006. PMID: 12799929.

21. Popescu C. Cluster-Like Headache Revealing Polycythemia Vera: A Case Report. *Case Rep Neurol.* 2020 Jun 10;*12*(2):184–8. doi: 10.1159/000508356.

22. Cervantes F. Management of essential thrombocythemia. *Hematology Am Soc Hematol Educ Program.* 2011;*2011*:215–21. doi: 10.1182/asheducation-2011.1.215. PMID: 22160037.

23. Rumi E, Passamonti F, Della Porta MG, et al. Familial chronic myeloproliferative disorders: clinical phenotype and evidence of disease anticipation. *J Clin Oncol.* 2007 Dec 10;*25*(35):5630–5. doi: 10.1200/JCO.2007.12.6896. Epub 2007 Nov 12. PMID: 17998545.

24. Rumi E, Harutyunyan AS, Pietra D, et al. Associazione Italiana per la Ricerca sul Cancro Gruppo Italiano Malattie Mieloproliferative Investigators. CALR exon 9 mutations are somatically acquired events in familial cases of essential thrombocythemia or primary myelofibrosis. *Blood.* 2014 Apr 10;*123*(15):2416–9. doi: 10.1182/blood-2014-01-550434. Epub 2014 Feb 19. PMID: 24553179.

25. Jabaily J, Iland HJ, Laszlo J, et al. Neurologic manifestations of essential thrombocythemia. *Ann Intern Med.* 1983;*99*:513–8.

26. Cassidy EM, Tomkins E, Dinan T, et al. Central 5-HT receptor hypersensitivity in migraine without aura. *Cephalalgia.* 2003 Feb;*23*(1):29–34. doi: 10.1046/j.1468-2982.2003.00441.x. PMID: 12534577.

27. Hanington E. Migraine: the platelet hypothesis after 10 years. *Biomed Pharmacother.* 1989;*43*(10):719–26. doi: 10.1016/0753-3322(89)90160-1. PMID: 2701286.

28. Michiels JJ. Acquired von Willebrand disease due to increasing platelet count can readily explain the paradox of thrombosis and bleeding in thrombocythemia. *Clin Appl Thromb Hemost.* 1999; *5*:147–151.

29. Rejto L, Huszka M, Káplár M, et al. Effects of in vitro platelet activation on platelet derived nitric oxide production in healthy humans and in chronic myeloproliferative diseases with elevated platelet counts. *Platelets.* 2003 Aug;*14*(5):283–6. doi: 10.1080/0953710031000123672. PMID: 14524361.

30. Griesshammer M, Bangerter M, van Vliet HH, et al. Aspirin in essential thrombocythemia: status quo and quo vadis. *Semin Thromb Hemost.* 1997; *23*: 371–377.

31. Vainchenker W, Kralovics R. Genetic basis and molecular pathophysiology of classical myeloproliferative neoplasms. *Blood.* 2017;*129*(6):667–679.

32. Arber DA, Orazi A, Hasserjian RP, et al. International Consensus Classification of myeloid neoplasms and acute leukemia: integrating morphological, Clinicalc, and genomic data. *Blood.* 2022;*140*(11):1200–28.

33. Visani G, Finelli C, Castelli U, et al. Myelofibrosis with myeloid metaplasia: clinical and haematological parameters predicting survival in a series of 133 patients. *Br J Haematol.* 1990 May;*75*(1):4–9. doi: 10.1111/j.1365-2141.1990.tb02609.x. PMID: 2375922.

34. Smith RE, Chelmowski MK, Szabo EJ. Myelofibrosis: a review of clinical and pathologic features and treatment. *Crit Rev Oncol Hematol.* 1990;*10*(4):305–14. doi: 10.1016/1040-8428(90)90007-f. PMID: 2278639.

35. Furia F, Canevini MP, Federici AB, et al. Unexpected Neurological Symptoms of Ruxolitinib: A Case Report. *J Hematol.* 2020 Dec;*9*(4):137–139. doi: 10.14740/jh642.

36. Birgegard G, Bjorkholm M, Kutti J, et al. Adverse effects and benefits of two years of anagrelide treatment for thrombocythemia in chronic myeloproliferative disorders. *Haematologica.* 2004;*89*:520–7.

37. Steurer M, Gastl G, Jedrzejczak W-W, et al. Anagrelide for thrombocytosis in myeloproliferative disorders. *Cancer*. 2004; *101*: 2239–46. doi: 10.1002/cncr.20646.

38. George JN, Nester CM. Syndromes of thrombotic microangiopathy. *N Engl J Med*. 2014 Aug 14;*371*(7):654–66. doi: 10.1056/NEJMra1312353. PMID: 25119611.

39. Joly BS, Coppo P, Veyradier A. Thrombotic thrombocytopenic purpura. *Blood*. 2017; *129* (21): 2836–46. doi: 10.1182/blood-2016-10-709857.

40. Mannucci PM, Canciani MT, Forza I, et al. Changes in health and disease of the metalloprotease that cleaves von Willebrand factor. *Blood*. 2001;*98*(9):2730–5.

41. Saultz JN, Wu HM, Cataland S. Headache prevalence following recovery from TTP and aHUS. *Ann Hematol*. 2015 Sep;*94*(9):1473–6. doi: 10.1007/s00277-015-2411-2. Epub 2015 Jun 11. PMID: 26063190.

42. Idiculla PS, Gurala D, Palanisamy M, et al. Cerebral Venous Thrombosis: A Comprehensive Review. *Eur Neurol*. 2020;*83*(4):369–79. doi: 10.1159/000509802. Epub 2020 Sep 2. PMID: 32877892.

43. Soffietti R, Rudā R, Mutani R. Management of brain metastases. J Neurol. 2002 Oct;*249*(10):1357–69. doi: 10.1007/s00415-002-0870-6. PMID: 12382150.

44. Esquenazi Y, Lo VP, Lee K. Critical Care Management of Cerebral Edema in Brain Tumors. *J Intensive Care Med*. 2017 Jan;*32*(1):15–24. doi: 10.1177/0885066615619618. Epub 2015 Dec 8. PMID: 26647408.

45. Barnholtz-Sloan JS, Sloan AE, Davis FG, et al. Incidence proportions of brain metastases in patients diagnosed (1973 to 2001) in the Metropolitan Detroit Cancer Surveillance System. *J Clin Oncol*. 2004 Jul 15;*22*(14):2865–72. doi: 10.1200/JCO.2004.12.149. PMID: 15254054.

46. Rostami R, Mittal S, Rostami P, et al. Brain metastasis in breast cancer: a comprehensive literature review. *J Neurooncol*. 2016 May;*127*(3):407–14. doi: 10.1007/s11060-016-2075-3. Epub 2016 Feb 24. PMID: 26909695.

47. Gavrilovic IT, Posner JB. Brain metastases: epidemiology and pathophysiology. *J Neurooncol*. 2005 Oct;*75*(1):5–14. doi: 10.1007/s11060-004-8093-6. PMID: 16215811.

48. Delattre JY, Krol G, Thaler HT, et al. Distribution of brain metastases. *Arch Neurol*. 1988 Jul;*45*(7):741–4. doi: 10.1001/archneur.1988.00520310047016. PMID: 3390029.

49. Sze G, Milano E, Johnson C, Heier L. Detection of brain metastases: comparison of contrast-enhanced MR with unenhanced MR and enhanced CT. *AJNR Am J Neuroradiol*. 1990 Jul-Aug;*11*(4):785–91.

50. Tabouret E, Chinot O, Metellus P, et al. Recent trends in epidemiology of brain metastases: an overview. *Anticancer Res*. 2012;*32*:4655–62.

51. Darlix A, Louvel G, Fraisse J, et al. Impact of breast cancer molecular subtypes on the incidence, kinetics and prognosis of central nervous system metastases in a large multicentre real-life cohort. *Br J Cancer*. 2019;*121*(12): 991–1000. doi: 10.1038/s41416-019-0619-y.

52. Terceiro LEL, Ikeogu NM, Lima MF, et al. Navigating the blood-brain barrier: Challenges and therapeutic strategies in breast cancer brain metastases. *Int J Mol Sci*. 2023 Jul 27;*24*(15):12034. doi: 10.3390/ijms241512034.

53. Kim YJ, Kim JS, Kim IA. Molecular subtype predicts incidence and prognosis of brain metastasis from breast cancer in SEER database. *J Cancer Res Clin Oncol*. 2018;*144*(9):1803–16. doi: 10.1007/s00432-018-2697-2.

54. Achrol AS, Rennert RC, Anders C, et al. Brain metastases. *Nat Rev Dis Primers*. 2019 Jan 17;*5*(1):5. doi: 10.1038/s41572-018-0055-y. PMID: 30655533.

55. Dhakal A, Van Swearingen AED, O'Regan R, et al. Systemic Therapy Approaches for Breast Cancer Brain and Leptomeningeal Metastases. *Curr Treat Options Oncol*. 2022 Oct;*23*(10):1457–76. doi: 10.1007/s11864-022-01011-w. Epub 2022 Sep 22. PMID: 36136177.

56. Wang N, Bertalan MS, Brastianos PK. Leptomeningeal metastasis from systemic cancer: Review and update on management. *Cancer*. 2018 Jan 1;*124*(1):21–35. doi: 10.1002/cncr.30911.

57. Villano JL, Durbin EB, Normandeau C, et al. Incidence of brain metastasis at initial presentation of lung cancer. *Neuro Oncol*. 2015 Jan;*17*(1):122–8. doi: 10.1093/neuonc/nou099. Epub 2014 Jun 2.

58. Johung KL, Yeh N, Desai NB, et al. Extended survival and prognostic factors for patients with ALK-rearranged non-small-cell lung cancer and brain metastasis. *J Clin Oncol*. 2016 Jan 10;*34*(2):123–9. doi: 10.1200/JCO.2015.62.0138.

59. Zhang I, Zaorsky NG, Palmer JD, et al. Targeting brain metastases in ALK-rearranged non-small-cell lung cancer. *Lancet Oncol*. 2015 Oct;*16*(13):e510–21. doi: 10.1016/S1470-2045(15)00013-3. PMID: 26433824.

60. Shin DY, Na II, Kim CH, et al. EGFR mutation and brain metastasis in pulmonary adenocarcinomas. *J Thorac Oncol*. 2014 Feb;*9*(2):195–9. doi: 10.1097/JTO.0000000000000069. PMID: 24419416.

61. Saleem K, Davar D. The role of systemic therapy in melanoma brain metastases: a narrative review. *Chin Clin Oncol*. 2022 Jun;*11*(3):24. doi: 10.21037/cco-22-1. PMID: 35818856.

62. Sun M, De Velasco G, Brastianos PK, et al. The Development of Brain Metastases in Patients with Renal Cell Carcinoma: Epidemiologic Trends, Survival, and Clinical Risk Factors Using a Population-based Cohort. *Eur Urol Focus.* 2019 May;*5*(3):474–481. doi: 10.1016/j.euf.2017.12.007. Epub 2018 Jan 5. PMID: 29311016.

63. Sperduto PW, Kased N, Roberge D, et al. Summary report on the graded prognostic assessment: an accurate and facile diagnosis-specific tool to estimate survival for patients with brain metastases. *J Clin Oncol.* 2012 Feb 1;*30*(4):419–25. doi: 10.1200/JCO.2011.38.0527.

64. Crisman CM, Patel AR, Winston G, et al. Clinical Outcomes in Patients with Renal Cell Carcinoma Metastases to the Choroid Plexus. *World Neurosurg.* 2020 Aug;*140*:e7–e13. doi: 10.1016/j.wneu.2020.03.125.

65. Shapira Y, Hadelsberg UP, Kanner AA, et al. The ventricular system and choroid plexus as a primary site for renal cell carcinoma metastasis. *Acta Neurochir (Wien).* 2014 Aug;*156*(8):1469–74. doi: 10.1007/s00701-014-2108-7. Epub 2014 May 9. PMID: 24809532.

66. van Maanen JM, Retèl J, de Vries J, et al. Mechanism of action of antitumor drug etoposide: a review. *J Natl Cancer Inst.* 1988 Dec 7;*80*(19):1526–33. doi: 10.1093/jnci/80.19.1526. PMID: 2848132.

67. Drug name: Etoposide - BC Cancer. (2020). *BC Cancer.* Retrieved December 18, 2023, from http://www.bccancer.bc.ca/drug-database-site/Drug%20Index/Etoposide_monograph.pdf

68. DailyMed - Etoposide injection. (2020). *U.S. National Library of Medicine.* National Institutes of Health. Retrieved December 18, 2023, from https://dailymed.nlm.nih.gov/dailymed/drugInfo.cfm?setid=4f850eb2-3542-43a0-90e8-bb37fa05cf15#:~:text=Two%20different%20-,Etoposide%20Injection%20USP%20has%20been%20shown%20to%20cause%20metaphase%20arrest,cells%20entering%20mitosis%20is%20observed.

69. Fields SZ, Budman DR, Young RR, et al. Phase I study of high-dose etoposide phosphate in man. *Bone Marrow Transplant.* 1996 Nov;*18*(5):851–6. PMID: 8932836.

70. Rai AC, Goyal A, Khurana AK, et al. Chemotherapy as cause of refractory severe headache in a case of small-cell lung cancer. *BMJ Case Rep.* 2021 Apr 28;*14*(4):e240654. doi: 10.1136/bcr-2020-240654.

71. Arca KN, Halker Singh RB. Dehydration and Headache. *Curr Pain Headache Rep.* 2021 Jul 15;*25*(8):56. doi: 10.1007/s11916-021-00966-z.

72. Bhatia M, Gupta R, Srivastava S. Migraine Associated with Water Deprivation and Progressive Myopia. *Cephalalgia.* 2006;*26*(6):758–760. doi:10.1111/j.1468-2982.2006.01083.x

73. Vail, D. M., & Withrow, S. J. (2007). Chapter 11 - Cancer Chemotherapy. In *Withrow & Macewen's small animal clinical oncology (fourth edition)* (pp. 163–192). Essay, W.B. Saunders.

74. HPRA Summary of Product Characteristics - Vincristine. (2007). *Vincristine sulfate 1MG/ML solution for injection or infusion.* Retrieved December 18, 2023, from https://www.hpra.ie/homepage/medicines/medicines-information/find-a-medicine/results/item?pano=PA0822%2F232%2F001

75. Fox LE. Carboplatin. *J Am Anim Hosp Assoc.* 2000 Jan-Feb;*36*(1):13–4. doi: 10.5326/15473317-36-1-13. PMID: 10667400.

76. Dille MF, Konrad-Martin D, Gallun F, et al. Tinnitus onset rates from chemotherapeutic agents and oto-toxic antibiotics: results of a large prospective study. *J Am Acad Audiol.* 2010 Jun;*21*(6):409–17. doi: 10.3766/jaaa.21.6.6.

77. Theriot J, Wermuth HR, Ashurst JV. Antiemetic Serotonin 5-HT3 Receptor Blockers. [Updated 2022 Nov 21]. In: StatPearls [Internet]. Treasure Island (FL): StatPearls Publishing; 2023 Jan-. Available from: https://www.ncbi.nlm.nih.gov/books/NBK513318/

78. Russell D, Kenny GN. 5-HT3 antagonists in postoperative nausea and vomiting. *Br J Anaesth.* 1992; *69*: 63S–8S.

79. Aggarwal M, Puri V, Puri S. Serotonin and CGRP in migraine. *Ann Neurosci.* 2012 Apr;*19*(2):88–94. doi: 10.5214/ans.0972.7531.12190210.

80. Finn AL. Toxicity and side effects of ondansetron. *Semin Oncol.* 1992 Aug;*19*(4 Suppl 10):53–60. PMID: 1387251.

81. Center for Drug Evaluation and Research. (2016). Updated information on 32 mg intravenous ondansetron dose. *U.S. Food and Drug Administration.* FDA. Retrieved December 18, 2023, from https://www.fda.gov/drugs/drug-safety-and-availability/fda-drug-safety-communication-updated-information-32-mg-intravenous-ondansetron-zofran-dose-and-pre

82. Aziz, F. Neurokinin-1 receptor antagonists for chemotherapy-induced nausea and vomiting. *Annals Palliative Med.* 2012; *1*(2), 130–136. doi:10.3978/j.issn.2224-5820.2012.07.10.

83. Ritchie MK, Kohli A. Aprepitant. [Updated 2022 Sep 22]. In: StatPearls [Internet]. Treasure Island (FL): StatPearls Publishing; 2023 Jan-. Available from: https://www.ncbi.nlm.nih.gov/books/NBK551588/

84. Rao KV, Faso A. Chemotherapy-induced nausea and vomiting: optimizing prevention and management. *Am Health Drug Benefits* 2012 Jul;*5*(4):232–40.

85. Yu F, Bender W. The mechanism of tamoxifen in breast cancer prevention. *Breast Cancer Res.* 2001;*3*(Suppl 1):A74. doi: 10.1186/bcr404.

86. Milani M, Jha G, Potter DA. Anastrozole use in early stage breast cancer of postmenopausal women. *Clin Med Ther.* 2009 Mar *31*;1:141–56. doi: 10.4137/cmt.s9.

87. Nappi RE, Tiranini L, Sacco S, et al. Role of Estrogens in Menstrual Migraine. *Cells.* 2022 Apr 15;*11*(8):1355. doi: 10.3390/cells11081355.

88. Somerville BW. The role of estradiol withdrawal in the etiology of menstrual migraine. *Neurology.* 1972 Apr;*22*(4):355–65. doi: 10.1212/wnl.22.4.355. PMID: 5062827.

89. Lichten EM, Lichten JB, Whitty A, et al. The confirmation of a biochemical marker for women's hormonal migraine: the depo-estradiol challenge test. *Headache.* 1996 Jun;*36*(6):367–71. doi: 10.1046/j.1526-4610.1996.3606367.x. PMID: 8707555.

90. Rangel-Méndez JA, Rubi-Castellanos R, Sánchez-Cruz JF, Moo-Puc RE. Tamoxifen side effects: pharmacogenetic and clinical approach in Mexican mestizos. *Transl Cancer Res.* 2019 Feb;*8*(1):23–34. doi: 10.21037/tcr.2018.12.27.

91. Higa GM, alKhouri N. Anastrozole: a selective aromatase inhibitor for the treatment of breast cancer. *Am J Health Syst Pharm.* 1998 Mar 1;*55*(5):445–52. doi: 10.1093/ajhp/55.5.445. PMID: 9522927.

92. Zhan M, Flaws JA, Gallicchio L, et al. Profiles of tamoxifen-related side effects by race and smoking status in women with breast cancer. *Cancer Detect Prev.* 2007;*31*(5):384–90. doi: 10.1016/j.cdp.2007.10.004. Epub 2007 Nov 26. PMID: 18023540.

93. Wilson AC, Meethal SV, Bowen RL, et al. Leuprolide acetate: a drug of diverse clinical applications. *Expert Opin Investig Drugs.* 2007 Nov;*16*(11):1851–63. doi: 10.1517/13543784.16.11.1851. PMID: 17970643.

94. Clinton TN, Woldu SL, Raj GV. Degarelix versus luteinizing hormone-releasing hormone agonists for the treatment of prostate cancer. *Expert Opin Pharmacother.* 2017 Jun;*18*(8):825–32. doi: 10.1080/14656566.2017.1328056.

95. Shields LBE, Seifert T, Shelton BJ, et al. Testosterone levels in men with chronic migraine. *Neurol Int.* 2019 Jun 19;*11*(2):8079. doi: 10.4081/ni.2019.8079.

96. Stillman MJ. Testosterone replacement therapy for treatment refractory cluster headache. *Headache.* 2006 Jun;*46*(6):925–33. doi: 10.1111/j.1526-4610.2006.00436.x. PMID: 16732838.

97. Gomez JA. Vascular endothelial growth factor-tyrosine kinase inhibitors: Novel mechanisms, predictors of hypertension and management strategies. *American Heart Journal Plus: Cardiology Research and Practice.* 2022; *17*(100144): 1–4.

98. Schmidinger M. Understanding and managing toxicities of vascular endothelial growth factor (VEGF) inhibitors. *EJC Suppl.* 2013 Sep;*11*(2):172–91. doi: 10.1016/j.ejcsup.2013.07.016.

99. Kanis JA, Cooper C, Rizzoli R, et al. Scientific Advisory Board of the European Society for Clinical and Economic Aspects of Osteoporosis (ESCEO) and the Committees of Scientific Advisors and National Societies of the International Osteoporosis Foundation (IOF). European guidance for the diagnosis and management of osteoporosis in postmenopausal women. *Osteoporos Int.* 2019 Jan;*30*(1):3–44. doi: 10.1007/s00198-018-4704-5. Epub 2018 Oct 15. Erratum in: Osteoporos Int. 2020 Jan;31(1):209. Erratum in: Osteoporos Int. 2020 Apr;31(4):801.

100. Ganesan K, Goyal A, Roane D. Bisphosphonate. [Updated 2023 Jul 3]. In: StatPearls [Internet]. Treasure Island (FL): StatPearls Publishing; 2023 Jan-. Available from: https://www.ncbi.nlm.nih.gov/books/NBK470248/

101. Rizzoli R, Reginster JY, Boonen S, et al. Adverse reactions and drug-drug interactions in the management of women with postmenopausal osteoporosis. *Calcif Tissue Int.* 2011 Aug;*89*(2):91–104. doi: 10.1007/s00223-011-9499-8.

102. Ganguly A, Michael M, Goschin S, et al. Cancer Pain and Opioid Use Disorder. *Oncology (Williston Park).* 2022 Sep 7;*36*(9):535–41. doi: 10.46883/2022.25920973. PMID: 36107782.

103. De Felice M, Ossipov MH, Porreca F. Update on medication-overuse headache. *Curr Pain Headache Rep.* 2011 Feb;*15*(1):79–83. doi: 10.1007/s11916-010-0155-1.

104. Bigal ME, Serrano D, Buse D, et al. Acute migraine medications and evolution from episodic to chronic migraine: a longitudinal population-based study. *Headache.* 2008 Sep;*48*(8):1157–68. doi: 10.1111/j.1526-4610.2008.01217.x. PMID: 18808500.

105. Johnson JL, Hutchinson MR, Williams DB, et al. Medication-overuse headache and opioid-induced hyperalgesia: A review of mechanisms, a neuroimmune hypothesis and a novel approach to treatment. *Cephalalgia.* 2013 Jan;*33*(1):52–64. doi: 10.1177/0333102412467512. Epub 2012 Nov 9. PMID: 23144180.

106. Koźmiński P, Halik PK, Chesori R, et al. Overview of Dual-Acting Drug Methotrexate in Different Neurological Diseases, Autoimmune Pathologies and Cancers. *Int J Mol Sci.* 2020 May 14;*21*(10):3483. doi: 10.3390/ijms21103483.

107. Faruqi A, Tadi P. Cytarabine. [Updated 2023 Aug 8]. In: StatPearls [Internet]. Treasure Island (FL): StatPearls Publishing; 2023 Jan-. Available from: https://www.ncbi.nlm.nih.gov/books/NBK557680/

108. Yarbro JW. Mechanism of action of hydroxyurea. *Semin Oncol.* 1992 Jun;*19*(3 Suppl 9):1–10. PMID: 1641648.

109. Jinna S, Khandhar PB. Hydroxyurea Toxicity. [Updated 2023 Aug 8]. In: StatPearls [Internet]. Treasure Island (FL): StatPearls Publishing; 2023 Jan-. Available from: https://www.ncbi.nlm.nih.gov/books/NBK537209/

110. Tefferi A, Silverstein MN, Petitt RM, et al. Anagrelide as a new platelet-lowering agent in essential thrombocythemia: mechanism of action, efficacy, toxicity, current indications. *Semin Thromb Hemost.* 1997;*23*(4):379–83. doi: 10.1055/s-2007-996112. PMID: 9263355.

111. Haq M, Adnan G. Ruxolitinib. [Updated 2023 Jun 5]. In: StatPearls [Internet]. Treasure Island (FL): StatPearls Publishing; 2023 Jan-. Available from: https://www.ncbi.nlm.nih.gov/books/NBK570600/

112. Schiff PB, Horwitz SB. Taxol stabilizes microtubules in mouse fibroblast cells. *Proc Natl Acad Sci U S A.* 1980 Mar;*77*(3):1561–5. doi: 10.1073/pnas.77.3.1561.

113. Koźmiński P, Halik PK, Chesori R, et al. Overview of Dual-Acting Drug Methotrexate in Different Neurological Diseases, Autoimmune Pathologies and Cancers. *Int J Mol Sci.* 2020 May 14;*21*(10):3483. doi: 10.3390/ijms21103483. PMID: 32423175; PMCID: PMC7279024.

114. Ifosfamide. (2005). *Uses, Interactions, Mechanism of Action | DrugBank Online.* Retrieved December 18, 2023, from https://go.drugbank.com/drugs/DB01181

115. Church DB, Maddison JE, Page SW. 2008. Chapter 15 - Cancer chemotherapy. In *Small animal clinical pharmacology (second edition)* (pp. 330–366). W B Saunders Company.

116. Salerni BL, Bates DJ, Albershardt TC, et al. Vinblastine induces acute, cell cycle phase-independent apoptosis in some leukemias and lymphomas and can induce acute apoptosis in others when Mcl-1 is suppressed. *Mol Cancer Ther.* 2010 Apr;*9*(4):791–802. doi: 10.1158/1535-7163.MCT-10-0028.

117. Soltau J, Drevs J. Mode of action and clinical impact of VEGF signaling inhibitors. *Expert Rev Anticancer Ther.* 2009 May;*9*(5):649–62. doi: 10.1586/era.09.19. PMID: 19445581.

118. Yu F, Bender W. The mechanism of tamoxifen in breast cancer prevention. *Breast Cancer Res.* 2001;*3*(Suppl 1):A74. doi: 10.1186/bcr404.

119. Wilson AC, Meethal SV, Bowen RL, et al. Leuprolide acetate: a drug of diverse clinical applications. *Expert Opin Investig Drugs.* 2007 Nov;*16*(11):1851–63. doi: 10.1517/13543784.16.11.1851. PMID: 17970643.

120. Clinton TN, Woldu SL, Raj GV. Degarelix versus luteinizing hormone-releasing hormone agonists for the treatment of prostate cancer. *Expert Opin Pharmacother.* 2017 Jun;*18*(8):825–32.

121. Aziz F. Neurokinin-1 receptor antagonists for chemotherapy-induced nausea and vomiting. *Ann Palliat Med.* 2012 Jul;*1*(2): 130–36.

122. Rodan GA, Reszka AA. Bisphosphonate mechanism of action. *Curr Mol Med.* 2002 Sep;*2*(6):571–7. doi: 10.2174/1566524023362104. PMID: 12243249.

123. Pathan H, Williams J. Basic opioid pharmacology: an update. *Br J Pain.* 2012 Feb;*6*(1):11–6. doi: 10.1177/2049463712438493.

Infectious Diseases for the Headache Practitioner

11

Rebecca Linfield and Elizabeth Thottacherry

LEARNING OBJECTIVES

1. Understand guidelines for infection screening in the general population
2. Generate a differential diagnosis for headache and infection, and first steps for diagnosis and treatment
3. Discuss CNS side effects of commonly prescribed antimicrobials
4. Create awareness of potential medication interactions between antimicrobials and headache therapies

---

Case 1

A 25-year-old female with episodic migraine presents to your clinic to establish care. She was born in Mexico. What infectious routine screening should she undergo as part of comprehensive care?

SCREENING

The US Preventive Services Task Force (USPSTF) recommends screening for certain infections for all patients, including those with a longitudinal primary headache condition.[1]

HIV

The USPSTF recommends that all patients, including those who are pregnant, be screened for human immunodeficiency virus (HIV) at least once during their lifetimes (ages 15–65).[2] This is most typically performed using a fourth-generation HIV screening test, which consists of testing antibodies to HIV-1 and HIV-2, and detecting the presence of the p24 antigen.[3] This can detect virus as early as 18 days into

DOI: 10.1201/b23330-11

infection.[3] An HIV-1 viral load can detect HIV infection as early as ten days into infection.[3] More frequent testing should be done for those at higher risk.

In 2023, the USPTSF also recommended pre-exposure prophylaxis (PrEP) for those who are at high risk of acquiring HIV.[4] Currently, PrEP consists of either a daily pill with tenofovir disoproxil-emtricitabine or tenofovir alafenamide emtricitabine, or a long-acting injectable cabotegravir. Note that the tenofovir-alafenamide formulation is not approved for receptive vaginal sex as it was not studied in this patient population.[5] Those who are at high risk of HIV include the following:[4]

- Sexually active adolescents and adults who have a partner who is HIV positive (especially with unknown or detectable viral load)
- Bacterial sexually transmitted infection in the past six months (syphilis, gonorrhea, or chlamydia)
- Inconsistent or no condom use
- People who inject drugs who share equipment
- Those who engage in transactional sex

Headache, nausea, and diarrhea can occur in those initiated on PrEP but usually resolve with time.[6] Headache medicine physicians can refer eligible patients to primary care or infectious diseases to initiate PrEP. Screening labs performed prior to PrEP initiation include HIV screening, basic metabolic panel, lipid panel, sexually transmitted infection screening, hepatitis screening, and assessment for signs and symptoms of HIV.[7]

Syphilis

The USPTSF recommends screening adolescents and adults who are at high risk for syphilis.[8] Similar to the recommendations for screening for HIV, those who are at high risk for syphilis include the following:

- Men who have sex with men
- People with HIV or other sexually transmitted infections
- People who use illicit drugs
- Those who engage in transactional sex
- Those who have been incarcerated
- Those who have served in the military
- Young adults

In clinical practice, we screen these high-risk patients every three to six months.

We now follow a reverse screening algorithm for syphilis. This is a two-step screening process consisting of an initial treponemal test followed by an automated reflex nontreponemal test. Discordant results are resolved with a second confirmatory treponemal test.[9] This has been implemented because many treponemal-specific tests are cheaper than the non-treponemal test rapid plasma reagin (RPR) and also identifies more patients whose RPR may have become negative due to a long untreated course of syphilis (Figure 11.1).[10]

DoxyPEP

A recent development, now endorsed by the Centers for Disease Control and Prevention (CDC), is "DoxyPEP" – postexposure prophylaxis for the acquisition of sexually transmitted infections, which consists of 200 mg of doxycycline taken within 24–72 hours of unprotected sex for those at higher risk. This has shown benefits for men who have sex with men and transgender women. In these two populations, the DoxyPEP randomized controlled trial published in 2023 in the *New England Journal of Medicine*

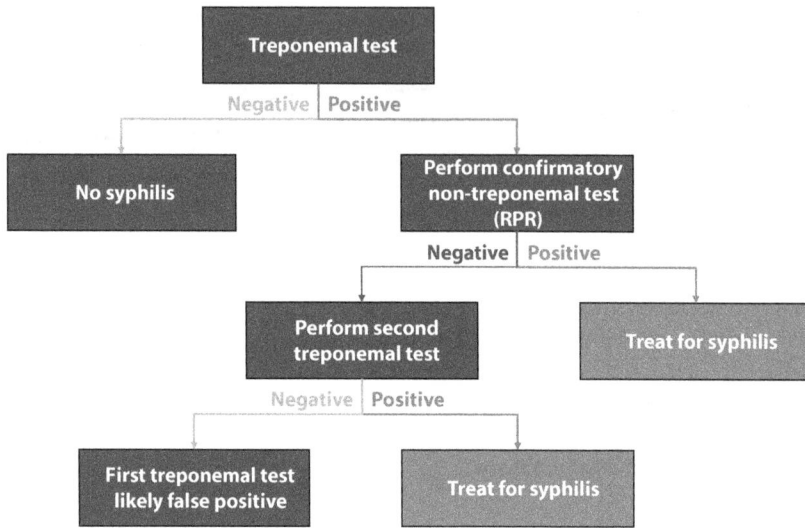

FIGURE 11.1   Syphilis screening algorithm.

showed that overall sexually transmitted infection (STI) rates were decreased in 65% compared to controls.[11] However, DoxyPEP was not effective in preventing STIs in women in a randomized control trial in Kenya, though follow-up testing revealed 44% of women in the intervention arm did not have doxycycline detected in hair testing.[12, 13]

Gonorrhea and Chlamydia

The USPSTF supports screening for gonorrhea and chlamydia in all women who are sexually active under 24 years of age, and in women over 25 years old at increased risk for infection.[14] Those who are at increased risk of infection include women who have multiple partners, a partner with an STI, inconsistent condom use if not in a mutually monogamous relationship, history of exchanging sex for money or drugs, or a history of incarceration.

The USPSTF says there is insufficient evidence to make recommendations regarding men. However, the CDC recommends that men with increased risks—e.g., those being seen in adolescent medicine services, prisons, STD clinics, or men who have sex with men—be tested on a more frequent basis. In clinical practice, patients on PrEP or those living with HIV usually obtain testing every three months. Testing should also be based on type of sex—e.g., pharyngeal, urethra/vaginal, and rectal swabs.[15]

Hepatitis Screening

In the United States, treatment of hepatitis B and C is now under the guidance of gastroenterology specialists. However, the USPSTF recommends that those at increased risk of hepatitis B be screened, and all adults ages 18 to 79 be screened for hepatitis C at least once in their lifetime.[16, 17] Those who are at increased risk of hepatitis B include those born in an area with high prevalence of hepatitis B infection (>2% of the population) including Asia, Africa, the Pacific Islands, and parts of South America.[16] In addition, if US citizens were not vaccinated against hepatitis B as an infant and have parents born in those areas of the world, they are also at increased risk of maternal-fetal transmission of hepatitis B.[16] The other high-risk populations for hepatitis B are those at risk for other infections, including those with HIV, people who inject drugs, men who have sex with men, and sexual partners or household contacts of people living with hepatitis B.[16] Those populations may need to be screened more frequently. Those who use injection drugs should be screened more often for both hepatitis B and C, though there is not enough evidence to suggest a definite frequency.[16, 17]

Latent Tuberculosis

Tuberculosis (TB) is caused by *Mycobacterium tuberculosis* (MTB) and is spread through airborne transmission from those with active pulmonary disease. Thirty percent of people exposed to active TB will develop latent tuberculosis, a state in which the mycobacterium is contained by the body's immune system.[18] Unfortunately, ~5%–10% of those with latent TB will develop active tuberculosis without treatment of latent TB due to their bodies' decreased ability to contain the mycobacterium.[18] Thus, the USPSTF recommends screening those at risk for latent TB so that those individuals can be treated to prevent progression to active tuberculosis.[18] Factors vary across regions, but known risk factors include the following:[18]

- Born in a high-risk area outside the United States, which includes most countries except Canada, Australia, New Zealand, or Western and Northern European Countries
- Having a family member with active tuberculosis
- Incarceration
- Homelessness
- Use of illicit drugs
- Working in a health-care setting

The CDC recommends an interferon-gamma release assay (IGRA) over the older tuberculin skin test (TST).[19] Prior to the widespread use of IGRA, the TST was the standard screening test. However, it was much more cumbersome for patients, as the protein derivative is injected underneath the skin and the test is read 48–72 hours later, meaning that the patient would have to return for evaluation.[19] The TST also cross-reacts with the BCG vaccine.[19] Both the T-spot and QuantiFERON TB Gold are types of IGRA tests used as screening tools for latent tuberculosis.[20] There can be false negative tests due to a variety of factors, including immune suppression.[21] If active tuberculosis is suspected, sputum testing should be obtained per public health department regulations, and any other suspected site of infection should be biopsied and cultured, with MTB polymerase chain reaction (PCR) testing as appropriate.[22]

Latent TB treatment can prevent progression to active disease in ~90% of cases.[23] Recommendations regarding latent TB treatments have changed. The newest recommendations consist of four months of rifampin monotherapy versus three months of daily isoniazid and rifampin, versus three months of weekly isoniazid and rifapentine.[24] The older regimen of six to nine months of isoniazid is less preferred due to the length of therapy, which increases the risk of noncompletion of therapy and the risk of hepatotoxicity.[24] Tuberculosis meningitis, as well as interactions of rifampin and isoniazid with headache medications, will be discussed later in this chapter.

Case 2

A 30-year-old male of Filipino ancestry who works as a grape harvester in the San Joaquin Valley in California presents with weeks of fevers, headaches, nausea, and vomiting. What next steps should be taken and what disease does he likely have?

CNS INFECTIONS

Central nervous system (CNS) infections can include headache as a presenting or continuing symptom. Overall, CNS infection usually reflects systemic disease, and so the treatments are also systemic, though

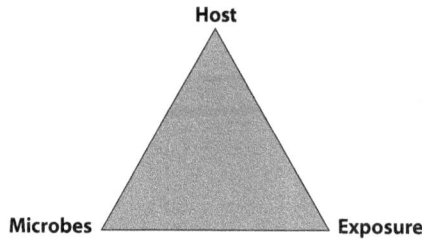

FIGURE 11.2   The infectious diseases triad.

many systemic therapies have poor cerebrospinal fluid (CSF) penetration. Infectious Diseases physicians usually think of a triad of factors contributing to the risk of disease in any patient, including in CNS infections (Figure 11.2).

With regard to the host – is the patient immunocompromised in some way? This can be from multiple causes, most commonly including diabetes, pregnancy, HIV, cancer, chemotherapy, or immunosuppressant medications for transplant or other diseases. With respect to microbes – what organisms can cause this clinical syndrome? E.g., a chronic process is usually not caused by rapidly growing bacteria but rather by slow-growing mycobacterium, fungus, or parasites. Lastly, exposures – what environmental risk factors may the patient have been exposed to? E.g., recent surgery or hospital stay leads to a higher risk of *S. aureus* or *Pseudomonas* infection, or birthplace in another country leads to higher exposure to TB. In the next section, we will discuss common presenting scenarios in CNS infections. A general approach to diagnosing and managing CNS infections includes taking a detailed history; doing an appropriate physical exam, including a neurologic exam; and then performing appropriate microbiological testing, which usually includes blood cultures and a lumbar puncture with opening pressure to evaluate CSF. CSF studies include the following:

- Cell counts
- Protein
- Glucose
- Gram stain and bacterial cultures

Depending on the clinical scenario, the following tests could also be ordered:

- BioFire meningitis/encephalitis PCR panel
- Fungal cultures
- Acid-fast bacilli (AFB) cultures
- MTB PCR
- Venereal Disease Research Laboratory (VDRL) test for neurosyphilis
- Cryptococcal antigen
- HIV-1 or HIV-2

Acute Bacterial Meningitis

Acute bacterial meningitis is the quintessential CNS infection that practitioners will encounter during inpatient clinical practice. These patients present with fever, neck stiffness, headache, photophobia, and sometimes altered mental status.[25] The duration between onset of symptoms and seeking care is usually less than five days.[25] However, the headache caused by acute bacterial meningitis should be adequately treated by intravenous antimicrobials, so a patient with acute bacterial meningitis is unlikely to see a headache physician for this condition. Obtaining a lumbar puncture with CSF cell count, protein, glucose, gram stain bacterial cultures, and usually a BioFire meningoencephalitis panel is paramount. CT head is needed prior to lumbar puncture if increased intracranial pressure is suspected, and blood cultures can also be helpful.[26] The most common pathogens causing bacterial meningitis in order of prevalence are *Strep pneumoniae, Neisseria meningitidis, Group B streptococcus, Haemophilus influenzae, Listeria monocytogenes*, and *E. Coli.*[27, 28]

The BioFire meningitis/encephalitis panel has improved our ability to classify the cause of meningitis/encephalitis. As of the time of publication, the BioFire test employs rapid polymerase chain testing for 14 pathogens, including the 6 most common bacteria noted earlier, as well as the following viruses: cytomegalovirus (CMV), enterovirus, herpes simplex virus 1 (HSV-1), herpes simplex virus 2 (HSV-2), human herpesvirus 6 (HHV-6), human parechovirus (HPeV), and varicella virus (VZV).[29] BioFire also tests for *Cryptococcus*, though there are other tests that can be sent for that, discussed later in this chapter. Vaccination has decreased rates of *S. pneumoniae, N. meningitidis*, and *H. influenzae* bacterial meningitis.[30–33] Vancomycin and ceftriaxone, with the addition of ampicillin if the patient is over 50 years, are usually appropriate therapies to cover community-acquired meningitis pathogens before diagnostics result.[26]

Diagnosing and treating health-care-associated meningitis and ventriculitis is more complicated. It is usually related to prior surgical intervention, and the Infectious Diseases and Neurosurgery teams should be consulted for management.[34]

Encephalitis

Encephalitis is a process of brain inflammation due to direct infection, post-infectious process, or noninfectious condition.[35] A 2013 Consensus Statement by the International Encephalitis Consortium presented the major criteria as patients with altered mental status with no alternative cause identified, and with three minor criteria required for probable or confirmed encephalitis, including fever >38.0°F, seizures not fully attributable to a prior seizure disorder, new focal neurologic findings, CSF WBC $\geq 5/$ mm^3, new abnormality of brain parenchyma on imaging suggestive of encephalitis, or electroencephalography consistent with encephalitis.[35] Of note, only ~50% of hospitalizations for encephalitis found an etiology, based on a study of 263,352 encephalitis-associated hospitalizations in the United States from 1998–2010 as part of the Nationwide Inpatient Sample Survey.[36] This same type of finding was found in the California Encephalitis Project, which attempted to find etiologies of encephalitis in California from 1998–2000.[37] The study enrolled 334 patients and found that 9% of patients had a probable viral cause, 3% had a likely bacterial cause, and 1% had a likely parasitic cause. 10% of cases had a noninfectious etiology identified. A possible etiology was identified in 12% of cases, and a non-encephalitis infection was found in 3%. However, 62% of cases of encephalitis were unexplained.

In the California Encephalitis Project, most patients with viral encephalitis had either enterovirus identified or one of the herpes viruses, including VZV, HSV-1, HSV-2, and CMV.[37] HSV classically attacks the temporal lobe(s).[38] The 2008 Infectious Diseases Society of America (IDSA) guidelines for the management of encephalitis recommended empirically starting all patients with encephalitis on high-dose acyclovir until further diagnostic results, as acyclovir treats VZV, HSV-1, and HSV-2.[39] Unfortunately, there is no treatment for arboviruses that can cause viral encephalitis, such as West Nile Virus or St. Louis Encephalitis Virus. Influenza can sometimes cause encephalitis and be treated with antivirals.[40] The IDSA guidelines also recommend empiric doxycycline for rickettsial or ehrlichia infection based on epidemiologic risk factors.[39] The differential is larger for immunocompromised patients—e.g., CMV, HHV-6, JC virus, aspergillus, and other pathogens—and we recommend consulting an infectious diseases physician specializing in immunocompromised patients.[40]

Focal CNS Infections

Focal CNS infections develop from contiguous spread from adjacent structures (e.g., sinusitis, otitis media); hematogenous spread, such as in bacterial endocarditis; or trauma.[41] Focal infections include brain abscess, subdural empyema, epidural abscess, as well as skull base osteomyelitis. Symptoms can include headache, along with nausea, vomiting, or focal neurologic findings.[41] MRI can be helpful in diagnosis, with more advanced imaging sometimes needed for skull-based osteomyelitis.[41, 42] The microbiologic agent depends on the source; some common examples include strep species from otitis media or *S. aureus* in bacterial endocarditis.[41] Treatment is dependent upon location and whether the lesion is causing increased intracranial pressure and/or loss of neurologic function; ideally, surgical drainage would be obtained, along with cultures, and the patient treated with targeted antimicrobials with CNS penetration.[41]

Subacute or Chronic Meningitis

Subacute (5–30 days from onset to presentation) or chronic (30+ days from symptom onset) meningitis has a broad differential, including infectious and noninfectious etiologies. We will discuss TB meningitis, neurosyphilis, common types of fungal meningitis, and neurocysticercosis. However, we will not discuss other infectious etiologies, such as neurobrucellosis, that can be on the differential, as well as noninfectious etiologies, including vasculitis, sarcoidosis, multiple sclerosis, neuro-Behçet's, other autoimmune disorders, paraneoplastic disorders, and oncologic metastases.[43]

Besides an MRI of the brain, common tests in the diagnosis of subacute or chronic meningitis include lumbar puncture with CSF testing as follows:

- Cell count and differential, protein, glucose
- Bacterial gram stain and culture
- Fungal culture
- Flow cytometry to evaluate for malignancy
- VDRL test for neurosyphilis
- CSF cryptococcal antigen
- Aspergillus galactomannan antigen
- MTB PCR
- Other endemic fungi testing, such as for *Coccidioides*, depends on exposure history.[44]

Serologic tests can include an HIV test, syphilis screening test, and antibodies to Coccidioides, histoplasma, toxoplasma, and brucella.[44] Eosinophilic meningitis (>10% eosinophils in CSF leukocyte count) is usually caused by parasitic infection, including *T. solium*, *A. cantonensis*, and *G. spinigerum*.[45] Additional testing often depends on environmental exposures and risk factors.

TB Meningitis

TB meningitis can be a complication of disseminated MTB infection. While patients usually have abnormal CSF results on lumbar puncture, MRI can be normal or have small lesions in central sulci.[44] CSF nucleic acid testing (MTB PCR) is likely the fastest and most sensitive test, with the Xpert Ultra machine having 70% sensitivity compared to a case definition.[46] However, acid-fast stains and AFB cultures should also be sent. If the patient has clinical symptoms or imaging findings consistent with pulmonary tuberculosis, additional pulmonary testing with AFB and MTB-PCR sputum sampling should be performed.[44]

In those in endemic areas and with symptoms, empiric treatment with rifampin, isoniazid, pyrazinamide, and ethambutol (HRZE) can be considered, as there is high morbidity and mortality without treatment.[44] TB meningitis often occurs in patients with advanced HIV. Current World Health Organization (WHO) guidelines recommend delaying antiretroviral therapy for HIV by four weeks after initiating antituberculosis therapy.[47] This is due to earlier initiation of ART being associated with an inflammatory response (termed Immune Reconstitution Inflammatory Syndrome) leading to increased morbidity and mortality for those with TB meningitis.[48] IRIS can also be seen with cryptococcal meningitis, as described in Section *Cryptococcal Meningitis*.

Neurosyphilis

We discussed general testing for syphilis in the prior section on infectious disease screening.

Syphilis is caused by the bacterial spirochete *treponema pallidum*. We refer you to the CDC guidelines on STIs for further discussion of primary, secondary, and tertiary syphilis.[15]

Neurosyphilis can occur at any stage of syphilis disease. Ocular syphilis and otosyphilis can present with isolated clinical findings or in conjunction with neurosyphilis. Symptoms of ocular syphilis can be quite broad, with common findings being pan-uveitis, and the involvement of ophthalmologists is helpful.[49] Otosyphilis usually involves hearing loss, tinnitus, or vertigo and requires evaluation by otolaryngologists.[50] All patients with symptoms concerning ocular syphilis or otosyphilis should undergo a full cranial nerve exam, and if abnormalities are noted, a lumbar puncture (LP) evaluation, as detailed next. Neurosyphilis can involve the CSF, meninges, and cerebrospinal vasculature in early stages and later involve the brain with psychiatric manifestations or the spinal cord with tabes dorsalis.[51-53] Ischemic stroke in a young person can be a manifestation of syphilis vasculitis, and the patient may have headache, dizziness, or personality changes preceding the stroke.[53] LP evaluation should consist of cell counts, glucose, protein, and CSF VDRL, along with a serum RPR.[53] If there are CSF abnormalities, they can include a lymphocytic pleocytosis, elevated protein, and a reactive CSF-VDRL test. However, since these studies can be negative, clinical judgment is needed on whether to treat for neurosyphilis. The management of ocular syphilis, otosyphilis, and neurosyphilis consists of 10–14 days of IV penicillin, a much more cumbersome burden for patients, so careful consideration must be made in interpreting the clinical picture and laboratory studies.[15]

After treatment of neurosyphilis, repeat testing is needed every three to six months with a neurological exam and LP. The CSF white blood cell count should decrease, and the CSF-VDRL titer should decrease fourfold (e.g., from 1:64 to 1:16) within one year.[53]

Fungal Meningitis

Coccidioides meningitis

Clinicians in California and Arizona are familiar with an endemic fungus that can lead to chronic fungal meningitis – that is, *Coccidioides immitis* and *Coccidioides posadasii*. In endemic areas, primarily the San Joaquin Valley of Central California, as well as in Arizona, *Coccidioides* is endemic in the soil and patients are exposed by inhaling the spores. Most patients are asymptomatic or present with mild to moderate pneumonia, which may not require antifungal therapy.[54] However, patients with certain immunocompromising risk factors (diabetes, transplant, pregnancy, etc.) or race/ethnicity risk factors (such as of African American or Filipino descent) are at risk for disseminated disease, the most serious of which is coccidioidal meningitis, colloquially known as cocci meningitis.[54] Before the advent of modern antifungals, cocci meningitis was a uniformly fatal diagnosis. Mortality rates decreased to ~30% when intrathecal amphotericin came onto market.[55] A recent case series out of UCSF Fresno reported a 23% mortality rate using mostly systemic azoles such as fluconazole, posaconazole, and itraconazole.[56]

Treatment of cocci meningitis requires an interdisciplinary discussion between infectious diseases specialists, neurologists, rheumatologists, and neurosurgeons, as patients can develop CNS vasculitis and/or obstructive hydrocephalus from cocci meningitis.[54] For this disease, headache may be a useful parameter, along with CSF studies, neuroimaging, and serologic markers to track disease burden.[54] In our clinical experience, most patients' headaches can be treated with acetaminophen, ibuprofen, or oxycodone. More research is needed on whether triptans are safe given the increased risk of stroke with those medications and the high burden of stroke in cocci meningitis patients.

Cryptococcal meningitis

Cryptococcal meningitis is caused by *Cryptococcus neoformans* and *Cryptococcus gattii*.[44] Cryptococcal meningitis is often seen in patients with an impaired immune system, such as those with uncontrolled HIV.

CSF cultures obtained by LP can take days to weeks to turn positive; thus, a CSF cryptococcal antigen can provide a more rapid answer.[44] In patients with uncontrolled HIV and symptomatic cryptococcal disease, serum cryptococcal antigen (serum CrAg) is considered to be as sensitive as CSF cryptococcal antigen and can be used in those who cannot undergo an LP.[57] Serum CrAg is also a sensitive screening tool in those with advanced immunosuppression.[58]

For patients with cryptococcal meningitis and HIV, the WHO recommends delaying initiation of anti-retroviral therapy for four to six weeks after beginning treatment for Cryptococcus due to clinical trials showing increased mortality with early ART initiation.[59, 60] Amphotericin B and flucytosine are corner-stones of initial therapy, along with serial lumbar punctures to decrease intracranial pressure.[57]

Postprocedural fungal meningitis

Patients can develop fungal meningitis post-procedurally due to contaminated materials used during the procedure. There was a fungal meningitis outbreak in 2023 from patients who underwent epidural anes-thesia in Matamoros, Mexico.[61] Clinicians should have a low index of suspicion to perform an LP to investigate potential CNS infections and report it to their local public health department or to the CDC.

Neurocysticercosis

Neurocysticercosis (NCC) is a parasitic infection caused by the larval cysts of the pork tapeworm *Taenia Solium*.[62] Contrary to popular belief, patients do not contract this disease by eating undercooked pork with the tapeworm, as that only causes the tapeworm to take up residence in the patient's gut (taenia-sis).[62] However, if someone then swallows the eggs that are excreted in the feces of someone with the tapeworm, when those eggs hatch, the larva can hatch and migrate elsewhere in the body, primarily musculature and the CNS.[62] Neurocysticercosis is endemic across much of the world, with a high burden in South America, Africa, and Asia.[63] The primary manifestation of NCC is seizure and/or elevated intra-cranial pressure due to the cysts.[64] The disease is diagnosed based on imaging findings with confirmatory serologic testing performed with enzyme-linked immunoelectrotransfer blot.[64] CSF testing for antigen and *T. solium* PCR is also now available through the US National Institutes of Health and can be used for both diagnosis and monitoring response to treatment.[65, 66] Albendazole with or without praziquantel is the mainstay of therapy, and duration depends on whether the disease is parenchymal or extraparenchy-mal.[64] Management of seizure, elevated intracranial pressure with a ventriculoperitoneal shunt, and anti-inflammatory therapy due to the inflammatory effect of degenerating cysts may also be needed before or during treatment.[64]

ANTIMICROBIAL CNS EFFECTS

Case 3

A 65-year-old male is hospitalized with fevers, chills, and severe burning with urination, along with increased urinary urgency and frequency. He is found to have 3+ leukocyte esterase and nitrates in his dipstick urine. He is started empirically on ceftriaxone but fails to improve. His urine grows >100,000 CFU/ml of drug-resistant E. Coli (including resistance to ceftriaxone), and he is switched to ertapenem. However, he wants to be discharged home without a peripherally inserted central catheter, so he is placed on fosfomycin to finish out his course at home. He now presents to your clinic with a new headache and dizziness. Which medication(s) could have caused his headaches?

TABLE 11.1   Antimicrobial rates of headache

ANTIMICROBIAL	RATE OF HEADACHE
Metronidazole	18%
Fluconazole (antifungal)	2%–13%
Fosfomycin	4%–10%
Linezolid	6%–9%
Vancomycin (IV)	7%
Nitrofurantoin	6%
Bictegravir/emtricitabine/tenofovir alafenamide (antiretroviral)	4%–5%
Ciprofloxacin	1%–3%
Trimethoprim-sulfamethoxazole	Not defined
Cephalexin	Not defined
Rifampin	Not defined

Beta-lactam antibiotics are notorious for their CNS side effects, including encephalopathy and seizure, usually associated with renal dysfunction.[67] However, other antimicrobials are also associated with headache. Usually, discontinuation of the antibiotic results in cessation of the headache.

Table 11.1 presents selected antimicrobials with reported rates of headache >1%.[68, 69]

ANTIMICROBIAL INTERACTIONS WITH HEADACHE MEDICATIONS

Case 4

A 43-year-old female who is undergoing treatment for latent tuberculosis presents to your clinic for evaluation of chronic migraine. She is on daily rifampin, planned for four months. Her CSF and imaging studies are negative for tuberculous meningitis. What acute and preventative medications for headache are safe to use?

Providers should be aware of medication interactions between headache treatments, both preventative and acute, and antimicrobials, especially if patients require long-term antimicrobials. Selected medication interactions are listed in Table 11.2, but clinicians should always search for drug interactions before prescribing new medications.

The main locus of interaction is for CYP3A4 inhibition or induction. For instance, carbamazepine, an antiepileptic that can be used to treat trigeminal neuralgia, is a CYP3A4 inducer, so it can increase the metabolism of some antimicrobials, such as the antifungals itraconazole and isavuconazonium.[69] Likewise, rifampin, which is used in both TB treatment and for staph aureus infections, is a CYP3A4 inducer and so increases the metabolism and decreases the concentration of some headache medications, such as sertraline or rimegepant. On the other hand, all the azole antifungals are CYP3A4 inhibitors and so can increase the concentrations of many headache medications metabolized by that pathway.[69]

There are also polymorphisms in CYP activity, most notably CYP2C19, in which ~15% of Asians are poor metabolizers versus 3%–5% of those of Caucasian or Black ancestry.[70] Thus, with antifungal azole medications fluconazole and voriconazole, which are CYP2C19 inhibitors, one must be extra cautious

TABLE 11.2 Notable antimicrobial interactions with headache medications

	ANTIBIOTICS						ANTIFUNGALS	ANTI-TUBERCULOSIS		ARVS[a]
	BETA LACTAMS (AMOXICILLIN, CEPHALEXIN)	FLUOROQUINOLONE (CIPROFLOXACIN)	MACROLIDES (AZITHROMYCIN)	OXAZOLIDINONE (LINEZOLID)	SULFONAMIDES (TMP-SMX)	TETRACYCLINE (DOXYCYCLINE)	AZOLES (FLUCONAZOLE, POSACONAZOLE, ITRACONAZOLE, VORICONAZOLE, ISAVUCONAZONIUM)	RIFAMPIN	ISONIAZID	BICTEGRAVIR, EMTRICITABINE & TENOFOVIR ALAFENAMIDE
Acute medications										
Acetaminophen								CYP1A2 indu.	CYP2E1 indu.	
NSAIDs[b]							CYP2C9 inh.	CYP2C9 indu.		AKI
Triptans				MAOI inh.			CYP3A4 inh.			
Gepants			P-gp inh.				CYP3A4 inh.	CYP34A indu.	CYP3A4 inh.	
Preventative medications										
Anti-CGRP										
Beta Blockers		CYP1A2 inh.					P-gp inh.	Many[c]		
Calcium Channel Blockers							CYP3A4 inh.	CYP34A indu.		
Other anti-HTN		QTc pr., HyperK	QTc pr.		HyperK		QTc pr.			
Tricyclic Antidepressants		QTc pr.	QTc pr.	MAOI inh.						
SSRI		QTc pr.	QTc pr.	MAOI inh.			CYP2C19 inh.	CYP34A indu.		
SNRI		QTc pr.	QTc pr.	MAOI inh.			CYP2C19 inh.			
Anti-Seizure				MAOI inh.			CYP3A4 inh.	CYP34A indu.	CYP3A4 inh.	

a   Antiretrovirals

b   Non-Steroidal Anti-Inflammatory Drugs

c   For rifampin-beta blocker interactions, it is believed that rifampin induces many CYP pathways for metabolism of propranolol (CYP1A2, CYP2C19, CYP3A4). The mechanism by which rifampin induces metoprolol metabolism is unknown. For nadolol, rifampin is a p-gyloprotein inducer.

with medications metabolized by that pathway, which includes many antidepressants such as amitriptyline, escitalopram, fluoxetine, and venlafaxine.

Clinicians should note certain other interactions:

- **Risk of serotonin syndrome**: Linezolid is an MAOI inhibitor and thus runs the risk of inducing serotonin syndrome with many classes of antidepressants, including SSRIs, SNRIs, and TCAs. Carbamazepine may decrease the metabolism of linezolid and thus lead to increased MAOI inhibition. Empirically, however, there is some real-world evidence that the risk of serotonin syndrome remains low with the concurrent administration of linezolid and antidepressants.[71] Note that the oxazolidinone tedizolid is a weak inhibitor of MAOI and thus can sometimes be used in cases where linezolid is indicated but too many drug interactions exist.[72]
- **Acute kidney injury**: There is a risk of acute kidney injury if nonsteroidal anti-inflammatory drugs (NSAIDs) are used in conjunction with bictegravir/emtricitabine/tenofovir alafenamide, the most prescribed antiretroviral for HIV. This is due to a nephrotoxic interaction between NSAIDs and tenofovir.[69]
- **Hepatotoxicity**: Rifampin and isoniazid, the backbone of drug-susceptible TB therapy, can already lead to hepatotoxicity in patients, and current guidelines recommend pausing or stopping those agents if patients develop abdominal pain or jaundice with LFTs three times the upper limit of normal, or if asymptomatic, five times the upper limit of normal.[24] With regard to headache, the main medication interaction is with acetaminophen. Rifampin is thought to induce CYP1A2, increasing the metabolism of acetaminophen into toxic metabolites, and likewise, isoniazid is thought to induce CYP2E1, which increases the metabolism of acetaminophen into toxic metabolites.[69]

FURTHER RESOURCES

The infectious diseases practitioner, or anyone who encounters infectious diseases, is constantly learning. Resources that are quite helpful as of publication time are the following:

1. IDSA Guidelines
2. USPST Guidelines
3. CDC guidelines
4. UpToDate – Fairly current overview of a range of infections
5. Sanford Guide – Includes quick bullet points on infections, as well as antibacterial spectrum
6. NIH HIV website
7. Local hospital antibiogram regarding antibiotic susceptibilities

SUMMARY

- All adults should be screened at least once for HIV and hepatitis C during their lifetimes. High-risk groups should be screened for syphilis, gonorrhea/chlamydia, hepatitis B, and latent tuberculosis. PrEP for HIV and postexposure prophylaxis for sexually transmitted infections (DoxyPEP) can help decrease infection burden.
- Headache can be the presenting symptom of a wide range of CNS infectious diseases, including the syndromes of acute meningitis or encephalitis, focal CNS infection, and chronic meningitis.

Careful attention should be given to epidemiologic risk factors, host immunity, and potential microbiologic agents. LP is usually essential to help with diagnosis.

- Many antimicrobials can cause headache in patients, which usually resolves with cessation of the antibiotics.
- There are potential medication interactions between antimicrobials and headache medications.

REFERENCES

1. Recommendation topics [Internet]. U.S. Preventive Services Taskforce; [cited 2023 Nov 3]. Available from: https://www.uspreventiveservicestaskforce.org/uspstf/recommendation-topics
2. Human immunodeficiency virus (HIV) infection: Screening [Internet]. US Preventive Services Taskforce; 2019 [cited 2023 Nov 3]. Available from: https://www.uspreventiveservicestaskforce.org/uspstf/recommendation/human-immunodeficiency-virus-hiv-infection-screening
3. Which HIV tests should I use? [Internet]. Centers for Disease Control and Prevention; 2023 [cited 2023 Nov 3]. Available from: https://www.cdc.gov/hiv/clinicians/screening/tests.html
4. Prevention of acquisition of HIV: Preexposure prophylaxis [Internet]. US Preventive Services Taskforce; 2023 [cited 2023 Nov 3]. Available from: https://www.uspreventiveservicestaskforce.org/uspstf/recommendation/prevention-of-human-immunodeficiency-virus-hiv-infection-pre-exposure-prophylaxis
5. Descovy for PrEP (emtricitabine/tenofovir alafenamide) clinical data in cisgender women [Internet]. Gilead Medical Information; 2019 [cited 2023 Nov 3]. Available from: https://www.askgileadmedical.com/docs/truvada/descovy-for-prep-clinical-data-in-cisgender-women
6. About PrEP [Internet]. Centers for Disease Control and Prevention; 2022 [cited 2023 Nov 3]. Available from: https://www.cdc.gov/hiv/basics/prep/about-prep.html
7. Krakower D, Mayer KH. *HIV pre-exposure prophylaxis*. UpToDate. Gulick RM, Mitty J, editors. 2023.
8. Syphilis infection in nonpregnant adolescents and adults: Screening [Internet]. US Preventive Services Taskforce; 2022 [cited 2023 Nov 3]. Available from: https://www.uspreventiveservicestaskforce.org/uspstf/recommendation/syphilis-infection-nonpregnant-adults-adolescents-screening
9. Hicks CB, Clement M. *Syphilis: Screening and Diagnostic Testing*. UptoDate. Marrazzo J, Mitty J, editors. 2022.
10. Centers for Disease Control and Prevention (CDC). Syphilis testing algorithms using treponemal tests for initial screening–four laboratories, New York City, 2005–2006. MMWR. Morbidity and mortality weekly report. 2008 Aug 15;57(32):872–875.
11. Luetkemeyer AF, Donnell D, Dombrowski JC, Cohen S, Grabow C, Brown CE, Malinski C, Perkins R, Nasser M, Lopez C, Vittinghoff E. Postexposure doxycycline to prevent bacterial sexually transmitted infections. *The New England Journal of Medicine* 2023 Apr 6;388(14):1296–306.
12. Stewart J, Oware K, Donnell D, et al. Conference on Retroviruses and Opportunistic Infections. In Seattle; 2023 [cited 2023 Nov 3]. Available from: https://www.croiconference.org/abstract/doxycycline-postexposure-prophylaxis-for-prevention-of-stis-among-cisgender-women/
13. Stewart et al. DPEP ISSTDR July 2023.
14. Chlamydia and gonorrhea: Screening [Internet]. US Preventive Services Taskforce; 2021 [cited 2023 Nov 3]. Available from: https://www.uspreventiveservicestaskforce.org/uspstf/recommendation/chlamydia-and-gonorrhea-screening
15. STI treatment guidelines [Internet]. Centers for Disease Control and Prevention; 2021 [cited 2023 Nov 3]. Available from: https://www.cdc.gov/std/treatment-guidelines/chlamydia.htm
16. Hepatitis B virus infection in adolescents and adults: Screening [Internet]. US Preventive Services Taskforce; 2020 [cited 2023 Nov 3]. Available from: https://www.uspreventiveservicestaskforce.org/uspstf/recommendation/hepatitis-b-virus-infection-screening
17. Hepatitis C virus infection in adolescents and adults: Screening [Internet]. US Preventive Services Taskforce; 2020 [cited 2023 Nov 3]. Available from: https://www.uspreventiveservicestaskforce.org/uspstf/recommendation/hepatitis-c-screening
18. Latent tuberculosis infection in adults: Screening [Internet]. US Preventive Services Taskforce; 2023 [cited 2023 Nov 3]. Available from: https://www.uspreventiveservicestaskforce.org/uspstf/recommendation/latent-tuberculosis-infection-screening

19. Testing for TB infection [Internet]. Centers for Disease Control and Prevention; 2016 [cited 2023 Nov 3]. Available from: https://www.cdc.gov/tb/topic/testing/tbtesttypes.htm

20. IGRAs– Blood Tests for TB Infection Fact Sheet [Internet]. Centers for Disease Control and Prevention; 2016 [cited 2023 Nov 3]. Available from: https://www.cdc.gov/tb/publications/factsheets/testing/igra.htm

21. Yamasue M, Komiya K, Usagawa Y, Umeki K, Nureki SI, Ando M, Hiramatsu K, Nagai H, Kadota JI. Factors associated with false negative interferon-γ release assay results in patients with tuberculosis: a systematic review with meta-analysis. *Scientific Reports* 2020 Jan 31;*10*(1):1607.

22. Fitzgerald DW, Sterling TR, Haas DW. Mycobacterium tuberculosis. In: Bennett JE, Dolin R, Blaser MJ, editors. *Mandell, Douglas, and Bennett's Principles and Practice of Infectious Diseases.* 9th ed. Philadelphia, PA: Elsevier; 2020. p. 2985–3021.

23. Huaman MA, Sterling TR. Treatment of latent tuberculosis infection—an update. *Clinics in Chest Medicine* 2019 Dec 1;*40*(4):839–848.

24. Tuberculosis (TB) [Internet]. Centers for Disease Control and Prevention; 2023 [cited 2023 Nov 5]. Available from: https://www.cdc.gov/tb/default.htm

25. Hasbrun R and Tunkel AR. Approach to the Patient With Central Nervous System Infection. In: Bennett JE, Dolin R, Blaser MJ, editors. *Mandell, Douglas, and Bennett's Principles and Practice of Infectious Diseases.* 9th ed. Philadelphia, PA: Elsevier; 2020. p. 1176–1182.

26. Tunkel AR, Hartman BJ, Kaplan SL, Kaufman BA, Roos KL, Scheld WM, Whitley RJ. Practice guidelines for the management of bacterial meningitis. *Clinical Infectious Diseases.* 2004 Nov 1;*39*(9):1267–84.

27. Castelblanco RL, Lee M, Hasbun R. Epidemiology of bacterial meningitis in the USA from 1997 to 2010: a population-based observational study. *The Lancet Infectious Diseases* 2014 Sep 1;*14*(9):813–9.

28. Bacterial meningitis [Internet]. Centers for Disease Control and Prevention; 2021 [cited 2023 Nov 3]. Available from: https://www.cdc.gov/meningitis/bacterial.html

29. The biofire® FilmArray® meningitis/encephalitis (ME) panel [Internet]. Biomerieux; 2023 [cited 2023 Nov 3]. Available from: https://www.biofiredx.com/products/the-filmarray-panels/filmarrayme/

30. Mbaeyi S, Pondo T, Blain A, Yankey D, Potts C, Cohn A, Hariri S, Shang N, MacNeil JR. Incidence of meningococcal disease before and after implementation of quadrivalent meningococcal conjugate vaccine in the United States. *JAMA Pediatrics* 2020 Sep 1;*174*(9):843–51.

31. Dawson KG, Emerson JC, Burns JL. Fifteen years of experience with bacterial meningitis. *The Pediatric Infectious Disease Journal* 1999 Sep 1;*18*(9):816–22.

32. Makwana N, Riordan FA. Bacterial meningitis: the impact of vaccination. *CNS Drugs* 2007 May;*21*:355–66.

33. Whitney CG, Farley MM, Hadler J, Harrison LH, Bennett NM, Lynfield R, Reingold A, Cieslak PR, Pilishvili T, Jackson D, Facklam RR. Decline in invasive pneumococcal disease after the introduction of protein–polysaccharide conjugate vaccine. *The New England Journal of Medicine* 2003 May 1;*348*(18):1737–46.

34. Tunkel AR, Hasbun R, Bhimraj A, Byers K, Kaplan SL, Scheld WM, van de Beek D, Bleck TP, Garton HJ, Zunt JR. 2017 Infectious Diseases Society of America's clinical practice guidelines for healthcare-associated ventriculitis and meningitis. *Clinical Infectious Diseases.* 2017 Mar 15;*64*(6):e34–65.

35. Venkatesan A, Tunkel AR, Bloch KC, Lauring AS, Sejvar J, Bitnun A, Stahl JP, Mailles A, Drebot M, Rupprecht CE, Yoder J. Case definitions, diagnostic algorithms, and priorities in encephalitis: consensus statement of the international encephalitis consortium. *Clinical Infectious Diseases.* 2013 Oct 15;*57*(8):1114–28.

36. Vora NM, Holman RC, Mehal JM, Steiner CA, Blanton J, Sejvar J. Burden of encephalitis-associated hospitalizations in the United States, 1998–2010. *Neurology* 2014 Feb 4;*82*(5):443–51.

37. Glaser CA, Gilliam S, Schnurr D, Forghani B, Honarmand S, Khetsuriani N, Fischer M, Cossen CK, Anderson LJ. In search of encephalitis etiologies: diagnostic challenges in the California Encephalitis Project, 1998—2000. *Clinical Infectious Diseases.* 2003 Mar 15;*36*(6):731–42.

38. Barnett EM, Jacobsen G, Evans G, Cassell M, Perlman S. Herpes simplex encephalitis in the temporal cortex and limbic system after trigeminal nerve inoculation. *The Journal of Infectious Diseases* 1994 Apr 1;*169*(4):782–6.

39. Tunkel AR, Glaser CA, Bloch KC, Sejvar JJ, Marra CM, Roos KL, Hartman BJ, Kaplan SL, Scheld WM, Whitley RJ. The management of encephalitis: clinical practice guidelines by the Infectious Diseases Society of America. *Clinical Infectious Diseases.* 2008 Aug 1:303–27.

40. Beckham JD and Tyler KL. Encephalitis. In: Bennett JE, Dolin R, Blaser MJ, editors. *Mandell, Douglas, and Bennett's Principles and Practice of Infectious Diseases.* 9th ed. Philadelphia, PA: Elsevier; 2020. p. 1226–1247.

41. Tunkel, AR. Subdural Empyema, Epidural Abscess, and Suppurative Intracranial Thrombophlebitis. In: Bennett JE, Dolin R, Blaser MJ, editors. *Mandell, Douglas, and Bennett's Principles and Practice of Infectious Diseases.* 9th ed. Philadelphia, PA: Elsevier; 2020. p. 1262–1271.

42. Auinger AB, Dahm V, Stanisz I, Schwarz-Nemec U, Arnoldner C. The challenging diagnosis and follow-up of skull base osteomyelitis in clinical practice. *European Archives of Oto-Rhino-Laryngology* 2021 Dec 1:1–8.

43. Marrodan M, Bensi C, Alessandro L, Muggeri AD, Farez MF. Chronic and subacute meningitis: differentiating neoplastic from non-neoplastic etiologies. *Neurohospitalist.* 2018 Oct;*8*(4):177–82.

44. Bennett JE and Hoover SE. Chronic Meningitis. In: Bennett JE, Dolin R, Blaser MJ, editors. *Mandell, Douglas, and Bennett's Principles and Practice of Infectious Diseases.* 9th ed. Philadelphia, PA: Elsevier; 2020. p. 1220–1225.

45. Sawanyawisuth K, Chotmongkol V. Eosinophilic meningitis. *Handbook of Clinical Neurology* 2013 Jan 1;*114*:207–15.

46. Bahr NC, Nuwagira E, Evans EE, Cresswell FV, Bystrom PV, Byamukama A, Bridge SC, Bangdiwala AS, Meya DB, Denkinger CM, Muzoora C. Diagnostic accuracy of Xpert MTB/RIF Ultra for tuberculous meningitis in HIV-infected adults: a prospective cohort study. *The Lancet Infectious Diseases.* 2018 Jan 1;*18*(1):68–75.

47. Updated recommendations on HIV prevention, infant diagnosis, antiretroviral initiation and monitoring [Internet]. World Health Organization; [cited 2023 Nov 5]. Available from: https://www.who.int/publications/i/item/9789240022232

48. Török ME, Yen NT, Chau TT, Mai NT, Phu NH, Mai PP, Dung NT, Chau NV, Bang ND, Tien NA, Minh NH. Timing of initiation of antiretroviral therapy in human immunodeficiency virus (HIV)–associated tuberculous meningitis. *Clinical Infectious Diseases.* 2011 Jun 1;*52*(11):1374–83.

49. Moradi A, Salek S, Daniel E, Gangaputra S, Ostheimer TA, Burkholder BM, Leung TG, Butler NJ, Dunn JP, Thorne JE. Clinical features and incidence rates of ocular complications in patients with ocular syphilis. American Journal of Ophthalmology 2015 Feb 1;*159*(2):334–43.

50. Yimtae K, Srirompotong S, Lertsukprasert K. Otosyphilis: a review of 85 cases. *Otolaryngology and Head and Neck Surgery* 2007 Jan;*136*(1):67–71.

51. Marra CM, Maxwell CL, Smith SL, Lukehart SA, Rompalo AM, Eaton M, Stoner BP, Augenbraun M, Barker DE, Corbett JJ, Zajackowski M. Cerebrospinal fluid abnormalities in patients with syphilis: association with clinical and laboratory features. *The Journal of Infectious Diseases.* 2004 Feb 1;*189*(3):369–76.

52. Timmermans M, Carr J. Neurosyphilis in the modern era. *Journal of Neurology, Neurosurgery, and Psychiatry* 2004 Dec 1;*75*(12):1727–30.

53. Marra, CM. *Neurosyphilis.* UptoDate. Gonzalez-Scarano F, Marrazzo J, Wilterdink J, editors. 2020.

54. Galgiani JN, Ampel NM, Blair JE, Catanzaro A, Geertsma F, Hoover SE, Johnson RH, Kusne S, Lisse J, MacDonald JD, Meyerson SL. 2016 Infectious Diseases Society of America (IDSA) clinical practice guideline for the treatment of coccidioidomycosis. *Clinical Infectious Diseases.* 2016 Sep 15;*63*(6):e112–46.

55. Ho J, Fowler P, Heidari A, Johnson RH. Intrathecal amphotericin B: a 60-year experience in treating coccidioidal meningitis. *Clinical Infectious Diseases.* 2017 Feb 15;*64*(4):519–24.

56. Sivasubramanian G, Kadakia S, Kim JM, Pervaiz S, Yan Y, Libke R. Challenges in the Long-term Management of Patients with Coccidioidal Meningitis: A Retrospective Analysis of Treatment and Outcomes. *In Open Forum Infectious Diseases 2023 Jun* (Vol. 10, No. 6, p. ofad243). US: Oxford University Press.

57. Perfect JR. Cryptococcosis (Cryptococcus neoformans and Cryptococcus gattii). In: Bennett JE, Dolin R, Blaser MJ, editors. *Mandell, Douglas, and Bennett's Principles and Practice of Infectious Diseases.* 9th ed. Philadelphia, PA: Elsevier; 2020. p. 3146–61.

58. Cryptococcosis: NIH [Internet]. HIV.gov; 2021 [cited 2023 Nov 5]. Available from: https://clinicalinfo.hiv.gov/en/guidelines/hiv-clinical-guidelines-adult-and-adolescent-opportunistic-infections/cryptococcosis.

59. Guidelines for diagnosing, preventing and managing cryptococcal disease among adults, adolescents and children living with HIV [Internet]. World Health Organization; 2022 [cited 2023 Nov 5]. Available from: https://www.who.int/publications/i/item/9789240052178

60. Boulware DR, Meya DB, Muzoora C, Rolfes MA, Huppler Hullsiek K, Musubire A, Taseera K, Nabeta HW, Schutz C, Williams DA, Rajasingham R. Timing of antiretroviral therapy after diagnosis of cryptococcal meningitis. *The New England Journal of Medicine* 2014 Jun 26;*370*(26):2487–98.

61. Fungal meningitis outbreak associated with procedures performed under epidural anesthesia in Matamoros, Mexico [Internet]. Centers for Disease Control and Prevention; 2023 [cited 2023 Nov 5]. Available from: https://www.cdc.gov/hai/outbreaks/meningitis-epidural-anesthesia.html

62. CDC - cysticercosis [Internet]. Centers for Disease Control and Prevention; 2023 [cited 2023 Nov 5]. Available from: https://www.cdc.gov/parasites/cysticercosis/

63. WHO taenia solium endemicity map – 2022 update [Internet]. World Health Organization; 2022 [cited 2023 Nov 5]. Available from: https://www.who.int/publications/i/item/who-wer9717-169-172

64. White Jr AC, Coyle CM, Rajshekhar V, Singh G, Hauser WA, Mohanty A, Garcia HH, Nash TE. Diagnosis and treatment of neurocysticercosis: 2017 clinical practice guidelines by the Infectious Diseases Society of America (IDSA) and the American Society of Tropical Medicine and Hygiene (ASTMH). *Clinical Infectious Diseases*. 2018 Apr 15;*66*(8):e49–75.

65. O'Connell EM, Harrison S, Dahlstrom E, Nash T, Nutman TB. A novel, highly sensitive quantitative polymerase chain reaction assay for the diagnosis of subarachnoid and ventricular neurocysticercosis and for assessing responses to treatment. *Clinical Infectious Diseases*. 2020 Apr 15;*70*(9):1875–81.

66. Corda M, Sciurba J, Blaha J, Mahanty S, Paredes A, Garcia HH, Nash TE, Nutman TB, O'Connell EM. A recombinant monoclonal-based Taenia antigen assay that reflects disease activity in extra-parenchymal neurocysticercosis. *PLoS Neglected Tropical Diseases* 2022 May 26;*16*(5):e0010442.

67. Wanleenuwat P, Suntharampillai N, Iwanowski P. Antibiotic-induced epileptic seizures: mechanisms of action and clinical considerations. *Seizure* 2020 Oct 1;*81*:167–74.

68. Mohsen S, Dickinson JA, Somayaji R. Update on the adverse effects of antimicrobial therapies in community practice. *Canadian Family Physician* 2020 Sep 1;*66*(9):651–9.

69. Lexicomp: Evidence-Based Drug Referential Content. Wolters Kluwer accessed 5 Nov 2023.

70. Scott SA, Sangkuhl K, Stein CM, Hulot JS, Mega JL, Roden DM, Klein TE, Sabatine MS, Johnson JA, Shuldiner AR. Clinical Pharmacogenetics Implementation Consortium guidelines for CYP2C19 genotype and clopidogrel therapy: 2013 update. *Clinical Pharmacology and Therapeutics* 2013 Sep;*94*(3):317–23.

71. Bai AD, McKenna S, Wise H, Loeb M, Gill SS. Association of linezolid with risk of serotonin syndrome in patients receiving antidepressants. *JAMA Network Open*. 2022 Dec 1;*5*(12):e2247426.

72. Flanagan S, Bartizal K, Minassian SL, Fang E, Prokocimer P. In vitro, in vivo, and clinical studies of tedizolid to assess the potential for peripheral or central monoamine oxidase interactions. *Antimicrobial Agents and Chemotherapy* 2013 Jul;*57*(7):3060–6.

Nephrology Comorbidities in the Treatment of Headache

12

Nivetha Subramanian and Shuchi Anand

CLINICAL CASE 1

The patient is a 48-year-old male with a history of dyslipidemia on atorvastatin who presents for evaluation of headache. He reports that he had episodic migraine with visual and sensory aura during college but has not had any headache until three years prior when the episodes began to return. He now endorses having ten days per month of migraine, preceded by 45 minutes of rainbows in his vision. The physical exam is reassuring. His blood pressure is 144/92, and this remains elevated after five minutes of resting comfortably. He then conveys that he has checked his blood pressure at his local pharmacy on occasion when picking up his atorvastatin each month, and it has been similarly high.

Preventive medications are discussed, and the patient expresses a strong interest in starting candesartan. A basic metabolic panel is performed prior to initiation with normal potassium and creatinine of 1.01 mg/dL. Triptans are avoided given his uncontrolled hypertension, and he is instead started on lasmiditan for the treatment of acute migraine.

Two weeks later, the patient has a repeat basic metabolic panel performed that is normal except for an increased creatinine to 1.12. He also conveys that lasmiditan has made him dizzy and he is switched to rimegepant.

One month after, repeat creatinine has decreased to 1.02, and his blood pressure is now 134/82. He has been on the full dose of candesartan for three weeks after an initial up-titration period and states that he has noticed that his headache frequency has started to decrease, with only one headache day the past month and a notable decrease in severity in his headaches, which respond to his rimegepant.

DOI: 10.1201/b23330-12

HYPERTENSION AND HEADACHE

Headache and blood pressure present a synergistic relationship: hypertension can trigger headache, while pain can activate the sympathetic nervous system, leading to further elevated blood pressure. Affecting about 45% of the adult population, or over one billion adults worldwide, hypertension is common, and when left untreated, it results in the development of cardiovascular disease and CKD progression.[1–6] Patients with CKD are among the largest group of patients with difficult to manage blood pressure, and many will present with symptomatic elevated blood pressure. Several studies have suggested an association between hypertension and various types of headaches, including migraine and tension-type headache.[7–10] We will next discuss the diagnosis, workup and management of hypertension, highlighting data relevant to patients with concomitant headache with and without accompanying chronic kidney disease (CKD).

Equal to the product of cardiac output and systemic vascular resistance, blood pressure is a mechanism by which the body sustains adequate perfusion. Through the renin-angiotensin-aldosterone system (RAAS), the kidneys play a key role in maintaining blood pressure.[13] The afferent arteriole of each glomerulus contains juxtaglomerular cells that synthesize renin.[13] Hypotension, hypovolemia, or general renal hypoperfusion restricts sodium chloride delivery to the macula densa, triggering renin release from the kidneys.[13] Renin then cleaves angiotensinogen, which is released by the liver, to angiotensin I.[13] The angiotensin-converting enzyme (ACE) converts angiotensin I to angiotensin II.[13] Angiotensin II promotes aldosterone secretion from the adrenal glands, which act on the kidneys, leading to reabsorption of renal sodium and systemic blood pressure rise. Angiotensin II is also a potent vasoconstrictor, acting on the smooth muscle of arterioles.[13] Vasopressin also known as antidiuretic hormone, released by the hypothalamus, also helps with fluid retention and increasing blood pressure.[13] The aforementioned pathways also simultaneously activate the sympathetic system, causing elevated blood pressure. Figure 12.1 provides a schematic of the pathways.

Hypertension can be divided into two categories: primary or secondary hypertension.[6, 14] Primary or essential hypertension is defined as hypertension for which a secondary cause has not been identified. Risk factors for essential hypertension include age, family history, and race but also more modifiable characteristics, many of which may coalesce in a single individual. These include alcohol consumption, high sodium diet, insufficient sleep, physical inactivity, and stress. Social determinants of health also contribute to either undiagnosed risk factors or less intensive management of blood pressure.[3, 12] Secondary hypertension is caused by a specific identifiable etiology, including medications such as nonsteroidal anti-inflammatory drugs (NSAIDs) and oral contraceptives, renal artery stenosis, obstructive sleep apnea, primary hyperaldosteronism, pheochromocytoma, or pain.[11] Since the treatment of secondary hypertension often involves treating the underlying etiology, it is important to distinguish this category of hypertension from essential hypertension.

Lifestyle management is a first step toward blood pressure reduction for mildly elevated pressures and can be prescribed in tandem with pharmacotherapy in people with higher pressures. A large meta-analysis analyzing 105 trials found that salt restriction to 4–6 grams/day was associated with 3.6 mmHg reduction in systolic blood pressure. In comparison, the Kidney Disease Improving Global Outcomes (KDIGO) provides a class 2C recommendation for reducing dietary sodium to less than 2 grams, acknowledging difficulty with dietary adherence.[15] Similarly, the meta-analysis found that a diet with a reduction in fat and more fruits and vegetables was associated with an average of 5 mmHg reduction in systolic pressures.[16] Exercise and alcohol intake reduction were similarly associated with modest reductions in blood pressure, although the interventions varied widely in the trials.[16] In addition to reducing blood pressure, lifestyle modifications, including reducing sodium and following a DASH diet, have been associated with fewer migraines.[17]

The widely accepted American College of Cardiology/American Heart Association (ACC/AHA) defines hypertension as systolic blood pressure exceeding 130 mmHg and diastolic blood pressure over 80

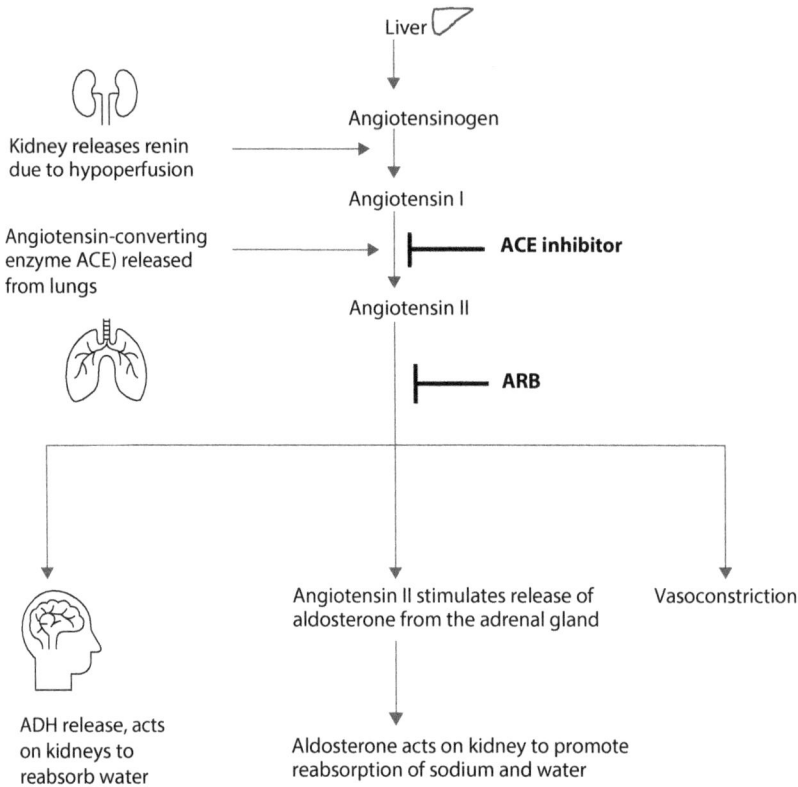

FIGURE 12.1   RAAS pathway.

mmHg.[11] For individuals diagnosed with hypertension, the guidelines recommend shared decision-making and weighing the risks and benefits of drug initiation. In individuals who are otherwise healthy with systolic blood pressure between 130–140 mmHg or diastolic blood pressure between 80–90 mmHg, the ACC/AHA recommends calculating the atherosclerotic CVD (ASCVD) risk through the Pooled Cohort Equation to estimate the ten-year risk of atherosclerotic cardiovascular disease.[11] In individuals who are 65 years or older, with type 2 diabetes, CKD, known cardiovascular disease, or an estimated ten-year ASCVD risk of 10% or higher, pharmacotherapy is recommended.[11] Individuals with systolic blood pressure of 140 mmHg or higher or diastolic blood pressure of 90 mmHg or higher should also initiate pharmacotherapy.[11]

Patients with hypertension and CKD should be followed by a nephrologist who can identify the etiology of CKD, closely monitor kidney function, and initiate early pharmacotherapy to reduce the progression of kidney disease. National guidelines from the KDIGO group recommend targeting a systolic blood pressure goal of less than 120 mm Hg in individuals with CKD.[12] However, the trials analyzed typically excluded frail and elderly individuals for whom the risk and benefit ratio for stringent blood pressure control may be different.[12] For example, individuals with limited life expectancy, severe symptomatic orthostatic hypotension, or frequent falls may benefit from more relaxed blood pressure targets. Interestingly, guidelines recommending optimal blood pressure for adults with a kidney transplant are not as clear. KDIGO recommends maintaining blood pressure less than 130/80, possibly due to increased need for perfusion of the transplant.[12]

In patients with migraine, hypertension, and CKD with or without albuminuria, a potential medication to target all three conditions would be an ACE inhibitor or angiotensin II receptor blocker (ARB). Used for migraine prevention, ACE inhibitors and ARBs are also used frequently in CKD patients for their antihypertensive and proteinuria-reducing effects.[18–20] In fact, several studies have demonstrated that ACE inhibitors and ARBs can reduce protein loss by 30%–35% and prevent further decline in renal function among diabetic and nondiabetic patients with CKD.[21–28] By dilating efferent and afferent arterioles, these medications can reduce intraglomerular pressure, leading to a reduction in protein loss and preservation of the glomerulus. Patients with CKD often have cardiovascular disease as well, and both medications may also reduce the risk of harmful cardiac remodeling.[24] ACE inhibitors and ARBs need to be monitored closely in patients with CKD due to possible side effects, including hyperkalemia and further reduction in glomerular filtration rate (GFR).[29] There is increasing evidence that these medications can be continued safely should patients experience progressive or advancing renal disease.[30] In patients with advanced CKD, typically a GFR less than 30 mL/min/1.73 m², initiating these medications may lead to hyperkalemia, and thus specialist care, typically under the supervision of a nephrologist, is recommended. After starting an ACE inhibitor or ARB, it is not uncommon to see a transient rise in creatinine. Typically, a repeat serum creatinine, potassium, and blood pressure should be checked within two weeks of initiating therapy. If the creatinine rise is less than 30%, it is reasonable to continue using the medication with gentle titration of the ACE inhibitor or ARB every few weeks while closely monitoring renal function and electrolytes. In addition to hyperkalemia and reduction in GFR, side effects from ACE inhibitors include dry cough, which is estimated to affect 10%–20% of all users, and much less commonly, angioedema.[31] Patients on dialysis generally can be safely initiated and maintained on nondialyzable ACE inhibitors or ARBs.

Other agents commonly used to treat both hypertension and migraine include beta-blockers and calcium channel blockers.[32] Although these agents lack antiproteinuric effect, their use is often necessary to control blood pressure in patients with CKD, as an adjunct therapy to the cornerstone of ACE inhibitor or ARB.[32, 33]

Although most cases of hypertension can be managed in the outpatient setting, there are some exceptions. Hypertensive emergency, defined as severely elevated blood pressure typically exceeding 180/120 mmHg with end-organ damage, requires prompt assessment and treatment.[34] Neurologic end-organ damage can include hemorrhagic or ischemic stroke. A distinct etiology associated with malignant hypertension is posterior reversible encephalopathy syndrome (PRES).[35, 36] This condition can present with several neurologic symptoms, including constant headache, altered mental status, visual disturbances, and seizures.[35, 36] Although an estimated 70% of cases present with severe hypertension, others occur in normotensive or mildly elevated blood pressure and may result from fluctuations and sudden, steep rises in blood pressure.[36] Underlying renal disease, autoimmune conditions such as lupus, and use of immunosuppressive medications, including tacrolimus or cyclosporine, have all been associated with PRES.[35–37] Several mechanisms have been postulated. Similar to preeclampsia, a systemic inflammatory process may contribute to endothelial dysfunction, impairing the integrity of the blood–brain barrier and causing vasogenic edema.[35, 36] Another theory is that severe hypertension disrupts cerebral blood flow autoregulation, leading to hyperperfusion and subsequent blood–brain barrier damage.[35, 36] When it is suspected, imaging becomes crucial to the diagnosis. Brain magnetic resonance imaging (MRI) is preferred and typically shows increased signal in T2-weighted images and increased white matter edema in the posterior cerebral hemispheres, usually but not exclusively in the occipital and parietal lobes.[36] Prompt treatment with discontinuation of any culprit medications and reduction of blood pressure by no more than 25% is essential. Abrupt, aggressive blood pressure reduction can propagate cerebral, cardiac, and renal ischemia. In many cases, treatment of PRES usually reverses symptoms and imaging findings within a few days.

CLINICAL CASE 2

The patient is a 74-year-old female with a history of diabetes, hypertension, and end-stage renal disease who presents for evaluation of worsening headache. The patient started hemodialysis one month prior and states that with every session, she will have a severe headache that begins roughly two hours after initiation of dialysis. The pain is holocephalic and throbbing with associated nausea but no photophobia or phonophobia. While she understands the necessity of continuing dialysis, she has had increasing doubts about this as a viable option given the extent of her headaches. She is off of antihypertensives, but her blood pressure was previously controlled on hydrochlorothiazide, amlodipine, and lisinopril. Her diabetes is controlled with long-acting and short-acting insulin.

In discussion with the patient, she is amenable to considering onabotulinumtoxinA for prevention of her headaches with a chronic migraine phenotype but requests to try preventive remote electrical neuromodulation first.

Two months later, the patient returns to clinic and reports that she immediately started using the remote electrical neuromodulation device every other day, typically in the hour before she starts dialysis, and that this has greatly decreased the severity of her headaches. She continues to have her headaches with dialysis, but they are tolerable, and she declines starting onabotulinumtoxinA treatment at this time.

HEADACHE ASSOCIATED WITH DIALYSIS

Over 550,000 people are on dialysis in the United States. Many of them suffer high morbidity and mortality, and thus, there is an increasing recognition in the field to undertake patient-oriented interventions that improve quality of life. Dialysis headache can be debilitating and impede an individual's ability to tolerate hemodialysis sessions. Dialysis headache is thought to affect 27%–73% of all individuals on hemodialysis.[38] Challenging to treat, these headaches require early collaboration between nephrologists and headache specialists.

In 1972, Bana et al. first described dialysis-related headaches among a cohort of patients on hemodialysis in Boston, Massachusetts.[39] The authors noted that these headaches typically commenced after the start of dialysis or changed characteristics if the person was experiencing headache prior to the start of dialysis.[39] The authors described the headache as a mild bifrontal ache that would crescendo into a more intense throbbing headache, become worse when reclined, and often associated with nausea and vomiting.[38, 39] In 2013, the Headache Classification Committee of the International Headache Society (IHS) defined diagnostic criteria for dialysis headaches.[40] Dialysis headaches occur during hemodialysis and improve within 72 hours after cessation of dialysis.[40] They meet the following criteria:[40]

1. At least three episodes of acute headache fulfilling Criteria C
2. Patient is on hemodialysis
3. Evidence of causation demonstrated by at least two of the following:
   - Each headache has developed during a session of hemodialysis
   - Either or both of the following:
     - Each headache has worsened during dialysis
     - Each headache has resolved within 72 hours
   - Headache episodes cease altogether after kidney transplantation or termination of hemodialysis
4. Not accounted for by an alternative *International Classification of Headache Disorders, 3rd Edition* diagnosis

Dialysis headache is associated with blood pressure fluctuations, more commonly with hypotension, which triggers the RAAS pathway and causes cerebral vasoconstriction. They can also be associated with dialysis disequilibrium syndrome—a serious neurologic phenomenon characterized by severe headache and altered mental status, which can progress to obtundation.[41] Dialysis disequilibrium is often caused by rapid shifts in blood urea and pH (relative to cerebrospinal fluid), leading to cerebral edema, although other osmotic shifts may also be implicated.

Other risk factors for dialysis headache include high serum sodium and low serum magnesium. Caffeine removal on dialysis leading to caffeine withdrawal, acetate dialysis, intradialytic hypertension, and hypotension triggering RAS activation and concomitantly cerebral vasoconstriction have been postulated mechanisms.[42] Individuals with higher blood urea levels and elevated predialysis blood pressure are at a higher risk of developing a headache as well, pointing to electrolyte and water shifts as a potential etiology.[43]

There are no clear guidelines on how to treat dialysis headache. Case reports have suggested success with using amitriptyline and nondialyzable ACE inhibitors. Botulinum toxin may be an option in this cohort.[43] Reports also suggest improvement in headache and response to magnesium and chlorpromazine prior to dialysis and the use of non-dialyzable ACE inhibitors, nortriptyline, and magnesium oxide for prevention. Modifications to the dialysis prescription with a reduction in blood flow and ultrafiltration rate and adjustment of the sodium level in the dialysate bath may also be trialed.

AUTOSOMAL DOMINANT POLYCYSTIC KIDNEY DISEASE

Aneurysms affect 3%–6% of the population, and one-third of all patients with unruptured aneurysms report a headache.[44] About 10%–12% of patients with autosomal dominant polycystic kidney disease (ADPKD), one of the most common genetic conditions involving the kidneys, have intracranial aneurysms compared to 2%–3% of the general population. The aneurysms typically occur in the anterior circulation of the circle of Willis.[41–48] Ruptured aneurysms confer a 40%–60% risk of morbidity and mortality. Patients with ADPKD may also experience other types of headaches. In a study examining the distribution of pain in 171 patients with ADPKD, 48.5% reported headaches, typically frontal (19.3%), whole head (13.3%), and localized to one side (12%).[49]

ADPKD affects about 1 in 1,000 births, although it is postulated that more people have the disease and remain without clinical manifestations during their lifetime.[47] A majority of individuals with ADPKD have mutations in the PKD1 or PKD2 genes, although there is a subset of patients who also have defects in transporter proteins (e.g., GANAB and DNAJB11 genes). Individuals with PKD2 tend to have less severe manifestations of the disease than PKD1, developing cysts and progressing to end-stage kidney disease (ESKD) at a later age (mean age 74 years compared to 54 years).[50] However, all individuals who have PKD1 and PKD2 mutations develop renal cysts.

Clinical manifestations include renal dysfunction, headache, hypertension, palpable kidneys with the presence of cysts, hematuria, proteinuria, and flank pain. Genetic testing is typically reserved in cases where imaging is not definitive or patients have atypical manifestations, such as severe ADPKD diagnosed at an early age, variation in disease between kidneys, kidney failure without renal enlargement, or lack of family history. One study examining the leading cause of death in 129 patients with ADPKD found that cardiac causes were most common (36%), followed by infection (24%) and a neurologic event (12%).[51] Neurologic-related mortality was due to ruptured intracranial aneurysm (6%), hypertensive intracerebral hemorrhage (5%), or ischemic stroke (1%).[51]

ADPKD patients with a family history of intracranial aneurysm or subarachnoid hemorrhage have about 21%–22% prevalence of intracerebral aneurysm. People with ADPKD and a personal or family history of subarachnoid hemorrhage or intracranial aneurysm should be screened using MRA with time of flight without contrast (KDIGO).[52] Individuals with ADPKD should be referred to nephrology early as there are several strategies used to prevent the progression of renal dysfunction, including tolvaptan, a Food and Drug Administration (FDA) approved potent vasopressin receptor antagonist that reduces cyst progression.

HEADACHE IN KIDNEY TRANSPLANT PATIENTS

Headache among individuals with kidney transplants has not been well studied. A study analyzing 83 kidney transplant recipients in Italy found that 45% of individuals experienced headaches, with migraine as the most common type.[53, 54] Although patients with kidney transplants also experience similar headaches to the general population, additional etiologies should be considered because of immunosuppression. Kidney transplant patients are two to three times more likely than the general population of the same age and sex to experience malignancy, with the risk increasing the longer patients have a kidney transplant.[54, 55] The greatest risk is from non-melanoma skin cancers, viral-associated malignancies such as Kaposi's sarcoma, and posttransplant lymphoproliferative disease.[54]

Patients who are experiencing red flag symptoms, including abrupt onset of headaches, long-standing headache with recent change in pattern, weight loss, or neurologic deficits, should obtain additional neuroimaging to rule out an intracranial process.[56] An estimated 5%–10% of kidney transplant recipients may experience CNS-related infections, which can also manifest as headache. These infectious complications include meningitis, encephalitis, or focal brain infections, including toxoplasma gondii, nocardia asteroids, or fungal processes such as mucormycosis and bacterial meningitis.[58] If transplant patients are diagnosed with cancer or infection, there should be ongoing discussions with their transplant nephrologist to reduce immunosuppression.[57, 58]

CLINICAL CASE 3

The patient is a 65-year-old female with a history of CKD and hypertension who presents for follow-up of headache management. The patient has a long history of chronic migraine, currently well controlled on verapamil 240 mg daily for prevention and almotriptan 12.5 mg for acute treatment. She is concerned because her nephrologist has just let her know that her kidney function has decreased, and she now has a creatinine clearance of 25 mL/min.

Renal dosing is discussed with the patient, and her verapamil is left unchanged while her almotriptan is decreased to 6.25 mg per dose, with a maximum of 12.5 mg per 24 hours. She messages two months later that the lower dosage of almotriptan is working similarly to her higher previous dose.

MEDICATION DOSING

Adjustment of medication dosing is essential among individuals with CKD since many classes of medications are cleared by the kidneys. Inadequate drug dosing can be problematic, leading to drug toxicity and poor outcomes.[59] CKD can affect renal clearance of medications by impairing glomerular filtration, tubular secretion and reabsorption, and drug metabolism.[59] Dose adjustment becomes more complicated during situations such as acute kidney injury, when renal function is in flux, or in ESKD when dialysis clears the drugs from the blood. For individuals with acute kidney injury (AKI), it becomes important to consider loading dose dynamics while also minimizing nephrotoxic medications to reduce the risk of ongoing nephrotoxicity. Early discussion between nephrology, neurology, and primary care can be helpful in identifying therapies to safely and effectively treat headaches while preventing further renal decline.

There are many ways to estimate renal function, each with its own strengths and limitations. During the initial drug pharmacokinetic trials, the FDA used the Cockcroft-Gault equation to guide drug clearance.[60, 61] Since that time, several alternative equations have emerged with greater accuracy in certain populations.[60, 62–67] The Kidney Disease Outcomes Quality Initiative's (KDOQI) 2011 guidelines advocate that clinicians use the formula that provides the most accurate assessment of GFR among their patients.[68] Similarly, in its Drug Dosage guidelines released in 2020, the FDA recognizes various equations that have emerged since these initial studies and recommend following an equation that most accurately captures the GFR of the individual.[69] Nephrologists and headache specialists can discuss appropriate dosing of medications for their individual patients.

NSAIDs

NSAIDs are often used in the treatment of headache but can be associated with adverse renal effects. One study found that 1%–5% of all NSAID users develop AKI, and another found that even otherwise healthy individuals without renal dysfunction are at risk for adverse renal events.[70, 71] They are not recommended in individuals with kidney disease or with kidney transplants given their propensity to cause an acute reduction in GFR, increase sodium and potassium retention, and promote hypertension.[72, 73] These effects are primarily mediated by inhibiting cyclooxygenase (COX) enzymes, thereby reducing prostaglandin release.[72, 73] As a vasodilator, prostaglandin normally helps the kidneys autoregulate blood flow.[72, 73] Inhibition of prostaglandins can prevent afferent arteriolar vasodilatation, causing a reduction in GFR and leading to renal ischemia.[72, 73] Risk factors for NSAID-induced AKI include the presence of CKD, volume depletion, older age, and certain medications.[73–75] In an observational study of 1,522 patients with CKD Stages 3–5, discontinuing NSAIDs was associated with an increase in GFR with the greatest magnitude of improvement among patients with more severe CKD at baseline.[74] Hemodynamic injury with NSAIDs may occur during volume-depleted states or among patients with concomitant use of NSAIDs and medications such as ACE inhibitors, ARBs, diuretics, or calcineurin inhibitors.[75]

NSAIDs can increase the risk of cardiovascular mortality and gastrointestinal bleeding by inhibiting the protective effects of prostaglandins on gastric and intestinal mucosa.[76–78] In addition to patients with Stage 4–5 CKD, NSAIDs should be avoided in adults over 75 years of age, patients on concomitant anticoagulant or antiplatelet agents, or among individuals taking corticosteroids since these also increase the risk of bleeding.[79–83]

Other common headache medications with dosing considerations are shown in Table 12.1.

TABLE 12.1   Common migraine medications and renal considerations[84]

MEDICATION	EXAMPLE MEDICATIONS	RENAL DOSING	DIALYZABLE
Preventive Medications			
Anti-CGRP	*Erenumab Fremanezumab Atogepant*	Not studied but not expected to be affected by kidney impairment Atogepant CrCl < 30 mL/min: avoid use for chronic use Prevention: 10 mg once daily	Atogepant: consider 10 mg dosing after hemodialysis on hemodialysis days
Beta-blockers	*Atenolol Metoprolol Nadolol Propanol*	Atenolol CrCl < 10 mL/min: maximum dose 25 mg daily CrCl 10–30 mL/min: maximum dose 50 mg Nadolol CrCl 10-30 mL/min: dosing every 24–48 hours Metoprolol and Propanol are not dose adjusted	Atenolol is estimated 20%–50% dialyzable Metoprolol is dialyzable (consider dosing after dialysis) Nadolol can be administered three times a week after hemodialysis Propanolol is not significantly dialyzed
Calcium channel blockers	*Verapamil*	Typically well tolerated. No dose adjustment needed	Not significantly dialyzed in hemodialysis or peritoneal dialysis due to large protein-bound state
ACEI ARB	*Lisinopril Candesartan*	Be cautious with initiation CrCl < 30 mL/min due to hyperkalemia	Lisinopril is 50% dialyzable; alternate fosinopril is not significantly dialyzed Candesartan is not significantly dialyzed

(Continued)

TABLE 12.1 (Continued) Common migraine medications and renal considerations[84]

MEDICATION	EXAMPLE MEDICATIONS	RENAL DOSING	DIALYZABLE
Acute Medications			
Tricyclic Antidepressant	*Amitryptyline* *Nortriptyline*	No dosing adjustment required, but use with caution	Unlikely to be dialyzed, monitor closely for QTc prolonging effects
NSAIDs	*Celecoxib* *Diclofenac* *Ibuprofen* *Indomethacin* *Ketorolac*	Avoid if CrCl <30 mL/min CrCl 30–60 mL/min, consider the lowest dose. Avoid use if possible	Unlikely to be significantly dialyzed due to high protein-bound state. Avoid due to higher risk of bleeding, cardiovascular events, and loss of residual renal function
Triptans	*Almotriptan* *Eletriptan* *Frovatriptan* *Naratriptan* *Rizatriptan* *Sumatriptan*	Almotriptan CrCl ≤ 30 mL/minL 6.25 mg as single dose. Maximum dose 12.5 mg in 24 hours Naratriptan 1 mg and max dose 2.5 mg in 24 hours	Naratriptan is contraindicated CrCl <15 mL/min

CONCLUSION

Patients with headache may develop de novo kidney disease due either to sympathetic surges or treatment with medications such as NSAIDs. At the same time, patients with kidney disease commonly have uncontrolled blood pressure, which will contribute to headache, but also may have specific conditions (e.g., ADPKD, kidney transplant, or need for dialysis), which will relate to distinct headache etiologies requiring further workup. Prophylactic treatment of headaches can involve medications with renal protective benefits. When treating individuals with kidney disease, neurologists and nephrologists should collaborate early to safely treat headaches while reducing the progression of renal disease. There are some additional considerations for certain patient populations with kidney disease and headaches.

1. Individuals with migraines are at higher risk of hypertension. Patients with CKD, headaches, and hypertension would benefit from the initiation of ACE inhibitors or ARBs for both headache prophylaxis and renal protective effects.
2. Dialysis headache typically occurs right after starting dialysis. Although no definitive cause for this headache has been found, consider early discussion with nephrology to adjust the prescription during dialysis and trial therapeutics.
3. ADPKD is a typically inherited condition with an increased risk of aneurysms. Consider early involvement of nephrology if ADPKD is suspected. Individuals with ADPKD should be screened for intracranial aneurysm if they have a personal or family history of subarachnoid hemorrhage or intracranial aneurysm.
4. Kidney transplant recipients are at higher risk of malignancies and infections. Consider a broad differential, including infectious and malignancy-related etiologies of headache, when evaluating this cohort.
5. Medications should be dosed based on renal function using the formula that is most appropriate for the individual. Certain medications commonly used for headache management, such as NSAIDs, should be avoided in advanced kidney disease, while other medications should be dosed-adjusted for renal function.

REFERENCES

1. Jha V, Garcia-Garcia G, Iseki K, et al. Chronic kidney disease: global dimension and perspectives. *The Lancet.* 2013;*382*(9888):260–272. doi:10.1016/S0140-6736(13)60687-X

2. Chronic Kidney Disease Initiative. https://www.cdc.gov/kidneydisease/publications-resources/ckd-national-facts.html

3. Xie Y, Bowe B, Mokdad AH, et al. Analysis of the Global Burden of disease study highlights the global, regional, and national trends of chronic kidney disease epidemiology from 1990 to 2016. *Kidney International.* 2018;*94*(3):567–581. doi:10.1016/j.kint.2018.04.011

4. Tackling G, Borhade MB. Hypertensive Heart Disease. In: *StatPearls.* StatPearls Publishing: 2023. Accessed October 6, 2024. https://www.ncbi.nlm.nih.gov/books/NBK539800/

5. Horowitz B, Miskulin D, Zager P. Epidemiology of Hypertension in CKD. *Adv Chronic Kidney Dis* 2015;*22*(2):88–95. doi: 10.1053/j.ackd.2014.09.004

6. Iqbal AM, Jamal SF. Essential Hypertension. In: *StatPearls.* StatPearls Publishing; 2023. Accessed October 12, 2023. http://www.ncbi.nlm.nih.gov/books/NBK539859/

7. Entonen AH, Suominen SB, Korkeila K, et al. Migraine predicts hypertension--a cohort study of the Finnish working-age population. *The European Journal of Public Health.* 2014;*24*(2):244–248. doi:10.1093/eurpub/ckt141

8. Gardener H, Monteith T, Rundek T, Wright CB, Elkind MSV, Sacco RL. Hypertension and Migraine in the Northern Manhattan Study. *Ethn Dis.* 2016;*26*(3):323–330. doi:10.18865/ed.26.3.323

9. Rist PM, Winter AC, Buring JE, Sesso HD, Kurth T. Migraine and the risk of incident hypertension among women. *Cephalalgia.* 2018;*38*(12):1817–1824. doi:10.1177/0333102418756865

10. Pietrini U, De Luca M, De Santis G. Hypertension in headache patients? A clinical study. *Acta Neurol Scand.* 2005;*112*(4):259–264. doi:10.1111/j.1600-0404.2005.00476.x

11. Whelton PK, Carey RM, Aronow WS, et al. 2017 ACC/AHA/AAPA/ABC/ACPM/AGS/APhA/ASH/ASPC/NMA/PCNA guideline for the prevention, detection, evaluation, and management of high blood pressure in adults: a report of the American College of Cardiology/American Heart Association Task Force on Clinical Practice Guidelines. *Hypertension.* 2018;*71*(6). doi:10.1161/HYP.0000000000000065

12. Cheung AK, Chang TI, Cushman WC, et al. Executive summary of the KDIGO 2021 clinical practice guideline for the management of blood pressure in chronic kidney disease. *Kidney International.* 2021;*99*(3):559–569. doi:10.1016/j.kint.2020.10.026

13. Fountain JH, Kaur J, Lappin SL. Physiology, Renin Angiotensin System. In: *StatPearls.* StatPearls Publishing; 2023. Accessed October 12, 2023. http://www.ncbi.nlm.nih.gov/books/NBK470410/

14. Hegde S, Ahmed I, Aeddula NR. Secondary Hypertension. In: *StatPearls.* StatPearls Publishing; 2023. Accessed October 12, 2023. http://www.ncbi.nlm.nih.gov/books/NBK544305/

15. Dickinson BD. Reducing the population burden of cardiovascular disease by reducing sodium intake: a report of the council on science and public health. *Arch Intern Med.* 2007;*167*(14):1460. doi:10.1001/archinte.167.14.1460

16. Dickinson HO, Mason JM, Nicolson DJ, et al. Lifestyle interventions to reduce raised blood pressure: a systematic review of randomized controlled trials. *Journal of Hypertension.* 2006;*24*(2):215–233. doi:10.1097/01.hjh.0000199800.72563.26

17. Amer M, Woodward M, Appel LJ. Effects of dietary sodium and the DASH diet on the occurrence of headaches: results from randomised multicentre DASH-Sodium clinical trial. *BMJ Open.* 2014;*4*(12):e006671. doi:10.1136/bmjopen-2014-006671

18. Tronvik E, Stovner LJ, Helde G, Sand T, Bovim G. Prophylactic Treatment of Migraine With an Angiotensin II ReceptorBlocker: A Randomized Controlled Trial. *JAMA.* 2003;*289*(1):65. doi:10.1001/jama.289.1.65

19. Schrader H, Stovner LJ, Helde G, Sand T, Bovim G. Prophylactic treatment of migraine with angiotensin converting enzyme inhibitor (lisinopril): randomised, placebo controlled, crossover study. *BMJ.* 2001;*322*(7277):19–22. doi:10.1136/bmj.322.7277.19

20. Stovner LJ, Linde M, Gravdahl GB, et al. A comparative study of candesartan versus propranolol for migraine prophylaxis: A randomised, triple-blind, placebo-controlled, double cross-over study. *Cephalalgia.* 2014;*34*(7):523–532. doi:10.1177/0333102413515348

21. Gansevoort RT, Sluiter WJ, Hemmelder MH, de Zeeuw D, de Jong PE. Antiproteinuric effect of blood-pressure-lowering agents: a meta-analysis of comparative trials. *Nephrol Dial Transplant.* 1995;*10*(11):1963–1974.

22. Jafar TH. Angiotensin-Converting Enzyme Inhibitors and Progression of Nondiabetic Renal Disease: A Meta-Analysis of Patient-Level Data. *Ann Intern Med.* 2001;*135*(2):73. doi:10.7326/0003-4819-135-2-200107170-00007

23. Jafar TH, Stark PC, Schmid CH, et al. Progression of Chronic Kidney Disease: The Role of Blood Pressure Control, Proteinuria, and Angiotensin-Converting Enzyme Inhibition: A Patient-Level Meta-Analysis. *Ann Intern Med.* 2003;*139*(4):244. doi:10.7326/0003-4819-139-4-200308190-00006

24. Xie X, Liu Y, Perkovic V, et al. Renin-Angiotensin System Inhibitors and Kidney and Cardiovascular Outcomes in Patients With CKD: A Bayesian Network Meta-analysis of Randomized Clinical Trials. *American Journal of Kidney Diseases.* 2016;*67*(5):728–741. doi:10.1053/j.ajkd.2015.10.011

25. Agodoa LY. Effect of Ramipril vs Amlodipine on Renal Outcomes in Hypertensive NephrosclerosisA Randomized Controlled Trial. *JAMA.* 2001;*285*(21):2719. doi:10.1001/jama.285.21.2719

26. Maione A, Navaneethan SD, Graziano G, et al. Angiotensin-converting enzyme inhibitors, angiotensin receptor blockers and combined therapy in patients with micro- and macroalbuminuria and other cardiovascular risk factors: a systematic review of randomized controlled trials. *Nephrology Dialysis Transplantation.* 2011;*26*(9):2827–2847. doi:10.1093/ndt/gfq792

27. The GISEN Group. Randomised placebo-controlled trial of effect of ramipril on decline in glomerular filtration rate and risk of terminal renal failure in proteinuric, non-diabetic nephropathy. The GISEN Group (Gruppo Italiano di Studi Epidemiologici in Nefrologia). *Lancet.* 1997;*349*(9069):1857–1863.

28. Wright, Jr JT. Effect of Blood Pressure Lowering and Antihypertensive Drug Class on Progression of Hypertensive Kidney Disease Results From the AASK Trial. *JAMA.* 2002;*288*(19):2421. doi:10.1001/jama.288.19.2421

29. Raebel MA. Hyperkalemia Associated with Use of Angiotensin-Converting Enzyme Inhibitors and Angiotensin Receptor Blockers: Hyperkalemia with ACEI and ARB. *Cardiovascular Therapeutics.* 2012;*30*(3):e156–e166. doi:10.1111/j.1755-5922.2010.00258.x

30. Bhandari S, Mehta S, Khwaja A, et al. Renin–Angiotensin System Inhibition in Advanced Chronic Kidney Disease. *N Engl J Med.* 2022;*387*(22):2021–2032. doi:10.1056/NEJMoa2210639

31. Goyal A, Cusick AS, Thielemier B. ACE Inhibitors. In: *StatPearls.* StatPearls Publishing; 2023. Accessed October 12, 2023. http://www.ncbi.nlm.nih.gov/books/NBK430896/

32. Limmroth V, Michel MC. The prevention of migraine: a critical review with special emphasis on beta-adrenoceptor blockers. *Br J Clin Pharmacol.* 2001;*52*(3):237–243. doi:10.1046/j.0306-5251.2001.01459.x

33. Markley HG. Verapamil and migraine prophylaxis: mechanisms and efficacy. *The American Journal of Medicine.* 1991;*90*(5):S48–S53. doi:10.1016/0002-9343(91)90486-H

34. Alley WD, Schick MA. Hypertensive Emergency. In: *StatPearls.* StatPearls Publishing; 2023. Accessed October 12, 2023. http://www.ncbi.nlm.nih.gov/books/NBK470371/

35. Fugate JE, Claassen DO, Cloft HJ, Kallmes DF, Kozak OS, Rabinstein AA. Posterior reversible encephalopathy syndrome: associated clinical and radiologic findings. *Mayo Clin Proc.* 2010;*85*(5):427–432. doi:10.4065/mcp.2009.0590

36. Hobson EV, Craven I, Blank SC. Posterior reversible encephalopathy syndrome: a truly treatable neurologic illness. *Perit Dial Int.* 2012;*32*(6):590–594. doi:10.3747/pdi.2012.00152

37. Hinchey J, Chaves C, Appignani B, et al. A reversible posterior leukoencephalopathy syndrome. *N Engl J Med.* 1996;*334*(8):494–500. doi:10.1056/NEJM199602223340803

38. Sousa Melo E, Carrilho Aguiar F, Sampaio Rocha-Filho PA. Dialysis Headache: A Narrative Review. *Headache.* 2017;*57*(1):161–164. doi:10.1111/head.12875

39. Bana DS, Yap AU, Graham JR. Headache During Hemodialysis. *Headache.* 1972;*12*(1):1–14. doi:10.1111/j.1526-4610.1972.hed1201001.x

40. Headache Classification Committee of the International Headache Society (IHS). The International Classification of Headache Disorders, 3rd edition (beta version). *Cephalalgia.* 2013;*33*(9):629–808. doi:10.1177/0333102413485658

41. Zepeda-Orozco D, Quigley R. Dialysis disequilibrium syndrome. *Pediatr Nephrol.* 2012;*27*(12):2205–2211. doi:10.1007/s00467-012-2199-4

42. Nikić PM, Zidverc-Trajković J, Andrić B, Milinković M, Stojimirović B. Caffeine-withdrawal headache induced by hemodialysis. *J Headache Pain.* 2009;*10*(4):291–293. doi:10.1007/s10194-009-0119-1

43. Levin M. Resident and Fellow Section. *Headache: The Journal of Head and Face Pain.* 2013;*53*(1):181–185. doi:10.1111/head.12019

44. Schwedt TJ, Gereau RW, Frey K, Kharasch ED. Headache outcomes following treatment of unruptured intracranial aneurysms: a prospective analysis. *Cephalalgia.* 2011;*31*(10):1082–1089. doi:10.1177/0333102411398155

45. Anzai Y. MRI Screening for Cerebral Aneurysm in Adult Polycystic Kidney Disease: Is the Money Worth Spending? *Radiology.* 2019;*291*(2):409–410. doi:10.1148/radiol.2019190179

46. Flahault A, Joly D. Screening for Intracranial Aneurysms in Patients with Autosomal Dominant Polycystic Kidney Disease. *Clin J Am Soc Nephrol.* 2019;*14*(8):1242–1244. doi:10.2215/CJN.02100219

47. Kuo IY, Chapman A. Intracranial Aneurysms in ADPKD: How Far Have We Come? *Clin J Am Soc Nephrol.* 2019;*14*(8):1119–1121. doi:10.2215/CJN.07570719

48. Rozenfeld MN, Ansari SA, Shaibani A, Russell EJ, Mohan P, Hurley MC. Should patients with autosomal dominant polycystic kidney disease be screened for cerebral aneurysms? *AJNR Am J Neuroradiol.* 2014;*35*(1):3–9. doi:10.3174/ajnr.A3437

49. Bajwa ZH, Sial KA, Malik AB, Steinman TI. Pain patterns in patients with polycystic kidney disease. *Kidney International.* 2004;*66*(4):1561–1569. doi:10.1111/j.1523-1755.2004.00921.x

50. Grantham JJ. Autosomal Dominant Polycystic Kidney Disease. *N Engl J Med.* 2008;*359*(14):1477–1485. doi:10.1056/NEJMcp0804458

51. Fick GM, Johnson AM, Hammond WS, Gabow PA. Causes of death in autosomal dominant polycystic kidney disease. *Journal of the American Society of Nephrology.* 1995;*5*(12):2048–2056. doi:10.1681/ASN.V5122048

52. Chapman, AB et al. Autosomal-dominant polycystic kidney disease (ADPKD): executive summary from a Kidney Disease: Improving Global Outcomes (KDIGO) Controversies Conference. *Kidney Int.* 2015;*88*, 17–27.

53. Maggioni F, Mantovan MC, Rigotti P, et al. Headache in kidney transplantation. *J Headache Pain.* 2009;*10*(6):455–460. doi:10.1007/s10194-009-0148-9

54. Wong G, Chapman JR, Craig JC. Death from cancer: a sobering truth for patients with kidney transplants. *Kidney International.* 2014;*85*(6):1262–1264. doi:10.1038/ki.2013.494

55. Fuhrmann JD, Valkova K, Von Moos S, Wüthrich RP, Müller TF, Schachtner T. Cancer among kidney transplant recipients >20 years after transplantation: post-transplant lymphoproliferative disorder remains the most common cancer type in the ultra long-term. *Clinical Kidney Journal.* 2022;*15*(6):1152–1159. doi:10.1093/ckj/sfac013

56. Wijeratne T, Wijeratne C, Korajkic N, Bird S, Sales C, Riederer F. Secondary headaches - red and green flags and their significance for diagnostics. *eNeurologicalSci.* 2023;*32*:100473. doi:10.1016/j.ensci.2023.100473

57. Ponticelli C, Campise MR. Neurological complications in kidney transplant recipients. *J Nephrol.* 2005;*18*(5):521–528.

58. Wright AJ, Fishman JA. Central Nervous System Syndromes in Solid Organ Transplant Recipients. *Clinical Infectious Diseases.* 2014;*59*(7):1001–1011. doi:10.1093/cid/ciu428

59. Munar MY, Singh H. Drug dosing adjustments in patients with chronic kidney disease. *Am Fam Physician.* 2007;*75*(10):1487–1496.

60. Stevens LA, Nolin TD, Richardson MM, et al. Comparison of drug dosing recommendations based on measured GFR and kidney function estimating equations. *Am J Kidney Dis.* 2009;*54*(1):33–42. doi:10.1053/j.ajkd.2009.03.008

61. Cockcroft DW, Gault H. Prediction of Creatinine Clearance from Serum Creatinine. *Nephron.* 1976;*16*(1):31–41. doi:10.1159/000180580

62. Levey AS. A More Accurate Method To Estimate Glomerular Filtration Rate from Serum Creatinine: A New Prediction Equation. *Ann Intern Med.* 1999;*130*(6):461. doi:10.7326/0003-4819-130-6-199903160-00002

63. Levey AS, Stevens LA, Schmid CH, et al. A new equation to estimate glomerular filtration rate. *Ann Intern Med.* 2009;*150*(9):604–612. doi:10.7326/0003-4819-150-9-200905050-00006

64. Levey AS, Coresh J, Greene T, et al. Expressing the Modification of Diet in Renal Disease Study Equation for Estimating Glomerular Filtration Rate with Standardized Serum Creatinine Values. *Clinical Chemistry.* 2007;*53*(4):766–772. doi:10.1373/clinchem.2006.077180

65. Shlipak MG, Matsushita K, Ärnlöv J, et al. Cystatin C versus Creatinine in Determining Risk Based on Kidney Function. *N Engl J Med.* 2013;*369*(10):932–943. doi:10.1056/NEJMoa1214234

66. Inker LA, Eneanya ND, Coresh J, et al. New Creatinine- and Cystatin C–Based Equations to Estimate GFR without Race. *N Engl J Med.* 2021;*385*(19):1737–1749. doi:10.1056/NEJMoa2102953

67. Inker LA, Schmid CH, Tighiouart H, et al. Estimating Glomerular Filtration Rate from Serum Creatinine and Cystatin C. *N Engl J Med.* 2012;*367*(1):20–29. doi:10.1056/NEJMoa1114248

68. Matzke GR, Aronoff GR, Atkinson AJ, et al. Drug dosing consideration in patients with acute and chronic kidney disease-a clinical update from Kidney Disease: Improving Global Outcomes (KDIGO). *Kidney Int.* 2011;*80*(11):1122–1137. doi:10.1038/ki.2011.322

69. FDA. Pharmacokinetics in Patients with Impaired Renal Function- Study Design, Data Analysis, and Impact on Dosing.

70. Whelton A. Nephrotoxicity of nonsteroidal anti-inflammatory drugs: physiologic foundations and clinical implications. *The American Journal of Medicine.* 1999;*106*(5):13S–24S. doi:10.1016/S0002-9343(99)00113-8

71. Nelson DA, Marks ES, Deuster PA, O'Connor FG, Kurina LM. Association of Nonsteroidal Anti-inflammatory Drug Prescriptions With Kidney Disease Among Active Young and Middle-aged Adults. *JAMA Netw Open.* 2019;*2*(2):e187896. doi:10.1001/jamanetworkopen.2018.7896

72. Dixit M, Doan T, Kirschner R, Dixit N. Significant Acute Kidney Injury Due to Non-steroidal Anti-inflammatory Drugs: Inpatient Setting. *Pharmaceuticals (Basel).* 2010;*3*(4):1279–1285. doi:10.3390/ph3041279

73. Baker M, Perazella MA. NSAIDs in CKD: Are They Safe? *American Journal of Kidney Diseases.* 2020;*76*(4):546–557. doi:10.1053/j.ajkd.2020.03.023

74. Wei L, MacDonald TM, Jennings C, Sheng X, Flynn RW, Murphy MJ. Estimated GFR reporting is associated with decreased nonsteroidal anti-inflammatory drug prescribing and increased renal function. *Kidney International.* 2013;*84*(1):174–178. doi:10.1038/ki.2013.76

75. Lapi F, Azoulay L, Yin H, Nessim SJ, Suissa S. Concurrent use of diuretics, angiotensin converting enzyme inhibitors, and angiotensin receptor blockers with non-steroidal anti-inflammatory drugs and risk of acute kidney injury: nested case-control study. *BMJ.* 2013;*346*(12 Jan 08):e8525–e8525. doi:10.1136/bmj.e8525

76. Varga Z, Sabzwari SRA, Vargova V. Cardiovascular Risk of Nonsteroidal Anti-Inflammatory Drugs: An Under-Recognized Public Health Issue. *Cureus.* 2017;*9*(4):e1144. doi:10.7759/cureus.1144

77. Taubert KA. Can Patients With Cardiovascular Disease Take Nonsteroidal Antiinflammatory Drugs? *Circulation.* 2008;*117*(17). doi:10.1161/CIRCULATIONAHA.107.749135

78. Goldstein JL, Cryer B. Gastrointestinal injury associated with NSAID use: a case study and review of risk factors and preventative strategies. *Drug Healthc Patient Saf.* 2015;*7*:31–41. doi:10.2147/DHPS.S71976

79. Wongrakpanich S, Wongrakpanich A, Melhado K, Rangaswami J. A Comprehensive Review of Non-Steroidal Anti-Inflammatory Drug Use in The Elderly. *Aging and disease.* 2018;*9*(1):143. doi:10.14336/AD.2017.0306

80. American Geriatrics Society 2015 Beers Criteria Update Expert Panel. American Geriatrics Society 2015 updated beers criteria for potentially inappropriate medication use in older adults. *J American Geriatrics Society.* 2015;*63*(11):2227–2246. doi:10.1111/jgs.13702

81. Schjerning Olsen AM, Gislason GH, McGettigan P, et al. Association of NSAID Use With Risk of Bleeding and Cardiovascular Events in Patients Receiving Antithrombotic Therapy After Myocardial Infarction. *JAMA.* 2015;*313*(8):805. doi:10.1001/jama.2015.0809

82. Narum S, Westergren T, Klemp M. Corticosteroids and risk of gastrointestinal bleeding: a systematic review and meta-analysis. *BMJ Open.* 2014;*4*(5):e0d04587. doi:10.1136/bmjopen-2013-004587

83. Paternoster M, Steichen O, Lapeyre-Mestre M, et al. Risk of Bleeding Associated With Nonsteroidal Anti-inflammatory Drug Use in Patients Exposed to Antithrombotic Therapy: A Case-Crossover Study. *The Journal of Clinical Pharma.* 2022;*62*(5):636–645. doi:10.1002/jcph.2003

84. Uptodate. www.uptodate.com

Neurologic Comorbidities in Patients with Headache Disorders

13

Liza Smirnoff, Jocelyn Jiao, Lisa Surowiec, Yensea M. Costas Encarnación, Nina Massad, and Leticia Tornes

---

LEARNING OBJECTIVES

1. Identify neurological comorbidities that may impact the treatment of headache disorders such as stroke, multiple sclerosis, epilepsy, movement disorders, and other neurological disorders
2. Understand when headaches may be a presenting feature of other neurologic conditions
3. Understand treatment paradigms that can serve as concomitant treatment of headache disorders and comorbid neurologic conditions

---

STROKE AND MIGRAINE MANAGEMENT

Introduction

Stroke is a known possible complication of migraine, with studies reporting a two- to threefold increase in ischemic stroke risk and a 50% increased risk of hemorrhagic stroke in migraine patients, with higher numbers of ischemic stroke seen in women with migraine with aura [1, 2]. Active migraine and increased

DOI: 10.1201/b23330-13

attack frequency increase the risk of ischemic stroke [3]. Migraine with aura is an important stroke risk factor for women younger than 45, active smokers, and those who use oral contraceptives containing estrogen [4–6]. Migrainous infarction is a rare complication of prolonged aura lasting more than 60 minutes in patients with migraine with aura, accounting for 0.2%–0.5% of all ischemic strokes [7]. During the migraine aura, the brain undergoes cortical spreading depression (the electrophysiologic aspect of the migraine), which can cause severe hypoperfusion with correlated lesions on brain imaging [8]. The majority, 65%–82%, of migraine infarctions are located in the posterior circulation, mostly in the cerebellum, where typical aura symptoms initiate [9]. Migraine with aura is associated with traditionally known stroke risk factors, including hypertension, hyperlipidemia, diabetes mellitus, cigarette smoking, atrial fibrillation, and patent foramen ovale [10].

Given the known increased risk of stroke in migraine patients, as well as coexisting stroke and migraine, we may see patients in our poststroke clinic for concurrent migraine management [11]. In addition, poststroke patients may have worsening of migraines and limited treatment options given the risk factors associated with common medications for migraine.

Pathophysiology

Multiple mechanisms have been attributed to the complex association between stroke and migraine. Some implicate the central nervous system, while others involve the vasculature (vasospasm, arterial dissection, endothelial dysfunction, venous thrombosis), heart (patent foramen ovale), and blood (hypercoagulability). Cortical spreading depression (CSD) is the electrophysiological phenomenon occurring in migraine with aura and consists of a self-propagating, short-lasting depolarization wave that traverses the cortex from the posterior cortices anteriorly [12]. This process leads to an initial increase in blood flow (hyperemia) accompanied by hypoperfusion (oligemia), and that can potentially lead to an ischemic event if prolonged [13]. CSD spreads at a rate of 3–5 mm/min and is associated with toxic alterations in transmembrane ion gradients, including influx of sodium, calcium, and efflux of potassium, protons, glutamate, adenosine triphosphate (ATP), as well as neurotransmitters and other substances with vasoactive and inflammatory properties that are thought to propagate the wave contiguously by affecting adjacent cells [14]. Biomarkers of endothelial dysfunction, particularly von Willebrand and other cytokines are elevated in migraine patients, particularly during the aura phase [15]. Furthermore, persons with migraine, in comparison to controls, have a higher percentage of patent foramen ovale (PFO). In one study, PFO was found in 33/61 (54%) patients with migraine with aura compared to 15/60 (25%) migraine without aura and 16/65 (25%) control subjects [16]. These mechanisms suggest some common mechanisms between stroke and migraine.

MRI changes

White matter hyperintensities (WMHs) are MRI T2 flair hyperintensities that are commonly thought to be nonspecific but occur commonly in people with migraine. WMHs are present in 43.1% of migraine patients [17]. The CAMERA study findings strongly suggest that patients affected by migraine are independently at increased risk for subclinical brain lesions, and the association between migraine and subclinical infarctions was independent of cardiovascular risk factors and was significant in the subgroup with migraine without aura [9]. WMHs are typically located in the periventricular areas or within the deep white matter and mainly distributed in the frontal lobe (30 patients, 78.9%), limbic system (23 patients, 60.5%), and parietal lobe (11 patients, 28.9%) [9, 18]. A meta-analysis showed that the risk of WMHs in patients with migraine with aura was nearly twice of that of persons in the healthy control group [19]. WMHs being associated with low, rather than high, intracranial artery resistance suggests that WMH formation in migraine patients may have a distinct pathophysiology relative to that in small vessel diseases [20].

Previously, there was no direct evidence to support that prophylactic migraine treatment would reduce future stroke risk [21]. However, certain risk factors are associated with WMH and migraine, including older age, longer disease duration, frequent attacks, and high serum homocysteine level [22]. In individuals of older age with vascular risk factors and migraines, studies found that migraine lesions were typically in lobar regions and were more commonly under 3 mm in diameter. Periventricular WMHs were uncommon, as were basal ganglia and infratentorial WMHs, especially in the absence of frontal WMHs [23]. These characteristics may be helpful in differentiating MRI findings from migraine vs. other vascular risk factors. There are proposed etiologic mechanisms underlying WMLs that include ischemic microvascular disturbances with subsequent focal hypoperfusion of the cerebral parenchyma (seen with decreased cerebral perfusion in migraine attacks). This further impairs clearance of embolic particles as well as increased levels of vasoconstrictive neurotransmitters at particularly vulnerable to hypoperfusion-related border zone ischemic lesion formation, which are typical sites for WMH in migraines [24]. The data is not clear on whether treating these lesions with secondary stroke prevention is necessary at this time.

Therapy

According to predefined criteria, stroke-attributed headache was reported in 7.2% (16/222) of patients, with tension-type-like headache in 50.0%, migraine-like in 31.3%, and medication overuse in 6.25% of patients [25]. More than half of patients experienced moderate to severe pain [25]. Furthermore, after an ischemic stroke, the treatment options for migraine reduce due to the concern for vasoconstrictive effects. For acute migraine attacks, nonvasoconstrictive agents are typically used, such as acetylsalicylic acid and nonsteroidal anti-inflammatory drugs. Lasmiditan (a selective 5–HT_{1F} receptor agonist) has no vasoconstrictive properties and can therefore be used for the treatment of acute migraine attacks in patients with a recent history of TIA or stroke [26].

Calcitonin gene-related peptide (CGRP) is involved in nociception and neurogenic inflammation in migraine and is a strong vasodilator. Monoclonal antibodies (CGRP mAbs) that bind to the CGRP ligand or the receptor, as well as oral medications and nasal sprays that directly block the receptor (gepants) have been used for preventative as well as abortive treatments. There are no clinical trials that have shown that CGRP inhibitors are associated with ischemic stroke; however, there have been case reports of ischemic stroke associated with these medications. There is one case reported of a patient with a posterior circulation ischemic stroke 34 days after the initiation of erenumab; however, the patient had other risk factors and was simultaneously using a triptan [27]. Given the known vasoactive properties of CGRP and animal studies showing delayed wound healing, there is concern (particularly for the monoclonal antibodies) that they may worsen recovery in patients immediately poststroke and may cause uncontrolled hypertension, potentially leading to vascular events [28]. At this time, the risk remains largely theoretical but should be considered particularly for patients with high stroke risk, or immediately poststroke being considered particularly for therapy with erenumab given the reported case and preferential binding to the CGRP receptor versus other CGRP therapies binding to the ligand.

Use of migraine prophylactic agents such as beta-blockers, calcium channel blockers, antiepileptics, antidepressants, and nutraceuticals for persistent poststroke headache with migrainous features may be warranted but should take stroke mechanism and comorbidities into account [29]. Beta-blockers and calcium channel blockers can be used and can improve comorbid hypertension. Selective serotonin reuptake inhibitors (SSRIs) in poststroke patients have been found to be effective in treating depression and improving anxiety, motor function, cognitive function, and independence [30]. Serotonin norepinephrine reuptake inhibitors (SNRIs), specifically duloxetine, have been shown to reduce poststroke depression [31]. In chronic migraine, onabotulinumtoxinA can be safely used. As part of secondary stroke prevention, the daily dose of acetylsalicylic acid can be increased from 81 to 300 or 325 mg for migraine prophylaxis [32]. An important consideration is that some secondary stroke prevention medications have been shown to cause migraine-type headaches. The antiplatelet, cilostazol, a drug that inhibits phosphodiesterase three and has vasodilatory activity, has been shown to cause bilateral pulsatile headaches in healthy individuals, as well as trigger typical headache features in persons with migraine [33].

As discussed previously, migraines have been associated with PFO and one proposed underlying mechanism of WMH has been associated with reduced clearance of micro-emboli, therefore leading to an ongoing debate on whether these patients should have PFO closure. The MIST trial did not achieve the primary efficacy endpoint of cessation of headache attacks during three or six months after the PFO closure [34]. In the PREMIUM trial, there was no difference in responder rate (defined as 50% reduction in migraine attacks and adverse events) between the PFO closure group and controls [35]. At this time, the decision of PFO closure should be based on stroke prevention and not on potential beneficial effects on migraine [36].

CADASIL, arteriopathies and migraine

Cerebral autosomal dominant arteriopathy with subcortical infarcts and leukoencephalopathy (CADASIL) is an inherited disease of the small blood vessels characterized by recurrent ischemic strokes, progressive cognitive decline, and psychiatric manifestations. Of note, 50%–75% of patients with CADASIL experience migraine. For many, migraine and, more commonly, migraine with aura is the presenting feature of CADASIL [37–39]. CADASIL is characterized by early onset of ischemic strokes: variable white matter lesions on MRI that, with time, become bilateral and confluent. In suspected patients, genetic testing for the NOTCH3 (*Notch homolog 3*) gene and a thorough review of family history are recommended.

When considering migraine management in patients with known CADASIL or similar arteriopathies, we must consider similar factors in treating other poststroke patients, as well as some special considerations. In terms of abortive options for migraine, although clinical evidence of stroke post triptan use has not been seen, given the small numbers of studies and small numbers of patients with CADASIL, they are relatively contraindicated given known small risk of stroke in migraine patients using triptans [40, 41]. Nonsteroidal anti-inflammatory drugs (NSAIDs), acetaminophen, and lasmiditan are safe considerations given lack of association with stroke risk.

Although one recent study did not find interictal serum CGRP differences in CADASIL patients with and without migraine [42], others have suggested potential stroke risk with CGRP blocking agents given the role of CGRP in maintaining cardiovascular hemostasis [37]. This data notably does not differentiate between monoclonal antibody therapies against CGRP and direct receptor blockers (gepants), and further data is needed on the safety of gepants and stroke risk. Therefore, given significant stroke risk in CADASIL patients and limited data, we recommend using alternative therapies for migraine management in patients with known CADASIL or other arteriopathies, including acetazolamide, sodium valproate, lamotrigine, topiramate, beta-blockers, calcium channel blockers, tricyclic antidepressants (TCAs), SNRIs and onabotulinumtoxinA, which have all been shown to have good long-term safety data in terms of stroke risk [37, 43].

Special considerations for procedure planning in postsurgical patients

In certain patients with diseases such as moyamoya vasculopathy who have undergone multiple craniotomies, special planning is required when using onabotulinumtoxinA or nerve blocks for the management of their migraines. The PHASE III Research Evaluating Migraine Prophylaxis Therapy (PREEMPT) protocol may not be appropriate in these patients given the disruption of multiple muscle groups by prior surgery [41]. In patients with prior suboccipital craniotomies without bone replacement, we recommend omitting the paraspinal injections. The authors recommend planning onabotulinumtoxinA therapy in these patients depending on the surgical sites with the goal to match PREEMPT dosing per muscle, with avoidance of any areas where bone has not been replaced [44]. For example, for a more complex postsurgical site, such as after a subtemporal craniotomy, the authors recommend placing one injection anterior to the first scar line, two between the two scar lines, and one posteriorly (Figure 13.1).

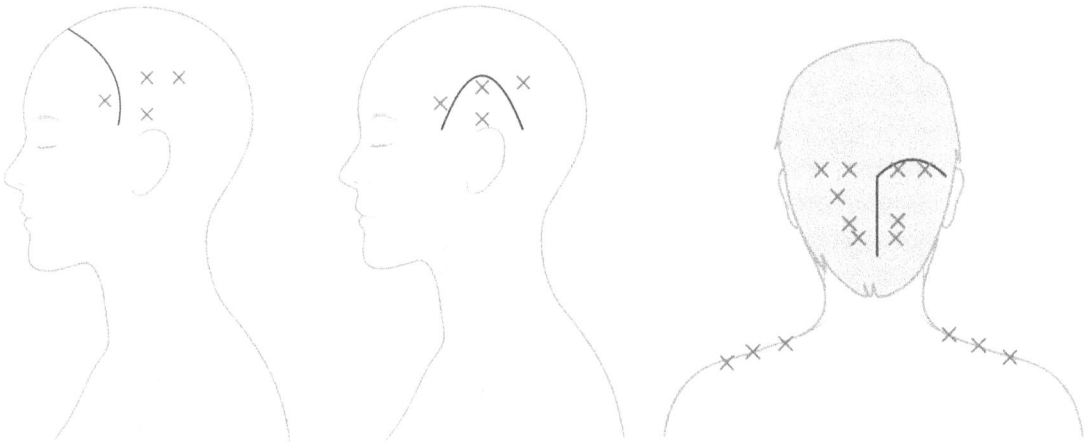

FIGURE 13.1   Recommended location of onabotulinumtoxinA injections (X) based on location of prior surgical scars. Recommended avoiding injecting onabotulinumtoxinA into scar lines and in areas where the patient has not had replacement of skull tissue (Image constructed in Bioender.com).

Likewise, occipital nerve blocks should only be considered with ultrasound guidance by a trained provider in patients with known posterior fossa bone defects given the risk of subarachnoid injection [45].

Neuroimmunology

Epidemiology of multiple sclerosis

Multiple sclerosis (MS) is a chronic, inflammatory, neurodegenerative disorder of the central nervous system that may cause a variety of symptoms ranging from cognitive, visual, motor, sensory, fatigue, and pain. There is an association between MS and headaches, particularly migraines; however, the etiology and clinical implications of this association remain poorly understood. The headache disorder may frequently predate MS disease onset but can also be seen during an MS relapse or throughout the disease course. Both MS and migraine individually have clinical and social impacts that may significantly burden the patient's quality of life and, when they exist comorbidly, increase disability further. It will be important to identify the exact pathogenesis of the MS and migraine association to determine if migraine is a risk factor, comorbidity, symptom, or an independent process.

Studies have consistently shown a heightened prevalence of migraines in MS patients compared to the general population. For instance, a systematic review reported migraine prevalence rates in MS patients between 20% and 45% [46]. A meta-analysis from 2023 involving over 250,000 MS patients found that the prevalence of migraine was 24%, with a nearly twofold increase in odds compared to healthy individuals [47].

Neurobiology of MS in migraines

There have been several hypotheses regarding the pathophysiology underlying migraine in MS patients. One theory is the disruption of migraine-associated pathways by the inflammatory demyelinating lesions [48]. This theory is supported by several case reports of patients with new onset migraine, cluster headache, and occipital neuralgia emerging concurrently with brainstem or upper cervical MS lesions [48]. Furthermore, retrospective studies indicate a fourfold increase in migraine in patients with brainstem lesions compared to those MS patients without brainstem lesions [49, 50].

Conversely, migraine may predispose one to MS. One theory suggests that permeability in the blood–brain barrier (BBB) causes exposure of circulating T cells to CNS antigens that may contribute to their sensitization of myelin [51]. Migraine involves activation of matrix metalloproteins, leading to the increase in permeability of the BBB and may favor an inflammatory cytokine profile in a way that can predispose to autoimmune reaction in CNS. Lastly, IL-10 and TNF-alpha have been overexpressed in both migraines and MS relapses [51].

Diagnostic challenges

It may be challenging to differentiate between an MS relapse and migraine aura. To diagnose MS, the McDonald criteria uses clinical and radiologic findings to meet diagnostic criteria [52]. As we currently have no biomarkers to diagnose MS, a detailed history and neurologic examination, as well as a review of MRI findings, is critical to ensure proper diagnosis. A 2016 review of 110 cases found that about 22% of cases initially diagnosed as MS were later determined to be migraine [53]. The main reasons for the misdiagnosis were using the migraine aura as a clinical event and using nonspecific T2 hyperintensities to count as brain MS lesions [53].

The clinical events for migraine and MS differ mostly in timing; migraine aura is typically minutes to hours, whereas MS clinical events can last days to weeks. Radiographically, MS lesions are ovoid, periventricular, juxtacortical, and infratentorial, and they can be enhancing. Migraine MRI lesions as nonspecific in subcortical areas, not periventricular, and nonenhancing. Spinal imaging can be helpful, as MS patients may have spinal cord involvement, whereas migraine patients do not. Findings on neurologic examination such as abnormal eye movements, increased tone, asymmetric reflexes, or positive Babinski sign can also help with MS diagnosis, as migraine patients should have a normal neurologic exam.

Migraine treatment

As in all patients with neurologic conditions, appropriate counseling on conservative measures should be provided. Counseling on proper hydration with electrolytes, especially if out in the heat or after intense exercise; proper nutrition; regular meals; consistent caffeine intake; exercise; and proper sleep should be addressed. If a patient snores or has other sleep-related comorbidities, such as insomnia or nocturia, those should be addressed to avoid headache exacerbations. Dietary supplements such as magnesium and riboflavin can be considered in those patients who have no contraindications (avoid magnesium in myasthenia gravis). Food and Drug Administration–approved noninvasive neuromodulation devices for preventive and acute treatment of migraine can be considered, especially in patients with polypharmacy, to avoid the addition of further medications [54]. In the appropriate patients, acupuncture can also be used as there is evidence that it can be used to decrease frequency of tension headaches and migraine [55]. In patients who do not have improvement with the above measures, preventive medication may be required to prevent headaches. The individual patient's needs, comorbid conditions, and current medications should all be considered when selecting the appropriate class of medication. In patients with hypertension, blood pressure medications can be considered; in those with neuropathic pain or mood disorders, antiseizure or antidepressants may be best. In general, these medication classes are safe to use with the MS disease-modifying therapies (DMTs). OnabotulinumtoxinA (onabotA) is safe and commonly used in patients with MS to treat chronic migraine, overactive bladder, and spasticity [56]. One area that has not been studied are the new CGRP mAbs and gepants in patients on monoclonal DMTs. However, there is no data at the present time suggesting they should not be used in MS patients on DMTs.

Trigeminal neuralgia

Secondary trigeminal neuralgia (TN) is common in MS. Patients with MS have a 20-fold increased risk of TN; the general population has a prevalence of 0.16%–0.3%, while MS patients can have up to 4% [57, 58].

Data from the North American Research Committee on MS found that 9.5% of MS patients had an episode of TN during their MS course [57]. The study also found that a TN diagnosis predated the MS diagnoses in 15% of cases [57]. In general, TN can be difficult to treat and debilitating. Traditional medications used to treat primary TN and neuropathic pain are used. Surgical methods are less effective in TN from MS and should be reserved for refractory cases [58].

Conclusions

Migraine, tension headache, and TN are more common in MS patients than in the general population. In some studies, migraines can predate the MS diagnosis, and there are theories as to the pathophysiology of their bidirectional relationship. In general, conservative measures should be used as first line to avoid polypharmacy. In patients who require acute medications, consider a medication that would treat other conditions the MS patient may have.

Special Considerations for the Movement Disorders Patient

Within neurology practices, movement disorders are known to commonly co-occur with headache. One study showed a correlation between essential tremor and migraine, with 36% of patients with ET with comorbid migraine versus 18% in controls [59]. Another study reported 49% of patients with Parkinson's disease had headache, with 17% specifically reporting migraine [60]. Several considerations should guide the selection of agents in the treatment of primary headache for people living with movement disorders. Particularly, agents utilized in the acute and preventive treatment of migraine can ameliorate, precipitate, and exacerbate abnormal movements. These considerations can be approached by moving through the classes of abnormal movements.

Tremor

Tremor is characterized by the involuntary rhythmic oscillation of a part of the body around one or more joints [61]. Numerous medications can precipitate, exacerbate, and ameliorate tremor. Beta-blockers are considered a first-line therapy option for the treatment of essential tremor, the most common adult movement disorder, which primarily manifests with postural and kinetic tremor of the limbs, head, voice, and sometimes trunk [62]. Propranolol reduces limb tremor (level A evidence) and, to a more modest degree, reduces head tremor, while atenolol, sotalol, and topiramate can also reduce limb tremor (level B evidence) [63]. Therefore, for patients with migraine and essential tremor, it would be reasonable to trial propranolol as a first-line therapy before moving onto topiramate, which is also used in the treatment of essential tremor as a second-line agent [64].

Numerous centrally acting medications are associated with medication-induced tremor. Medication-induced tremor is more commonly postural and kinetic, though certain medications (valproic acid [VPA], dopamine blocking agents, lithium) are associated with rest tremor as well. Lithium-induced tremor is one of the most commonly encountered medication-induced tremors in practice, affecting 27% of pooled patients in one review [65]. One meta-analysis noted an overall incidence of 14% of tremor in patients receiving valproic acid therapy. Doses <1,500 mg/daily of VPA and a VPA treatment duration <12 months led to a higher risk of tremor compared to other drugs, as did higher doses and longer treatment times [66]. TCAs and SNRIs (such as duloxetine or venlafaxine) have also all been associated with medication-induced tremor [67–69]. Lamotrigine use has also been associated with the development of tremor (affecting up to 4% of patients [70]), as well as other abnormal movements, including tics, myoclonus, and chorea [71]. Meanwhile, beta-blockers can be utilized in the treatment of medication-induced tremor for patients in whom these medications are the most effective treatment option for primary headache disorders, particularly in those with trigeminal autonomic cephalalgias.

Parkinsonism

Parkinsonism is a hypokinetic movement disorder characterized by rigidity, bradykinesia, and, at times, tremor caused by functionally impaired dopaminergic circuits in the brain. It is a prominent feature of idiopathic Parkinson's disease, the second-most common neurodegenerative condition in the United States. Parkinsonism is also a feature of other less common parkinsonian disorders: progressive supranuclear palsy, multiple systems atrophy, dementia with Lewy bodies, and vascular parkinsonism.

Prochlorperazine and metoclopramide are both commonly used acute headache medications with dopaminergic-blocking properties. As they can worsen parkinsonian symptoms, they and other dopaminergic-blocking medications (such as first-generation antipsychotics) should be particularly avoided in idiopathic Parkinson's disease and other parkinsonian disorders. Additionally, several studies since the 1970s have noted an association between the use of valproic acid and the development of drug-induced parkinsonism, which typically presents as a symmetric akinetic-rigid syndrome with postural, action, and rest tremor [72].

Steroids, which can be used in short courses for status migrainosus, should also be considered carefully in patients with parkinsonism, as many of the parkinsonian disorders are associated with mild to severe cognitive impairment; a short course of steroids in these cognitively vulnerable individuals can precipitate insomnia, disturbed sleep-wake cycles, and delirium. Acute options for patients with parkinsonism should therefore be limited to those categories that are less likely to precipitate delirium and/or exacerbate a hypodopaminergic state: triptans, anti-CGRP medications, lasmiditan, dihydroergotamine, and NSAIDs. Specifically, NSAIDs as a category can be considered concomitantly as abortive agents in treating headache and musculoskeletal pain, which is the most common type of pain affecting people living with Parkinson's disease [73].

Headache Disorders in Patients with Epilepsy

More than 45 million people throughout the world have active epilepsy. The lifetime prevalence of headache disorders is 52% greater in people with epilepsy than in the general population. The most common headache type is tension headache, followed by migraine. Therefore, regular screening for headache in this population should be performed, as they are often underreported, despite migraine leading to notable disability in patients during their most productive years [74, 75]. Here we will focus on headache disorders co-occurring with epilepsy and special considerations for treatment strategies, antiseizure medications (ASMs), side effects, and contraindications [76, 77].

When the clinician begins their assessment of headache in epilepsy patients, it is important to understand the distinction between headaches that coexist with epilepsy versus headaches with a special correlation to the ictus. Headaches that temporally correlate to the ictus are classified as pre-ictal, ictal, or post-ictal headaches. Post-ictal headaches are most common, occurring in 15%–65% of patients, while pre-ictal and ictal headaches are relatively rare, with pre-ictal headaches occurring in 4%–26% of patients [74, 78, 79].

A critical next step is assessing whether ASMs are contributing to or causing the headaches. A thorough medication review is highly valuable, as this may reveal a drug-induced headache, medication interaction, or medications with similar mechanisms of actions, which may lead to potentiation of side effects. Headache is one of the most frequent and nonspecific side effects of ASMs. For example, 14% of patients in the initial levetiracetam studies reported headache as a side effect [80]. Conversely, some ASMs can be helpful in certain pain conditions, such as the use of carbamazepine and oxcarbazepine in TN. ASMs are also used for prevention of chronic migraine. Among them, valproate and topiramate have FDA approval for migraine prophylaxis with level A evidence. As with any migraine prophylaxis agent, ASMs should be chosen based on level of evidence, comorbidities, and with special precautions in mind.

Antiseizure medications for chronic migraine prevention

Both valproate (or divalproex sodium) and topiramate are well-known broad-spectrum agents approved for many seizure types due to their multimodal mechanisms of actions, which include but are not limited to, GABA potentiation, voltage-gated sodium channel modulation/blockage, and reduction in the excitatory neurotransmitters such as glutamate. Unique to valproate is the modulation of dopaminergic and serotonergic transmission. Valproate also reduces the action of CGRP [78, 81].

Topiramate offers a uniquely treatment-favorable profile for headache secondary to idiopathic intracranial hypertension (IIH, formerly known as pseudotumor cerebri) [82]. It is a weak carbonic anhydrase isoenzyme inhibitor, an enzyme found in multiple organs, but specifically within the renal tubular system and the central nervous system. Inhibition of carbonic anhydrase leads to a diuretic effect and to decreased production of cerebrospinal fluid (CSF) within the choroid plexus, therefore providing modest therapeutic benefit to patients suffering from IIH. An additional beneficial side effect is weight loss, which at times can lead to remission of IIH [83].

Drug-Drug interactions

Both valproate and topiramate have important medication interactions to consider.

The combination of valproate and topiramate can potentially lead to severe hyperammonemia, even in patients without previous liver dysfunction [79]. Valproate is a CYP450 enzyme and UDP-glucuronosyltransferases (UGTs) inhibitor, so drug-drug interactions must be considered. One example is the need to immediately reduce the dose of lamotrigine by 50% once starting valproate due to inhibition of UGTs, doubling the half-life of lamotrigine, which may precipitate toxicity [79, 81].

Similarly, care must be taken when adding topiramate to a patient already on carbamazepine or phenytoin, as these drugs double the clearance of topiramate and decrease its half-life by half, requiring careful dose adjustments, particularly in patients with known epilepsy [84]. The use of topiramate in combination with other diuretics can lead to an increased risk of renal stone formation and metabolic alkalosis given the same carbonic anhydrase inhibition previously discussed [81, 83, 84].

Special consideration in women of childbearing age and pregnancy

Antiseizure medications used both for epilepsy and headache management hold teratogenic risk that should be discussed in this patient population, even if patients do not desire to become pregnant during the initial discussion. Valproate is considered unsafe in pregnancy, given its well-studied association with neural tube defects and long-term cognitive problems in children. Topiramate is also considered unsafe in pregnancy due to its association with cleft lip and cleft palate malformations. Therefore, a discussion on the need for contraception and teratogenic risk should be held. Of importance, doses of 200 mg/day or greater of topiramate can lead to contraceptive failure, specifically in oral contraceptive agents involving estrogen and progestin [84, 85].

Trigeminal neuralgia and antiseizure medications

TN is a disorder of recurrent, stimulus-elicited, unilateral, brief electrical shock-like pain within the trigeminal nerve distribution [86]. Sodium channel blockers, particularly carbamazepine (800–1,200 mg/d) and oxcarbazepine (600 mg–1,800 mg/d) in divided doses, are considered first-line therapy in preventative treatment of this disorder [87, 88].

In patients who have exhibited significant relief with carbamazepine or oxcarbazepine but are limited by undesirable side effects (dizziness, hyponatremia, somnolence), consideration should be given to eslicarbazepine. This medication offers more selective interaction with the inactive state of voltage-gated sodium channels in combination with single daily dosing and overall better tolerance [89]. In refractory cases, second-line prophylactic agents may include other antiepileptic medications such as lamotrigine, gabapentin, and phenytoin [82, 87, 88, 90].

While acute preventative treatment is of main importance, patients may present with acute exacerbation of excruciating pain, which, depending on the affected trigeminal dermatomes, may prevent them from even being able to ingest their medications [91].

While no large-scale randomized controlled trial (RCT) has been performed using these medications, there have been retrospective studies that have investigated the response of intravenous lacosamide and phenytoin with a positive response. One such study by Pinto et al. compared IV lacosamide (average dose of 200 mg) to IV phenytoin (average dose of 744 mg), showing higher responder rate among the lacosamide group, as well as less overall readmission and reported side effects [92].

Special considerations in the epilepsy patient

We will shift focus to special considerations in specific epilepsy syndromes or types. Until the epileptic syndrome has been properly classified, we recommend broad-spectrum agents as narrow-spectrum agents can potentially worsen or precipitate seizures in patients with generalized epilepsies—for example, juvenile absence epilepsies, juvenile myoclonic epilepsies, or generalized tonic-clonic epilepsy [85]. Furthermore, in patients with myoclonic seizures, such as juvenile myoclonic epilepsy or Lennox-Gastaut syndrome, ASMs with sodium channel blocker mechanisms (e.g., carbamazepine, oxcarbazepine, lamotrigine) can lead to worsening of myoclonic seizures. In patients with Dravet syndrome in which there is an underlying channelopathy, sodium channel blockade can also precipitate seizures [93].

Other special considerations include the mitochondrial epilepsies, particularly myoclonic epilepsy with ragged-red fibers (MERFF). MERFF is the only progressive myoclonic epilepsy in which valproate is strictly contraindicated, as it may precipitate liver failure. ASMs of choice within this epilepsy syndrome include levetiracetam, topiramate, clobazam, zonisamide, and potentially lamotrigine (keeping in mind that if the mitochondrial syndrome features myoclonic seizures, these may worsen) [94].

Neurocritical Care

Headache commonly occurs in the neuroscience critical care unit (NSICU) with a variety of underlying causes. While primary headache in the NSICU is typically less common, it may occasionally warrant ICU admission in select cases for specialized therapies such as continuous ketamine or lidocaine infusion in some centers for refractory cases. Much more commonly, secondary headaches, as classified by the *International Classification of Headache Disorders, 3rd Edition (ICHD-3)*, are seen [8]. Development or worsening of headache in the NSICU can also signal a change requiring urgent evaluation and treatment.

A comprehensive assessment of the headache should include relevant history and details regarding severity, onset, and quality. Concurrent symptoms such as nausea, vomiting, change in level of alertness or any focal neurologic deficit should raise concern. Context is especially important, as the patient's presenting pathology, procedural or surgical course in the hospital can contribute heavily to the development of headache.

Regarding common headache presentations for NSICU patients, the *thunderclap* headache is often invoked in several serious neurologic emergencies including aneurysmal subarachnoid hemorrhage, venous sinus thrombosis, vasculopathies such as reversal cerebral vasoconstriction syndrome (RCVS), and dissection. Thunderclap headaches typically present with a sudden onset of a maximally severe holocephalic pain that can persist for minutes to days, depending on underlying etiology, and can wax and wane.

Subarachnoid hemorrhage

The initial presentation of subarachnoid hemorrhage (SAH) is often characterized by an excruciating maximally severe headache commonly described as "the worst headache of my life." The onset of pain is abrupt, correlating with initial aneurysmal rupture, and can persist for at least a week to several weeks following initial presentation. Less commonly, patients can present with sentinel headache preceding a major hemorrhagic event, typically signaling aneurysmal wall changes leading to leakage or minor bleeding.

The contributors to headache in SAH are multifactorial: presence of blood in the subarachnoid space leading to chemical and mechanical irritation of the meninges, involvement of the trigemino-vascular system, complications such as vasospasm, and, finally, interventions (both surgical and endovascular) that may contribute to headache [95]. Headache is a major treatment concern for ICU patients admitted with SAH. Most commonly, acetaminophen is first line based on surveying providers, followed by opioids as the second-most used medication. Both antiseizure medication and corticosteroids are also used, along with gabapentin in a combination approach; nonsteroidal anti-inflammatory drugs are seldom used due to safety concerns about bleeding risk, although there is limited evidence for this [96, 97]. Although opioids continue to be used frequently, recent efforts have been made to introduce an opioid-sparing approach and other novel options for pain management, such as occipital and supraorbital peripheral nerve blocks, as well as sphenopalatine ganglion block [98, 99].

Vasculopathies, vascular malformations and headache

A common disease entity presenting with headache is RCVS, a condition involving reversible multifocal narrowing of cerebral arteries. Typically, patients present with a severe thunderclap headache, and because of segmental arterial narrowing, patients can additionally exhibit focal neurologic deficits due to complications such as ischemic stroke, cortical subarachnoid hemorrhage, changes related to cerebral edema, and seizure. RCVS is frequently associated with serotonergic medications; discontinuation of these medications along with supportive care is typically the first-line approach, although calcium channel blockers and intraarterial vasodilatory therapy can be used, but evidence is inconsistent for these interventions [95].

While patients with unruptured vascular malformations can develop headache, these typically do not result in presentation to the ICU unless rupture occurs or the patient presents following elective intervention.

Intracranial pressure-related headache

Cerebral venous sinus thromboses frequently present with headache, often thunderclap in quality, that tends to worsen with supine position, Valsalva, or other maneuvers that may increase intracranial pressure [42]. Treatment focuses on management of the underlying process with anticoagulation. Low-pressure headache can also be seen in the NSICU, more commonly following neurosurgical intervention. Transsphenoidal surgery is often a risk factor for the development of CSF leak leading to low-pressure headache, and CSF leak precautions along with close pain monitoring should be done in the days immediately following surgery [100]. Other contributors include post-lumbar puncture or spinal surgery. Spontaneous intracranial hypotension is another low-pressure etiology of headache in the inpatient setting and is typically accompanied by diffuse pachymeningeal enhancement and brain sagging [101]. Treatment initially involves conservative therapy with bed rest, caffeine, and intravenous hydration; however, in cases of refractory pain, epidural blood patches can be considered.

Acute ischemic stroke

Another common cause of secondary headache and under the larger umbrella of vascular etiologies is ischemic stroke or TIA, thought to be related to abrupt changes in both systemic and cerebral pressure. Typically, headache occurs in approximately 30% of patients [95]. Development of new or worsened headache following thrombolytic administration should warrant emergent evaluation with imaging to evaluate for thrombolytic-associated bleeding potentially requiring medication reversal. Additionally, postendovascular therapy headache may be seen; however, a significantly worsened headache may suggest cerebral *hyperperfusion syndrome*. Patients with large ischemic strokes at risk of worsening edema may also develop worsening headache related to inflammation and meningeal irritation. With some strokes presenting with headache as a prominent symptom, initial studies suggest that headache as a presenting symptom may favor improved functional outcomes [102]. Beyond the acute period, a proportion of patients (up to 10% following stroke) develop poststroke headache syndrome, which is often phenotypically like a primary headache disorder, and often requires long-term management and monitoring. A study from Hansen et al. demonstrated that up to 13% of patients with headache in the acute stroke phase had persistent headaches six months following the event [25, 103]. Consideration should be made regarding preventive therapies in these patients, and in situations of comorbid hypertension or cardiac disease, medications that might be beneficial for both, such as beta-blockers, angiotensin receptor blockers, or calcium channel blockers should be considered.

Postoperative pain

Finally, postoperative pain is a common cause of headache in the NSICU. This is typically worse 24 to 48 hours following surgery; however, it can also persist for longer. There is evidence to suggest that a proportion of patients who experience headache after neurosurgical intervention will continue to have headache even a year postoperatively. In the acute time frame, headache in postneurosurgical patients may indicate complications such as infection or ventriculitis in the setting of extraventricular drain, CSF leakage, and pneumocephalus, among other etiologies, and attention should be taken to identify if postoperative pain may indicate an acute change or complication requiring additional treatment. A multimodal opioid-sparing approach to postoperative pain has become more commonly practiced, as this can help reduce opioid side effects and improve pain scores. In addition to acetaminophen, use of gabapentinoids, alpha-2-agonists such as dexmedetomidine, NMDA antagonists such as ketamine and magnesium, and occipital nerve blocks are all becoming popular adjuncts to more traditional postoperative pain management [96, 104].

Neuro-oncology

Headache is rarely a first presenting feature of brain tumors unless complicated by intracranial hypertension. It is important to note that in most patients presenting with symptoms of primary headache, the relative risk of intracranial neoplasm is very low, and the risk only becomes slightly more notable at 0.28% in patients over the age of 50 with undifferentiated headaches. Notably, red flags such as clear worsening with Valsalva, abnormal neurological exam, headache causing arousal from sleep, new headache in an older patient, progressively worsening headaches, or those that are atypical should warrant imaging, especially when concerning features are present in combination [105].

Many patients undergoing or who have undergone therapy for intracranial tumors are referred for headache management. It is important to evaluate for and rule out the possibility of intracranial hypertension, which can be caused by tumor growth or associated edema, chemotherapy, radiation, or associated infections. These patients require therapy for the underlying cause of their headaches, which typically improves headaches as well [106].

In those presenting for headache management after definitive therapy for their cerebral neoplasm, headache care can be determined based on the phenotype of the headache, with many patients presenting with headaches similar to primary headaches. In addition, cutaneous entrapment or damage of peripheral nerves can cause significant pain and headaches in postsurgical patients [107]. These patients may benefit from topical anesthetics, antiseizure medications such as gabapentin and pregabalin, TCAs and SNRIs, muscle relaxants, injections, and, in intractable cases, surgical revision.

A complication of radiation therapy can also be headache, which may present early into radiation therapy or years after as a delayed reaction. In these patients, imaging is important to evaluate for complications such as radiation-related necrosis, and supportive care of headaches are other symptoms [108].

Postradiation SMART syndrome

SMART (stroke-like migraine attacks after radiation therapy) syndrome is a reversible neurological complication that occurs months to years after radiation of brain tumor. Recognition of this syndrome can reduce unneeded and potentially high-risk testing, such has brain biopsy. Modified criteria have been established and include remote history of external beam cranial radiation, prolonged signs and symptoms that may be reversible or persistent and attributable to a unilateral cortical region with (migraine-type headaches with and without aura, seizures, confusion, stroke-like hemiparesis, aphasia), reversible or sustained gyriform enhancement in the irradiated area, and no definitive evidence of residual tumor [109]. Doses higher than 50 Gy of radiation have been found to be associated with SMART syndrome [110]. Currently, there are no clear guidelines on effective approaches to treatment; however, steroid therapy may hasten recovery and improve signal abnormalities on MRI, patients are often times placed on antiseizure medications, especially those that address both the seizure and the comorbid headache (e.g., topiramate and valproate) [111].

OTHER NEUROLOGIC COMORBIDITIES

Idiopathic Intracranial Hypertension

IIH is a disorder of CSF pressure that occurs sporadically, with an annual incidence of 0.9/100,000 persons and 3.5/100,000 in women 15 to 44 years of age and is characterized by increased intracranial pressure without a secondary cause that often occurs in obese women of childbearing age [91, 112]. Additional risk factors can include use of high-dose vitamin A compounds, pregnancy, and use of oral contraceptives. Common symptoms include headache, transient visual obscurations, pulsatile tinnitus, and signs can include papilledema, with or without retinal hemorrhages, folds, cotton wool spots, and exudates, although notably, papilledema is not required for the diagnosis. The modified Dandy criteria can be used for the diagnosis (Table 13.1) [113].

Common radiographic features include empty sella turcica, dilation and tortuosity of the optic nerve sheaths, posterior globe flattening, and, more rarely, enhancing swollen optic discs and acquired cerebellar tonsillar descent. All patients with presumed IIH should have an MR venogram to rule out venous sinus thrombosis, particularly those with rapid or fulminant IIH [114].

If untreated, papilledema can result in progressive and irreversible vision loss with optic atrophy, with visual loss often not evident to the patient due to slow progression in many cases. Therefore, appropriate ophthalmologist evaluation and management is necessary and should be expedited in patients with present papilledema. Additionally, given the known relationship between obesity, weight gain, and IIH, a multimodal approach to weight management should be undertaken, as a reported 15%–24% weight loss will

TABLE 13.1   Modified Dandy criteria for the diagnosis of IIH

1	Awake and alert patient
2	Symptoms and signs of increased intracranial pressure (nausea, vomiting, transient obscurations of vision, papilledema)
3	Absence of focal signs on neurologic examination (although sixth and seventh nerve palsies are permitted)
4	Normal diagnostic studies (i.e., neuroimaging and CSF evaluation), except for evidence of increased intracranial pressure (i.e., a CSF opening pressure greater than 20 cm H_2O with signs of increased intracranial pressure on neuroimaging)
5	No other etiology for increased intracranial pressure identified

cause remission of IIH in obese patients [115]. Multidisciplinary approaches should be undertaken, including nutrition counseling, exercise programs, and often referral to a weight loss center. In some patients, medical or surgical management of obesity may be necessary, with the glucagon-like peptide 1 (GLP-1) agonists, commonly used for weight management now, having a potential additional benefit of reducing CSF secretion in vitro and intracranial pressure (ICP) in rodents [116]. Further studies in humans are necessary to evaluate this additional benefit.

Headache, meanwhile, is the most common symptom, present in 85% of patients in one study [117], and is often worst in the mornings and aggravated by Valsalva-like maneuvers. For many, it can mimic primary headache disorders, so it should be considered in patients with refractory headache disorders not improved with multiple headache therapies. Notably, many patients may not experience headache relief with treatment of ICP, and more so, patients with comorbid migraine or with migraine phenotype are less likely to experience headache relief with management [118]. In the same study headache improved most in those who had 5% or more weight loss, reiterating the importance of weight loss in this population group.

Furthermore, given the unclearly defined etiology, management for IIH is focused on reducing ICP, with the mainstay focused on carbonic anhydrase inhibitors, including acetazolamide and methazolamide. Topiramate, given its weak carbonic anhydrase activity, is also equally effective in mild to moderate IIH and can treat comorbid migraine, so it may be a more appropriate choice in patients with a migrainous phenotype. Other diuretics, such as furosemide, can also be used along or in combination. In those who fail to improve despite maximum medical therapy or are unable to tolerate medications, surgical interventions may be warranted [91]. However, a recent study has also shown erenumab is effective in improving IIH-related head pain, contributing to the thought that head pain in IIH may be CGRP mediated [119]. Additional preventive therapies targeted at the headache phenotype should likewise be utilized to decrease overuse of analgesics in this population, with at least half of IIH patients reporting regular use of analgesics for headache [120]. In some patients whose headaches do not improve with medication, cerebrospinal diversion shunting or cerebral venous sinus stenting may improve headaches.

Restless leg syndrome

Restless leg syndrome (RLS) is a chronic condition, thought to have an autosomal dominant pattern of inheritance, that is characterized by uncomfortable sensations that can feel like crawling or simply restlessness in the legs, paired with an irresistible urge to move [121]. Symptoms can spread to the arms and tend to resolve or improve with activity. Known risk factors include iron and folate deficiencies for which patients should be screened. RLS is known to be comorbid with migraine, occurring at nearly three times higher rates than the general population [122]. While many patients with RLS may benefit from behavioral interventions and vibration therapy, many may still require medication therapy. Common therapies include dopamine agonists such as ropinirole, pramipexole, and rotigotine patches [123].

Notably, TCAs and SNRIs that are commonly used for migraine can worsen or exacerbate symptoms, so use should be limited in patients with significant RLS symptoms. Avoidance of caffeine, nicotine, and alcohol is also recommended. Likewise, consideration should be given to the use of dopamine antagonists for migraine in this patient group, given the likely exacerbation of RLS symptoms with medications such as prochlorperazine, promethazine, and metoclopramide. Meanwhile, medications such as gabapentin and pregabalin, which can be used as second-line agents for RLS may also be used for certain headache disorders that thus could be considered for concomitant treatment [123].

Myasthenia gravis

Myasthenia gravis is an antibody-mediated, T-cell dependent autoimmune condition of the neuromuscular junction, which causes fluctuating weakness in ocular, bulbar, and limb muscles, and in some patients, causes myasthenic crisis, a critical exacerbation of symptoms of weakness which can be accompanied by respiratory weakness and compromise [124]. While some patients may present with mild symptomatology, such as ocular muscle weakness alone, some may have profound, difficult-to-control weakness, which can require intubation and mechanical ventilation. Treatment for myasthenia includes pyridostigmine, a reversible acetylcholinesterase inhibitor, steroid therapy, intravenous immunoglobulin therapies (IVIg), multiple DMTs, and now anti-FcRn therapies. Notably, 25% of patients receiving IVIG experience headache, and they occur more commonly in women and those with a baseline history of migraine, and typically occur in the first 72 hours following infusion. For management, patients can benefit from pretreatment with triptans, NSAIDs, or a prophylactic glucocorticoid to limit the recurrence of headaches with future treatments [125]. Meanwhile, for primary headache disorders co-occurring with myasthenia, it is important to avoid medications that may exacerbate myasthenia symptoms. Commonly used medications for headaches that are known to worsen myasthenia symptoms include beta-blockers, calcium channel blockers, magnesium supplements, and steroids. Medications such as carbamazepine and gabapentin should be used with caution. Likewise, special considerations for the location of weakness should be taken when using onabotulinumtoxinA, with avoidance of cervical paraspinal injections in most patients with non-ocular myasthenia [126].

CONCLUSIONS

There is significant crossover between patients with headache disorders and other neurologic conditions. A shared pathogenesis may be present between certain conditions, such as potential overlap of CSD in migraine and epilepsy and known increased stroke risk in patients with migraine with aura, as well as comorbid MS and migraine. While there is limited literature on treatment of comorbid headache disorders in neurology, given the high prevalence of headache disorders, many patients with headache disorders and comorbid neurological conditions require a tailored management plan to treat both conditions with therapies that do not exacerbate either of them. Considerations for safety, as well as implications in special populations (geriatrics/women of childbearing age), must also be accounted for.

Key Takeaways

- Headache in IIH often does not resolve with treatment of ICP and often requires additional management geared toward the headache phenotype.
- In patients with a history of prior stroke or significant stroke risk factors, medications such as triptans and ergotamines should be avoided as part of secondary stroke prevention.
- When considering procedural management of patients with prior neurosurgical interventions, consider moving the location of onatobulinumtoxinA injections to cover the same muscle groups as in the PREEMPT protocol.
- Occipital nerve blocks should be avoided in patients with prior suboccipital decompressive surgeries.
- Medications that can exacerbate myasthenia gravis, such as beta-blockers, calcium channel blockers, magnesium, and steroids, should be avoided for headache management when possible.
- Patients with known brain neoplasm must evaluated for signs of increased ICP when presenting with new or atypical headache.
- Sodium channel blockers such as carbamazepine or oxcarbazepine should be used with caution in patients with TN who have comorbid partial epilepsy.
- Counseling on conservative measures such as regular diet, consistent sleep, hydration, and exercise is important in patients with headache and comorbid neurologic disorders and may reduce the need for pharmacological management.

REFERENCES

1. Etminan, M., et al., *Risk of ischaemic stroke in people with migraine: systematic review and meta-analysis of observational studies.* BMJ, 2005. **330**(7482): p. 63.
2. Ornello, R., et al., *Migraine and hemorrhagic stroke: data from general practice.* J Headache Pain, 2015. **16**: p. 8.
3. Oie, L.R., et al., *Migraine and risk of stroke.* J Neurol Neurosurg Psychiatry, 2020. **91**(6): p. 593–604.
4. Monteith, T.S., et al., *Migraine and risk of stroke in older adults: Northern Manhattan Study.* Neurology, 2015. **85**(8): p. 715–21.
5. Goldstein, L.B., et al., *Guidelines for the primary prevention of stroke: a guideline for healthcare professionals from the American Heart Association/American Stroke Association.* Stroke, 2011. **42**(2): p. 517–84.
6. Li, L., et al., *Age-specific association of migraine with cryptogenic TIA and stroke: Population-based study.* Neurology, 2015. **85**(17): p. 1444–51.
7. Lee, M.J., C. Lee, and C.S. Chung, *The Migraine-Stroke Connection.* J Stroke, 2016. **18**(2): p. 146–56.
8. *Headache Classification Committee of the International Headache Society (IHS) The International Classification of Headache Disorders, 3rd edition.* Cephalalgia, 2018. **38**(1): p. 1–211.
9. Kruit, M.C., et al., *Migraine is associated with an increased risk of deep white matter lesions, subclinical posterior circulation infarcts and brain iron accumulation: the population-based MRI CAMERA study.* Cephalalgia, 2010. **30**(2): p. 129–36.
10. Tietjen, G.E. and E.F. Maly, *Migraine and Ischemic Stroke in Women. A Narrative Review.* Headache, 2020. **60**(5): p. 843–863.
11. Alhazzani, A. and R.P. Goddeau, *Migraine and stroke: a continuum of association in adults.* Headache, 2013. **53**(6): p. 1023–7.
12. Tietjen, E.G., *Migraine and ischaemic heart disease and stroke: potential mechanisms and treatment implications.* Cephalalgia, 2007. **27**(8): p. 981–7.
13. Gryglas, A. and R. Smigiel, *Migraine and Stroke: What's the Link? What to Do?* Curr Neurol Neurosci Rep, 2017. **17**(3): p. 22.
14. Lai, J. and E. Dilli, *Migraine Aura: Updates in Pathophysiology and Management.* Curr Neurol Neurosci Rep, 2020. **20**(6): p. 17.
15. Tietjen, G.E., *Circulating microparticles in migraine with aura: cause or consequence, a link to stroke.* Cephalalgia, 2015. **35**(2): p. 85–7.
16. Domitrz, I., J. Mieszkowski, and A. Kaminska, *Relationship between migraine and patent foramen ovale: a study of 121 patients with migraine.* Headache, 2007. **47**(9): p. 1311–8.
17. Negm, M., et al., *Relation between migraine pattern and white matter hyperintensities in brain magnetic resonance imaging.* Egypt J Neurol Psychiatr Neurosurg, 2018. **54**(1): p. 24.
18. Gaist, D., et al., *Migraine with aura and risk of silent brain infarcts and white matter hyperintensities: an MRI study.* Brain, 2016. **139**(Pt 7): p. 2015–23.
19. Bashir, A., et al., *Migraine and structural changes in the brain: a systematic review and meta-analysis.* Neurology, 2013. **81**(14): p. 1260–8.
20. Cheng, C.Y., et al., *White matter hyperintensities in migraine: Clinical significance and central pulsatile hemodynamic correlates.* Cephalalgia, 2018. **38**(7): p. 1225–1236.
21. Sacco, S. and T. Kurth, *Migraine and the risk for stroke and cardiovascular disease.* Curr Cardiol Rep, 2014. **16**(9): p. 524.
22. Al-Hashel, J.Y., et al., *Risk factors of white matter hyperintensities in migraine patients.* BMC Neurol, 2022. **22**(1): p. 159.
23. Chong, C.D., et al., *The Characteristics of White Matter Hyperintensities in Patients With Migraine.* Front Pain Res (Lausanne), 2022. **3**: p. 852916.
24. Eikermann-Haerter, K. and S.Y. Huang, *White Matter Lesions in Migraine.* Am J Pathol, 2021. **191**(11): p. 1955–1962.
25. Hansen, A.P., et al., *Development of persistent headache following stroke: a 3-year follow-up.* Cephalalgia, 2015. **35**(5): p. 399–409.
26. Shapiro, R.E., et al., *Lasmiditan for acute treatment of migraine in patients with cardiovascular risk factors: post-hoc analysis of pooled results from 2 randomized, double-blind, placebo-controlled, phase 3 trials.* J Headache Pain, 2019. **20**(1): p. 90.

27. Aradi, S., E. Kaiser, and B. Cucchiara, *Ischemic Stroke Associated With Calcitonin Gene-Related Peptide Inhibitor Therapy for Migraine: A Case Report.* J Stroke Cerebrovasc Dis, 2019. **28**(10): p. 104286.

28. Schoenen, J., et al., *Ten open questions in migraine prophylaxis with monoclonal antibodies blocking the calcitonin-gene related peptide pathway: a narrative review.* J Headache Pain, 2023. **24**(1): p. 99.

29. Plecash, A.R., et al., *Updates in the Treatment of Post-Stroke Pain.* Curr Neurol Neurosci Rep, 2019. **19**(11): p. 86.

30. Kalbouneh, H.M., et al., *Safety and Efficacy of SSRIs in Improving Poststroke Recovery: A Systematic Review and Meta-Analysis.* J Am Heart Assoc, 2022. **11**(13): p. e025868.

31. Zhang, L.S., et al., *Prophylactic effects of duloxetine on post-stroke depression symptoms: an open single-blind trial.* Eur Neurol, 2013. **69**(6): p. 336–43.

32. Diener, H.C., *The Risks or Lack Thereof of Migraine Treatments in Vascular Disease.* Headache, 2020. **60**(3): p. 649–653.

33. Guo, S., J. Olesen, and M. Ashina, *Phosphodiesterase 3 inhibitor cilostazol induces migraine-like attacks via cyclic AMP increase.* Brain, 2014. **137**(Pt 11): p. 2951–9.

34. Dowson, A., et al., *Migraine Intervention With STARFlex Technology (MIST) trial: a prospective, multi-center, double-blind, sham-controlled trial to evaluate the effectiveness of patent foramen ovale closure with STARFlex septal repair implant to resolve refractory migraine headache.* Circulation, 2008. **117**(11): p. 1397–404.

35. Tobis, J.M., et al., *Percutaneous Closure of Patent Foramen Ovale in Patients With Migraine: The PREMIUM Trial.* J Am Coll Cardiol, 2017. **70**(22): p. 2766–2774.

36. Kurth, T. and H.C. Diener, *Migraine and stroke: perspectives for stroke physicians.* Stroke, 2012. **43**(12): p. 3421–6.

37. de Boer, I., A. MaassenVanDenBrink, and G.M. Terwindt, *The potential danger of blocking CGRP for treating migraine in CADASIL patients.* Cephalalgia, 2020. **40**(14): p. 1676–1678.

38. Chabriat, H., et al., *CADASIL: yesterday, today, tomorrow.* Eur J Neurol, 2020. **27**(8): p. 1588–1595.

39. Tan, R.Y. and H.S. Markus, *CADASIL: Migraine, Encephalopathy, Stroke and Their Inter-Relationships.* PLoS One, 2016. **11**(6): p. e0157613.

40. Roberto, G., et al., *Adverse cardiovascular events associated with triptans and ergotamines for treatment of migraine: systematic review of observational studies.* Cephalalgia, 2015. **35**(2): p. 118–31.

41. Albieri, V., T.S. Olsen, and K.K. Andersen, *Risk of Stroke in Migraineurs Using Triptans. Associations with Age, Sex, Stroke Severity and Subtype.* EBioMedicine, 2016. **6**: p. 199–205.

42. Goldstein, E.D., et al., *CGRP, Migraine, and Brain MRI in CADASIL: A Pilot Study.* Neurologist, 2023. **28**(4): p. 231–236.

43. Forteza, A.M., et al., *Acetazolamide for the treatment of migraine with aura in CADASIL.* Neurology, 2001. **57**(11): p. 2144–5.

44. Aurora, S.K., et al., *OnabotulinumtoxinA for chronic migraine: efficacy, safety, and tolerability in patients who received all five treatment cycles in the PREEMPT clinical program.* Acta Neurol Scand, 2014. **129**(1): p. 61–70.

45. Sprenger, T. and C.L. Seifert, *Coma after greater occipital nerve blockade in a patient with previous posterior fossa surgery.* Headache, 2013. **53**(3): p. 548–50.

46. Mirmosayyeb, O., et al., *The prevalence of migraine in multiple sclerosis (MS): A systematic review and meta-analysis.* J Clin Neurosci, 2020. **79**: p. 33–38.

47. Mohammadi, M., et al., *The association between multiple sclerosis and migraine: A meta-analysis.* Mult Scler Relat Disord, 2023. **79**: p. 104954.

48. Applebee, A., *The clinical overlap of multiple sclerosis and headache.* Headache, 2012. **52 Suppl 2**: p. 111–6.

49. Gee, J.R., et al., *The association of brainstem lesions with migraine-like headache: an imaging study of multiple sclerosis.* Headache, 2005. **45**(6): p. 670–7.

50. Qubty, W. and I. Patniyot, *Migraine Pathophysiology.* Pediatr Neurol, 2020. **107**: p. 1–6.

51. Kister, I., et al., *Increased risk of multiple sclerosis among women with migraine in the Nurses' Health Study II.* Mult Scler, 2012. **18**(1): p. 90–7.

52. Thompson, A.J., et al., *Diagnosis of multiple sclerosis: 2017 revisions of the McDonald criteria.* Lancet Neurol, 2018. **17**(2): p. 162–173.

53. Solomon, A.J., et al., *The contemporary spectrum of multiple sclerosis misdiagnosis: A multicenter study.* Neurology, 2016. **87**(13): p. 1393–9.

54. Blech, B. and A.J. Starling, *Noninvasive Neuromodulation in Migraine.* Curr Pain Headache Rep, 2020. **24**(12): p. 78.

55. Li, Y.X., et al., *Effectiveness and Safety of Acupuncture for Migraine: An Overview of Systematic Reviews.* Pain Res Manag, 2020. **2020**: p. 3825617.
56. Safarpour, Y., T. Mousavi, and B. Jabbari, *Botulinum Toxin Treatment in Multiple Sclerosis-a Review.* Curr Treat Options Neurol, 2017. **19**(10): p. 33.
57. Husain, F., G. Pardo, and M. Rabadi, *Headache and Its Management in Patients With Multiple Sclerosis.* Curr Treat Options Neurol, 2018. **20**(4): p. 10.
58. Di Stefano, G., S. Maarbjerg, and A. Truini, *Trigeminal neuralgia secondary to multiple sclerosis: from the clinical picture to the treatment options.* J Headache Pain, 2019. **20**(1): p. 20.
59. Kuiper, M., S. Hendrikx, and P.J. Koehler, *Headache and Tremor: Co-occurrences and Possible Associations.* Tremor Other Hyperkinet Mov (N Y), 2015. **5**: p. 285.
60. Angelopoulou, E., et al., *Migraine, Tension-Type Headache and Parkinson's Disease: A Systematic Review and Meta-Analysis.* Medicina (Kaunas), 2022. **58**(11): p. 1684.
61. Hess, C.W. and S.L. Pullman, *Tremor: clinical phenomenology and assessment techniques.* Tremor Other Hyperkinet Mov (N Y), 2012. **2**.
62. Pal, P.K., *Guidelines for management of essential tremor.* Ann Indian Acad Neurol, 2011. **14**(Suppl 1): p. S25–8.
63. Zesiewicz, T.A., et al., *Practice parameter: therapies for essential tremor: report of the Quality Standards Subcommittee of the American Academy of Neurology.* Neurology, 2005. **64**(12): p. 2008–20.
64. Chang, K.H., S.H. Wang, and C.C. Chi, *Efficacy and Safety of Topiramate for Essential Tremor: A Meta-Analysis of Randomized Controlled Trials.* Medicine (Baltimore), 2015. **94**(43): p. e1809.
65. Gelenberg, A.J. and J.W. Jefferson, *Lithium tremor.* J Clin Psychiatry, 1995. **56**(7): p. 283–7.
66. Zhang, C.Q., et al., *Risk of Valproic Acid-Related Tremor: A Systematic Review and Meta-Analysis.* Front Neurol, 2020. **11**: p. 576579.
67. Morgan, J.C., et al., *Insights into Pathophysiology from Medication-induced Tremor.* Tremor Other Hyperkinet Mov (N Y), 2017. **7**: p. 442.
68. Baizabal-Carvallo, J.F. and J.C. Morgan, *Drug-induced tremor, clinical features, diagnostic approach and management.* J Neurol Sci, 2022. **435**: p. 120192.
69. Diaz-Martinez, A., et al., *A randomized, open-label comparison of venlafaxine and fluoxetine in depressed outpatients.* Clin Ther, 1998. **20**(3): p. 467–76.
70. Rissardo, J.P. and A.L. Fornari Caprara, *Lamotrigine-Associated Movement Disorder: A Literature Review.* Neurol India, 2021. **69**(6): p. 1524–1538.
71. Morgan, J.C. and K.D. Sethi, *Drug-induced tremors.* Lancet Neurol, 2005. **4**(12): p. 866–76.
72. Rissardo, J.P., A.L.F. Caprara, and I. Durante, *Valproate-associated Movement Disorder: A Literature Review.* Prague Med Rep, 2021. **122**(3): p. 140–180.
73. Janssen, S., B.R. Bloem, and B.P. van de Warrenburg, *The clinical heterogeneity of drug-induced myoclonus: an illustrated review.* J Neurol, 2017. **264**(8): p. 1559–1566.
74. Bauer, P.R., et al., *Headache in people with epilepsy.* Nat Rev Neurol, 2021. **17**(9): p. 529–544.
75. Diseases, G.B.D. and C. Injuries, *Global burden of 369 diseases and injuries in 204 countries and territories, 1990-2019: a systematic analysis for the Global Burden of Disease Study 2019.* Lancet, 2020. **396**(10258): p. 1204–1222.
76. Cilliler, A.E., H. Guven, and S.S. Comoglu, *Epilepsy and headaches: Further evidence of a link.* Epilepsy Behav, 2017. **70**(Pt A): p. 161–165.
77. Nunes, J.C., et al., *Headache among mesial temporal lobe epilepsy patients: a case-control study.* J Neurol Sci, 2011. **306**(1–2): p. 20–3.
78. Duko, B., M. Ayalew, and A. Toma, *The epidemiology of headaches among patients with epilepsy: a systematic review and meta-analysis.* J Headache Pain, 2020. **21**(1): p. 3.
79. Kim, D.W. and S.K. Lee, *Headache and Epilepsy.* J Epilepsy Res, 2017. **7**(1): p. 7–15.
80. *From the FDA: FDA approves Keppra.* J Am Osteopath Assoc, 1999. **99**(12): p. 608a.
81. Johannessen, S.I. and C.J. Landmark, *Antiepileptic drug interactions - principles and clinical implications.* Curr Neuropharmacol, 2010. **8**(3): p. 254–67.
82. Lambru, G., J. Zakrzewska, and M. Matharu, *Trigeminal neuralgia: a practical guide.* Pract Neurol, 2021. **21**(5): p. 392–402.
83. Dodgson, S.J., R.P. Shank, and B.E. Maryanoff, *Topiramate as an inhibitor of carbonic anhydrase isoenzymes.* Epilepsia, 2000. **41**(S1): p. 35–9.
84. Bialer, M., et al., *Pharmacokinetic interactions of topiramate.* Clin Pharmacokinet, 2004. **43**(12): p. 763–80.

85. Kanner, A.M. and M.M. Bicchi, *Antiseizure Medications for Adults With Epilepsy: A Review.* JAMA, 2022. **327**(13): p. 1269–1281.

86. Finnerup, N.B., R. Kuner, and T.S. Jensen, *Neuropathic Pain: From Mechanisms to Treatment.* Physiol Rev, 2021. **101**(1): p. 259–301.

87. Bendtsen, L., et al., *Advances in diagnosis, classification, pathophysiology, and management of trigeminal neuralgia.* Lancet Neurol, 2020. **19**(9): p. 784–796.

88. Bendtsen, L., et al., *European Academy of Neurology guideline on trigeminal neuralgia.* Eur J Neurol, 2019. **26**(6): p. 831–849.

89. Alcantara Montero, A. and C.I. Sanchez Carnerero, *Eslicarbazepine acetate for neuropathic pain, headache, and cranial neuralgia: Evidence and experience.* Neurologia (Engl Ed), 2019. **34**(6): p. 386–395.

90. Munoz-Vendrell, A., et al., *Intravenous lacosamide and phenytoin for the treatment of acute exacerbations of trigeminal neuralgia: A retrospective analysis of 144 cases.* Cephalalgia, 2022. **42**(10): p. 1031–1038.

91. Thurtell, M.J., *Idiopathic Intracranial Hypertension.* Continuum (Minneap Minn), 2019. **25**(5): p. 1289–1309.

92. Pinto, M.J., et al., *Treatment of acute exacerbations of trigeminal neuralgia in the emergency department: A retrospective case series.* Headache, 2022. **62**(8): p. 1002–1006.

93. Wirrell, E.C., *Treatment of Dravet Syndrome.* Can J Neurol Sci, 2016. **43 Suppl 3**: p. S13–8.

94. Lopriore, P., et al., *Mitochondrial Epilepsy, a Challenge for Neurologists.* Int J Mol Sci, 2022. **23**(21): p. 13216.

95. Dhakal, L.P., et al., *Headache and Its Approach in Today's NeuroIntensive Care Unit.* Neurocrit Care, 2016. **25**(2): p. 320–34.

96. Maciel, C.B., et al., *Acute Headache Management for Patients with Subarachnoid Hemorrhage: An International Survey of Health Care Providers.* Neurocrit Care, 2023. **38**(2): p. 395–406.

97. Morad, A.H., R.J. Tamargo, and A. Gottschalk, *The Longitudinal Course of Pain and Analgesic Therapy Following Aneurysmal Subarachnoid Hemorrhage: A Cohort Study.* Headache, 2016. **56**(10): p. 1617–1625.

98. Ogunlaja, O.I. and R. Cowan, *Subarachnoid Hemorrhage and Headache.* Curr Pain Headache Rep, 2019. **23**(6): p. 44.

99. Rajagopalan, S., et al., *Safety and efficacy of peripheral nerve blocks to treat refractory headaches after aneurysmal subarachnoid hemorrhage - A pilot observational study.* Front Neurol, 2023. **14**: p. 1122384.

100. Doglietto, F., et al., *CSF leak in transsphenoidal surgery.* J Neurosurg, 2015. **123**(4): p. 1108–9.

101. Beyhan, M., E. Gokce, and S.F. Ocak Karatas, *Magnetic resonance imaging findings of intracranial hypotension.* Neurol Sci, 2022. **43**(5): p. 3343–3351.

102. Chen, P.K., et al., *Onset headache predicts good outcome in patients with first-ever ischemic stroke.* Stroke, 2013. **44**(7): p. 1852–8.

103. Hansen, A.P., et al., *Pain following stroke: a prospective study.* Eur J Pain, 2012. **16**(8): p. 1128–36.

104. Ahmad, S., et al., *Efficacy of an opioid-sparing analgesic protocol in pain control after less invasive cranial neurosurgery.* Pain Rep, 2021. **6**(3): p. e948.

105. Kahn, K. and A. Finkel, *It IS a tumor -- current review of headache and brain tumor.* Curr Pain Headache Rep, 2014. **18**(6): p. 421.

106. Forst, D.A., *Palliative and Supportive Care in Neuro-oncology.* Continuum (Minneap Minn), 2020. **26**(6): p. 1673–1685.

107. Charipova, K., et al., *A Comprehensive Review and Update of Postsurgical Cutaneous Nerve Entrapment.* Curr Pain Headache Rep, 2021. **25**(2): p. 11.

108. Dietrich, J., *Neurotoxicity of Cancer Therapies.* Continuum (Minneap Minn), 2020. **26**(6): p. 1646–1672.

109. Ota, Y., et al., *Comprehensive Update and Review of Clinical and Imaging Features of SMART Syndrome.* AJNR Am J Neuroradiol, 2023. **44**(6): p. 626–633.

110. Singh, A.K., et al., *Stroke-like migraine attacks after radiation therapy syndrome: Case report and review of the literature.* Neuroradiol J, 2017. **30**(6): p. 568–573.

111. Dominguez, M. and R. Malani, *Stroke-Like Migraine Attacks After Radiation Therapy (SMART) Syndrome: A Comprehensive Review.* Curr Pain Headache Rep, 2021. **25**(5): p. 33.

112. Chen, J. and M. Wall, *Epidemiology and risk factors for idiopathic intracranial hypertension.* Int Ophthalmol Clin, 2014. **54**(1): p. 1–11.

113. Smith, J.L., *Whence pseudotumor cerebri?* J Clin Neuroophthalmol, 1985. **5**(1): p. 55–6.

114. Agid, R., et al., *Idiopathic intracranial hypertension: the validity of cross-sectional neuroimaging signs.* Neuroradiology, 2006. **48**(8): p. 521–7.

115. Hoffmann, J., *Clinical Significance and Therapeutic Management of Weight Loss in Patients With Idiopathic Intracranial Hypertension.* Neurology, 2022. **99**(11): p. 451–452.

116. Mollan, S.P., A.A. Tahrani, and A.J. Sinclair, *The Potentially Modifiable Risk Factor in Idiopathic Intracranial Hypertension: Body Weight.* Neurol Clin Pract, 2021. **11**(4): p. e504–e507.

117. Wall, M., et al., *The idiopathic intracranial hypertension treatment trial: clinical profile at baseline.* JAMA Neurol, 2014. **71**(6): p. 693–701.

118. Bsteh, G., et al., *Idiopathic intracranial hypertension presenting with migraine phenotype is associated with unfavorable headache outcomes.* Headache, 2023. **63**(5): p. 601–610.

119. Yiangou, A., et al., *Erenumab for headaches in idiopathic intracranial hypertension: A prospective open-label evaluation.* Headache, 2021. **61**(1): p. 157–169.

120. Mollan, S.P., O. Grech, and A.J. Sinclair, *Headache attributed to idiopathic intracranial hypertension and persistent post-idiopathic intracranial hypertension headache: A narrative review.* Headache, 2021. **61**(6): p. 808–816.

121. Miyasaki, J.M. and A. Aldakheel, *Movement disorders in pregnancy.* Continuum (Minneap Minn), 2014. **20**(1 Neurology of Pregnancy): p. 148–61.

122. Valente, M., et al., *Prevalence of Restless Legs Syndrome in Migraine Patients: A Case-Control Study. Analysis of Risk Factors for Restless Legs Syndrome in Migraine Patients.* Headache, 2017. **57**(7): p. 1088–1095.

123. Buchfuhrer, M.J., *Strategies for the treatment of restless legs syndrome.* Neurotherapeutics, 2012. **9**(4): p. 776–90.

124. Ciafaloni, E., *Myasthenia Gravis and Congenital Myasthenic Syndromes.* Continuum (Minneap Minn), 2019. **25**(6): p. 1767–1784.

125. Hasirci Bayir, B.R., et al., *IVIg-induced headache: prospective study of a large cohort with neurological disorders.* Neurol Sci, 2023. **44**(8): p. 2871–2881.

126. Sheikh, S., et al., *Drugs That Induce or Cause Deterioration of Myasthenia Gravis: An Update.* J Clin Med, 2021. **10**(7): p. 1537.

Headache and Pulmonary Disease

14

Rahul Gomez, Neha Bijjala, and Pamela Resnikoff

LEARNING OBJECTIVES

1. Identify the mechanisms behind pulmonary comorbidities and their effects on headache disorders
2. Identify the implications of specific pulmonary diseases on the development and treatment of headaches
3. Apply concepts of the pulmonary-headache relationship to some clinical cases

---

MECHANISMS UNDERLYING THE RELATIONSHIP BETWEEN HEADACHE AND PULMONARY DISEASES

The majority of pulmonary patients with headache have one of the following findings: cough, hypoxia, sleep disturbance (sleep apnea), or medication-related side effects. Patients can also have overlapping mechanisms. Much of the data presented for the underlying mechanisms is under study and not fully explored.

Mechanisms of Cough-Related Headaches

According to a systematic review from 2018, cough is one of the most common chief complaints for which patients present to their primary care provider.[1] The underlying mechanism of cough involves a complex interplay between cough receptors and various triggers. These cough receptors are distributed not only in the respiratory tract but also within the pericardium, esophagus, stomach, and diaphragm. Triggers for these receptors include changes in pressure, temperature, or acidity, as well as the presence of chemical irritants or ion channel activators.

Acute (≤ 3 weeks), subacute (3–8 weeks), and chronic cough (> 8 weeks) are associated with many disorders, both pulmonary and nonpulmonary. Acute cough is most often caused by acute infection, with viral being more common than bacterial, although it can be related to other causes, such as asthma and COPD. Some of the more common pulmonary causes of subacute to chronic cough include asthma,

DOI: 10.1201/b23330-14

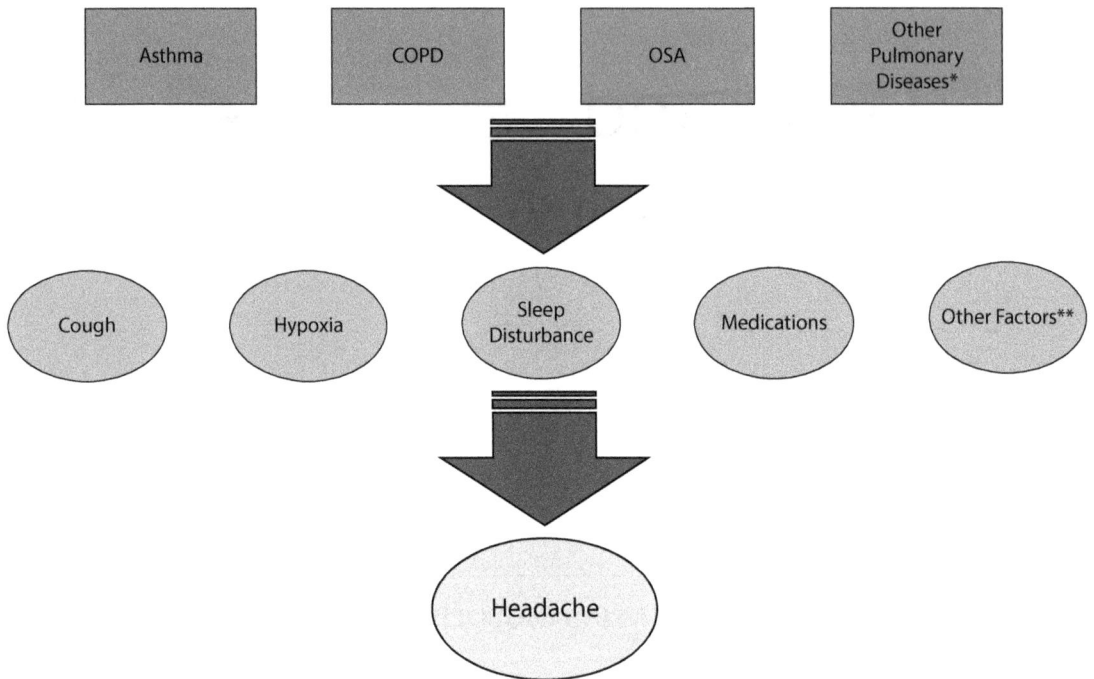

FIGURE 14.1 Relationship between pulmonary diseases and headache. (*Other pulmonary diseases such as pulmonary hypertension, interstitial lung diseases, and bronchiectatic lung diseases). (**The range of other factors that may precipitate headaches is broad, but specifically, the pulmonary microbiome will be addressed in this chapter.)

COPD, diffuse parenchymal lung diseases such as sarcoidosis and pulmonary fibrosis, and bronchiectatic diseases such as cystic fibrosis (CF). Coughing paroxysms are most frequent in patients who produce large amounts of sputum daily, but a dry cough can also be troubling and persistent. Common nonpulmonary causes of chronic cough include gastroesophageal reflux disease (GERD), laryngopharyngeal reflux (LPR), and upper airway cough syndrome (UACS) secondary to sinusitis, allergies, or nonallergic rhinitis. It can also be a side effect of angiotensin-converting enzyme (ACE) inhibitors and occasionally angiotensin receptor blockers (ARBs). Less often, cough can result from a mass lesion pressing on or occupying an airway, such as a tumor or lodged foreign body (see Table 14.1 for additional information on common causes of cough).

Regardless of the etiology of the cough, the mechanism remains the same. It typically involves a sudden, forceful contraction of the thoracic and abdominal muscles against a closed glottis, which suddenly opens to expel air and foreign matter from the lungs. This action results in a sharp increase in the pressure gradients throughout the thoracic and abdominal cavities.

Although the exact mechanism of the relationship between coughing and headache has not been established, several theories have been proposed. One such theory posits that the increased intrathoracic and intra-abdominal pressures are transmitted to the cerebrospinal fluid (CSF), as well as the venous structures. Pascual et al.[2] demonstrated that this resulting pressure wave can transiently obstruct the CSF outflow through the foramen magnum, resulting in increased intracranial pressure as observed through the use of computed tomography (CT) myelography performed during coughing. This is identical to the effects seen during a Valsalva maneuver. Nociceptors throughout the dura and pia mater can be activated by the resulting increased tension, producing the headache. Roughly half of patients in that study who presented with cough headaches had no other contributing factors, but others were found to have structural abnormalities, the most common of which was a Chiari type I malformation at the level of the foramen magnum.[2]

TABLE 14.1   Common etiologies of cough, based on chronicity

CHRONICITY OF COUGH	CAUSES OF COUGH	ADDITIONAL COMMENTS
Acute Cough	Upper or lower respiratory tract infections	Most commonly viral infections but may also be bacterial
	Exacerbation of underlying chronic pulmonary disease (asthma, COPD, bronchiectasis, congestive heart failure, rhinosinusitis)	Most frequently triggered by infection or exposure to triggering agents
Subacute Cough	Postinfectious cough	This may last several weeks beyond the infectious period
	Pertussis	Bacterial infection with Bordetella pertussis
Chronic Cough	Asthma	Cough is a prominent feature in cough-variant asthma (CVA); however, it can be present in other forms of uncontrolled asthma
	COPD (chronic bronchitis, emphysema)	Cough in COPD can be triggered or worsened in acute exacerbations
	Reflux disorders (GERD, laryngopharyngeal reflux)	Can be due to chronic recurrent microaspiration
	Upper airway cough syndrome	Multifactorial, due to postnasal drip, secondary to multiple underlying etiologies
	Congestive heart failure	Typically accompanied by other clinical signs of heart failure not discussed here
	Bronchiectasis	A chronic productive cough with daily sputum production
	Interstitial lung disease	Dry cough, accompanied by dyspnea
	Nonasthmatic eosinophilic bronchitis	Signs of atopy with airway eosinophilia, in the absence of airway hyperresponsiveness
	Lung cancer	Somewhat rare as a sole cause of cough
	Smoldering infection/prolonged postinfectious cough	Can be due to mycobacterial, fungal, parasitic, or nocardia infections or lung abscesses
	Aspiration	Often due to oropharyngeal dysphagia, GERD, or LPR
	Vagal nerve irritation	Typically a separate disease process irritating or compressing the vagus nerve
	Somatic cough disorder/chronic refractory cough	Diagnosis of exclusion once other etiologies have been ruled out
	Medication-related	ACE inhibitors most commonly

Another proposed mechanism for the relationship between cough and headache describes a phenomenon known as the "bloodless brain." This theory posits that the high intrathoracic pressures generated during a coughing paroxysm are transmitted into the valveless sinus system, which carries cerebrospinal fluid and ultimately causes compression of cranial vessels, leading to a transient loss of blood flow, which can manifest as a headache, a hemiplegic migraine or even syncope.[4] Rao et al. reported on a series of two cases of CF who experienced neurological symptoms such as altered level of consciousness, dizziness, blurry vision, presyncope, headache, and hemiplegia shortly after a severe coughing paroxysm that resolved within a few minutes. Both of the patients underwent an extensive workup for evaluation of the hemiplegia, but given the lack of abnormalities on head CT, electroencephalogram, brain magnetic resonance imaging (MRI), and echocardiography for assessment of atrial shunt, the symptoms were attributed to a sporadic hemiplegic migraine.[4]

Another study conducted by the French Society for the Study of Migraine and Headache looked at a small cohort of patients with primary cough headaches, which, based on the *International Classification of Headache Disorders* (*ICHD*) classification, is diagnosed after patients have at least two sudden-onset headaches brought on by coughing, straining, or other Valsalva maneuver lasting between one second and two hours.[5] Each patient underwent brain MRI, magnetic resonance angiography, and magnetic resonance venography to assess for vascular stenosis as a predisposition for primary cough headaches. The control group was composed of 36 patients with no history of chronic headache conditions, and the experimental group was composed of patients with primary cough, primary exertional, and primary headaches associated with sexual activity. No patients in the control group had evidence of vascular stenosis on MRI. In the group with primary cough headaches, however, five of the seven patients were noted to have some form of vascular abnormality, which consisted of unilateral, bilateral transverse sinus, or jugular venous stenosis. This study suggests that certain individuals might be at higher risk for headaches from intracranial pressure (ICP) changes during Valsalva maneuvers, such as coughing, because they have cerebral vascular abnormalities that predispose them to headaches. However, it is unclear whether the stenosis seen in patients with primary cough headaches is the primary cause or a secondary outcome of long-term chronic headaches.

Treatment of cough requires identification of the etiology of the cough, which could necessitate a pulmonary and/or otolaryngology consultation, as the diagnosis can be elusive, and patients may have multiple coexisting conditions (Table 14.1). However, in addition to specific management, antitussive medications can be very helpful, such as guaifenesin, an expectorant that works by loosening secretions by increasing the water content of the mucus. This is particularly helpful in those affected by productive cough with increased sputum production. In patients with either productive or dry cough, agents with low risk of side effects may be used more liberally, such as dextromethorphan (usually comes in elixir combined with guaifenesin) and benzonatate. Other agents with dependency issues, such as codeine, hydrocodone, and promethazine, should be used more sparingly and for brief periods for severe symptoms. Palliation of cancer or other end-stage disease-related cough can be achieved with more liberal use of these agents.

In addition to pharmacologic interventions, it is important to utilize pulmonary hygiene therapies in patients who have difficulty clearing secretions. These include the use of flutter valves, chest physiotherapy vests, airway suctioning, and nebulized medications used for asthma and COPD, as well as hypertonic saline or even nebulized lidocaine. Often, a referral to a pulmonary specialist can be helpful. Palliative care specialists are also familiar with these tools for patients with terminal diseases.

Mechanisms of Hypoxia-Related Headaches

Hypoxia is a hallmark of many pulmonary diseases and has a longstanding association with migraine with aura. For example, it is well described in high-altitude populations. The etiology of migraine with aura is believed to be secondary to a cortical spreading depression, which is described as a "self-propagating wave of depolarization"[6] that spreads across the entire cerebral cortex. It has been theorized that hypoxia decreases the threshold for the cortical spreading depression, thus increasing the incidence of migraine with aura in patients with hypoxia, but the exact physiology behind the proposed decreased threshold is not well understood. One proposed mechanism is a possible correlation between lactate and glutamate concentrations in brains exposed to hypoxia or due to hypoxia-induced vasodilation of the cranial arteries. This was investigated in a 2016 study published in *Brain*[7] in which researchers performed a randomized, double-blind crossover study to assess the possible mechanism behind hypoxia-mediated headaches. Fifteen patients with a history of migraine with aura and a control group of 15 patients with no prior history were exposed to normobaric hypoxia. Eight of the 15 patients with a migraine history developed a migraine when exposed to hypoxia compared to only one of the control group members. However, magnetic resonance spectroscopy analysis noted that the glutamate levels, which have long been thought to be a potential mediator of hypoxia-induced headaches, remained unchanged after exposure to hypoxia. Additionally, patients in the control and experimental groups both had a relatively equal increase in lactate levels and cranial artery dilatation. The study authors thus hypothesized that patients with a history of migraine are more sensitive to arterial vasodilation or, perhaps, to mediators of arterial vasodilation, such as nitric oxide.

The idea that nitric oxide and other mediators of cerebral arterial flow might influence hypoxia-associated headaches is not novel. A 2002 study published in the *Journal of Applied Physiology* looked at the potential effect of nitric oxide on changes in cerebral blood flow associated with hypoxia and/or hypercapnia.[8] The study involved a small cohort (n=8) of healthy male volunteers without a history of smoking, alcohol abuse, hypertension, diabetes mellitus, cardiovascular disease, or any blood gas, physical exam, electrocardiogram, or MRI brain abnormalities. Each patient's cerebral blood flow was estimated based on dynamic end-tidal forcing (DEF) via MRI. DEF involves the rapid alteration of the partial pressures of inspired gasses to rapidly set the end-tidal oxygen and carbon dioxide to the desired level. These patients were exposed to hypercapnia or hypoxia via DEF, both with and without a nitric oxide synthetase inhibitor. Healthy volunteers did have changes in cerebral blood flow associated with hypoxia and hypercapnia; however, this was independent of the presence of the inhibitor, suggesting that cerebral vasodilation is not mediated by nitric oxide. Of note, this study was done on healthy male subjects, and it is not known whether this data can be applied to pulmonary patients with headaches.

While the exact mediators of hypoxia-induced headaches are not well defined, there is a correlation between the two. This begs the question of whether oxygen therapy could help mitigate symptoms of hypoxia-associated headaches in patients with chronic hypoxia. However, there is very little data on oxygen therapy in patients with headaches. In a 2021 systematic review published in *Brain*, the authors conducted a meta-analysis of six studies that looked at the use of oxygen therapy for the treatment of primary headaches, which in this case were defined as migraines, cluster, and tension-type headaches.[9] The meta-analysis looked at the use of oxygen by high-flow nasal cannula and found no statistically significant benefit in headache symptoms in patients receiving oxygen therapy. It is important to note that this study focused on patients with a primary headache disorder who did not have chronic hypoxia. We were unable to find data on whether oxygen therapy improves headaches in patients with chronic hypoxic respiratory failure and chronic migraine. This would be an important area for further study. The use of oxygen for the acute treatment of cluster headache is beyond the scope of this chapter.

Although evidence is lacking, it seems prudent to monitor headache patients with pulmonary disease for hypoxia and treat as clinically indicated, in the hope that it will not only improve pulmonary outcomes but also reduce headache symptoms. Pulmonary patients on home oxygen often obtain their own finger pulse oximeters and are instructed to keep oxygen saturations above 90%. In addition, pulmonary function labs can assess resting and ambulatory oxygen saturations and titrate supplemental oxygen to a target saturation. Nocturnal oximetry can also be obtained by durable medical equipment companies that supply oxygen to patients at home.

Mechanisms of Sleep Disorders and Headache

Several pulmonary diseases, such as obstructive sleep apnea and obesity hypoventilation syndrome, are associated with headaches. Sleep disorders often coexist with migraine. Several studies have presented evidence that patients with a past medical history of migraine often have worse sleep quality than those without a history of migraine.[10] Although it is unclear whether migraine contributes to sleep disturbances, vice versa, or perhaps both, their relationship is well established. Mechanistic hypotheses for sleep disturbances causing headaches have ranged from hypoxia-induced headaches to disturbances in REM sleep; however, no underlying pathway has yet been identified.

In a retrospective study conducted by the Baystate Medical Center in 2006, investigators assessed a cohort of 52 patients with polysomnography-confirmed obstructive sleep apnea who were also undergoing treatment for headache. Of this patient group, 40% of the patients who were able to tolerate and were adherent to their continuous positive airway pressure (CPAP) therapy reported improvement in headache symptoms, suggesting that adherence to CPAP therapy can help alleviate sleep/hypoxia-associated headaches often seen in patients with sleep apnea.[11]

Sleep apnea is underdiagnosed in the United States.[12] For this reason, clinicians should maintain a high index of suspicion for possible sleep pathology in any patient presenting with headache. Patients suffering from headache should be evaluated for coexistent sleep disorders with a thorough history and physical exam, including oropharyngeal assessment and neck circumference. We encourage the routine use of a standardized screening questionnaire such as the STOP-Bang questionnaire, the Berlin questionnaire, or the Sleep Apnea Clinical Score (SACS). When indicated by the results of the screening questionnaire, history, and physical exam, patients should be referred to a sleep specialist to undergo polysomnography and subsequent management. Additionally, all mission-critical workers with any suspicion of sleep apnea, regardless of screening questionnaire results, should also be referred to a sleep specialist.

Mechanisms of Medication-Induced Headaches

As discussed earlier, hypoxia-induced migraine headaches are thought to result from cerebral arterial vasodilation. Nitric oxide may play some role, though research has not shown any definitive evidence of this. Interestingly, the pulmonary medications most often associated with the side effects of migraine are first-line treatments for group 1 pulmonary hypertension (pulmonary arterial hypertension): phosphodiesterase-5 inhibitors, such as sildenafil; prostacyclin vasodilators and their analogs, such as treprostanil; and guanylate cyclase inhibitors, such as riociguat. The underlying mechanism for the benefit of these medications is pulmonary vasodilation. However, some degree of systemic vasodilation also occurs. As a result, a common side effect of these medications, migraine, is thought to be mediated by vasoactive peptides.

In 1996, a group of researchers conducted a study in which patients with angina pectoris were randomized to a high or a low dose of nitrate therapy. Notably, both dosages demonstrated a similar efficacy in the resolution of anginal symptoms.[13] Additionally, the patients in the high-dose group were three times as likely to develop a headache as those in the low-dose group, suggesting that headache mediated by nitric oxide has a dose-response relationship.

Headache has also been reported in the postmarketing analysis of endothelin receptor antagonists (ERAs), such as bosentan, sitaxentan, macitentan, and ambrisentan. Despite this, ERAs have not been shown to cause a statistically significant increase in headache incidence in clinical trials. In fact, Wei et al. showed a relative risk of 1.09 (95% confidence interval (CI) 0.93–1.29) in a meta-analysis of 4,894 patients across 24 double-blind, placebo-controlled studies of ERAs.[36]

Headache, as will be discussed further in this chapter, is a common adverse effect reported with the use of other pulmonary medications, notably inhaled corticosteroids (ICS), beta-2 agonists, and leukotriene antagonists. Although this is a frequent complaint, sometimes necessitating medication changes, clinical trials for the latter two have not shown a consistent relationship, as seen in a meta-analysis conducted by Chauhan and Ducharme, which did not demonstrate an increased frequency of headaches in patients using these medications.[14] Interestingly, multiple case reports have linked ICS use with increased intraocular pressure and headache. This was thought to be primarily a result of small amounts of aerosolized droplets of corticosteroids coming in contact with the eye surface. The proposed mechanism behind the increased intraocular pressure was attributed to upregulation and accumulation of polymerized glycosaminoglycosides, which increase production of collagen, elastin, and fibronectin in the extracellular network.

As headache is frequently reported with common pulmonary medications, when working with a headache patient taking these medications, it is reasonable to make clinically appropriate changes in medication without adversely affecting their pulmonary status to see if headache can be avoided. For example, at times, asthma patients have intermittent symptoms and can reduce their medications when their disease is less active. In some cases, muscarinic antagonists such as ipratropium and tiotropium can be substituted for beta-agonists in asthma and COPD patients with little impact on their pulmonary symptoms. Referral to a pulmonary specialist can help optimize management when such constraints occur.

Miscellaneous

While the gut microbiome has been explored extensively in many disease states, the role of the pulmonary microbiome in the development of headaches is an emerging area of study. It has been hypothesized that the pulmonary flora of the lung may play a role in the level of immune reactivity within the brain. For example, fungal species may directly infect or inflame the meninges through hematogenous spread or the spread of affected macrophages. Additionally, bacterial or viral components may enter the blood in the form of vesicles or even as direct bacterial elements, such as lipopolysaccharides. These elements have been shown to then cross the blood–brain barrier, where they increase the prevalence of proinflammatory cytokines, several of which are implicated in headaches.[19, 20, 21]

RELATIONSHIP BETWEEN SPECIFIC PULMONARY DISEASES AND HEADACHE

Based on the association between pulmonary symptoms, findings, and the development of headache described so far, it is worthwhile to turn to specific pulmonary conditions and address the intersection between pulmonary therapies and headache management. Although we are focusing on the most common pulmonary conditions, the strategies presented here should also apply to other less common pulmonary diseases as well.

Asthma

Asthma, more than any of the other pulmonary diseases, appears to have the strongest correlation with migraine, so much so that asthma at one point was called the "pulmonary migraine." In 2018, Sayyah et al. conducted a meta-analysis[15] exploring the relationship between the two and the potential causality. From an extensive literature review, he gathered eight studies with a total of approximately 400,000 participants. A statistical analysis of pooled estimates demonstrated the odds ratio for the prevalence of migraines in patients with asthma when compared to patients without asthma was 1.62 (95% CI 1.43–1.82). The currently accepted connection is that both asthma and migraines have a common denominator of inflammation leading to smooth muscle activation. It remains unclear whether one triggers the other or if they both share common genetic factors that result in their coexistence.

One of the most accepted mechanisms is the "atopy theory," which notes that both migraine and asthma have similar atopic pathophysiology, also referred to as type 2 inflammation. This involves the release of allergen-specific immunoglobulin E (IgE) antibodies, resulting in mast cell degranulation upon exposure to the allergen.[15] This, in turn, leads to parasympathetic hyperactivity, a common feature of both asthma and migraine headaches.

In a cross-sectional study, Graif et al. looked at the association between asthma and migraine in adolescents and conducted a subgroup analysis in patients with asthma and allergic rhinitis.[16] They found an increased prevalence of migraine headaches in patients with both asthma and allergic rhinitis (OR 3.18; 95% CI 2.8–3.63), thus supporting the atopy theory.

Mast cells play a role in allergic rhinitis, asthma, and migraine. Upon stimulation, they release important inflammatory mediators, which include histamine, tryptase, and prostaglandins. Additionally, intracranial mast cell degranulation specifically can trigger a "prolonged state of excitation of the meningeal nociceptors," which can activate the pain pathway of migraine headaches.[17] Intracranial mast cells also release vasodilatory molecules in response to corticotropin-releasing hormone, which can lead to migraine.

It has also been theorized that leukotrienes play a role in the association between migraine and headache. In asthma, they are known to mediate smooth muscle contraction of the airway and result in bronchospasm. Earlier in this chapter, we discussed that migraine, specifically those triggered by hypoxia, are thought to occur as a likely result of nitric oxide. However, leukotrienes may also play a role, though the exact mechanism is unclear, possibly relating to platelet hyperactivity or cerebral arterial vasodilation.[18] Ince et al. performed a randomized controlled trial measuring urinary levels of leukotriene E4 (LT-E4) in 64 pediatric patients with at least a 6-month history of migraine and a control group of 50 patients. The urinary LT-E4 levels were notably higher in the patient group during periods of headache, suggesting leukotrienes might play a role in migraines.

The Global Initiative for Asthma (GINA) publishes guidelines annually with updates on asthma management. ICS, beta 2 agonists, and leukotriene antagonists are fundamental elements of asthma treatment, and headache is a commonly reported side effect of these medications. However, as noted earlier, several studies found no significant association between the use of these medications and increased headache frequency compared with controls,[19] with the possible exception of ICS medications. In fact, these studies showed a correlation between poor asthma control and increased frequency of migraine, suggesting that optimizing asthma therapy is more important for headache management than changing medications over concern for medication-associated headaches. There are also many therapeutic options available for managing severe persistent asthma, including initiating biologic therapies such as anti-IgE, anti-IL-5, anti-IL-4R, and anti-thymic stromal lymphopoietin (anti-TSLP) antibodies in appropriately selected patients. A referral to a pulmonary specialist is recommended in cases of difficult-to-manage asthma.

COPD

While the underlying pathophysiology of obstructive lung disease has some notable overlap with asthma, COPD differs from asthma, not only in symptoms, timing, and etiology but also in the disease progression, associated comorbidities, and medications. Asthma is characterized by *reversible* airway obstruction due to airway hyperreactivity from bronchoconstriction and acute inflammation. COPD is associated with *fixed* airway obstruction due to chronic inflammation as well as smooth muscle bronchoconstriction, resulting in lung hyperinflation limiting chest wall movement, and at the end stages, pulmonary cachexia with generalized muscle weakness. COPD should be suspected in all tobacco users, although not all smoking individuals develop COPD. It is more likely in those with more than 20 pack years of smoking, especially in those with a chronic cough.

Mechanistically, there is little data to directly correlate the underlying disease processes involved in COPD with the development of headache; however, Minen et al. performed a study utilizing data from the 2013–2015 National Health Interview Survey, which did show a statistically significant correlation between COPD and severe headaches and migraine.[32] HajGhanbari et al. found that patients suffering from COPD reported 2.5 times greater pain levels than those in an age and sex-matched healthy cohort.[23] As seen in asthma, the systemic inflammatory pathway may also play a part in COPD patients by increasing the sensitivity of nociceptors in the brain and throughout the body. This may result in increased headache directly or via other pain disorders leading to headache, such as neck and shoulder musculoskeletal pain.

These other musculoskeletal pain syndromes may contribute to the development of headache through other mechanistic ways in COPD as well. With increased lung volumes due to hyperinflation in chronic obstructive disease, rib motion is decreased, resulting in stiffness and loss of thoracic kyphosis, which produces muscular pain in the postural and paravertebral musculature of the thoracic and even cervical regions. Chronic pain and inflammation in these regions can produce increased frequency and severity of headaches.[23, 29]

Another major factor in COPD patients is the presence of concomitant sleep disturbances. As patients with COPD are more likely to suffer from concomitant disturbances in REM sleep, it has been proposed that this may play a role. Özge et al. showed in a study of 119 COPD patients that over 30% of these patients suffered from headaches, and among these, over half also suffered from sleep disorders, including sleep apnea.[31] The mechanistic pathway in these patients with headaches is likely similar to obstructive sleep apnea (OSA); however, headache is more prevalent in the COPD population.

Chronic hypercapnia has also been hypothesized to play a role. Physiologically, the presence of high levels of dissolved CO_2 leads to vascular smooth muscle relaxation resulting in intracerebral vasodilation and headache. As mentioned in the section on hypoxia-related headaches earlier, Wise et al. were able to demonstrate intracerebral vasodilation in the presence of hypercapnia.[8] This relationship was even tested outside the Earth's atmosphere when Law et al. studied the relationship between CO_2 levels and reported headache frequency in the crew of the International Space Station.[24] For every 1 mm Hg increase in ambient CO_2, the likelihood of headache doubled.

As mentioned earlier, hypoxemia is known to correlate with headache in patients with a variety of pulmonary disorders. The study performed by Argim et al. showed a correlation between exposure to hypoxia and the development of migraine.[7] As COPD is a common pulmonary disease causing hypoxia, this is an integral component of the disease process to address when controlling headaches in this population. In addition to hypoxia, Özge et al. found that measures of lung function, the FEV1 and FEV1/FVC ratio, were inversely related to the development of headache.[31] For these reasons, we encourage optimizing COPD management, including cessation of tobacco use.

The approach to patients with COPD is summarized in the Global Initiative for Chronic Obstructive Lung Disease (GOLD) guidelines for COPD management.[35] Adequate symptom control and avoidance of exacerbations is paramount, and will likely improve headache outcomes as well. Medications and therapies for the optimal treatment of cough and dyspnea, the use of oxygen when indicated, and tobacco cessation should reduce the manifestations of COPD and hopefully reduce or prevent associated headaches. The avoidance of air trapping improves chest wall mobility and reduces musculoskeletal pain, which may also be helpful. With treatment of the underlying obstruction, patients are less likely to suffer from associated sleep disturbances and have less CO_2 retention, which can also help with headaches.

Tobacco, the underlying primary risk factor for the development of COPD, has separately been shown to be associated with headaches. A study performed on 980 patients in New Zealand showed an odds ratio of 2.16 (95% CI 1.39–3.35) during mid-adolescence for smokers developing frequent headaches, as compared to nonsmokers. Interestingly, this risk did not carry forward to adulthood in this population.[25] More recently, Gan et al. studied a US cohort of 8,399 adults, showing an odds ratio of 1.38 (95% CI 1.17–1.62) in smokers for the development of migraine, as compared to nonsmokers.[22]

The mechanism by which tobacco use worsens migraine is poorly understood and poorly described. Some theorize that the pituitary adenylate cyclase-activating polypeptide may be implicated, as it has been linked to the development of both migraines and nicotine dependence in animal models.[26] Additionally, smoking has deleterious effects on the cardiovascular system, partially through inflammation. This same mechanism may play a role in increasing the likelihood of developing migraines.[27]

Obstructive Sleep Apnea

OSA is a common disorder, affecting 25%–30% of males and 9%–17% of females in the North American population.[3] Historically associated with OSA, the presence of morning headaches should prompt clinicians to consider screening for OSA utilizing one of several widely accepted screening tools, as mentioned earlier. While the relationship between OSA and headaches is well established, the underlying mechanism is not.

Most frequently, OSA has been associated with the development of tension-type headaches. Chiu et al. studied 4,759 participants with OSA confirmed by polysomnography. They found that patients with OSA had a statistically significant increased incidence of tension-type headaches when compared to a matched population of non-OSA patients.[30] The development of tension-type headache can be attributed to a decrease in serum levels of serotonin. Özge et al. describe that sleep disturbances may also lead to dysfunction of pain modulation in regions such as the dorsolateral pontine tegmentum, the rostral ventromedial medulla, and the periaqueductal gray matter.[31] Disruption of these regions is postulated to play a role in developing morning headaches after sleep disturbances.[31] This decrease in serotonin is driven by disturbances in sleep patterns and can be brought on by many sleep disorders.

The timing of headaches may also play a role in identifying OSA as a potential cause. As mentioned earlier, the presence of morning headaches in particular should raise suspicion for the presence of OSA. Spałka et al. showed that 25.9% of 1,009 patients with OSA were found to suffer from morning headache. Interestingly, however, the severity of OSA was not directly related to the severity of morning headaches in these patients. In fact, this study showed an inverse correlation in that headaches were associated with less severe OSA, as manifested by lower arousal indices.[33] We were unable to find any further data exploring the relationship between the severity of OSA and headaches.

However, there are data to suggest that treatment of OSA decreases the frequency of headaches in these patients, as noted earlier. Johnson et al. demonstrated a statistically significant decrease in the frequency and severity of headaches reported in patients with OSA who were adherent to the use of CPAP.[37] For this reason, we recommend appropriate screening and early initiation of CPAP therapy in all eligible patients found to have OSA. Additionally, Park et al. were able to demonstrate that the use of oral appliance treatment decreased the frequency of headaches in OSA patients, with 62% reporting a greater than 30% reduction in frequency of headache symptoms.[34] However, due to a small sample size, they were unable to describe consistent reduction in migraine severity, defined in the study as a decrease of >50% Migraine Disability Assessment Questionnaire Score. Finally, weight loss can also reduce or even eliminate OSA and should be recommended.

Miscellaneous Disorders

In addition to more common pulmonary disorders, there are implications for other diseases, including bronchiectatic diseases (including CF and primary ciliary dyskinesia), interstitial lung diseases, and pulmonary arterial hypertension, which may lead to headaches. As described previously, there are multiple modalities through which pulmonary diseases may manifest headache, including hypoxemia, cough, and medication side effects.

Patients suffering from bronchiectatic diseases will likely present with increased sputum production and an associated productive cough. In addition, these patients may suffer from baseline hypoxemia, both of which may potentially significantly worsen during acute flares. Any patient identified as suffering from chronic, progressive, or congenital bronchiectatic diseases should be co-managed with the help of a pulmonary specialist, who will help guide disease-specific and symptomatic management and monitoring. These patients should have routine follow-up, and if not already done so, the underlying cause of their bronchiectatic disease should be identified through imaging and lab work, including sweat chloride and gene testing.

Interstitial lung disease (ILD) can cause progressive hypoxic respiratory failure and cough. Typically characterized by a progressive, dry cough, ILD may be accompanied by cough-associated headache and hypoxia-induced headaches. Once again, given the complexity and progressive nature of these diseases, these patients should be co-managed with a pulmonary specialist and potentially a multidisciplinary team, including rheumatology and palliative care medicine. Any patients presenting with chronic, progressive respiratory symptoms and/or CT findings concerning ILD should be referred to a pulmonary specialist for management.

Pulmonary hypertension patients frequently suffer from headaches, often as a result of their medical regimen, as described earlier. These medications commonly rely on underlying vasodilatory pathways, and this same pathophysiology can result in headaches when active within the brain. Patients with pulmonary hypertension typically present with progressive dyspnea on exertion, which may worsen dyspnea at rest. This patient population should be co-managed with either a pulmonologist or a cardiologist with expertise in pulmonary hypertension. While headaches may complicate the process of titrating the vasodilatory medications, expectation setting can be beneficial in this population to improve compliance with the medication regimen.

Impact of Headache Management on Pulmonary Disorders

While this chapter has focused on the various implications of pulmonary diseases on headaches, it is important to also be familiar with the opposite relationship. Some of the medications used to manage headache conditions have well-documented effects on lung function. Beta-blocker medications, for example, have been shown to increase airway reactivity and blunt responsiveness to beta-agonist inhalers used to control reactive airway disease. In a cohort of 35,502 patients, Morales et al. showed that noncardioselective beta-blockers increased the risk for moderate and even severe asthma exacerbations, while cardioselective beta-blockers did not confer the same risks.[28] We, therefore, recommend the careful titration and close monitoring of patients initiated on nonselective beta-blockers with concomitant reactive airway disease.

CLINICAL EXAMPLES

1. **30-year-old F with moderate persistent asthma who also has episodic migraine**

   Ms. T is a 30-year-old female with a history of moderate persistent asthma who presents for evaluation of headache. She reports the onset of severe headaches after puberty that occur on ten days of the month and are characterized by unilateral throbbing pain and nausea but no photophobia or phonophobia. Her headaches last for 12–24 hours and often require her to leave work early or miss important social functions. Of note, the patient developed asthma in her late teens, which has slowly worsened over time, and she now has some wheezing every day and had to give up playing squash due to it frequently exacerbating her asthma. One month prior, she was started on a combination low-dose inhaled corticosteroid with formoterol and has noticed some improvement in these symptoms.

   The patient's headaches are consistent with episodic migraine with aura. Given that her headache frequency is ten days per month, and it has greatly interfered with her daily activities, she was interested in starting a daily preventive medication. She was previously prescribed as-needed propranolol, but unfortunately, the beta antagonistic effect of the medication resulted in exacerbation of her asthma, and this had to be discontinued. Topiramate was agreed to be the best option for her for prevention, and after three months of use, her headache frequency decreased to four days per month, which responded well to her as-needed zolmitriptan. She did report that she initially had some bothersome peripheral paresthesias after starting the topiramate, but these resolved a couple of weeks into the course.

2. **64-year-old M with OSA and worsening daily headaches**

   Mr. K is a 64-year-old male with a past medical history of diabetes and hypertension who presents for evaluation of worsening headaches. The patient reports that over the past three years, he has had progressively more frequent and worse headaches that occur solely in the morning. He notes that on roughly 25 days of the month, he will wake up with holocephalic and pressure-like pain. These episodes are not associated with any nausea, photophobia, or phonophobia. He does report that after he goes through his morning routine and leaves for his job as a computer programmer, his headaches are mostly resolved. He is currently taking metformin and empagliflozin for his diabetes, as well as chlorthalidone and losartan for hypertension. He notes that he recently started an exercise program to lose weight to lower his current body mass index (BMI) of 34. On further discussion, he reports that his husband tells him that he is constantly snoring, and Mr. K then tells you that he is constantly fatigued throughout the day despite sleeping for eight hours each night.

Mr. K's headaches are likely secondary to OSA. This patient was referred to a sleep medicine clinic and underwent polysomnography. This test showed 31 respiratory events per hour of sleep. He was started on CPAP and after a couple of weeks noted only minor headaches in the morning. After multiple months of supervised exercise, his BMI decreased to 31, and he noted resolution of the headaches when he used his CPAP.

3. **74-year-old F with chronic migraine and a COPD exacerbation**

Ms. I is a 74-year-old female with a history of chronic migraine who follows up with you for her quarterly onabotulinumtoxinA treatment and notes that she was recently hospitalized for a COPD exacerbation. Her headache burden is currently back at her baseline of 10 days per month, which responds to her as-needed rizatriptan. In addition to the onabotulinumtoxinA, she uses daily candesartan and memantine for control of her headaches. During her hospitalization for COPD, she received multiple rounds of albuterol and was started on a course of glucocorticoids with improvement in respirations. On the second hospitalization day, the patient was noted to have a severe migraine that was not responsive to her usual rizatriptan. The Pain Medicine Team was consulted and performed an occipital nerve block for the patient with improvement in her headache.

CONCLUSION

In this chapter, we discussed the relationship between headache and pulmonary medicine. We noted a direct connection between specific clinical features, such as cough, hypoxia, and sleep disturbances, as well as common pulmonary disorders, such as asthma, COPD, and ILD. Cough, one of the most common chief complaints seen in primary care offices, can directly cause primary cough headache that can be managed symptomatically with antitussives. Other causes of cough should be identified and treated appropriately. Hypoxia, a common feature in most pulmonary diseases, has long been thought to be associated with headaches. Although there is insufficient evidence for oxygen therapy to treat headaches in patients with chronic hypoxia, it is important to monitor for and treat hypoxia appropriately. Headaches in patients with OSA are thought to be secondary to sleep disturbances and hypoxia, and several studies have demonstrated improvement in both sleep and headaches when patients adhere to CPAP therapy. OSA is often underdiagnosed in the United States, and screening is important in patients with chronic headaches.

Headache is commonly reported as an adverse reaction to many medications commonly used for the treatment of pulmonary diseases, although formal studies have not always shown a clear relationship. In addition, headache medicines can exacerbate pulmonary diseases, such as beta-blockers in asthma. Medication changes to improve headache symptoms should be made carefully to avoid adversely affecting the underlying pulmonary disease. For example, poor asthma control has been shown to worsen headaches.

In summary, while the exact pathophysiologic relationship between headaches and pulmonary diseases is complex and remains largely unknown, the correlation is clear, and it is, therefore, important for clinicians to evaluate and manage both appropriately. Collaboration with pulmonary specialists can help optimize management in patients with pulmonary disease and headaches.

REFERENCES

1. Finley CR, Chan DS, Garrison S, Korownyk C, Kolber MR, Campbell S, Eurich DT, Lindblad AJ, Vandermeer B, Allan GM. What are the most common conditions in primary care? Systematic review. *Can Fam Physician.* 2018 Nov;*64*(11):832–40. PMID: 30429181; PMCID: PMC6234945.

2. Pascual J, Iglesias F, Oterino A, Vázquez-Barquero A, Berciano J. Cough, exertional, and sexual headaches: an analysis of 72 benign and symptomatic cases. *Neurology.* 1996 Jun;*46*(6):1520–4. doi: 10.1212/wnl.46.6.1520. PMID: 8649540.

3. Slowik JM, Sankari A, Collen JF. Obstructive Sleep Apnea. [Updated 2022 Dec 11]. In: StatPearls [Internet]. Treasure Island (FL): StatPearls Publishing; 2023 Jan-. Available from: https://www.ncbi.nlm.nih.gov/books/NBK459252/

4. Rao DS, Infeld MD, Stern RC, Chelimsky TC. Cough-induced hemiplegic migraine with impaired consciousness in cystic fibrosis. *Pediatr Pulmonol.* 2006 Feb;*41*(2):171–6. doi: 10.1002/ppul.20309. PMID: 16372353.

5. Donnet A, Valade D, Houdart E, Lanteri-Minet M, Raffaelli C, Demarquay G, Hermier M, Guegan-Massardier E, Gerardin E, Geraud G, Cognard C, Levrier O, Lehmann P. Primary cough headache, primary exertional headache, and primary headache associated with sexual activity: a clinical and radiological study. *Neuroradiology.* 2013 Feb;*55*(3):297–305. doi: 10.1007/s00234-012-1110-0. Epub 2012 Nov 2. PMID: 23117256.

6. Cui Y, Kataoka Y, Watanabe Y. Role of cortical spreading depression in the pathophysiology of migraine. *Neurosci Bull.* 2014 Oct;*30*(5):812–22. doi: 10.1007/s12264-014-1471-y. Epub 2014 Sep 28. PMID: 25260797; PMCID: PMC5562594.

7. Arngrim N, Schytz HW, Britze J, Amin FM, Vestergaard MB, Hougaard A, Wolfram F, de Koning PJ, Olsen KS, Secher NH, Larsson HB, Olesen J, Ashina M. Migraine induced by hypoxia: an MRI spectroscopy and angiography study. *Brain.* 2016 Mar;*139* (Pt 3):723–37. doi: 10.1093/brain/awv359. Epub 2015 Dec 16. PMID: 26674653

8. Wise RG, Pattinson KT, Bulte DP, Chiarelli PA, Mayhew SD, Balanos GM, 'Connor DF, Pragnell TR, Robbins PA, Tracey I, Jezzard P. Dynamic forcing of end-tidal carbon dioxide and oxygen applied to functional magnetic resonance imaging. *J Cereb Blood Flow Metab.* 2007 Aug; *27*(8):1521–32. doi: 10.1038/sj.jcbfm.9600465. Epub 2007 Apr 4. PMID: 17406659

9. Ciarambino T, Sansone G, Menna G, Para O, Signoriello G, Leoncini L, Giordano M. Oxygen therapy in headache disorders: A systematic review. *Brain Sci.* 2021 Mar 17;*11*(3):379. doi: 10.3390/brainsci11030379. PMID: 33802647; PMCID: PMC8002555

10. Tiseo C, Vacca A, Felbush A, Filimonova T, Gai A, Glazyrina T, Hubalek IA, Marchenko Y, Overeem LH, Piroso S, Tkachev A, Martelletti P, Sacco S. European Headache Federation School of Advanced Studies (EHF-SAS). Migraine and sleep disorders: a systematic review. *J Headache Pain.* 2020 Oct 27;*21*(1):126. doi: 10.1186/s10194-020-01192-5. PMID: 33109076; PMCID: PMC7590682

11. Johnson KG, Ziemba AM, Garb JL. Improvement in headaches with continuous positive airway pressure for obstructive sleep apnea: a retrospective analysis. *Headache.* 2013 Feb;*53*(2):333–43. doi: 10.1111/j.1526-4610.2012.02251.x. Epub 2012 Sep 10. PMID: 22963547

12. Motamedi KK, McClary AC, Amedee RG. Obstructive sleep apnea: a growing problem. *Ochsner J.* 2009 Fall;*9*(3):149–53. PMID: 21603432; PMCID: PMC3096276.

13. Cleophas TJ, Niemeyer MG, van Der Wall EE. Nitrate-induced headache in patients with stable angina pectoris: beneficial effect of starting on a low dosage. *Am J Ther.* 1996 Dec; *3*(12):802–6. doi: 10.1097/00045391-199612000-00003. PMID: 11862241.

14. Chauhan BF, Ducharme FM. Addition to inhaled corticosteroids of long-acting beta2-agonists versus anti-leukotrienes for chronic asthma. *Cochrane Database Syst Rev.* 2014 Jan 24;*2014*(1):CD003137. doi: 10.1002/14651858.CD003137.pub5. PMID: 24459050; PMCID: PMC10514761.

15. Sayyah M, Saki-Malehi A, Javanmardi F, Forouzan A, Shirbandi K, Rahim F. Which came first, the risk of migraine or the risk of asthma? A systematic review. *Neurol Neurochir Pol.* 2018 Sep-Oct;*52*(5):562–9. doi: 10.1016/j.pjnns.2018.07.004. Epub 2018 Aug 3. PMID: 30119907]

16. Graif Y, Shohat T, Machluf Y, Farkash R, Chaiter Y. Association between asthma and migraine: A cross-sectional study of over 110 000 adolescents. *Clin Respir J.* 2018 Oct;*12*(10):2491–6. doi: 10.1111/crj.12939. Epub 2018 Oct 4. PMID: 30004178.

17. Levy D, Burstein R, Kainz V, Jakubowski M, Strassman AM. Mast cell degranulation activates a pain pathway underlying migraine headache. *Pain.* 2007 Jul;*130*(1–2):166–76. doi: 10.1016/j.pain.2007.03.012. Epub 2007 Apr 24. PMID: 17459586; PMCID: PMC2045157.

18. Ince H, Aydin ÖF, Alaçam H, Aydin T, Azak E, Özyürek H. Urinary leukotriene E4 and prostaglandin F2a concentrations in children with migraine: a randomized study. *Acta Neurol Scand.* 2014 Sep;*130*(3):188–92. doi: 10.1111/ane.12263. Epub 2014 May 15. PMID: 24828386.

19. Li C, Chen W, Lin F, Li W, Wang P, Liao G, Zhang L. Functional two-way crosstalk between brain and lung: The brain-lung axis. *Cell Mol Neurobiol.* 2023 Apr;*43*(3):991–1003. doi: 10.1007/s10571-022-01238-z. Epub 2022 Jun 9. PMID: 35678887; PMCID: PMC9178545.

20. Ousman Bajinka, Lucette Simbilyabo, Yurong Tan, John Jabang & Shakeel Ahmed Saleem. Lung-brain axis, *Crit Rev Microbiol;*2022;*48*:3, 257–69. doi: 10.1080/1040841X.2021.1960483

21. Kim JH, Lee Y, Kwon YS, Sohn JH. Clinical Implications of the Association between Respiratory and Gastrointestinal Disorders in Migraine and Non-Migraine Headache Patients. *J Clin Med.* 2023 May 12;*12*(10):3434. doi: 10.3390/jcm12103434. PMID: 37240541; PMCID: PMC10219163.

22. Gan WQ, Estus S, Smith JH. Association between overall and mentholated cigarette smoking with headache in a nationally representative sample. *Headache.* 2016 Mar;*56*(3):511–8. doi: 10.1111/head.12778. Epub 2016 Mar 1. PMID: 26926358.

23. HajGhanbari, B., Holsti, L., Road, J. D., & Darlene Reid, W. (2012). Pain in people with chronic obstructive pulmonary disease (COPD). *Respiratory Medicine,* 106(7), 998–1005. https://doi.org/10.1016/j.rmed.2012.03.004

24. Law, Jennifer, Van Baalen, Mary, Foy, Millennia, Mason, Sara S., Mendez, Claudia, Wear, Mary L., Meyers, Valerie E., Alexander, David. Relationship between carbon dioxide levels and reported headaches on the international space station. *J Occup Environ Med* 2014 May;*56*(5):477–83. doi: 10.1097/JOM.0000000000000158

25. Waldie KE, McGee R, Reeder AI, Poulton R. Associations between frequent headaches, persistent smoking, and attempts to quit. Headache. 2008 Apr;*48*(4):545–52. doi: 10.1111/j.1526-4610.2007.01037.x. Epub 2008 Jan 23. PMID: 18218010.

26. Moody TW, Jensen RT. Pituitary adenylate cyclase-activating polypeptide/vasoactive intestinal peptide [Part 1]: biology, pharmacology, and new insights into their cellular basis of action/signaling which are providing new therapeutic targets. *Curr Opin Endocrinol Diabetes Obes.* 2021 Apr 1;*28*(2):198–205. doi: 10.1097/MED.0000000000000617. PMID: 33449573; PMCID: PMC7957349.

27. Weinberger AH, Seng EK. The Relationship of tobacco use and migraine: A narrative review. *Curr Pain Headache Rep.* 2023 Apr;*27*(4):39–47. doi: 10.1007/s11916-023-01103-8. Epub 2023 Mar 11. PMID: 36905552; PMCID: PMC10006570.

28. Morales DR, Lipworth BJ, Donnan PT, Jackson C, Guthrie B. Respiratory effect of beta-blockers in people with asthma and cardiovascular disease: population-based nested case control study. *BMC Med.* 2017 Jan 27;*15*(1):18. doi: 10.1186/s12916-017-0781-0. PMID: 28126029; PMCID: PMC5270217.

29. van Dam van Isselt EF, Groenewegen-Sipkema KH, Spruit-van Eijk M, et al. Pain in patients with COPD: a systematic review and meta-analysis. *BMJ Open* 2014;*4*:e005898. doi: 10.1136/bmjopen-2014-005898

30. Chiu YC, Hu HY, Lee FP, Huang HM. Tension-type headache associated with obstructive sleep apnea: a nationwide population-based study. J *Headache Pain.* 2015 Apr 21;*16*:34. doi: 10.1186/s10194-015-0517-5. PMID: 25896615; PMCID: PMC4408303.

31. Özge, A., Özge, C., Kaleagasi, H. et al. Headache in patients with chronic obstructive pulmonary disease: effects of chronic hypoxaemia. *J Headache Pain* 2006;*7*:37–43. https://doi.org/10.1007/s10194-006-0264-8

32. Minen MT, Weissman J, Tietjen GE. The relationship between migraine or severe headache and chronic health conditions: A cross-sectional study from the national health interview survey 2013-2015. *Pain Med.* 2019 Nov 1;*20*(11):2263–71. doi: 10.1093/pm/pnz113. PMID: 31127846; PMCID: PMC7963202.

33. Spałka J, Kędzia K, Kuczyński W, Kudrycka A, Małolepsza A, Białasiewicz P, Mokros Ł. Morning headache as an obstructive sleep apnea-related symptom among sleep clinic patients-a cross-section analysis. *Brain Sci.* 2020 Jan 19;*10*(1):57. doi: 10.3390/brainsci10010057. PMID: 31963788; PMCID: PMC7016602.

34. Park JW, Mehta S, Fastlicht S, Lowe AA, Almeida FR. Changes in headache characteristics with oral appliance treatment for obstructive sleep apnea. *Sci Rep.* 2021 Jan 28;*11*(1):2568. doi: 10.1038/s41598-021-82041-6. PMID: 33510288; PMCID: PMC7843638.

35. Agustí A, Celli BR, Criner GJ, Halpin D, Anzueto A, Barnes P, Bourbeau J, Han MK, Martinez FJ, Montes de Oca M, Mortimer K, Papi A, Pavord I, Roche N, Salvi S, Sin DD, Singh D, Stockley R, López Varela MV, Wedzicha JA, Vogelmeier CF. Global initiative for chronic obstructive lung disease 2023 report: GOLD executive summary. *Eur Respir J.* 2023 Apr 1;*61*(4):2300239. doi: 10.1183/13993003.00239-2023. PMID: 36858443; PMCID: PMC10066569.

36. Wei A, Gu Z, Li J, Liu X, Wu X, Han Y, Pu J. Clinical adverse effects of endothelin receptor antagonists: Insights from the meta-analysis of 4894 patients from 24 randomized double-blind placebo-controlled clinical trials. *J Am Heart Assoc*. 2016 Oct 26;5(11):e003896. doi: 10.1161/JAHA.116.003896. PMID: 27912207; PMCID: PMC5210319.

37. Johnson KG, Ziemba AM, Garb JL. Improvement in headaches with continuous positive airway pressure for obstructive sleep apnea: a retrospective analysis. *Headache*. 2013 Feb;53(2):333–43. doi: 10.1111/j.1526-4610.2012.02251.x. Epub 2012 Sep 10. PMID: 22963547.

Psychiatric Comorbidities in the Treatment of Headache

15

Sarah Erdelyan and Liza Smirnoff

LEARNING OBJECTIVES

1. Identify psychiatric comorbidities that commonly affect patients with headache disorders, learn common screening tools, and understand typical treatment strategies
2. Understand appropriate evaluation and management of headaches in a patient with significant psychiatric comorbidity
3. Learn the facets of multidisciplinary management for headache and psychiatric disorders

---

INTRODUCTION

In headache management, we often come across patients with comorbid psychiatric disorders who require thoughtful consideration in managing their headache disorder while not exacerbating their psychiatric illness and vice versa. In one population study of migraine, up to 47% of patients had comorbid depression, and 58% had comorbid anxiety.[1] In one study of new persistent daily headache (NDPH), 92% of participants met criteria for generalized anxiety disorder (GAD), and another 90% met criteria for depression.[2] Likewise, a study evaluating patients with bipolar disorder and schizophrenia showed a 23% prevalence of migraine in the bipolar group and 16% in the schizophrenia group.[3]

In patients with significant mental health disorders, management may be challenging due to delay in diagnosis from competing demands of the patient's comorbid psychiatric disorder, limited ability to fully elaborate on their comorbid disorder, the headache physician's comfort with treating the comorbid headache disorder in the patient with a significant psychiatric illness, or concerns for potential medication side effects, interactions, or possibility of worsening the comorbid psychiatric illness.

DOI: 10.1201/b23330-15

In both less severe and more significant psychiatric illnesses, migraine and other headache disorders are likely underrecognized and require more thorough attention and collaboration with the patient's other providers.

MOOD DISORDERS

Mood is defined as a pervasive and sustained feeling tone that is endured internally, and that impacts nearly all aspects of a person's behavior in the external world. Mood disorders or affective disorders are described by marked disruptions in emotions (severe lows called depression or highs called hypomania or mania). These are common psychiatric disorders leading to an increase in morbidity and mortality.[4] According to the *Diagnostic and Statistical Manual of Mental Disorders, Fifth Edition, Text Revision (DSM-5-TR)*, mood disorders have been broadly categorized as bipolar and related disorders and depressive disorders. Bipolar disorders are further categorized as bipolar I disorder, bipolar II disorder, cyclothymic disorder, bipolar and related disorder to another medical condition, substance/medication-induced bipolar and related disorder, other specified bipolar and related disorder, and unspecified bipolar and related disorder.[5]

Bipolar I disorder is defined as a syndrome in which a complete set of mania symptoms (elevated mood with three or more of the following symptoms: increased goal-directed activity, grandiosity, a diminished need for sleep, distractibility, racing thoughts, increased/pressured speech, and reckless behaviors) has occurred, lasting for at least one week or required hospitalization. If the mood is irritable instead of elevated, four or more of the aforementioned symptoms are needed to meet the criteria for a manic episode.

Bipolar II disorder consists of current or past major depressive episodes interspersed with current or past hypomanic periods of at least four days duration.

Cyclothymia is defined as a subthreshold bipolar trait or temperament with low-grade affective manifestations of the subthreshold major depression and mild hypomania. It is diagnosed in adults who experience at least two years of both hypomanic and depressive periods without ever meeting the criteria for mania, hypomania, or major depression. For a child or an adolescent to be diagnosed with cyclothymia, these episodes should last over one year.

Hypomania is defined as a nonpsychotic, milder, or subthreshold manic state of short duration lasting for at least four consecutive days and without marked social and occupational impairment. It requires elevated mood with (three or more symptoms) or irritable mood (with four or more of the following symptoms: increased goal-directed activity, grandiosity, a diminished need for sleep, distractibility, racing thoughts, increased/pressured speech, and reckless behaviors).

Major depressive disorder is diagnosed by the presence of five out of the nine symptoms of sad mood, insomnia, feelings of guilt, decreased energy levels, decreased concentration, decreased appetite, decrease in pleasurable activities (anhedonia), increased or decreased psychomotor activity, and recurrent suicidal ideation/acts of self-harm/suicide attempt existing over a period of two weeks.

A meta-analysis of data from 12 studies on migraine and depression found that the incidence of depression in patients with migraine is highly variable, ranging from 8.6% to 47.9%.[6] People with migraine are three times more likely to suffer from bipolar disorder or depression than the general population and vice versa.[7] Furthermore, a recent study using single nucleotide polymorphism (SNP) and gene-based analysis of genome-wide association study (GWAS) found significant overlap between migraine and major depressive disorder (MDD). This study suggested pathways of signaling and ion channel regulation to be involved in the pathophysiology of both disorders.[8]

Evaluation

Headaches, particularly migraine and chronic daily headaches, have high rates of comorbidity with psychiatric mood and anxiety disorders. There is evidence that mood or anxiety disorders have contributory roles in headache chronicity and refractoriness to treatment.[9] Pharmacological interventions targeting both headache and comorbid depressive or anxiety disorders can lead to better headache treatment outcomes. Such interventions are implemented within a comprehensive program of treatment that integrates treatment of the psychiatric disorder with behavioral, educational, and pharmacological headache treatments. Provisional guidelines have been proposed:[10]

- Headache patients should be screened for anxiety and depression due to high rates of comorbidity.
- When a screening instrument identifies a patient with a potential psychiatric diagnosis, the diagnosis should be confirmed according to valid and reliable diagnostic criteria.
- Treatment for a comorbid mood or anxiety disorder can include medication that has established dual efficacy for both the psychiatric disorder and the patient's type of headache to minimize polypharmacy.
- Mood or anxiety disorder medications can have side effects, including worsening of headache frequency or severity. Additionally, headache medications can potentially worsen mood or anxiety symptoms. Both should be monitored clinically.
- Adherence to treatment recommendations can be poor when headaches and mood or anxiety disorders are comorbid, emphasizing a need for patient education about both disorders.
- Clinicians should be sensitive and anticipate that a psychiatric diagnosis may carry potential stigma for patients and address these concerns in an empathetic and nonjudgmental manner.

A detailed longitudinal and in-depth family history, followed by a thorough mental status examination, is crucial for early diagnosis of mood disorders. Mood disorders secondary to substance abuse require a urine drug test. Specific rating scales are also available for the evaluation of mood disorders. Hamilton Rating Scale for Depression (HAM-D) and the Montgomery-Asberg Depression Rating Scale (MADRS) are for depression, and the Young Mania Rating Scale (YMRS) is for mania.[11]

HAM-D is a 17-item depression rating scale administered by the clinician. It rates depressed mood, sleep difficulties, the ability to concentrate, guilt, suicidality, anxiety symptoms, and somatic symptoms on a 3- or 5-point scale. A score of 0 to 7 is considered normal; a score of more than 20 needs intervention.

MADRS is a questionnaire administered by the clinician for the diagnosis of depression. It assesses sadness, inner tension, appetite, sleep, thoughts of self-harm, and suicide on a scale of 0 to 60. Scores between 0 to 6 are considered normal, 7 to 19 as mild depression, 20 to 34 as moderate depression, and a score of more than 34 is categorized as severe depression.

YMRS is a clinician-administered scale for mania. It is an 11-item scale with 4 items (irritability, speech, thought content, and disruptive behavior) graded on a 0 to 8 scale, and the remaining items (elevated mood, increase in motor activity, libido, sleep, appearance, and insight) are graded on a 0 to 4 scale. Scores less than 12 indicate remission, 13 to 25 as moderate, and 38 to 60 as severe mania.

Commonly used screening tools include the Patient Health Questionnaire (PHQ), which is a 3-page questionnaire that can be entirely self-administered by the patient.[12] The PHQ-9 is the nine-item depression module from the full PHQ. Major depression is diagnosed if five or more of the nine depressive symptom criteria have been present at least "more than half the days" in the past two weeks, and one of the symptoms is depressed mood or anhedonia. Other depression is diagnosed if two, three, or four depressive symptoms have been present at least "more than half the days" in the past two weeks, and one of the symptoms is depressed mood or anhedonia. One of the nine symptom criteria ("thoughts that you would be better off dead or of hurting yourself in some way") counts if present at all, regardless of duration.[13]

Medication Considerations

Selective serotonin reuptake inhibitors (SSRIs) and serotonin-norepinephrine reuptake inhibitors (SNRIs) are considered first-line treatments for depressive disorders.[14] A 2015 Cochrane Review looked at studies evaluating five SSRIs (citalopram, sertraline, fluoxetine, paroxetine, fluvoxamine) and one SNRI (venla-faxine) for efficacy in prevention of chronic tension-type headache but concluded that the use of SSRIs and venlafaxine for the prevention of chronic tension-type headache is not supported by evidence.[15] Venlafaxine is the only SNRI to have Level B evidence (probably effective and should be considered for migraine prevention) to support its use.[16]

Divalproex sodium, sodium valproate, topiramate, metoprolol, propranolol, and timolol are effective for migraine prevention and should be offered to patients with migraine to reduce migraine attack frequency and severity (Level A).[17] Despite widespread assertions that beta-blockers exacerbate or cause depression, a large review by the *Journal of American Medical Association* that looked at 45 years of trials showed that this does not appear to be true.[18] Divalproex sodium and sodium valproate are commonly used as mood-stabilizing medications and may be useful in managing comorbid psychiatric illness if appropriate.

The acute treatment of bipolar disorder often involves antipsychotic medications, such as olanzapine or quetiapine, and mood-stabilizing medications. Lithium has the strongest evidence for long-term relapse prevention and, notably, is also seen to be efficacious in the management of cluster headaches, as well as multiple other trigeminal autonomic cephalalgias.[19] The evidence for anticonvulsant mood-stabilizing medications such as divalproex and lamotrigine is less robust.[20]

Tricyclic antidepressants, or TCAs, such as amitriptyline, are often also used for migraine prophy-laxis. While these medications can also be effective treatments for depression, the doses needed for treat-ment of depressive disorders are typically much higher than those used for migraine prophylaxis. Therapeutic doses generally range from 100 to 300 mg per day, but some patients find it difficult to reach these doses due to sedation and other common side effects such as dry mouth, constipation, and dizzi-ness.[21] Caution should be exercised in administering antidepressants such as SSRIs, SNRIs, and TCAs to patients with bipolar disorder, as they are associated with an increased risk of hypomania or mania.[22]

In 2006, the US Food and Drug Administration (FDA) issued an alert regarding a potential risk of developing serotonin toxicity as a result of concomitant use of SSRI or SNRI antidepressants with triptans. Since then, the literature has been largely critical of the FDA's position. Subsequent analyses of the case reports on which the FDA alert was based have found that a number of them did not actually meet diag-nostic criteria for serotonin toxicity. A position paper from the American Headache Society in 2010 found that the quality of evidence supporting the FDA's recommendation was poor and that there was insufficient evidence to support limiting the dual prescription of SSRIs/SNRIs and triptans.[23]

Antidepressant Medications and Sexual Function

A commonly reported complaint among patients taking antidepressant medications is sexual dysfunction, defined as a disruption in one of the three sequential aspects of the normal sexual response cycle: sexual desire, arousal (including clitoral engorgement and lubrication in women and erectile function in men), and orgasm. Studies vary greatly in the prevalence of sexual side effects in patients taking antidepres-sant medications, with some reporting up to 80% of patients taking an antidepressant with a serotonergic mechanism potentially affected.[24] This is further complicated by patients' tendency to underreport these symptoms unless directly and specifically asked by the treating clinician and by the fact that sexual dys-function can often be associated with mood and anxiety disorders even when untreated.

Medication-induced sexual dysfunction is a potentially distressing adverse effect of antidepressants and a leading cause of medication nonadherence. Sexual function should be actively assessed at baseline, at regular intervals during treatment, and after treatment cessation. Trials comparing the risk of sexual dysfunction with individual antidepressants are inadequate, but it is reasonable to conclude that the risk is greatest with antidepressant medications, which are strongly selective for serotonin. This includes SSRIs and SNRIs, and it occurs less commonly with tricyclic antidepressants (except clomipramine) and mir-tazapine, and least with bupropion.[25] Managing sexual dysfunction attributable to these agents requires a patient-centered, individualized approach, which may include switching agents, dosage adjustments, aug-menting agents (bupropion is commonly used and showed favorable evidence, at a starting dose of 150mg, though clinicians should be aware that adding bupropion may worsen anxiety levels in some patients[26]), and nonpharmacological treatments, such as cognitive behavioral therapy (CBT).

ANXIETY DISORDERS

Anxiety disorders (GAD, social anxiety disorder, panic disorder, specific phobia, and others) are the most prevalent psychiatric disorders and are associated with a high burden of illness. Anxiety disorders are often underrecognized and undertreated in primary care. Treatment is indicated when a patient shows marked distress or suffers from complications resulting from the disorder.[27]

More than 50% of patients with migraine will meet the criteria for at least one anxiety disorder in their lifetime. Anxiety disorders are two to five times more prevalent in patients with migraine than in the general population and up to two times more common in patients with migraine than in patients with depression.[28] Notably, migraine pain can contribute to anxiety due to severity, unpredictability, and uncontrollable occurrences, which can all lead to catastrophizing, despair, and compounded disability.[29]

Evaluation

The Generalized Anxiety Disorder (GAD-7) Questionnaire is a seven-item, self-report anxiety questionnaire designed to assess the patient's health status during the previous two weeks. The items inquire about the degree to which the patient has been bothered by feeling nervous, anxious, or on edge, not being able to stop or control worrying, worrying too much about different things, having trouble relaxing, being so restless that it is hard to sit still, becoming easily annoyed or irritable and feeling afraid as if something might happen.[30]

Medication Considerations

SSRIs and SNRIs are the preferred initial pharmacotherapy in the treatment of GAD. SSRIs such as sertraline and escitalopram have been shown to be effective in the treatment of anxiety symptoms associated with GAD. SSRIs and SNRIs have less propensity to cause sedation or cognitive side effects than other antidepressant options (e.g., TCAs) and less risk of dependence than benzodiazepines.[31]

NEURODEVELOPMENTAL DISORDERS

Autism

Autism spectrum disorder (ASD) is a complex neurobehavioral and neurodevelopmental condition characterized by difficulties in social interaction and communication; restricted and repetitive patterns of behavior, interests, and activities; and altered sensory processing.[32]

Though autism and migraine are common neurological conditions, there are few studies that examine comorbidity and implications for treatment. These studies, despite small sample sizes, indicate a high rate of migraine symptomatology in patients with ASD. Individuals with autism frequently have altered pain sensitivity that could distort their perception of headaches. There is also concern that social expression related to pain in autism (facial expression changes, verbal activity, posture, movement, and behavior) could be impaired, leading to potential underrecognition or reporting of pain. For example, in certain patients, head banging or repetitive self-soothing movements could indicate ongoing migrainosus or other headache pain. Caregivers should be encouraged to keep headache diaries, including propensity to headache symptoms such as nausea, which could be displayed as a lack of interest in food or in vomiting; photophobia, which may present as avoidance of light; or phonophobia, with patients often covering their ears.

Autism and migraine share common pathophysiological changes, including dysregulation of neurotransmission, especially within the serotoninergic system. Both autism and migraine are characterized by serotonergic abnormalities and by a hyperexcitable cortex.[33] However, ASD is characterized by insufficient or excessive serotonin signaling, which may suggest a bidirectional serotonin involvement.[34] Research supports that both conditions share an altered immune response causing neurogenic neuroinflammation, abnormal findings, especially in the cortical minicolumn organization and in the dysfunctional gut–brain axis, and shared susceptibility genes.[35] Treatment should focus on symptoms reported by the patient and caregiver, if applicable, with headache diaries, including nonverbal symptom cues.

Attention Deficit Hyperactivity Disorder

There is limited research available on the association of headache and attention deficit hyperactivity disorder (ADHD) or on the effects of ADHD medications in childhood. In 2022, the first systematic review and meta-analysis on the association between headache and ADHD was published by Pan et al. The results indicated that pediatric patients with ADHD have a doubled risk compared to those without ADHD to experience headaches, with a pooled prevalence of 26.6%.[36] Short-term randomized control trials of ADHD medications showed an increased risk of headache with atomoxetine, guanfacine, and methylphenidate compared to placebo. No statistically significant associations of headache with amphetamine, bupropion, clonidine, or modafinil were found, but it must be noted that these studies have been very limited. It is considered premature to draw conclusions about ADHD medication's effects on headaches at this stage, and further research is warranted.

OBSESSIVE-COMPULSIVE AND RELATED DISORDERS

Obsessive-compulsive disorder (OCD) is characterized by the presence of obsessions or compulsions, or commonly of both. OCD is the fourth most common mental disorder after depression, alcohol/substance misuse, and social phobia, with a lifetime prevalence in the community of 1.6%.[37]

Evaluation

Obsessive-compulsive symptom severity levels are most commonly defined by the Yale-Brown Obsessive-Compulsive Scale (Y-BOCS), a widely used clinician-administered measure that assesses the severity of obsessive-compulsive symptoms over the past week. The ten items that comprise the Y-BOCS Severity Scale assess time occupied, associated distress, impairment, resistance, and control of obsessions and compulsions.[38]

Medication Considerations

Epidemiological studies indicate that psychiatric comorbidities can be a risk factor for the evolution of episodic headache into chronic headache.[39] Moreover, the presence of poorly controlled psychiatric symptoms appears to predict relapse and poor response to treatment, favoring the persistence of medication-overuse headache (MOH) and complicating headache management.[40] MOH is defined as headache lasting ≥15 days per month for more than 3 months and is due to a regular overuse of symptomatic drugs (≥10–15 days per month).[41]

There is a higher prevalence of psychiatric comorbidity (anxiety and mood disorders) in the group of patients with MOH compared with controls, episodic migraine, and chronic migraine. Among anxiety disorders, there is a higher prevalence of subclinical OCD in MOH.[42] Patients who are highly dependent on medication and display drug-seeking behaviors share the compulsive quality of this behavior with OCD. Involvement of the striato-thalamo-orbitofrontal circuit has been postulated for both OCD and drug-seeking behaviors.[42]

It has been hypothesized that certain behaviors and psychological states (i.e., fear of headache, anticipatory anxiety, obsessive drug-taking behaviors, and psychological drug dependence) are particularly important in prompting and sustaining the overuse of headache medication.[43]

There is limited research on using nondrug coping skills to address MOH. Behavioral treatments require patient investment in learning and practicing, and some patients may be disheartened when they are not sensing an immediate reduction in headache sensation as is associated with a triptan, ergot, or analgesic. However, patients undergoing biofeedback and behavioral therapy can learn to restructure their cognitive approach to pain, tolerate discomfort, reduce pain-related emotional distress, stop overly frequent pharmacological preemptive treatment of an impending headache, and reduce limbic escalation of the pain experience. If reinforced and maintained over time, learning these behavioral skills can help reduce dependency or overuse of pain medication and MOH relapse and should be considered in addition to pharmacological measures.[44]

PERSONALITY DISORDERS

Personality disorders affect roughly 10% of the general population[45] and represent enduring patterns of inflexible behavior that present in adolescence or young adulthood, cause clinically significant impairment, and are typically refractory to standard pharmacologic and behavioral interventions. The *Diagnostic and Statistical Manual of Mental Disorders, 5th edition (DSM-5)* lists ten personality disorders that are divided into three clusters, clusters A, B, and C.

Limited studies have investigated the relationship between headache and personality disorders. One study found that 26% of inpatients with chronic daily headache have been diagnosed with a personality disorder, most commonly the cluster B personality disorders, which include borderline, antisocial, narcissistic, and histrionic personality disorders.[46]

Existing literature has primarily focused on the comorbidity of chronic headache and borderline personality disorder (BPD). Over half of BPD patients report symptoms consistent with migraine.[47] BPD is a cluster B disorder that is characterized by hypersensitivity to rejection and resulting instability of interpersonal relationships, self-image, affect, and behavior.[48] Additional studies show that avoidant personality disorder and obsessive-compulsive personality disorder are also associated with headache.

Studies have indicated an association between BPD and female gender, more pervasive headache, greater migraine-related disability, a higher prevalence of MOH, more unscheduled visits for acute headache treatment, a higher prevalence of moderate-to-severe depression, and a lower likelihood of responding to pharmacologic treatment intended for migraine prophylaxis.[49]

When BPD is present, the treating clinician should consider referring the patient for psychiatric comanagement; psychotherapy combined with psychopharmacologic treatment may impact BPD positively and may as a result impact headache management.[50, 51] Clinically, setting consistent limits is essential to avoid iatrogenic harm and to encourage the learning of coping skills that help these patients better tolerate distress and increase their capacity for self-regulation.[52]

POST-TRAUMATIC STRESS DISORDER

Post-traumatic stress disorder (PTSD) is a prevalent disorder that adversely affects 6.1 to 8.3% of US adults. Rates of PTSD are higher among veterans and others whose vocation increases the risk of traumatic exposures (e.g., police, firefighters, emergency medical personnel).[52] The *DSM-5-TR* requires that a person experience or witness a major traumatic event (exposure to actual or threatened death, serious injury, or sexual violence) (Criterion A). After experiencing or witnessing such an event, four symptom clusters become present. First, one needs to have at least one of the following reexperiencing symptoms: intrusive distressing memories, recurrent distressing dreams, dissociative reactions (e.g., flashbacks), intense or prolonged psychological distress at exposure to reminders of the trauma, marked physiological reactions to internal or external cues symbolizing or resembling an aspect of the traumatic event (Criterion B).

Second, one is required to have active avoidance of internal (e.g., thoughts, memories) and/or external (e.g., situations, conversations) reminders of the trauma (Criterion C).

Third, at least two "alterations in cognitions and mood" symptoms are needed, including inability to remember an important aspect of the traumatic event, persistent and exaggerated negative thoughts about oneself or the world, persistent distorted cognitions about the cause or consequences of the event, pervasive negative emotions, markedly diminished interest, feeling detached or estranged from others, persistent inability to experience positive emotions (Criterion D).

Finally, one has to present at least two of the following arousal symptoms: irritable behavior and angry outbursts, reckless or self-destructive behavior, hypervigilance, exaggerated startle response, problems with concentration, or sleep disturbance (Criterion E). Symptoms must be present for more than one month after trauma exposure to make the diagnosis of PTSD in order to minimize the pathologizing of normal stress reactions. When these symptoms are present between three days and up to a month in duration (but not longer than one month), the *DSM* defines this as acute stress disorder.[53]

Evaluation

Although there are many self-reporting instruments for assessing PTSD, the PCL is the most widely used self-reporting instrument used in research and clinical settings for the assessment of PTSD. There are three versions of the PCL: the PCL-C (civilian version, referring to "stressful experiences"), the PCL-M (military version, referring to "stressful military experiences"), and the PCL-S (specific version, referring to a specific identified "stressful experience"). Because it is framed most generally, the PCL-C has been the most widely used form of the PCL, even in military or Veterans Administration settings.[54]

Medication Considerations

The neurobiological mechanism by which PTSD is associated with migraine is not known. However, of those with episodic migraine and PTSD, 69% reported symptoms related to PTSD before the onset of severe or frequent headache.[55] Hypotheses for the possible mechanisms contributing to the PTSD–migraine association include dysfunction of the autonomic system and the hypothalamic-pituitary-adrenal (HPA) axis. Serotonin and norepinephrine levels have been demonstrated to be lower in both those with PTSD and those with migraine, which may support the presence of sympathetic dysfunction.[56]

Diagnosis of PTSD in patients with migraine is intrinsically linked to management of migraine, considering that treating PTSD alone can improve the sense of well-being and significantly reduce pain and disability in patients with migraine.[57] Controlling the amount of stress may be crucial for headache management as migraine may also be associated with a dysfunctional coping style.[58] CBT is increasingly considered a fundamental part of migraine management. The aim of this treatment approach is to change dysfunctional behaviors that are significantly involved in maintaining depression and anxiety and involve the practice of stress management and coping techniques. The highest benefits of CBT are observed when combined with pharmacological treatment.[59]

Only two medications are currently approved by the US FDA for the treatment of PTSD: paroxetine and sertraline—both belonging to the same class of SSRIs.[60]

PSYCHOTIC DISORDERS

The psychotic disorders are defined by clinical syndromes rather than diseases and are distinguished from one another mainly by duration (e.g., ≥6 months for symptoms of schizophrenia and <1 month for a brief psychotic disorder), by symptom profile (e.g., various psychotic symptoms in schizophrenia and only delusions in delusional disorder), by the relationship between psychotic symptoms and episodes of disturbed mood (i.e., whether the psychotic symptoms occur during, or extend beyond, a mood disturbance, as seen in schizoaffective disorder), and by cause (i.e., whether psychotic symptoms are due to the use of such substances as stimulants or hallucinogens, or to medical conditions that affect the brain, such as epilepsy, autoimmune diseases, tumors, or dementias). In the current clinical nomenclature, "psychotic symptom" refers to the demonstration of cognitive or perceptual dysfunction, mainly delusions or hallucinations, whereas "psychotic disorder" refers to a condition in which psychotic symptoms meet specific diagnostic criteria for a disease.[61]

The key symptoms of schizophrenia include positive psychotic symptoms (i.e., delusions, hallucinations, disorganized thoughts, or disorganized/catatonic behavior) and negative symptoms, including avolition (diminished self-initiated activities); alogia (decreased speech output); anhedonia (reduced ability to experience pleasure); and asociality (a lack of interest in social interactions).[62]

Evaluation

The Positive and Negative Syndrome Scale (PANSS; Kay et al., 1987) was developed in order to provide a well-defined instrument to specifically assess both positive and negative symptoms of schizophrenia as well as general psychopathology. Eighteen items of the Brief Psychiatric Rating Scale (Overall and Gorham, 1962) and 12 items of the Psychopathology Rating Schedule (Singh and Kay, 1975) were combined in one scale, and all items were given a complete definition, as well as detailed anchoring criteria for all rating points. Strong psychometric properties in terms of reliability, validity, and sensitivity have been shown in a number of subsequent studies.[63]

Medication Considerations

Antipsychotic treatment of migraines is supported by the theory that dopaminergic hyperactivity leads to migraine. Antipsychotics have been used off-label in migraine patients who do not tolerate triptans or have status migrainosus—intense, debilitating migraine lasting >72 hours.[64] There is intermediate strength evidence for using chlorpromazine, droperidol, and prochlorperazine in migraine treatment. There is weak evidence in support of using haloperidol and very weak evidence for aripiprazole, olanzapine, quetiapine, and ziprasidone. In the treatment of cluster headache, there is weak evidence for the use of chlorpromazine and very weak evidence favoring clozapine or olanzapine. In migraine, patients are thought to be hypersensitive to dopamine agonists or dopamine transporter dysfunction. There is some evidence that the dopamine D2 (DRD2) gene is involved. In cluster headache, pain alleviation is possibly related to dopamine receptor antagonism.[65]

Clinical Case

A 64-year-old woman with a past history of diabetes, hypertension, and schizoaffective disorder complicated by tardive dyskinesia presents with a 40-year history of headaches. She reports typically unilateral, throbbing headaches, which last for seven to ten hours, are associated with significant nausea and sometimes vomiting, and photophobia. Headaches currently occur at 12 days per month. Her current medications include lithium, tetrabenazine, bupropion, and losartan. Diabetes is currently managed with diet and exercise. Due to prior difficulties with self-care, the patient has not had prior management for her headaches. What treatment recommendations should be made for this patient's headaches?

Answer: Based on the *International Classification of Headache Disorders, 3rd Edition* criteria, this patient meets the criteria for migraine, given throbbing unilateral headache lasting 4–72 hours, with associated nausea/vomiting and photophobia.[66] Although red flags cannot be clearly ruled out in this case, the history of headaches lasting for the past 40 years in similar phenotypes is reassuring. Additionally, given the patient's high headache frequency, there is concern for chronification or chronic migraine, so the patient should be started on preventive therapy.[67] In considering common preventive therapies for migraine, for antiseizure medications, valproate and topiramate may not be appropriate, as valproate may interact with her lithium, and topiramate is known to affect mood negatively, which may not be appropriate in this patient. Antihypertensives such as propranolol or verapamil may be appropriate, but blood pressure and heart rate should be evaluated. Notably, verapamil may increase lithium toxicity, so lithium levels should be monitored closely while on this medication.[68] In terms of antidepressants, any use of TCA's or SNRI's should be discussed with the patient's psychiatrist and may not be safe in a patient with known schizoaffective disorder given the possibility of provoking a manic episode. In terms of newer preventive therapies, calcitonin gene-related peptide (CGRP) antagonists and monoclonal antibodies are appropriate choices and could be considered in this patient. OnabotulinumA likewise may be an appropriate choice if the patient meets criteria for chronic migraine.

In terms of migraine abortive therapy, given the patient's known history of diabetes and hypertension, triptans can be appropriate for use but should be avoided in patients with uncontrolled hypertension or additional vascular risk factors. CGRP antagonists or selective serotonin blockers such as lasmiditan would be a safe option for this patient.[69] Given her known history of tardive dyskinesia, dopamine antagonists such as metoclopramide should not be used.

SUBSTANCE-USE DISORDERS

The essential feature of a substance-use disorder is a cluster of cognitive, behavioral, and physiological symptoms indicating that the individual continues using the substance despite significant substance-related problems. An important characteristic of substance-use disorders is an underlying change in brain circuitry that may persist beyond detoxification, particularly in individuals with severe disorders. Diagnostic criteria are organized into groupings of impaired control, social impairment, risky use, and pharmacologic criteria (e.g., tolerance and withdrawal).[70]

One study found that migraines were clearly more pronounced in patients using benzodiazepines, methylamphetamine, cocaine, heroin, and volatile solvents than in those taking cannabis and alcohol. It was also observed that the chronic use of cocaine influenced the evolution and symptomatology of MOH.

This suggests that more frequent presence of MOHs headaches could be associated with a motivation to self-medicate and an attempt to use analgesics compulsively as a result of a pattern of addictive behavior in this population.[71]

Substance abuse is associated with a variety of neurological complications, including headache.[72] There is no single, unifying, etiologic explanation for abuse and substance-use headache in patients who normally suffer from primary headache, such as migraine. Nonmigrainous headaches are not well represented in the literature in this population, so insight into their etiology is limited. It is likely that at least some substance-use headaches represent direct, chemically mediated irritative effects on trigeminal afferents, whereas others might act as triggers that produce excitation of cortical neurons and cause withdrawal of descending sensory inhibition originating in the brainstem.[73] Nonetheless, these hypotheses require further investigation (Table 15.1).

Motivational interviewing (MI) is a "collaborative conversation style for strengthening a person's own motivation and commitment to change."[74] Alternatively, it is defined as "a psychotherapeutic method commonly used for helping clients resolve ambivalence about changing problem behaviors."[75] MI comprises two principal components: MI spirit, a relational component, is described as a nonjudgmental, collaborative, evoking of the patient's perspectives and a guiding style supportive of autonomy that uses open questions and reflections. The technical component also employs open questions and reflective listening aimed at encouraging specific patient statements that are arguments for change in negative or self-destructive behaviors, known as "change talk." MI-training approaches have improved such that clinicians may want to consider MI training as a way to support their patients more effectively as they address behavioral health-related problems (e.g., tobacco use, drug use, other unhealthy behaviors).[76]

TABLE 15.1   Commonly prescribed medications for headache and psychiatric use

TREATMENT	PSYCHIATRIC COMORBIDITY USE	HEADACHE PREVENTION EFFECTIVENESS[77]
TCAs, e.g., amitriptyline	Effective for depression at high doses (but more likelihood of intolerable side effects)[78]	Effective for migraine prevention at low doses, with minimal side effects
SNRIs, e.g., venlafaxine	Effective for depression. Venlafaxine FDA approved for MDD, GAD, panic disorder, and social phobia. Duloxetine FDA approved for MDD and GAD[79]	Only venlafaxine has grade B evidence of efficacy for migraine prevention. Most recent Cochrane study did not find venlafaxine to be more effective than placebo for prevention of chronic migraines
SSRIs, e.g., sertraline	Effective for depression, anxiety, OCD, PTSD, bulimia nervosa, panic disorder, social anxiety disorder, premenstrual dysphoric disorder. Many off-label uses[79]	According to the Cochrane review, SSRIs were not better than placebo for migraine prevention
β-blockers, e.g., propranolol	May help with anxiety; there is some conflicting research about possible depressive symptoms. Also used to treat akathisia from neuroleptics[80]	Effective for migraine prevention
Anticonvulsants		
Topiramate	May help with mood stabilization but worsen depression	Effective for migraine prevention
Divalproex sodium	Used for mood stabilization, bipolar disorder	Effective for migraine prevention
Carbamazepine and oxcarbazepine	Used for mood stabilization, bipolar disorder	Effective for trigeminal neuralgia pain[81, 82]

CONCLUSIONS

Psychiatric comorbidities, particularly mood and anxiety disorders, are common in patients with headache disorders. Their management is imperative for the overall health of the patient and clinically often impacts the outcome of headache management. A multidisciplinary approach, including the physician treating the headaches, the psychiatrist, and/or psychologist, is important for best outcomes for these patients. In patients with more severe psychiatric illnesses where verbal communication is impaired, physical clues such as holding the head, other signs of distress, and avoidance of sensory stimuli can all cue the physician into the presence of headache. Forming therapeutic alliances with caregivers, when present, is also essential to the management of these patients.

Key Takeaways:

- Implement routine basic screenings for psychiatric conditions given high comorbidity with headache diagnoses.
- Treatment can incorporate medications with dual efficacy for both the psychiatric disorder and the patient's type of headache to minimize polypharmacy.
- Headache diaries in patients with significant autism or other cognitive disorders should focus on nonverbal cues such as head banging, covering ears, or food avoidance.
- In patients with substance abuse disorders, medication overuse may be particularly difficult to manage and requires a multidisciplinary approach.
- Nonpharmacologic treatment interventions (psychotherapy referrals, instruction on nondrug coping skills, MI) are an important consideration in a general approach to many comorbid psychiatric and headache diagnoses.

REFERENCES

1. Minen MT et al. Migraine and Its Psychiatric Comorbidities. *Journal of Neurology, Neurosurgery and Psychiatry* 2016;*87*(7):741–749.
2. Uniyal R, Paliwal VK, and Tripathi A. Psychiatric Comorbidity in New Daily Persistent Headache: A Cross-sectional Study. *Eur J Pain* 2017;*21*(6):1031–1038. Web.
3. ElGizy N et al. Migraine in Bipolar Disorder and Schizophrenia; The Hidden Pain. *Int J Psychiatry Med* 2023:912174231178483–. Print.
4. Sekhon S, Gupta V. Mood Disorder. [Updated 2023 May 8]. In: StatPearls [Internet]. Treasure Island (FL): StatPearls Publishing; 2023 Jan-. Available from: https://www.ncbi.nlm.nih.gov/books/NBK558911/#
5. American Psychiatric Association. (2022). Bipolar and Related Disorders. In *Diagnostic and statistical manual of mental disorders* (5th ed., text rev.).
6. Antonaci F, Nappi G, Galli F, et al. Migraine and psychiatric comorbidity: a review of clinical findings. *J Headache Pain* 2011;*12*:115–25.
7. Bahrami S, Hindley G, Winsvold BS, O'Connell KS, Frei O, Shadrin A, Cheng W, Bettella F, Rødevand L, Odegaard KJ, Fan CC, Pirinen MJ, Hautakangas HM, HUNT All-In Headache, Dale AM, Djurovic S, Smeland OB, Andreassen OA. Dissecting the shared genetic basis of migraine and mental disorders using novel statistical tools. *Brain*. 2022 Mar 29;*145*(1):142–153. doi: 10.1093/brain/awab267. PMID: 34273149; PMCID: PMC8967089.
8. Yang Y et al. Molecular Genetic Overlap Between Migraine and Major Depressive Disorder. *European Journal of Human Genetics: EJHG* 2018;*26*(8):1202–1216. Web.

9. Lake AE, Rains JC, Penzien DB, Lipchik GL. Headache and psychiatric comorbidity: Historical context, clinical implications, and research relevance. *Headache* 2005:*45*:493–506.

10. Griffith JL and Razavi M (2006), Pharmacological Management of Mood and Anxiety Disorders in Headache Patients. *Headache: The Journal of Head and Face Pain*, *46*:S133–S141. https://doi.org/10.1111/j.1526-4610.2006.00564.x

11. Furukawa TA. Assessment of mood: guides for clinicians. *J Psychosom Res* 2010 Jun;*68*(6):581–9.

12. Spitzer RL, Kroenke K, Williams JBW. Patient Health Questionnaire Study Group. Validity and utility of a self-report version of PRIME-MD: the PHQ Primary Care Study. *JAMA* 1999;*282*:1737–44.

13. Kroenke K, Spitzer RL, Williams JB. The PHQ-9: validity of a brief depression severity measure. *J Gen Intern Med* 2001 Sep;*16*(9):606–13. doi: 10.1046/j.1525-1497.2001.016009606.x. PMID: 11556941; PMCID: PMC1495268.

14. Dale E, Bang-Andersen B, Sánchez C. Emerging mechanisms and treatments for depression beyond SSRIs and SNRIs. *Biochem Pharmacol* 2015 May 15;*95*(2):81–97. doi: 10.1016/j.bcp.2015.03.011. Epub 2015 Mar 24. PMID: 25813654.

15. Banzi R, Cusi C, Randazzo C, Sterzi R, Tedesco D, Moja L. Selective serotonin reuptake inhibitors (SSRIs) and serotonin-norepinephrine reuptake inhibitors (SNRIs) for the prevention of tension-type headache in adults. *Cochrane Database Syst Rev* 2015(5);CD011681. DOI: 10.1002/14651858.CD011681.

16. Silberstein SD, Holland S, Freitag F, Dodick DW, Argoff C, Ashman E. Quality Standards Subcommittee of the American Academy of Neurology and the American Headache Society. Evidence-based guideline update: pharmacologic treatment for episodic migraine prevention in adults: report of the Quality Standards Subcommittee of the American Academy of Neurology and the American Headache Society. *Neurology* 2012 Apr 24;*78*(17):1337–45. doi: 10.1212/WNL.0b013e3182535d20. Erratum in: Neurology. 2013 Feb 26;80(9):871. PMID: 22529202; PMCID: PMC3335452.

17. Silberstein SD, Holland S, Freitag F, Dodick DW, Argoff C, Ashman E. *Neurology* 2012 Apr:*78*(17):1337–1345; DOI: 10.1212/WNL.0b013e3182535d20

18. Ko DT, Hebert PR, Coffee CS, et al. Beta-blocker therapy and symptoms of depression, fatigue, and sexual dysfunction. *JAMA* 2002;*288*:351–7.

19. Steiner, TJ et al. Double-Blind Placebo-Controlled Trial of Lithium in Episodic Cluster Headache. *Cephalalgia* 1997:*17*(6):673–675.

20. Geddes JR, Miklowitz DJ. Treatment of bipolar disorder. *Lancet* 2013 May 11;*381*(9878):1672–82. doi: 10.1016/S0140-6736(13)60857-0. PMID: 23663953; PMCID: PMC3876031.

21. Nelson JC. Tricyclic and tetracyclic drugs. In: *The American Psychiatric Association Publishing Textbook of Psychopharmacology*, Fifth Edition, Schatzberg AF, Nemeroff CB (Eds), American Psychiatric Association Publishing, Arlington, VA 2017. p. 305.

22. Tondo L, Vázquez G, Baldessarini RJ. Mania associated with antidepressant treatment: comprehensive meta-analytic review. *Acta Psychiatr Scand* 2010;*121*:404–414.

23. Jin G, Stokes P. Drug interaction between a selective serotonin reuptake inhibitor and a triptan leading to serotonin toxicity: a case report and review of the literature. *J Med Case Rep* 2021 Jul 26;*15*(1):371. doi: 10.1186/s13256-021-02946-8. PMID: 34304734; PMCID: PMC8311984.

24. Serretti A, Chiesa A. Treatment-Emergent Sexual Dysfunction Related to Antidepressants: A Meta-Analysis. *J Clin Psychopharmacol* 2009 June:*29*(3):259–266. I DOI: 10.1097/JCP.0b013e3181a5233f

25. Rothmore J. Antidepressant-induced sexual dysfunction. *Med J Aust* 2020 Apr;*212*(7):329–334. doi: 10.5694/mja2.50522. Epub 2020 Mar 15. PMID: 32172535.

26. Montejo AL, Prieto N, de Alarcón R, Casado-Espada N, et al. Management Strategies for Antidepressant-Related Sexual Dysfunction: A Clinical Approach. *J Clin Med.* 2019 Oct 7;*8*(10):1640. doi: 10.3390/jcm8101640. PMID: 31591339; PMCID: PMC6832699.

27. Bandelow B, Michaelis S & Wedekind D. Treatment of anxiety disorders, *Dialogues Clin Neurosci*, 2017:*19*(2), 93–107. DOI: 10.31887/DCNS.2017.19.2/bbandelow

28. Breslau N. Psychiatric comorbidity in migraine. *Cephalalgia* 1998;*18*(Suppl 22):56–8; discussion 58–61.

29. Fuller-Thomson E, Jayanthikumar J, Agbeyaka S. Untangling the Association Between Migraine, Pain, and Anxiety: Examining Migraine and Generalized Anxiety Disorders in a Canadian Population Based Study. *Headache* 2017;*57*(3): 375–390.

30. Williams N, The GAD-7 questionnaire, *Occup Med*, 2014 April:*64*(3):224, https://doi.org/10.1093/occmed/kqt161

31. Slee A, Nazareth I, Bondaronek P, et al. Pharmacological treatments for generalised anxiety disorder: a systematic review and network meta-analysis. *Lancet* 2019 Feb 23;*393*(10173):768–777. doi: 10.1016/S0140-6736(18)31793-8. Epub 2019 Jan 31. Erratum in: Lancet. 2019 Apr 27;393(10182):1698. PMID: 30712879.

32. American Psychiatric Association. (2022). *Diagnostic and statistical manual of mental disorders* (5th ed., text rev.). https://doi.org/10.1176/appi.books.9780890425787

33. Aggarwal M, Puri V, Puri S. Serotonin and CGRP in migraine. *Ann Neurosci* 2012;*19*:88–94. doi: 10.5214/ans.0972.7531.12190210.

34. Vetri L. Autism and Migraine: An Unexplored Association? *Brain Sci* 2020 Sep 6;*10*(9):615. doi: 10.3390/brainsci10090615. PMID: 32899972; PMCID: PMC7565535.

35. Vetri L. Autism and migraine: An unexplored association?. *Brain Sci*, 2020:*10*(9):615.

36. Pan P, Jonsson U, Şahpazoğlu Çakmak S, et al. Headache in ADHD as comorbidity and a side effect of medications: A systematic review and meta-analysis. *Psychol Med*, 2022:*52*(1):14–25. doi:10.1017/S0033291721004141

37. Kessler RC, Berglund P, Demler O, et al. Lifetime prevalence and age-of-onset distributions of DSM-IV disorders in the National Comorbidity Survey Replication. *Arch Gen Psychiatry* 2005;*62*:593–602.

38. Goodman WK, et al. The Yale-Brown Obsessive Compulsive Scale. I. Development, use, and reliability. *Arch Gen Psychiatry* 1989;*46*(11):1006–1011.

39. Radat F, Creac'h C, Swendsen JD, et al. Psychiatric comorbidity in the evolution from migraine to medication overuse headache. *Cephalalgia* 2005;*25*:519–522.

40. Migliore S, Paolucci M, Quintiliani L, et al. Psychopathological Comorbidities and Clinical Variables in Patients With Medication Overuse Headache. *Front Hum Neurosci* 2020 Nov 27;*14*:571035. doi: 10.3389/fnhum.2020.571035. PMID: 33328928; PMCID: PMC7728851.

41. Headache Classification Committee of the International Headache Society (IHS). The International Classification of Headache Disorders, 3rd edition (beta version). *Cephalalgia* 2013;*33*:629–808

42. Cupini LM, De Murtas M, Costa C, et al. Obsessive-compulsive disorder and migraine with medication-overuse headache. *Headache* 2009 Jul;*49*(7):1005–13. doi: 10.1111/j.1526-4610.2009.01457.x. Epub 2009 Jun 1. PMID: 19496831.

43. Ibid.

44. Saper JR, Hamel RL, Lake AE III. Medication overuse headache (MOH) is a biobehavioral disorder. *Cephalalgia* 2005;*25*:545–546.

45. Lake AE 3rd. Medication overuse headache: biobehavioral issues and solutions. *Headache*. 2006 Oct;*46* Suppl 3:S88–97. doi: 10.1111/j.1526-4610.2006.00560.x. PMID: 17034403.

46. Lenzenweger MF. Epidemiology of personality disorders. *Psychiatr Clin North Am* 2008:*31*:395–403.

47. Lake AE, Saper JR, Hamel RL Comprehensive inpatient treatment of refractory chronic daily headache. *Headache* 2009;*49*:555–562.

48. Hegarty AM. The prevalence of migraine in borderline personality disorder. *Headache* 1993;*33*:271.

49. Chapman J, Jamil RT, Fleisher C. Borderline Personality Disorder. [Updated 2023 Jun 2]. In: StatPearls [Internet]. Treasure Island (FL): StatPearls Publishing; 2023 Jan-. Available from: https://www.ncbi.nlm.nih.gov/books/NBK430883/

50. Rothrock J, Lopez I, Zweilfer R, Andress-Rothrock D, Drinkard R, Walters N. Borderline personality disorder and migraine. *Headache* 2007 Jan;*47*(1):22–6. doi: 10.1111/j.1526-4610.2007.00649.x. PMID: 17355490.

51. Linehan MM. Combining pharmacotherapy with psychotherapy for substance abusers with borderline personality disorder: Strategies for enhancing compliance. *NIDA Res Monogr* 1995:*150*:129–142.

52. Davis RE, Smitherman TA, Baskin, SM. Personality traits, personality disorders, and migraine: a review. *Neurol* Sci 2013:*34*(Suppl 1):7–10. https://doi.org10.1007/s10072-013-1379-8

53. American Psychiatric Association. *Diagnostic and Statistical Manual of Mental Disorders [text revision]*. 5th ed. American Psychiatric Publishing; 2022.

54. Bryant RA. Post-traumatic stress disorder: a state-of-the-art review of evidence and challenges. *World Psychiatry* 2019 Oct;*18*(3):259–269. doi: 10.1002/wps.20656.

55. Sonis, J. PTSD in Primary Care—An Update on Evidence-based Management. *Curr Psychiatry Rep 15*, 373 (2013). https://doi.org/10.1007/s11920-013-0373-4

56. Peterlin BL, Rosso AL, Sheftell FD, et al. Post-traumatic stress disorder, drug abuse and migraine: New findings from the national comorbidity survey replication (NCS-R). *Cephalalgia* 2011;*31*:235–244.

57. Peterlin BL, Nijjar SS, Tietjen GE. Post-traumatic stress disorder and migraine: epidemiology, sex differences, and potential mechanisms. *Headache* 2011 Jun;*51*(6):860–868. doi: 10.1111/j.1526-4610.2011.01907.x.

58. Peterlin BL, Tietjen GE, Brandes JL, Rubin SM, Drexler E, Lidicker JR et al. Posttraumatic stress disorder in migraine. *Headache* 2009:*49*(4):541–551.

59. Sances G, Galli F, Anastasi S, Ghiotto N, De Giorgio G, Guidetti V et al. Medication-overuse headache and personality: a controlled study by means of the MMPI-2. *Headache* 2010:*50*(2):198–209.

60. Dresler T, Caratozzolo S, Guldolf K et al., European Headache Federation School of Advanced Studies (EHF-SAS). Understanding the nature of psychiatric comorbidity in migraine: a systematic review focused on interactions and treatment implications. *J Headache Pain.* 2019 May 9;*20*(1):51. doi: 10.1186/s10194-019-0988-x.

61. Ehret M. Treatment of posttraumatic stress disorder: Focus on pharmacotherapy. *Ment Health Clin* 2019 Nov 27;*9*(6):373–382. doi: 10.9740/mhc.2019.11.373.

62. Lieberman JA, First MB. Psychotic Disorders. *N Engl J Med* 2018 Jul 19;*379*(3):270–280. doi: 10.1056/NEJMra1801490. PMID: 30021088.

63. American Psychiatric Association. *Diagnostic and Statistical Manual of Mental Disorders* [text revision]. 5th ed. American Psychiatric Publishing; 2022.

64. Leucht S, Kane JM, Kissling W, Hamann J, Etschel E, Engel RR. What does the PANSS mean? *Schizophr Res* 2005 Nov 15;*79*(2–3):231–238. doi: 10.1016/j.schres.2005.04.008. Epub 2005 Jun 27. PMID: 15982856.

65. Bigal M, Bordini CA, Speciali JG. Intravenous chlorpromazine in the emergency department treatment of migraines: a randomized controlled trial. *J Emerg Med* 2002;*23*(2):141–148.

66. Tripathi A, Macaluso M (2013). Antipsychotics for migraines, cluster headaches, and nausea. *Curr Psychiatr Ther, 12*(2), E1.

67. *Headache Classification Committee of the International Headache Society (IHS) The International Classification of Headache Disorders*, 3rd edition. Cephalalgia. 2018.

68. Loder E, Burch R, Rizzoli P. The 2012 AHS/AAN guidelines for prevention of episodic migraine: a summary and comparison with other recent clinical practice guidelines. *Headache* 2012 Jun;*52*(6):930–945. doi: 10.1111/j.1526-4610.2012.02185.x.

69. Brandt RB, Doesborg PGG, Haan J, Ferrari MD, Fronczek R. Pharmacotherapy for Cluster Headache. CNS Drugs. 2020.

70. Shapiro RE, et al. Lasmiditan for acute treatment of migraine in patients with cardiovascular risk factors: post-hoc analysis of pooled results from 2 randomized, double-blind, placebo-controlled, phase 3 trials. *J Headache Pain*, 2019. *20*(1): p. 90.

71. American Psychiatric Association. *Diagnostic and Statistical Manual of Mental Disorders [text revision].* 5th ed. American Psychiatric Publishing; 2022.

72. Beckmann YY, Seçkin M, Manavgat Aİ, Zorlu N. Headaches related to psychoactive substance use. *Clin Neurol Neurosurg* 2012 Sep;*114*(7):990–999. doi: 10.1016/j.clineuro.2012.02.041. Epub 2012 Mar 15. PMID: 22424726.

73. Panconesi A. Alcohol and migraine: trigger factor, consumption, mechanisms. A review. *J Headache Pain* 2008;*9*: 19–27.

74. Lambert GA, Zagami AS. The mode of action of migraine triggers: a hypothesis. *Headache* 2009;*49*:253–275.

75. Miller RM, Rollnick S. *Motivational Interviewing: Helping people change.* 3rd ed. New York: Guilford Press; 2013.

76. Moyers TB, Houck J, Glynn LH, Hallgren KA, Manuel JK. A randomized controlled trial to influence client language in sub stance use disorder treatment. *Drug Alcohol Depend* 2017, *172*: 43–50. doi: https://doi.org/10.1016/j.drugalcdep.2016.11.036.

77. Keeley R, Engel M, Reed A, Brody D, Burke BL. Toward an Emerging Role for Motivational Interviewing in Primary Care. *Curr Psychiatry Rep* 2018 May 18;*20*(6):41. doi: 10.1007/s11920-018-0901-3. PMID: 29777318.

78. Minen MT, Begasse De Dhaem O, Kroon Van Diest A, et al. Migraine and its psychiatric comorbidities. *J Neurol Neurosurg Psychiatry* 2016 Jul;*87*(7):741–749. doi: 10.1136/jnnp-2015-312233. Epub 2016 Jan 5. PMID: 26733600

79. Sansone RA, Sansone LA. Serotonin norepinephrine reuptake inhibitors: a pharmacological comparison. *Innov Clin Neurosci* 2014 Mar;*11*(3–4):37–42.

80. Chu A, Wadhwa R. Selective Serotonin Reuptake Inhibitors. [Updated 2023 May 1]. In: StatPearls [Internet]. Treasure Island (FL): StatPearls Publishing; 2023 Jan. Available from: https://www.ncbi.nlm.nih.gov/books/NBK554406/

81. Thippaiah SM, Fargason RE, Birur B. Struggling to find Effective Pharmacologic Options for Akathisia? B-CALM! *Psychopharmacol Bull* 2021 Jun 1;*51*(3):72–78.

82. Cruccu G, et al. AAN-EFNS Guidelines on Trigeminal Neuralgia Management. *Eur J Neurol* 2008:*15*10:1013–1028.

Comorbid Rheumatic Conditions in the Treatment of Headache

16

Hailey Baker and Joshua Bilsborrow

LEARNING OBJECTIVES

1. Recognize the most common rheumatic diseases that can be comorbid with headache disorders
2. Understand the clinical presentation, basic workup, and initial management of the most common rheumatic diseases
3. Appreciate symptoms that should raise concern for an underlying rheumatic disease and when to refer to a rheumatologist

OVERVIEW

Rheumatology focuses on the management of musculoskeletal diseases and systemic autoimmune and autoinflammatory conditions. Rheumatic diseases can affect any organ system in patients of any age, but this chapter will focus on rheumatological diseases in adults.

There are two main types of rheumatic diseases: autoinflammatory and autoimmune conditions. Autoinflammatory conditions result when overactivation of the innate immune system causes hyperinflammatory states that damage the body's tissues. Autoimmune conditions result when the adaptive immune system inappropriately attacks one's own tissues, typically through or along with the production of autoantibodies. The main categories of rheumatic diseases include inflammatory arthritides, connective tissue diseases, vasculitides, and noninflammatory pain syndromes, many of which can coexist with headache disorders.

It is important to recognize that rheumatic diseases can evolve over time. A patient may have some features of a rheumatic disease, but not meet diagnostic criteria until many years later. Similarly, a patient

DOI: 10.1201/b23330-16

may have one rheumatic diagnosis and later acquire additional rheumatic diagnoses. Therefore, it is essential to perform a thorough history and physical examination and follow patients over time to diagnose and manage any rheumatic disease. This chapter will outline classic presentations of the most common rheumatic diseases that, if recognized, should prompt referral to a rheumatologist.

Depending on the rheumatic condition, laboratory results and radiological studies may assist with the diagnosis. Generally, erythrocyte sedimentation rate (ESR) and C reactive protein (CRP) are expected to be elevated in the workup of many rheumatic diseases; if there is concern, checking the ESR and CRP is a good place to start. X-rays of symptomatic joints or the spine are also very helpful to collect prior to referral to a rheumatologist.

Treatment of rheumatic diseases generally involves anti-inflammatory medications and/or immunosuppression, but infection and malignancy need to be ruled out prior to starting immunosuppressive therapy, as these can often mimic rheumatic diseases. Steroids are often used to quickly control inflammation, and long-term steroid-sparing therapy is later initiated with a disease-modifying anti-rheumatic drug (DMARD). Each DMARD carries its own set of risks, but all immunosuppressing agents increase the risk for infection and patients should notify their rheumatologist immediately if there is concern for an infection.

Many patients with rheumatologic diseases have headache, whether as a direct symptom of their rheumatic condition, as in giant cell arteritis (GCA), or as a comorbid headache disorder. Studies have shown that the prevalence of migraine in patients with rheumatoid arthritis (RA) is 1.94 times higher than in patients without RA (1). Similarly, nearly 50% of patients with Sjögren's syndrome, 35% of patients with mixed connective tissue disease (MCTD), and 30% of patients with systemic sclerosis have migraine (2, 3). The link between headache and rheumatological conditions is not fully understood, but it is likely multifactorial. Chronic inflammation from rheumatological diseases involves the systemic release of proinflammatory cytokines (4). Levels of the proinflammatory cytokines IL-1β, IL-6, IL-8, and TNF-α have all been shown to be higher in patients with migraines (5). Higher levels of these cytokines likely contribute to neuroinflammation, which may increase the risk for development of migraines (6). In addition to chronic inflammation, many rheumatological diseases are also characterized by vascular abnormalities, particularly Raynaud's phenomenon. Raynaud's and migraines occur together frequently as both involve vascular dysfunction (7). The calcitonin gene-related peptide (CGRP) signaling pathway is involved in both Raynaud's and migraines, and therapies inhibiting CGRP signaling have been shown to cause Raynaud's at significantly higher rates than other migraine treatments (8). Management of rheumatological disease is complex, and living with these diseases can be physically and mentally taxing for patients (9). Stress is a well-known risk factor for migraine, and living with a rheumatological condition can contribute to this stress, potentially worsening headaches (10). Therefore, a multidisciplinary approach between rheumatology and neurology, in addition to other specialists, is essential to adequately treat patients with both rheumatic and headache disorders.

INFLAMMATORY ARTHRITIS

Arthralgia is joint pain without signs of inflammation. Conversely, arthritis is joint pain with evidence of inflammation, including swelling, warmth, and/or erythema. Inflammatory arthritis is caused by the body's immune system leading to inflammation in one or more joints, which contrasts with noninflammatory arthritis, such as osteoarthritis, which is caused by chronic degenerative joint damage and not the immune system causing joint damage. Inflammatory arthritis is characterized by joint pain that is worse in the morning with morning stiffness lasting greater than 30 minutes and that improves with activity and worsens with rest. This contrasts with noninflammatory arthritis, which is characterized by joint pain that is worse in the evenings, morning stiffness lasting less than 30 minutes, and pain that is worsened by activity but improves with rest.

Clinical Case 1

The patient is a 45-year-old female with no significant past medical history who presents for evaluation of daily headaches. The patient reports that over the past five years, her headache frequency has steadily increased from once monthly to now daily. She reports that these daily headaches are primarily holocephalic and dull, with absent nausea, photophobia, and phonophobia. On five days per month, she also has more severe unilateral headaches with nausea that are worse if she attempts to exercise, and she cancels work and social obligations. Further interview reveals that she has also had to increasingly use naproxen over this same interval due to recurrent pain and swelling in her metacarpophalangeal joints. She also notes morning stiffness in her joints lasting 90 minutes, as well as general fatigue. A diagnosis of medication-overuse headache (MOH) and probably chronic migraine is made. The patient is also referred to rheumatology, where rheumatoid factor and anti-cyclic citrullinated peptide antibody serologies return positive. A diagnosis of seropositive RA is made. The patient is started on methotrexate for the treatment of RA and nortriptyline for the prevention of chronic migraine. The patient is also counseled that these two treatments are in support not only of her underlying diseases but also to help her stop her naproxen, which is causing the MOH.

Three months later, the patient returns to clinic. She reports that one month after starting the methotrexate and nortriptyline, her joint pain has greatly improved, and she stopped the naproxen to treat her MOH. She has consequently been off of naproxen for two months and notes a significant improvement in her headache burden. She has only four headache days per month, and boasts that she has made it to every work happy hour during that time (but did not drink at them). She is started on as-needed rizatriptan for acute treatment of migraine.

Rheumatoid arthritis(RA) is the most common chronic inflammatory arthritis. RA is characterized by small joint symmetric arthritis lasting longer than six weeks that classically affects the hands, wrists, and feet but can affect the larger joints such as the elbows, shoulders, hips, and knees as well. Less commonly, it can also affect deep organs, like the lungs and the heart. It is a progressive disease that can lead to permanent joint damage, which makes early diagnosis and treatment essential to maintain mobility and quality of life. Risk factors for developing RA include both genetic and environmental influences. The most significant modifiable environmental risk factor is smoking, and a higher pack-year history directly correlates with a higher risk of RA (11–13).

RA is a clinical diagnosis, but most clinicians use the 2010 American College of Rheumatology (ACR)/European Alliance of Associations for Rheumatology (EULAR) RA classification criteria to help make a diagnosis, which includes duration of symptoms, number and types of joints affected, presence of autoantibodies, and inflammatory markers (14). Rheumatoid factor (RF) and anti-cyclic citrullinated peptide (anti-CCP) antibodies are the two autoantibodies that are used to aid in diagnosing RA, but the presence of these antibodies is neither essential nor sufficient for diagnosis. RA can be both seropositive (presence of RF and/or anti-CCP antibodies) or seronegative (neither RF nor anti-CCP antibodies present). Other important labs to order in the diagnosis of RA are ESR and CRP, which indicate levels of inflammation in the body and are typically elevated in active RA.

X-ray imaging of the hands and feet is helpful to look for evidence of bone erosions, joint destruction, or bony abnormalities. Once a diagnosis is made, a DMARD should be started to manage pain and prevent permanent joint destruction. Treatment decisions are made based on disease severity, but the mainstay of RA treatment is methotrexate with or without biologic DMARDs, such as anti-tumor necrosis factor drugs or others.

Spondyloarthritis (SpA) is a group of chronic inflammatory arthritides that includes ankylosing spondylitis (AS), psoriatic arthritis (PsA), enteropathic arthritis (associated with inflammatory bowel disease), reactive arthritis (ReA) (from an infection), and undifferentiated SpA. SpA can involve the axial skeleton, peripheral joints, and the entheses (where tendons and ligaments attach to the bones). Axial skeleton involvement can affect any part of the spine but classically involves inflammation of the sacroiliac (SI) joints, called sacroiliitis, which causes inflammatory lower back pain. Inflammatory back pain is characterized by pain and stiffness that is worse in the morning—morning stiffness lasting more than 30 minutes, which improves with activity and worsens with rest. Peripheral joint involvement is characterized by arthritis of any joint, large or small, and can be symmetric or asymmetric, which is in contrast to RA that classically manifests with symmetric small joint involvement. Extraarticular manifestations of SpA include dactylitis (inflammation of an entire finger or toe), uveitis (inflammation of the eye), psoriasis (an inflammatory skin condition), and inflammatory bowel diseases, such as Crohn's or ulcerative colitis.

There are no known autoantibodies associated with SpA, but genetic testing for the human leukocyte antigen (HLA)-B27 gene can increase the likelihood of a SpA diagnosis. However, HLA-B27 positivity is not essential nor sufficient for the diagnosis of SpA as up to 7% of the general United States population can be HLA-B27 positive, yet the prevalence of SpA is only approximately 1% (15, 16). X-rays of the SI joints and any affected peripheral joint can aid in the diagnosis. Once a diagnosis of SpA is made, targeted DMARD treatment depends on the type of SpA, but they are typically responsive to nonsteroidal anti-inflammatory drugs (NSAIDs) as initial therapy.

Crystalline arthritis is a group of acute and chronic inflammatory arthritides that result when the immune system responds to inappropriately deposited crystals in and around the joints. The two most common types of crystalline arthritis are gout and pseudogout.

Gout develops when elevated levels of uric acid in the blood lead to monosodium urate crystal deposition in and around the joints; the body then develops an inflammatory reaction to these crystals. Gout classically affects the first metatarsophalangeal joints, termed podagra, but can affect any joint in the body. Elevated levels of uric acid in the blood increase the risk of developing gout, but hyperuricemia alone without joint pain is not gout and does not require treatment. Risk factors for gout are chronic kidney disease, alcohol consumption (particularly purine-rich drinks such as beer), and consumption of purine-rich foods like shellfish or red meat.

Pseudogout, also known as calcium pyrophosphate deposition (CPPD) disease, develops when calcium pyrophosphate crystals are deposited in or around the joints, and the body develops an inflammatory reaction to these crystals. Risk factors for pseudogout are hyperparathyroidism, hypothyroidism, hemochromatosis, and hypomagnesemia, as well as advanced age. Both acute gout and pseudogout attacks are characterized by excruciating joint pain, swelling, warmth, and erythema of one or more joints. These symptoms can mimic septic arthritis, which classically affects only one joint at a time. Therefore, aspiration of joint fluid is typically performed to rule out infection and differentiate between gout and pseudogout.

Labs during an acute crystalline arthritis episode typically show elevated ESR and/or CRP levels, and leukocytosis. During an acute gout flare, uric acid can be inaccurately low and so should be repeated after the acute flare. There is no specific serological test for pseudogout. X-rays of affected joints can show erosions and/or tophi (accumulations of uric acid) in gout and chondrocalcinosis in pseudogout. Acute management of both gout and pseudogout flares involves NSAIDs, colchicine, and/or intraarticular or systemic steroids. Treatment choice depends on the severity of symptoms and the patient's comorbidities. Allopurinol lowers serum uric acid levels but is not necessary for every patient with gout. Starting allopurinol alone can precipitate a gout flare, so patients should also be on prophylaxis with either an NSAID, colchicine, or low-dose steroids to prevent allopurinol-induced gout attacks when initiating allopurinol. If gout or pseudogout attacks occur frequently, then long-term prophylaxis with colchicine or steroids may be considered.

RA, SpA, and crystalline arthritis are the three main categories of inflammatory arthritis that nonrheumatologists are most likely to see. There are other types of inflammatory arthritis, including infectious arthritis, and rarer diseases, such as adult-onset Still's disease. Other connective tissue diseases can also present with inflammatory arthritis as one manifestation. Overall, initial workup for any inflammatory arthritis should include ESR, CRP, X-rays of the affected joints, and referral to a rheumatologist to help with the diagnosis and management.

CONNECTIVE TISSUE DISEASES

Connective tissue diseases (CTDs) are a group of autoimmune disorders that primarily affect the connective tissues of the body. CTDs can affect any organ system in the body and can overlap with other autoimmune conditions, which means each patient presents differently, making these diseases diagnostically challenging. The most common CTDs are systemic lupus erythematosus (SLE), Sjögren's syndrome, systemic sclerosis, inflammatory myositis, mixed connective tissue disease (MCTD), and antiphospholipid syndrome. The same disease can present with mild manifestations in one patient and life-threatening end-organ failure in others, which makes management of these diseases complex and often necessitates involvement of multidisciplinary teams. Treatment ranges from simple symptomatic management to aggressive immunosuppression, which is individualized for each patient.

Clinical Case 2

The patient is a 38-year-old female with a history of depression and SLE who presents for evaluation of increasing headache frequency. She notes that over the past year, her headache frequency has steadily increased, and she now has 20 headache days per month, of which 12 have migrainous features. Her SLE is currently well controlled on hydroxychloroquine, and she is also taking venlafaxine for treatment of depression and migraine prevention. In the past, she has previously taken metoprolol and topiramate for migraine prevention but had to stop these medications due to bradycardia and weight loss, respectively.

Her headaches are now consistent with chronic migraine. While the venlafaxine has been helpful for her depression, it has not been effective for migraine prevention. Given that she had intolerable side effects on metoprolol and topiramate, a nonoral option is sought. The patient has seen advertisements for the CGRP monoclonal antibodies and is interested in starting one, but after discussion that CGRP monoclonal antibodies can potentially exacerbate autoimmune conditions, she elects to start preventive treatment with onabotulinumtoxinA instead and switch from her current sumatriptan to eletriptan for acute treatment.

Seven months later, after two rounds of onabotulinumtoxinA, the patient reports that she is feeling much better. She is down to ten headache days per month, only four of which have migrainous features and are severe enough such that she requires eletriptan. Her SLE has also remained stable throughout this time period.

Systemic lupus erythematosus (SLE) is a chronic autoimmune disease in which autoantibodies attack various organ systems in the body. SLE typically presents in young women but can affect patients of all ages, races, genders, and socioeconomic backgrounds. However, studies have consistently shown that black, Hispanic, Asian, and Native American patients with SLE have worse outcomes, particularly for lupus nephritis, which is one of the most severe complications (17–20).

SLE can present in many ways, but the most classic symptoms are a malar rash (AKA: "butterfly rash") on the cheeks sparing the nasolabial folds, photosensitivity, alopecia, oral or nasal ulcers, arthritis, myalgias, nephritis, and serositis. Kidney involvement is one of the most feared complications, as it can lead to end-stage renal disease requiring hemodialysis and renal transplantation, carrying significant morbidity and mortality. Patients with SLE are screened regularly for levels of proteinuria, and levels of random urine protein-to-creatinine ratios >0.5 should lead to urgent referral to nephrology for possible kidney biopsy. Presence of lupus nephritis warrants aggressive immunosuppression to prevent permanent kidney damage. Table 16.1 describes many of the manifestations and complications of SLE but is not exhaustive (21). Patients with SLE are typically young women who do not fit the expected phenotype of patients with cardiovascular or pulmonary disease, but cardiopulmonary symptoms should be taken seriously in patients with SLE given these limb- and life-threatening manifestations.

Diagnosis of SLE can be difficult given the variety of clinical manifestations, but it involves a combination of clinical features and laboratory results. The 2019 ACR/EULAR classification criteria require for

TABLE 16.1   Manifestations and complications of SLE

ORGAN/ORGAN SYSTEM INVOLVEMENT	MANIFESTATIONS AND COMPLICATIONS
Skin	Acute cutaneous lupus (AKA: malar/butterfly rash), subacute cutaneous lupus, chronic discoid lupus, skin ulceration, Raynaud's phenomenon, and permanent scarring alopecia
Eyes	Uveitis, retinal changes, optic atrophy, cataracts
Bone	Inflammatory arthritis, reversible arthropathy (called Jaccoud's arthropathy), deforming or erosive arthritis, osteoporosis, avascular necrosis leading to joint replacements
Muscle	Myalgias, myositis, muscular atrophy
Cardiovascular	Early coronary artery disease, myocardial infarction, cardiomyopathy, valvular disease, pericarditis, peripheral vascular disease leading to significant tissue loss, and even leading to the need for coronary artery bypass
Pulmonary	Pleurisy, pleural effusions, pulmonary hypertension, pulmonary or pleural fibrosis, shrinking lung, pulmonary infarction
Kidneys	Proteinuria, hematuria, pyuria, chronic kidney disease, end-stage renal disease requiring hemodialysis, kidney transplantation
Gastrointestinal System	Peritonitis, mesenteric insufficiency, GI strictures, pancreatic insufficiency, bowel infarction leading to bowel resection
Nervous System	Brain fog, cognitive impairment, psychosis, seizures, strokes, cranial or peripheral neuropathy, CNS vasculitis, transverse myelitis
Endocrine	Premature gonadal failure, diabetes
Hematology/Oncology	Venous thrombosis, malignancy, overlap with antiphospholipid syndrome

Note: This table outlines many of the manifestations and complications of SLE based on the Systemic Lupus International Collaborating Clinics/American College of Rheumatology (SLICC/ACR) Damage Index (21).

diagnosis of SLE to have a positive antinuclear antibody (ANA) of at least 1:80 (22). However, the presence of positive ANA alone is not sufficient for the diagnosis of SLE, as ANA can be positive in other autoimmune diseases and in up to 15% of healthy US adults (23). Other laboratory tests that aid in the diagnosis of SLE are anti-Smith antibodies, anti-RNP antibodies, anti-double stranded DNA antibodies, complement levels of C3 and C4, leukopenia, thrombocytopenia, proteinuria, and antiphospholipid antibodies (anti-cardiolipin antibodies, anti-beta 2 glycoprotein 1 antibodies, and lupus anticoagulant). All of these labs do not need to be abnormal to make a diagnosis of SLE, but the more that are abnormal the higher the likelihood of an SLE diagnosis.

Radiological imaging is generally not helpful for SLE diagnosis but can be used to assess organ involvement, as characterized in Table 16.1. Drug-induced lupus is a subset of SLE that can be caused by certain drugs, most commonly hydralazine, tumor necrosis factor (TNF) inhibitors such as infliximab and adalimumab, isoniazid, propylthiouracil, and sulfasalazine. Drug-induced lupus is typically characterized by the presence of either anti-histone antibodies or anti-chromatin antibodies. Management of SLE varies based on disease severity and organ involvement. In general, though, all SLE patients should be started on hydroxychloroquine early and continued without interruption if no contraindications exist, as hydroxychloroquine has been shown to reduce SLE flares and improve mortality (24, 25). If there is evidence of deep organ involvement, such as the kidneys, brain, or lungs, then more aggressive immunosuppression may be needed, including high-dose steroids, mycophenolate mofetil, azathioprine, belimumab, anifrolumab, rituximab, and/or cyclophosphamide.

Antiphospholipid syndrome (APS) is an autoimmune disease that is characterized by the presence of antiphospholipid antibodies in the blood and vascular thrombosis or pregnancy morbidity. APS can be a primary condition or secondary to other autoimmune diseases, typically SLE. Obstetrical APS is a subset of antiphospholipid syndrome that only manifests with pregnancy complications, including recurrent pregnancy loss, fetal growth restriction, preterm birth, and/or preeclampsia. Catastrophic APS (CAPS) is a rare but potentially life-threatening manifestation of APS that is characterized by thrombosis in three or more organ systems within one week and requires emergent treatment by a hematologist and rheumatologist. APS can present in many ways, as it can affect any organ in the body. In addition to vascular thrombosis and pregnancy complications, other clinical manifestations can include skin ulcerations, livedo reticularis, cardiac valve abnormalities, and/or organ ischemia. Diagnosis of APS requires the presence of both clinical manifestations (thrombosis and/or pregnancy loss) and laboratory abnormalities (anti-cardiolipin antibodies, anti-beta 2 glycoprotein 1 antibodies, and/or lupus anticoagulant) with abnormal labs persisting on two or more occasions at least 12 weeks apart (26). Management of APS focuses on minimizing risk factors for thrombosis, such as quitting smoking or discontinuing estrogen-containing medications and initiation of anticoagulation rather than immunosuppression. Warfarin is the standard of care for the treatment of APS as direct oral anticoagulants (DOACs) such as dabigatran or apixaban have shown increased risks of thrombosis in patients with APS (27).

Sjögren's syndrome is an autoimmune disease that causes inflammation of the salivary glands and tear ducts but can also affect the deep organs. Sjögren's can be a primary condition but also commonly overlaps with other autoimmune diseases such as SLE, RA, and scleroderma. Sjögren's is characterized by dry eyes and dry mouth, also known as sicca, which, if severe, can lead to corneal damage and dental complications such as accelerated tooth decay. Inflammation of parotid glands can lead to parotid gland enlargement. Parotid gland enlargement can also be seen in lymphoma and other inflammatory conditions, which should be ruled out as part of the Sjögren's workup. Extra-glandular manifestations of Sjögren's can include arthritis, rashes, interstitial lung disease, and peripheral neuropathy.

Diagnosis of Sjögren's syndrome includes both serological testing for anti-SSA (Ro) and anti-SSB (La) antibodies and objective determination of dry eyes or dry mouth or biopsy of the minor salivary glands showing inflammation (28). Treatment of Sjögren's depends on the severity of symptoms and organs involved. If the only manifestations are dry eyes and dry mouth, then treatment can be focused on symptomatic relief with artificial tears, oral rinses, oral hygiene, and cholinergic agonists for severe sicca, such as pilocarpine or cevimeline. Deep organ involvement of Sjögren's syndrome warrants immunosuppression with DMARDs as managed by a rheumatologist.

Systemic sclerosis (SSc), also known as scleroderma, is a complex autoimmune disease that typically involves the skin and deep internal organs. There are two main subtypes of SSc: limited and diffuse cutaneous systemic sclerosis. Limited cutaneous systemic sclerosis is defined as only involving the skin of the distal extremities (lower forearm, lower leg, and face), but not the torso. Limited cutaneous SSc is typically associated with the CREST syndrome, which stands for calcinosis, Raynaud's, esophageal dysmotility, sclerodactyly, and telangiectasias. Diffuse cutaneous SSc is defined as involving the skin of all of the extremities, distal and proximal, the face, and the torso.

Skin involvement is characterized by sclerosis, which is a tightening and hardening of the skin due to underlying skin fibrosis. Sclerosis of the hands and fingers, called sclerodactyly, can lead to severe motion restriction and impair patients' ability to perform activities of daily living. Sclerosis of the face and lips causes shrinking and hardening of the oral aperture, making eating and drinking difficult. Calcinosis manifests as hard calcium deposits under the skin that appear white and can be quite painful. Raynaud's phenomenon manifests as cold- or stress-induced color changes, red, white, or blue, of the fingers or toes due to vasoconstriction of the small digital arteries. Severe Raynaud's can lead to skin ulceration, tissue ischemia, and digital amputation, which is why it is critically important for patients with Raynaud's to keep their core, hands, and feet warm. Esophageal dysmotility is due to fibrosis of the esophageal muscles, which leads to food retention in the esophagus, increasing risk for aspiration. Telangiectasias are dilated blood vessels in the skin that do not cause significant morbidity, but high burden of telangiectasias can lead to profound skin spotting all over the body.

Deep organ involvement of SSc can include the lungs, heart, gastrointestinal tract, and kidneys. Deep organ involvement can manifest as interstitial lung disease (ILD), pulmonary arterial hypertension, heart failure, esophageal dysmotility, bowel malabsorption, and scleroderma renal crisis. Scleroderma renal crisis is characterized by elevated blood pressure, acute kidney injury, and microangiopathic hemolytic anemia.

Diagnosis of SSc is made based on both clinical features, as described earlier, and the presence of autoantibodies. Antinuclear antibodies are typically positive in patients with SSc. Other antibodies associated with SSc include anti-Scl-70, anti-centromere, anti-RNA polymerase III, and anti-PM/Scl antibodies.

Imaging studies are useful in screening for and monitoring of deep organ involvement. Pulmonary function tests and echocardiograms are performed yearly to monitor for ILD and pulmonary arterial hypertension. Esophageal manometry is helpful in assessing esophageal dysmotility.

Treatment of SSc depends on severity and organs involved. Raynaud's is treated with calcium channel blockers and/or phosphodiesterase inhibitors to promote vasodilation of the digits and reduce risk of digital ischemia. In general, glucocorticoids are used sparingly in patients with SSc as higher doses of glucocorticoids (above prednisone 15 mg daily or equivalent) can precipitate scleroderma renal crisis. Choice of immunosuppression with DMARDs depends on organs involved and severity of symptoms. Unfortunately, none of the DMARDs that are currently available prevent progression of sclerodactyly, which severely affects patients' quality of life. Overall, treatment of patients with SSc requires multidisciplinary collaboration given the many organ systems affected and the complexity of this disease.

Idiopathic inflammatory myositis (IIM) is a group of autoimmune diseases characterized by muscular inflammation and chronic, progressive proximal muscle weakness but can also involve the skin and other deep organs. Classic symptoms are an inability to climb stairs or stand from a seated position without pushing off with the arms. The two main types of IIM are dermatomyositis and polymyositis. **Dermatomyositis (DM)** is characterized by skin rashes, specifically Gottron's papules (plaques over the knuckles of the hands), heliotrope rash (periorbital rash; see Figure 16.1), and rashes on the chest and/or upper back (called the V-sign or shawl sign respectively), or upper thighs (Holster sign). Some patients have the classic skin rashes of DM but lack muscular weakness, which is called clinical amyopathic dermatomyositis (CADM). **Polymyositis (PM)** involves muscular weakness but lacks the skin findings of DM.

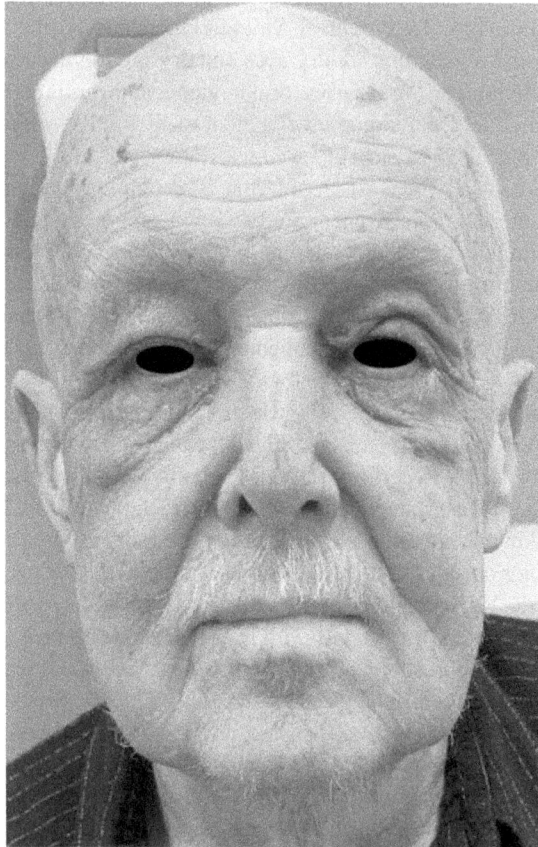

FIGURE 16.1   The heliotrope rash of dermatomyositis. The reddish-purplish rash involves the periorbital skin is characteristic of dermatomyositis (DM).

Immune-mediated necrotizing myositis (IMNM) is another subtype of inflammatory myositis that is caused in some cases by antibody formation to statins with anti-HMGCoA reductase antibodies. Anti-synthetase syndrome is another subtype of inflammatory myositis that is characterized by dry cracking hands ("mechanic's hands"), myositis, ILD, inflammatory arthritis, and Raynaud's phenomenon and is associated with anti-aminoacyl-transfer RNA (tRNA) synthetase antibodies, such as anti-Jo-1 antibodies. There are many other autoantibodies associated with IIM, many of which have clinical and therapeutic implications, which are outlined in Table 16.2. In adults, IIM can be associated with underlying malignancy, with anti-NXP2 and anti-TIF-1-gamma antibodies specifically being strongly associated with malignancy, so it is imperative to do a thorough malignancy workup in these patients. Other laboratory findings in IIM are elevated creatine kinase (CK) levels, and patients can also present with elevated liver transaminases and/or acute kidney injury. Workup of IIM typically involves electromyography (EMG), MRI of the thighs or biceps, and muscle biopsy. Management of IIM involves physical rehabilitation and immunosuppression with glucocorticoids, intravenous immunoglobulin (IVIG), and/or DMARDs.

Mixed connective tissue disease (MCTD) is a complex autoimmune disease characterized by the presence of ANA antibodies and anti-ribonucleoprotein (anti-RNP) antibodies. Classically, patients with MCTD should not be positive for any other autoantibodies other than ANA and anti-RNP. If there are other autoantibodies present, then this suggests more of an overlap syndrome of multiple autoimmune CTDs rather than MCTD. Manifestations of MCTD include Raynaud's, sclerodactyly, various skin rashes, sicca, arthritis, myositis, serositis, myocarditis, pleuritis, ILD, pulmonary arterial hypertension, glomerulonephritis, and many other symptoms, which means that every patient presents differently, making it a challenging diagnosis. Serologies are essential for the diagnosis and require anti-RNP positivity, but patients can also have other positive antibodies, as outlined in Table 16.2. Radiological studies are not required for diagnosis but rather are used to screen for deep organ involvement. Management of MCTD involves glucocorticoids and DMARDs, but specific treatment of choice depends on the disease manifestations, severity of symptoms, and which organs are involved.

Sarcoidosis is a granulomatous multisystem inflammatory disease characterized by noncaseating granuloma formation, which most commonly occurs in the lungs but can involve any organ in the body. Sarcoidosis can present in many ways given that it can affect any organ in the body and can present with asymptomatic to severe organ dysfunction. Classic manifestations of sarcoidosis are fever, hilar lymphadenopathy, erythema nodosum, uveitis, arthritis, and lung abnormalities. Labs that support the sarcoidosis diagnosis are elevated angiotensin-converting enzyme (ACE) levels, hypercalcemia, and elevated Vitamin D-1, 25, but these are not sensitive nor essential for diagnosis. Radiological studies are helpful in assessing organ involvement, specifically chest X-ray or CT chest, to evaluate lung involvement and other radiological imaging based on clinical manifestations. Ultimately, diagnosis is made by biopsy confirmation of noncaseating granulomas present in affected tissues. Treatment is not necessary for every patient with sarcoidosis. Patients who have mild symptoms without significant deep organ involvement can simply be monitored over time for progression of disease. Patients who have more significant organ involvement typically require multidisciplinary treatment with a combination of glucocorticoids and DMARD therapies, including methotrexate and/or TNF inhibitors.

VEXAS (vacuoles, E1 enzyme, X-linked, autoinflammatory, somatic) syndrome is a recently discovered disease, first described in 2020 by Beck et al. (29). VEXAS syndrome is a multisystem inflammatory disease that is caused by somatic mutations in the *UBA1* gene, which encodes the E1 ubiquitin-activating enzyme. Since it is somatic and X-lined, it predominantly presents in older men. VEXAS involves many organ systems, including the bone marrow, eyes, ears, connective tissues, skin, lungs, and blood vessels. Given the numerous organ systems involved, it can manifest with fevers, weight loss, macrocytic anemia, thrombocytopenia, myelodysplastic syndrome, multiple myeloma, inflammatory eye disease, sensorineural hearing loss, chondritis (see Figure 16.2), leukocytoclastic vasculitis, psoriasis, inflammatory arthritis, polymyalgia rheumatica, pleural effusions, vasculitis, and/or deep vein thrombosis (29–33). There are likely other manifestations that

TABLE 16.2 Summary table of autoantibodies

AUTOANTIBODY	DISEASE ASSOCIATION AND CLINICAL IMPLICATIONS
ANA	Highly sensitive for SLE, MCTD, SSc. Also, frequently positive with Sjögren's and IIM. Pattern of ANA can indicate certain rheumatic correlations
Anti-dsDNA	Aids in diagnosis of SLE; highly specific for SLE
Anti-Smith	Aids in diagnosis of SLE; highly specific for SLE
Anti-RNP	Aids in diagnosis of SLE and MCTD
Anti-SSA	Aids in diagnosis of SLE and Sjögren's syndrome
Anti-SSB	Aids in diagnosis of Sjögren's syndrome
Anti-Scl-70	Aids in diagnosis of the diffuse cutaneous variant of SSc
Anti-Centromere	Aids in diagnosis of the limited cutaneous variant of SSc
Anti-RNA polymerase III	Aids in diagnosis of SSc
Anti-Pm/Scl	Aids in diagnosis of SSc and IIM
Anti-HMG-CoA	Aids in diagnosis of IMNM related to statin exposure
Anti-SRP	Aids in diagnosis of IMNM
Anti-NXP2	Aids in diagnosis of IIM. Associated with increased risk of malignancy
Anti-TIF-1-gamma	Aids in diagnosis of IIM. Associated with increased risk of malignancy
Anti-MDA-5	Aids in diagnosis of IIM. Associated with increased risk of rapidly progressive ILD
Anti-Jo-1	Aids in diagnosis of IIM and anti-synthetase syndrome
RF	Aids in diagnosis of RA and Sjögren's syndrome. Low specificity as it is commonly elevated in inflammatory states, such as infections
Anti-CCP	Aids in diagnosis of RA; highly specific for RA
Lupus anticoagulant (LAC)	Aids in diagnosis of APS
Anti-cardiolipin	Aids in diagnosis of APS
Anti-beta 2 glycoprotein 1	Aids in diagnosis of APS
Anti-GBM	Aids in diagnosis of anti-glomerular basement membrane disease (AKA Goodpasture's disease)
C-ANCA	Aids in diagnosis of GPA. Associated with positivity for anti-PR3 antibodies
P-ANCA	Aids in diagnosis of MPA. Associated with positivity for anti-MPO antibodies
Atypical P-ANCA	Associated with inflammatory bowel disease and hepatobiliary disease
Anti-PR3	Aids in diagnosis of GPA. Associated with positivity for C-ANCA antibodies
Anti-MPO	Aids in diagnosis of MPA. Associated with positivity for P-ANCA antibodies

Note: This table lists the most commonly encountered antibodies and their associated rheumatic conditions with additional clinical correlations mentioned, when applicable. SLE = "Systemic Lupus Erythematosus"; SSc = "Systemic Sclerosis," also known as "Scleroderma"; IIM = "Idiopathic Inflammatory Myositis"; MCTD = "Mixed Connective Tissue Disease"; IMNM = "Immune-Mediated Necrotizing Myositis"; RA = "Rheumatoid Arthritis"; APS = "Antiphospholipid Syndrome"; GBM = "Glomerular basement membrane"; C-ANCA = "cytoplasmic antineutrophil cytoplasmic antibody"; P-ANCA = "perinuclear antineutrophil cytoplasmic antibody"; PR3 = "proteinase 3"; MPO = "myeloperoxidase".

have yet to be characterized given the recent discovery of this disease. Diagnosis of VEXAS is made through genetic testing for the *UBA1* gene mutation. Other relevant labs and radiological studies should be guided to work up each patient's clinical manifestations and to rule out other underlying etiologies, including malignancy and infection. There are currently no guidelines for the treatment of VEXAS given its recent discovery, but at this time, glucocorticoids are the mainstay of treatment in addition to DMARDs.

In summary, autoimmune CTDs are a complex group of disorders that can present in many ways. Early referral to a rheumatologist is appropriate for patients who have any of the symptoms outlined in

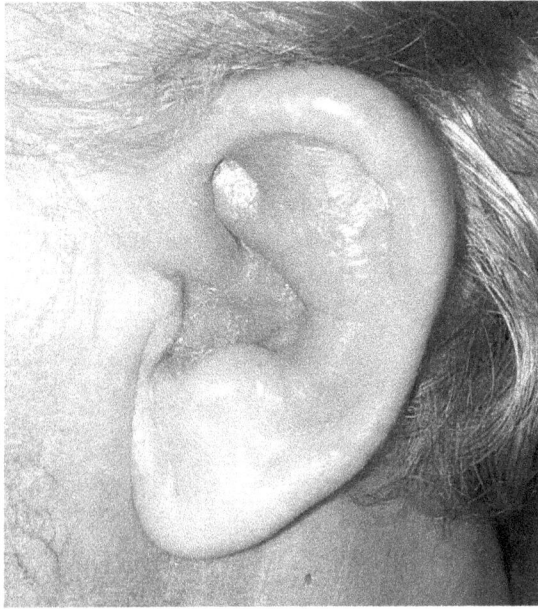

FIGURE 16.2   Chondritis of the ear manifesting as painful swelling of cartilaginous structures of the ear but classically sparing the earlobe, which does not contain cartilage.

Table 16.1, recurrent pregnancy losses, sclerodactyly, morning stiffness, or lab or radiological findings concerning an inflammatory disease. Diagnosis of any connective tissue disease involves a thorough history, physical exam, laboratory, and radiological workup. Specific serologies should be ordered based on clinical suspicion of a disease rather than ordering every possible autoantibody. Initially, some patients may present with certain features of a connective tissue disease, but do not fully meet criteria and are typically labeled as undifferentiated. These patients should be monitored closely over time for interval development of one of the aforementioned conditions.

VASCULITIS

Vasculitis is a group of complex autoimmune diseases characterized by inflammation of arteries and veins of various sizes and in different organs. Vasculitis is classified by the size of the blood vessels primarily affected: large, medium, or small. These can be primary conditions or secondary to an infection, drug, or another autoimmune disease. Treatment of vasculitis requires immunosuppression and if secondary, then treatment of the underlying cause.

Large vessel vasculitis (LVV) predominantly affects the aorta and its major branches. The two types of LVV are Takayasu arteritis and GCA, also known as temporal arteritis. GCA is within the same spectrum of disease as polymyalgia rheumatica (PMR), as outlined next.

- **Takayasu arteritis** (also known as pulseless disease) is an LVV that primarily affects young women. It is characterized by constitutional symptoms, weak or absent pulses, asymmetric blood pressures, limb claudication, angina, arterial bruits, aneurysms, and end-organ damage from chronic ischemia. Diagnosis requires a thorough history and physical examination with support of elevated inflammatory markers and imaging studies, as there are no specific autoantibodies for Takayasu arteritis nor for GCA. Imaging with CTA, MRA, and/or PET scan can also be helpful for diagnosing Takayasu arteritis (34).

- **Giant cell arteritis (GCA)** generally only affects individuals over 50 years of age. It classically presents with headaches, vision changes, scalp tenderness, jaw claudication, and/or other constitutional symptoms. The hallmark of GCA is an elevated ESR >50 mm/hour and CRP >10 mg/L in a patient with concerning symptoms (35). Since this is generally a disease of the elderly, it is important to remember that the normal reference range of ESR rises with age. For men, the upper limit of normal for their ESR is their age divided by two, and for women, their upper limit of normal for their ESR is their age plus ten divided by two (36). Gold standard for diagnosis is still temporal artery biopsy, but additional imaging with temporal artery ultrasound, CTA, or MRA of the chest, and/or PET scan can be helpful for diagnosis. Treatment of GCA involves immediate initiation of high-dose glucocorticoids (prednisone 1 mg/kg equivalent or pulse dose steroids if there is vision-threatening disease) and then initiation of tocilizumab as a steroid-sparing agent if no contraindications, such as diverticulitis (37).
- **Polymyalgia rheumatica (PMR)** is an inflammatory musculoskeletal disease that is thought to be on the same spectrum of disease as GCA. PMR is characterized by morning stiffness lasting over 30 minutes and joint and muscle pain, primarily in the shoulders, neck, hips, and low back. Peripheral joint pain is typically not present. The hallmark of PMR is an elevated ESR and/or CRP in a patient with concerning symptoms over 50 years of age. Additional laboratory workup to rule out other causes of inflammatory arthritis should be negative, specifically RF and anti-CCP antibodies (38). Radiological studies with ultrasound and/or MRI can be helpful to support the diagnosis and rule out other musculoskeletal conditions. PMR is exquisitely sensitive to glucocorticoids, and if symptoms do not quickly respond to moderate-dose steroids (prednisone 15 mg–20 mg daily or equivalent), then alternate diagnoses should be considered. Prednisone is tapered very slowly over months to prevent PMR recurrence. Patients are monitored closely over time to ensure response to treatment and monitor for the development of GCA, which is associated with PMR.

Medium vessel vasculitis (MVV) involves inflammation of the medium-sized arteries. The two main types of MVV are Kawasaki disease, which primarily only affects children, and polyarteritis nodosa (PAN).

- **Kawasaki's disease** primarily affects the coronary arteries in children and is characterized by fevers, rash, conjunctivitis, cervical lymphadenopathy, and "strawberry tongue." Vasculitis of the coronary arteries can cause coronary artery aneurysms in up to 25% of children, leading to potentially deadly complications later in life (39). Treatment with aspirin and/or IVIG is important early in the disease course to reduce the risk of negative outcomes (40).
- **Polyarteritis nodosa (PAN)** can occur spontaneously or can be triggered by hepatitis B or hepatitis C infections. PAN is characterized by constitutional symptoms (e.g., fevers, malaise, weight loss), subcutaneous nodules, arthritis, and/or abdominal pain. There are no autoantibodies associated with PAN, but if a biopsy of an affected area is collected, then that can aid in the diagnosis. Imaging with CTA, MRA, and/or PET scan can also be helpful in diagnosis.

Small vessel vasculitis (SVV) primarily affects small venules, arterioles, and capillaries. This class has the most diversity of diseases and includes immune complex SVV (anti-glomerular basement membrane [GBM] disease, cryoglobulinemic vasculitis, IgA vasculitis, and hypocomplementemic urticarial vasculitis) and anti-neutrophil cytoplasmic antibody (ANCA)-associated vasculitides (granulomatosis with polyangiitis [GPA, formerly Wegener's granulomatosis], microscopic polyangiitis [MPA], and eosinophilic granulomatosis with polyangiitis [EGPA, formerly Churg-Strauss]).

- **Anti-GBM vasculitis** (also called Goodpasture's disease) classically presents with hemoptysis secondary to pulmonary hemorrhage and hematuria secondary to glomerulonephritis in a young man, which is caused by anti-GBM antibodies leading to vasculitis of the pulmonary and renal capillaries.
- **Cryoglobulinemic vasculitis** is frequently associated with hepatitis C infection. Cryoglobulin immune complexes are deposited into the skin, causing palpable purpura (see Figure 16.3); into the kidneys, causing glomerulonephritis; and into the perineural blood vessels, causing neuropathy.
- **IgA vasculitis** (also known as Henoch-Schönlein purpura) occurs when IgA complexes deposit into the skin, causing palpable purpura (see Figure 16.3); into the gastrointestinal tract, causing abdominal pain/diarrhea/hematochezia; into the kidneys, causing glomerulonephritis, and into the joints causing arthritis.
- **Granulomatosis with polyangiitis (GPA)** primarily involves the sinuses, lungs, skin, and kidneys. Symptoms can be constitutional, and can include bloody nasal discharge, nasal crusting, nasal bridge collapse, hearing loss, shortness of breath, hemoptysis, and hematuria (41). Labs are positive for cytoplasmic ANCAs (C-ANCAs) and anti-proteinase 3 (PR3) antibodies. Imaging findings showing abnormal sinuses, pulmonary nodules, pulmonary masses, or pulmonary cavitation on imaging support the diagnosis. Pathology showing granulomas or giant cells of affected tissues and pauci-immune glomerulonephritis on kidney biopsy supports the diagnosis (41).

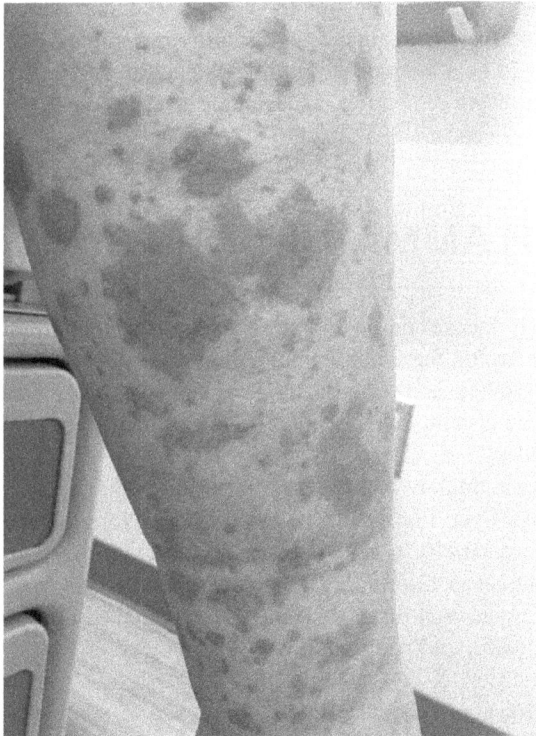

FIGURE 16.3   With inflammation of superficial blood vessels, the rash of vasculitis is raised over the surface of the surrounding skin and becomes palpable.

- **Microscopic polyangiitis (MPA)** primarily involves the skin, kidneys, and lungs, but notably not the sinuses. Symptoms can be constitutional and can include shortness of breath, hemoptysis, and hematuria. Labs are positive for perinuclear ANCAs (P-ANCAs) and anti-myeloperoxidase (MPO) antibodies. Imaging findings showing pulmonary fibrosis or ILD support the diagnosis. Similar to GPA, pathology showing pauci-immune glomerulonephritis on kidney biopsy supports the diagnosis (42).
- **Eosinophilic granulomatosis with polyangiitis (EGPA)** primarily affects the lungs, heart, skin, sinuses, and nerves. Symptoms can be constitutional and can include shortness of breath, coughing and wheezing, nasal congestion due to polyps, and neuropathy due to mononeuritis multiplex. Labs show eosinophilia $\geq 1.0 \times 10^9$/liter and positivity for P-ANCA and anti-MPO antibodies (in a minority of patients). Imaging may show transient or migratory pulmonary infiltrates and can help exclude other possible mimics (43).

There are also variable vessel vasculitides that can involve any size blood vessels, including Behçet's and Cogan's syndromes. **Behçet's syndrome** is characterized by inflammation of the eyes, oral and genital aphthous ulcers, erythema nodosum, acneiform dermatitis, thrombosis, neurological symptoms, and classical pathergy (44). **Cogan's syndrome** predominately involves anterior keratitis and sensorineural hearing loss.

Treatment for the primary vasculitides generally involves immediate initiation of glucocorticoids to quickly halt inflammation and then initiation of long-term, steroid-sparing agents. Dosing of glucocorticoids depends on whether there are organ or life-threatening manifestations, and steroids should be dosed in collaboration with a rheumatologist. Steroid-sparing agents used for maintenance therapy of vasculitis can include methotrexate, azathioprine, rituximab, and/or cyclophosphamide; the choice of steroid-sparing agent depends on the type of vasculitis, organs involved, and patient comorbidities. If vasculitis is secondary, then treating the underlying infection, removing the offending drug, or addressing the underlying autoimmune condition is the most important way to treat the secondary vasculitis, but patients may still require immunosuppression. Overall, treatment of vasculitis is complex and best initiated early in the disease course, so there should be a low threshold for consultation with a rheumatologist if a patient has signs or symptoms of any of the aforementioned vasculitides.

NONINFLAMMATORY PAIN SYNDROMES

While much of rheumatology focuses on the diagnosis and management of autoimmune and inflammatory conditions, as outlined earlier, these autoimmune diseases are relatively rare. Rheumatologists also commonly manage musculoskeletal and noninflammatory pain syndromes. Many more patients have noninflammatory causes of their musculoskeletal pain. The following are some of the most commonly seen noninflammatory pain disorders.

Osteoarthritis (OA) is a noninflammatory chronic arthritis that is caused by the degenerative destruction of joint cartilage and bone over time. OA is the most common form of arthritis in older adults and the leading contributing factor to disability in older persons (45). OA can affect any joint in the body, both the spine and the peripheral joints. Risk factors for OA are obesity, older age, and trauma.

General symptoms of OA are pain that is worsened by activity and improves with rest, morning stiffness lasting less than 30 minutes, and pain that is worse at the end of the day, which contrasts with the qualities of inflammatory arthritis. X-rays are helpful in diagnosing OA, showing degenerative changes, including joint space narrowing, subchondral sclerosis, and osteophytosis of the affected joints. Inflammatory markers, ESR and CRP, should generally be normal in OA and otherwise labs are generally not helpful in diagnosing OA, other than possibly to rule out concurrent inflammation. Treatment of OA involves physical therapy, acetaminophen, NSAIDs, intraarticular glucocorticoid injections, intraarticular hyaluronic acid injections, and/or surgical joint replacement.

Clinical Case 3: Fibromyalgia

The patient is a 43-year-old female with a history of migraine, depression and anxiety who presents for evaluation of headache and body pain. The patient was initially diagnosed with chronic migraine at the age of 27 and was started on daily topiramate, which decreased her headache frequency from 25 to ten days per month. She used sumatriptan on those days successfully. More recently, her headache frequency has increased to 22 days per month, and she now meets criteria for chronic migraine once again. She additionally notes that she has had terrible insomnia over the past few years, alongside worsening mood and difficulty with thinking and performing the daily activities of her accounting job. On physical examination, a number of tender points are noted.

A diagnosis of fibromyalgia and chronic migraine is made. A comprehensive management strategy is discussed. Referrals are placed to both pain psychology for cognitive behavioral therapy and physical therapy for help with developing a low-impact aerobic exercise plan. The patient is also started on daily duloxetine. While it is not clear that her topiramate has remained effective, after discussion, the patient elected to continue it while the duloxetine is up-titrated given that she has been on it for many years.

Three months later, the patient returns to clinic. While her pain is overall improved, it is still a work in progress. She continues to note daily body and head pain, though decreased in severity from treatment initiation. She also finds it hard to do the daily exercises as her fatigue has not gotten too much better. She continues to meet with her psychologist weekly.

Fibromyalgia is a chronic centralized pain disorder that is characterized by widespread noninflammatory musculoskeletal pain due to the central nervous system's misprocessing of painful stimuli (46). Symptoms of fibromyalgia are vast and nonspecific, including fatigue, insomnia, cognitive dysfunction/"brain fog," mood disturbances, and pain all over the body, commonly, though not exclusively, with particular tenderness at myofascial insertion points (47). Diagnosis of fibromyalgia requires a thorough history and physical examination to rule out other possible conditions. The ACR has created diagnostic criteria based on scoring of a widespread pain index and symptom severity score (48). Treatment includes both nonpharmacological and pharmacological therapies. Nonpharmacological treatments include cognitive behavioral therapy, exercise programs, and sleep hygiene. If nonpharmacological treatments are not enough to control symptoms, then pharmacological therapy can include selective serotonin-norepinephrine reuptake inhibitors (SNRIs) (such as duloxetine or milnacipran), tricyclic antidepressants (TCAs) (such as amitriptyline or nortriptyline), and/or gabapentinoids (such as gabapentin or pregabalin). Opioids are not recommended for treatment (47).

Complex regional pain syndrome (CRPS), also known as reflex sympathetic dystrophy and causalgia, is a chronic pain syndrome that is characterized by hyperalgesia, autonomic instability (color and temperature changes), limb swelling, sensory abnormalities, and motor dysfunction (49). CRPS typically only affects one limb or region of the body but occasionally can be bilateral and does not follow any dermatome or specific nerve distribution. CRPS typically occurs after an injury or trauma resulting in pain that is disproportionate to the inciting injury, but the underlying cause remains unknown. There are two types of CRPS described: Type I includes cases where there are no known specific nerve injuries, and Type II includes cases where there is a specific nerve injury identified (50). The severity of pain can be quite debilitating and interferes with patients' ability to perform activities of daily living.

Diagnosis of CRPS requires excluding other possible conditions and meeting diagnostic criteria from the International Association for the Study of Pain (IASP) task force (49). Labs can be used to rule out other inflammatory conditions, but there currently are not any specific lab tests for CRPS. Radiological studies can support the diagnosis, specifically triple-phase bone scans showing bone demineralization have a high specificity for CRPS (51). Treatment consists of a multidisciplinary approach with physical therapy, occupational therapy, behavioral therapy, pharmacotherapy, and pain management specialists. Pharmacotherapies have varying degrees of evidence, but mainstays of treatment include NSAIDs, bisphosphonates, TCAs, and gabapentinoids (52).

Overall, there are many causes of musculoskeletal pain, both inflammatory and noninflammatory. A comprehensive history, physical examination, and workup are necessary to narrow the differential diagnosis and rule out structural abnormalities. Treatment of noninflammatory pain syndromes can be challenging and requires multifactorial therapies and multidisciplinary collaboration.

SUMMARY

- Many patients with rheumatological diseases also experience headaches for a variety of reasons.
- Rheumatological conditions comprise a wide variety of diseases, including inflammatory arthritis, CTDs, vasculitis, and noninflammatory pain syndromes.
- Initial assessment of patients with possible rheumatic disease requires a thorough history and physical examination with a combination of various labs and radiological studies to support the diagnosis, but ESR and CRP are helpful in the initial workup of any rheumatological condition.
- Before a rheumatological diagnosis can be made, other conditions such as infection, malignancy, or structural musculoskeletal disorders need to be ruled out as possible etiologies of the symptoms.
- Once a rheumatological diagnosis is made, management typically involves a combination of anti-inflammatory and immunosuppressive medications but is individualized for every patient based on their specific clinical manifestations.
- All patients on immunosuppressive medications should be monitored regularly by a rheumatologist, and all members of their care team should be monitoring closely for signs and symptoms of infection or drug toxicities.

REFERENCES

1. Tian D, Zhao X, Ning Z, Gong Z, Wu J, Wang X. Migraine and risk of rheumatoid arthritis: A systematic review and meta-analysis of observational studies. *Heliyon*. 2023;9(8):e18430.
2. Pal B, Gibson C, Passmore J, Griffiths ID, Dick WC. A study of headaches and migraine in Sjogren's syndrome and other rheumatic disorders. *Ann Rheum Dis*. 1989;48(4):312–6.
3. Bronshvag MM, Pyrstowsky SD, Traviesa DC. Vascular headaches in mixed connective tissue disease. *Headache*. 1978;18(3):154–60.
4. Arend WP, Gabay C. Cytokines in the rheumatic diseases. *Rheum Dis Clin North Am*. 2004;30(1):41–67, v–vi.
5. Musubire AK, Cheema S, Ray JC, Hutton EJ, Matharu M. Cytokines in primary headache disorders: a systematic review and meta-analysis. *J Headache Pain*. 2023;24(1):36.
6. Edvinsson L, Haanes KA, Warfvinge K. Does inflammation have a role in migraine? *Nat Rev Neurol*. 2019;15(8):483–90.
7. Zahavi I, Chagnac A, Hering R, Davidovich S, Kuritzky A. Prevalence of Raynaud's phenomenon in patients with migraine. *Arch Intern Med*. 1984;144(4):742–4.
8. Gerard AO, Merino D, Van Obberghen EK, Rocher F, Destere A, Lanteri-Minet M, et al. Calcitonin gene-related peptide-targeting drugs and Raynaud's phenomenon: a real-world potential safety signal from the WHO pharmacovigilance database. *J Headache Pain*. 2022;23(1):53.
9. Walker JG, Littlejohn GO, McMurray NE, Cutolo M. Stress system response and rheumatoid arthritis: a multilevel approach. *Rheumatology (Oxford)*. 1999;38(11):1050–7.
10. Kelman L. The triggers or precipitants of the acute migraine attack. *Cephalalgia*. 2007;27(5):394–402.
11. Heliovaara M, Aho K, Aromaa A, Knekt P, Reunanen A. Smoking and risk of rheumatoid arthritis. *J Rheumatol*. 1993;20(11):1830–5.
12. Padyukov L, Silva C, Stolt P, Alfredsson L, Klareskog L. A gene-environment interaction between smoking and shared epitope genes in HLA-DR provides a high risk of seropositive rheumatoid arthritis. *Arthritis Rheum*. 2004;50(10):3085–92.

13. Hoovestol RA, Mikuls TR. Environmental exposures and rheumatoid arthritis risk. *Curr Rheumatol Rep.* 2011;*13*(5):431–9.

14. Aletaha D, Neogi T, Silman AJ, Funovits J, Felson DT, Bingham CO, 3rd, et al. 2010 Rheumatoid arthritis classification criteria: An American College of Rheumatology/European League Against Rheumatism collaborative initiative. *Arthritis Rheum.* 2010;*62*(9):2569–81.

15. Reveille JD, Hirsch R, Dillon CF, Carroll MD, Weisman MH. The prevalence of HLA-B27 in the US: data from the US National Health and Nutrition Examination Survey, 2009. *Arthritis Rheum.* 2012;*64*(5):1407–11.

16. Reveille JD. Epidemiology of spondyloarthritis in North America. *Am J Med Sci.* 2011;*341*(4):284–6.

17. Peschken CA, Esdaile JM. Systemic lupus erythematosus in North American Indians: a population based study. *J Rheumatol.* 2000;*27*(8):1884–91.

18. Costenbader KH, Desai A, Alarcon GS, Hiraki LT, Shaykevich T, Brookhart MA, et al. Trends in the incidence, demographics, and outcomes of end-stage renal disease due to lupus nephritis in the US from 1995 to 2006. *Arthritis Rheum.* 2011;*63*(6):1681–8.

19. Lim SS, Helmick CG, Bao G, Hootman J, Bayakly R, Gordon C, et al. Racial disparities in mortality associated with systemic lupus erythematosus - Fulton and DeKalb Counties, Georgia, 2002–2016. *MMWR Morb Mortal Wkly Rep.* 2019;*68*(18):419–22.

20. Aguirre A, Izadi Z, Trupin L, Barbour KE, Greenlund KJ, Katz P, et al. Race, ethnicity, and disparities in the risk of end-organ lupus manifestations following a systemic lupus erythematosus diagnosis in a multiethnic cohort. *Arthritis Care Res (Hoboken).* 2023;*75*(1):34–43.

21. Ghazali WSW, Daud SMM, Mohammad N, Wong KK. Slicc damage index score in systemic lupus erythematosus patients and its associated factors. *Medicine (Baltimore).* 2018;*97*(42):e12787.

22. Aringer M, Costenbader K, Daikh D, Brinks R, Mosca M, Ramsey-Goldman R, et al. 2019 European league against Rheumatism/American college of rheumatology classification criteria for systemic lupus erythematosus. *Arthritis Rheumatol.* 2019;*71*(9):1400–12.

23. Tan EM, Feltkamp TE, Smolen JS, Butcher B, Dawkins R, Fritzler MJ, et al. Range of antinuclear antibodies in "healthy" individuals. *Arthritis Rheum.* 1997;*40*(9):1601–11.

24. Cai T, Zhao J, Yang Y, Jiang Y, Zhang JA. Hydroxychloroquine use reduces mortality risk in systemic lupus erythematosus: A systematic review and meta-analysis of cohort studies. *Lupus.* 2022;*31*(14):1714–25.

25. Fanouriakis A, Kostopoulou M, Alunno A, Aringer M, Bajema I, Boletis JN, et al. 2019 update of the EULAR recommendations for the management of systemic lupus erythematosus. *Ann Rheum Dis.* 2019;*78*(6):736–45.

26. Miyakis S, Lockshin MD, Atsumi T, Branch DW, Brey RL, Cervera R, et al. International consensus statement on an update of the classification criteria for definite antiphospholipid syndrome (APS). *J Thromb Haemost.* 2006;*4*(2):295–306.

27. Pengo V, Denas G, Zoppellaro G, Jose SP, Hoxha A, Ruffatti A, et al. Rivaroxaban vs warfarin in high-risk patients with antiphospholipid syndrome. *Blood.* 2018;*132*(13):1365–71.

28. Shiboski CH, Shiboski SC, Seror R, Criswell LA, Labetoulle M, Lietman TM, et al. 2016 American College of Rheumatology/European League Against Rheumatism classification criteria for primary Sjogren's syndrome: A consensus and data-driven methodology involving three international patient cohorts. *Ann Rheum Dis.* 2017;*76*(1):9–16.

29. Beck DB, Ferrada MA, Sikora KA, Ombrello AK, Collins JC, Pei W, et al. Somatic Mutations in UBA1 and Severe Adult-Onset Autoinflammatory Disease. *N Engl J Med.* 2020;*383*(27):2628–38.

30. Ferrada MA, Sikora KA, Luo Y, Wells KV, Patel B, Groarke EM, et al. Somatic Mutations in UBA1 Define a Distinct Subset of Relapsing Polychondritis Patients With VEXAS. *Arthritis Rheumatol.* 2021;*73*(10):1886–95.

31. Grayson PC, Patel BA, Young NS. VEXAS syndrome. *Blood.* 2021;*137*(26):3591–4.

32. Patel BA, Ferrada MA, Grayson PC, Beck DB. VEXAS syndrome: An inflammatory and hematologic disease. *Semin Hematol.* 2021;*58*(4):201–3.

33. Beck DB, Bodian DL, Shah V, Mirshahi UL, Kim J, Ding Y, et al. Estimated prevalence and clinical manifestations of UBA1 variants associated with VEXAS syndrome in a clinical population. *JAMA.* 2023;*329*(4):318–24.

34. Grayson PC, Ponte C, Suppiah R, Robson JC, Gribbons KB, Judge A, et al. 2022 American College of Rheumatology/EULAR classification criteria for Takayasu arteritis. *Ann Rheum Dis.* 2022;*81*(12):1654–60.

35. Ponte C, Grayson PC, Robson JC, Suppiah R, Gribbons KB, Judge A, et al. 2022 American College of Rheumatology/EULAR Classification Criteria for Giant Cell Arteritis. *Arthritis Rheumatol.* 2022;*74*(12):1881–9.

36. Miller A, Green M, Robinson D. Simple rule for calculating normal erythrocyte sedimentation rate. *Br Med J (Clin Res Ed).* 1983;*286*(6361):266.

37. Stone JH, Tuckwell K, Dimonaco S, Klearman M, Aringer M, Blockmans D, et al. Trial of tocilizumab in giant-cell arteritis. *N Engl J Med.* 2017;*377*(4):317–28.

38. Dasgupta B, Cimmino MA, Maradit-Kremers H, Schmidt WA, Schirmer M, Salvarani C, et al. 2012 provisional classification criteria for polymyalgia rheumatica: a European League Against Rheumatism/American College of Rheumatology collaborative initiative. *Ann Rheum Dis.* 2012;*71*(4):484–92.
39. Burns JC, Glode MP. Kawasaki syndrome. *Lancet.* 2004;*364*(9433):533–44.
40. Murphy DJ, Jr., Huhta JC. Treatment of Kawasaki syndrome with intravenous gamma globulin. *N Engl J Med.* 1987;*316*(14):881.
41. Robson JC, Grayson PC, Ponte C, Suppiah R, Craven A, Judge A, et al. 2022 American College of Rheumatology/European Alliance of Associations for Rheumatology classification criteria for granulomatosis with polyangiitis. *Ann Rheum Dis.* 2022;*81*(3):315–20.
42. Suppiah R, Robson JC, Grayson PC, Ponte C, Craven A, Khalid S, et al. 2022 American College of Rheumatology/European Alliance of Associations for Rheumatology Classification Criteria for Microscopic Polyangiitis. *Arthritis Rheumatol.* 2022;*74*(3):400–6.
43. Grayson PC, Ponte C, Suppiah R, Robson JC, Craven A, Judge A, et al. 2022 American College of Rheumatology/European Alliance of Associations for Rheumatology Classification Criteria for Eosinophilic Granulomatosis With Polyangiitis. *Arthritis Rheumatol.* 2022;*74*(3):386–92.
44. International Team for the Revision of the International Criteria for Behcet's D. The International Criteria for Behcet's Disease (ICBD): a collaborative study of 27 countries on the sensitivity and specificity of the new criteria. *J Eur Acad Dermatol Venereol.* 2014;*28*(3):338–47.
45. Song J, Chang RW, Dunlop DD. Population impact of arthritis on disability in older adults. *Arthritis Rheum.* 2006;*55*(2):248–55.
46. Woolf CJ. Central sensitization: implications for the diagnosis and treatment of pain. *Pain.* 2011;*152*(3 Suppl):S2–S15.
47. Clauw DJ. Fibromyalgia: a clinical review. *JAMA.* 2014;*311*(15):1547–55.
48. Wolfe F, Clauw DJ, Fitzcharles MA, Goldenberg DL, Hauser W, Katz RS, et al. Fibromyalgia criteria and severity scales for clinical and epidemiological studies: a modification of the ACR Preliminary Diagnostic Criteria for Fibromyalgia. *J Rheumatol.* 2011;*38*(6):1113–22.
49. Harden RN, Bruehl S, Stanton-Hicks M, Wilson PR. Proposed new diagnostic criteria for complex regional pain syndrome. *Pain Med.* 2007;*8*(4):326–31.
50. Stanton-Hicks M, Janig W, Hassenbusch S, Haddox JD, Boas R, Wilson P. Reflex sympathetic dystrophy: changing concepts and taxonomy. *Pain.* 1995;*63*(1):127–33.
51. Wuppenhorst N, Maier C, Frettloh J, Pennekamp W, Nicolas V. Sensitivity and specificity of 3-phase bone scintigraphy in the diagnosis of complex regional pain syndrome of the upper extremity. *Clin J Pain.* 2010;*26*(3):182–9.
52. Duong S, Bravo D, Todd KJ, Finlayson RJ, Tran Q. Treatment of complex regional pain syndrome: an updated systematic review and narrative synthesis. *Can J Anaesth.* 2018;*65*(6):658–84.

Headache and Women's Health

17

Beverly Tse, Alexandra Loza, Stephanie Bakaysa, Amy Johnson, and Andrea Shields

---

LEARNING OBJECTIVES

1. Discuss headaches throughout the life phases of women and the effect of hormones
2. Review both primary and secondary diagnosis of headache in pregnancy and the postpartum period
3. Recognize headache diagnosis that may be specific to or exacerbated by pregnancy
4. Understand the evaluation and treatment of headache in pregnancy and the postpartum period
5. Review contraceptive management in patients with migraine headaches

---

INTRODUCTION

Migraine and severe headache affect one in five women and are the third leading cause of emergency department visits in reproductive-aged women.[1] It is well established that women are impacted more than men by headaches in regard to frequency, duration, and severity.[2, 3] Caring for women with headaches, especially migraine, requires special consideration of the unique life phases for women—menstruation, pregnancy, lactation, family planning, and menopause. The prevalence of migraine varies according to the life phase of a female, with prevalence increasing after menarche, during menstruation, postpartum, and during the perimenopause period. Conversely, the prevalence decreases in pregnancy, especially during the second and third trimester of pregnancy, and in postmenopausal women.[4–6]

Headache in women, especially migraine, is impacted by hormone fluctuations that vary throughout a woman's lifespan.[7] More specifically, it has been proposed that the withdrawal and decline in estrogen levels may be associated with migraine.[8] Estrogen may have a role in activating central pain pathways that cause headache through complex mechanisms that alter vascular inflammatory substances.[9, 10] There are relatively low estrogen levels before puberty, which correlates with the lower prevalence of migraine during this period. Estrogen levels begin to rise after puberty and with the start of menarche. Each menstrual cycle has a natural fluctuation in estrogen level, which rises during the follicular phase, or the first half of the menstrual cycle; peaks during the late follicular and early luteal phase; plateaus during the mid-luteal phase; and falls precipitously just prior to menstruation. As a result, 10%–20% of women will experience their first migraine at the beginning of menarche.[11] In the nonpregnant female, estrogen is produced primarily by the ovaries, with smaller quantities produced by the liver, adrenal gland, breasts, and adipocytes. Throughout pregnancy, estrogen is produced by the placenta. In addition, exogenous sources such as oral contraception pills, hormone replacement therapy for menopausal symptoms, hormones used as a part of in vitro fertilization cycles, and hormone therapy for transgender women may also impact estrogen levels.

Headache is responsible for a significant burden on quality of life, with children experiencing headache having poorer school attendance and school-related issues[12] and adults with headaches being more likely to have diminished health-related quality of life.[13] Women are impacted more than men, with an estimated number of bed rest days per year of 5.6 days compared to 3.8 days for men.[14] Given findings of increased severity of headache and the impact on quality of life, women are significantly more likely to seek medical attention for headache.[15] With the impact of headache on women, it is important for providers to consider unique factors such as menstruation, pregnancy, and menopause when caring for women throughout their life stages.

COMORBID CONDITIONS IN PREGNANCY AND IN THE POSTPARTUM PERIOD

Headache will impact about 35% of women during pregnancy[16] and 39% of women in the postpartum period.[17] Pregnancy is a unique clinical scenario in which the well-being of both the mother and fetus must be considered when assessing diagnostic and treatment options. In addition, diagnoses that are specific to pregnancy and the postpartum period, such as preeclampsia, must be considered. While many pregnant women are healthy, the average maternal age is rising.[18] Thus, the rates of coexisting medical conditions such as obesity, diabetes, and hypertension are increasing. The physiologic changes of pregnancy, including hypercoagulability, changes in the immune defense system, and hemodynamic changes, may cause pregnant women to be more susceptible to diagnoses that would typically be reserved for a population that is older or has more comorbidities. As a result, pregnancy may predispose women to serious and potentially life-threatening conditions that may present as headache.

The Approach to Headache in Pregnancy

Evaluating headache in pregnancy begins much like that for a nonpregnant individual, including gathering a history and physical exam with a specific assessment of neurologic status. Additional components of the history include gestational age, as well as pregnancy-related complications such as a hypertensive disorder of pregnancy. Ascertaining gestational age is essential since some diagnoses during pregnancy may only be present during specific trimesters. Moreover, due to fetal safety, diagnostic and treatment options such as medications or interventions may only be offered during specific trimesters.

Imaging may be required to assist in evaluating and diagnosing headache in pregnancy. The indications to consider imaging in pregnant women with headaches are like those of nonpregnant individuals, including change in baseline headache quality or severity for those with known headache disorders, sudden onset, accompanying abnormal neurologic exam or deficits, or seizures. While many women presenting with headaches will have a primary cause, such as migraine or tension headache, one study demonstrated that 27% of women who underwent magnetic resonance imaging (MRI) imaging had symptomatic pathological findings, including intracranial hemorrhage, cerebral venous thrombosis, stroke, and sinusitis.[19]

For the evaluation of headache, MRI and computed tomography (CT) are typically the imaging modalities utilized. MRI is typically the imaging modality of choice, as it does not expose the fetus to ionizing radiation, with data demonstrating no adverse fetal effects. According to the American College of Obstetrics and Gynecology, gadolinium contrast in pregnancy should be limited to situations where the benefits outweigh the risks given the uncertainty of possible fetal effects and ongoing theoretical concerns from animal studies.[20] There have been no reports of harm to an infant in a breastfeeding woman after receiving gadolinium contrast, and breastfeeding should continue after its administration.

Not all institutions have readily available MRIs, so CT is also an option in pregnancy. While ionizing radiation may concern patients and providers, the lowest clinically documented fetal radiation dose that may produce severe intellectual disability is 610 mGy,[21] and the risk of fetal anomalies, fetal growth restriction, or abortion has not been reported at less than 50 mGy.[22] A head or neck CT scan carries a fetal radiation dose of 1.0–10 mGy,[23] lower than the established thresholds for radiation to cause fetal harm. Thus, the American College of Obstetrics and Gynecology notes that if a CT scan or associated contrast materials are indicated, they should not be withheld from a pregnant woman following a discussion of risks and benefits.[20]

Lumbar puncture may also be safely performed during pregnancy to provide further diagnostic information if increased intracranial pressure or central nervous system infection is suspected or for treatment of conditions such as idiopathic intracranial hypertension.

Considerations Prior to Pregnancy

In reproductive-age women with chronic headache, it is important to discuss future childbearing plans and consider preconception counseling with an obstetric provider. Before conceiving, it is optimal for headaches to be well controlled and for medications to be reviewed with the patient to ensure they are compatible with pregnancy. In addition, certain medications, including antiepileptic medications, such as carbamazepine or valproic acid, [24, 25] can interfere with folic acid metabolism and frequently require supplemental folic acid to prevent fetal neural defects, if not preferably avoided outright. Ideally, folic acid supplementation should commence prior to conception and continue during the first trimester.

Headache Differential Diagnosis

The differential diagnosis for headaches in pregnancy can be divided into primary and secondary causes. Women who have had a diagnosis of headache prior to pregnancy may have headaches during pregnancy that are stable, improve, or worsen, depending on their etiology. It is also possible for pregnant women to be diagnosed with a primary headache disorder, though this occurs less frequently. When considering the differential for headache, characteristics that may prompt more immediate evaluation and intervention are like those of a nonpregnant individual. These characteristics include headaches with altered mental status, sudden onset of severe headaches, change in headache characteristics, headaches precipitated by head trauma or toxin exposure, suspected increase in intracranial pressure, or headaches unrelieved by patients' usual medication.

Primary headaches

The differential diagnosis for headaches in pregnancy includes those that providers are generally familiar with, including migraine, tension-type headache, and the trigeminal autonomic cephalalgias (TAC). Women who have a diagnosis of primary headache prior to pregnancy may continue to have headaches in pregnancy that are similar, and further diagnostic testing may not be necessary.

Tension headaches
The most common type of primary headache in pregnancy is a tension headache, characterized as pressure or tightness around the head. Tension headaches are not hormonally mediated and will improve in 28% of pregnant women, remain unchanged in 67%, and worsen and increase in 5%.[26] There are no known adverse effects to pregnancy in women with tension headaches. Physical and emotional stress can trigger tension headaches; thus, pregnant patients may be susceptible to tension headaches due to the physiologic changes of pregnancy and life stressors that may arise during the pregnancy.

CASE STUDY #1: CLINICAL CASE SCENARIO: WORSENING MIGRAINE HEADACHE IN A PREGNANT PATIENT

History: 36-year-old pregnant patient with migraine well controlled on daily propranolol and occasional use of sumatriptan for abortive therapy. Before pregnancy, she took gabapentin, propranolol, and onabotulinumtoxinA injections every 12 weeks. She reported using the calcitonin gene-related peptide (CGRP) antagonist rimegepant on average twice monthly. Before she conceived, her neurologist and her obstetrician advised her to discontinue the gabapentin and CGRP antagonist due to limited safety information during pregnancy. She was instructed to continue her beta-blocker therapy and use her triptan as needed. She had no other pertinent medical or surgical history and reported no medication allergies.

Clinical Presentation: She presented to labor and delivery at 32 weeks gestation with a 4-day history of a severe headache. She described her headache as her usual migraine headache, with subacute onset behind the right eye. The headache was associated with nausea, blurred vision, fatigue, and increased sensitivity to light. In the last two weeks, her headaches occurred every other day, were more intense (described as "8 out of 10" on a pain scale), and did not always respond to her sumatriptan. This current headache began four days prior, and while there was an initial response to her sumatriptan, her second dose had no effect. She has missed work for the last three days. Prior to that, she only missed, on average, three days of work per year due to her headaches. She denied other neurologic symptoms, fever, chills, abdominal pain, or vaginal bleeding.

Physical Examination: *Vital signs*: Blood pressure: 129/70 mmHg, Pulse rate: 105 beats per minute, Temperature: 98.6°F (37°C), Respiratory rate: 16 breaths per minute.

Neurological examination: Cranial nerves were intact, and no focal neurological deficits were observed. Bilateral DTRs were 2+.

Physical Exam: The patient was alert but appeared fatigued and covered her head with a blanket due to light sensitivity. Cardiac and respiratory exams were normal. The abdominal exam was normal without right upper quadrant pain, and her fundus was nontender. There was no calf tenderness or lower extremity edema. She was not contracting on the monitor, and her fetal status was reassuring.

Laboratory Results: Complete blood count including platelets, liver function tests, serum creatinine, and urine protein resulted normal.

Assessment: Based on her clinical presentation, examination, and laboratory results, she was diagnosed with status migrainosus. Given her symptoms were similar to her typical migraine and her blood pressures were normotensive with normal laboratory studies, including urine protein/creatinine, preeclampsia was excluded. Her symptoms were similar to typical migraine, and her blood pressures were normotensive with normal laboratory studies, including urine protein/creatinine, so preeclampsia was excluded.

Trigeminal autonomic cephalalgias, including cluster headache
Given that cluster headache is less prevalent in women, there is less data regarding cluster headaches and pregnancy outcomes. It is less likely that hormonal changes in pregnancy may impact cluster headaches, with one study suggesting that only 5% of women with cluster headaches will experience an attack during pregnancy.[27]

Migraine
Various factors present before or during pregnancy can affect migraine burden during pregnancy. Risk factors for worsening migraine in pregnancy include menstrual migraine, hyperemesis gravidarum, or a pathologic pregnancy course.[28] Other common exacerbating factors include stress, hormonal changes (such as fluctuations in estrogen levels), alcohol, lack of sleep, and sensory stimuli (bright lights, loud

noises).[8] The course of migraine during pregnancy can vary significantly from one patient to another.[29] For women with a history of migraine before pregnancy, 60%–70% will note improvement in their headache burden, and 20% will have migraine attacks disappear entirely during pregnancy.[30] Some patients experience a reduction in migraine frequency and severity during the first trimester due to hormonal changes, particularly a rise in estrogen levels, which can stabilize migraine patterns. Many patients find that their migraine continues to improve during the second trimester. Migraine may return or become more frequent and severe for some women in the third trimester. Hormonal fluctuations and the physical strain of pregnancy can contribute to these changes. After giving birth, migraine patterns can be unpredictable. Some patients experience a reduction in migraine, while others may have more frequent headaches, possibly due to hormonal fluctuations, sleep deprivation, and the stress of caring for a newborn.[29]

It is important to note that women with migraine disorder are at increased risk of developing hypertensive disorders of pregnancy, including gestational hypertension and preeclampsia. Evidence suggests that a history of migraine may be associated with an increased risk of low birth weight in infants and preterm birth. However, the evidence may not be as strong as that for hypertensive disorders.[31–33] This underscores the importance of close monitoring and early detection of hypertensive disorders in pregnant patients with a migraine history.

Pregnant patients should receive comprehensive information about migraine management during pregnancy, including lifestyle modifications and recognizing signs of worsening headaches that may not be due to migraine and require immediate medical attention. The decision to use medication should consider the severity of migraine, the impact on the patient's quality of life, the potential risks to the fetus, and the patient's specific needs and medical history. Communication and shared decision-making between the obstetrician, neurologist, and the patient are essential to achieve the best possible outcome while prioritizing both the mother's and the fetus' well-being.[34] Regular follow-up appointments are recommended with the neurologist and obstetrical team to assess the patient's response to treatment, monitor blood pressure, and watch for any signs of complications like preeclampsia. Overall, a patient-centered and multidisciplinary approach is crucial to address the unique challenges of managing migraine in pregnant patients while safeguarding both maternal and fetal health.

Treatment

The treatment of headache in pregnancy typically begins with simple lifestyle modifications and non-pharmacologic interventions, such as ensuring adequate sleep, adequate hydration, regular exercise, stress management, cognitive behavioral therapy, avoidance of any known triggers, and application of heat, ice, and massage.

Several medications may be considered during pregnancy for the treatment of headaches. The first line for treatment of an acute headache is acetaminophen, given its known fetal safety profile and the ability to be used throughout pregnancy and postpartum. Caffeine can also be utilized, though dosing should not exceed 200 mg daily. In addition, diphenhydramine and metoclopramide may be used as the first line.

Second-line treatment includes a single dose of nonsteroidal anti-inflammatory drugs (NSAID) such as aspirin, naproxen, or ibuprofen. The use of NSAID medications is limited to the second trimester to avoid premature constriction of the ductus arteriosus, a transient decrease in fetal renal function, persistent neonatal pulmonary hypertension, neonatal periventricular leukomalacia, intraventricular hemorrhage, and necrotizing enterocolitis that may occur with exposure during the first and third trimesters. Triptans, most often sumatriptan, may also be used for patients with persistent migraine headache and intractable emesis inadequately controlled by previously mentioned medications. Some headaches may also respond to intravenous magnesium sulfate, especially in migraine with aura. Noninvasive neuromodulator devices, such as remote electrical neuromodulation[35] and peripheral nerve blocks,[36] may also be considered.

Medications not recommended in pregnancy include ergot alkaloid-containing products, as they may stimulate strong uterine contractions.[37] Medications recently approved for treating migraine, including CGRP monoclonal antibodies and small molecule antagonists, have not been studied in pregnancy and are not currently recommended for use during pregnancy. The American College of Obstetrics and Gynecology also advises against using butalbital to treat headaches due to habituation and the risk of overuse headaches. The use of opioids to treat headaches is also discouraged.[38]

Secondary headaches due to pregnancy

Several pregnancy-related disorders may cause headaches in pregnancy. A secondary diagnosis should be considered in women with no known primary headache diagnosis or who experience a change in headache characteristics from their baseline.

Hyperemesis gravidarum

Pregnant women may commonly experience nausea and vomiting during the first trimester of pregnancy. A more severe form of nausea and vomiting in pregnancy is hyperemesis gravidarum, defined by vomiting multiple times a day, inability to tolerate oral intake, electrolyte abnormalities, and a 5% or more loss in prepregnancy body weight. Headache may be associated with hyperemesis gravidarum and the dehydration that can ensue. The mainstay of treatment for hyperemesis gravidarum includes fluid hydration, antiemetics, and supportive therapies.

Anemia of pregnancy

Dilutional physiologic anemia often occurs in pregnancy due to the more considerable increase in plasma volume than in red blood cell mass. Anemia in the first and third trimester is defined as a hemoglobin of less than or equal to 11 g/dL or a hematocrit of less than 33%. In the second trimester, anemia is a hemoglobin less than 10.5 g/dL or a hematocrit less than 32%. Besides the physiologic anemia that may occur, pregnant women are also at increased risk of nutritional deficiency anemias, such as iron, folic acid, and vitamin B12 deficiencies in addition to anemia from hemoglobinopathies. Anemia may present with headache in pregnancy and should be included in the differential diagnosis. Anemia in pregnancy may increase the risk of hypertension, diabetes, placental abruption, chorioamnionitis, need for blood transfusion, admission to the intensive care unit, preterm birth, and neonatal anemia.[39] Therefore, it is essential to identify and treat anemia that may present with headache.

Preeclampsia and eclampsia

Preeclampsia and eclampsia are conditions specific to pregnancy and are typically diagnosed at or beyond 20 weeks gestation and up to 12 weeks postpartum.

The exact pathophysiology of preeclampsia is unknown; however, endothelial dysfunction from abnormal placentation and spiral artery remodeling may contribute. Preeclampsia without severe features is a new onset blood pressure elevation in pregnancy, defined as systolic blood pressure ≥140 mmHg or diastolic blood pressure ≥90 mmHg accompanied by proteinuria. Proteinuria is defined as a random spot urine protein-to-creatinine ratio ≥0.3, 24-hour urine protein ≥300 mg, or a urine dip protein 2+. Preeclampsia with severe features can also be diagnosed due to maternal end-organ damage, even in the absence of proteinuria. Criteria include systolic blood pressure ≥160 mmHg or diastolic blood pressure ≥110 mmHg, thrombocytopenia, impaired liver function (defined as liver enzyme elevations to more than twice the upper limit of normal or severe persistent right upper quadrant or epigastric pain unresponsive to medication), renal insufficiency (defined as serum creatinine >1.1 mg/dL or a doubling of serum creatinine concentration in the absence of renal disease), pulmonary edema, new onset headache, and visual disturbances.[40]

In women with an underlying diagnosis of hypertension and known elevated blood pressures prior to pregnancy or before 20 weeks gestation, the diagnosis of superimposed preeclampsia is more nuanced and beyond the scope of this chapter. In patients with preeclampsia with severe features, IV magnesium sulfate is administered to prevent eclamptic seizures as an initial 4-gram bolus followed by 2-grams/hour continuous infusion. Blood pressure control with oral and IV medications for hypertensive urgency is paramount to preventing cerebral edema and hemorrhage.

Symptoms of preeclampsia may include neurologic manifestations, such as headache and visual disturbances (e.g., blurred vision or scotomata). While not all headache in the setting of elevated blood pressure may represent a manifestation of preeclampsia, it should be considered if the headache does not improve with medications, is severe, is new in onset, or has no alternative diagnosis to explain it. Headaches and scotomata in the setting of preeclampsia may be a precursor symptom for eclampsia; in one study,

80% of women experienced headache and 45% experienced visual disturbances prior to the seizure.[41] These seizures are typically self-limited, and magnesium sulfate is re-bolused during seizures to prevent further seizures. If an eclamptic seizure is refractory to intravenous magnesium sulfate, additional antiepileptics such as benzodiazepines or phenytoin may be utilized. In women with preeclampsia with headache accompanied by mental status changes, vomiting, or fever, reversible cerebral vasoconstriction syndrome and posterior reversible encephalopathy syndrome should be considered.

The definitive treatment for preeclampsia is delivery of the fetus and placenta, though some patients may be candidates for expectant management up to 34 weeks gestation. It is important to note that severe headache or visual changes due to preeclampsia preclude expectant management, and delivery is typically pursued. In women with elevated blood pressure and headache, preeclampsia should be included in the differential diagnosis, and a prompt obstetric consultation should be obtained.

Secondary headaches associated with conditions exacerbated by pregnancy

Given the physiologic changes associated with pregnancy and the risk of pregnancy-related diagnoses, such as preeclampsia, there are certain conditions that pregnant women are at risk for that may present with headaches.

Maternal stroke

Stroke impacts 34.2 per 100,000 deliveries, with death from stroke occurring in 1.4 per 100,000 deliveries.[42] The risk of stroke is highest during the delivery period and up to two weeks postpartum.[43, 44] This risk is in part due to a physiologic hypercoagulable state during pregnancy that protects women from excessive hemorrhage at delivery but may increase the risk of thromboembolic events, especially with underlying risk factors. In addition, cardiovascular hemodynamic adaptions, changes in coagulation factors, endothelial dysfunction, inflammation, and impaired cerebrovascular tone increase the risk of stroke.[45] Risk factors for stroke in pregnancy include preeclampsia and hypertensive disorders of pregnancy, African American race, age 35 years or older, systemic lupus erythematosus, receipt of blood transfusion in pregnancy, and migraine headaches.[46] Women with a history of stroke who desire future pregnancies should be counseled on their underlying risk factors and pregnancy management considerations based on the etiology of their prior stroke.

According to Western population studies, ischemic stroke is more frequent in pregnancy than hemorrhagic ones.[47] Ischemic stroke in reproductive-age women can result from cerebral venous thrombosis (CVT), with pregnancy being a transient but predisposing condition.[48] Headache is one of the most common symptoms of CVT, with 90% of patients reporting this symptom. The headache is typically described as diffuse and will become more severe over days to weeks.[49] Anticoagulation with subcutaneous LMWH or intravenous heparin is the mainstay of treatment. Neither of these medications crosses the placenta, and both are compatible with lactation, so they are safe during pregnancy and postpartum. Additional etiologies of ischemic stroke in pregnancy include antiphospholipid syndrome and paradoxical embolism.[46]

Hemorrhagic stroke, including subarachnoid or intracerebral hemorrhage, may occur due to vascular anomalies; preeclampsia/eclampsia; hemolysis, elevated liver enzymes, and low platelet (HELLP) syndrome; reversible cerebral vasoconstriction syndrome; and coagulopathy. Hemorrhagic strokes are associated with the poorest outcomes, including neurologic deficit and death. Preeclampsia, eclampsia, and HELLP syndrome are significant causes of hemorrhagic stroke during pregnancy, and rapid treatment of severe hypertension is the mainstay of prevention. In addition, disseminated intravascular coagulation (DIC) may cause hemorrhagic stroke; pregnant women are at increased risk of developing DIC due to postpartum hemorrhage, placental abruption, preeclampsia, amniotic fluid embolism, or intrauterine fetal demise.

Idiopathic intracranial hypertension

Idiopathic intracranial hypertension (IIH) impacts predominantly women of reproductive age with higher body mass indices. It is characterized by headache, transient visual obscuration, diplopia, and pulsatile tinnitus due to increased intracranial pressure. Most IIH cases are diagnosed outside of pregnancy, with only 1.6% of cases diagnosed during pregnancy. IIH may be associated with papilledema and visual loss during pregnancy.[50] However, patients diagnosed with IIH prior to pregnancy have similar longitudinal outcomes compared to patients who do not become pregnant. Thus, pregnancy does not need to be avoided in all patients with IIH, but disease and symptoms should be well managed and controlled before conceiving. In addition, acetazolamide may also be used in women with IIH.[51] Women with IIH are candidates for neuraxial anesthesia during labor but with special considerations regarding epidural bolus or continuous spinal analgesia in order to avoid abrupt increases in intracranial pressure.[52]

Infection

Common infections in pregnancy that present with headache include viral respiratory infections, sinusitis, and meningitis.

Headache can be a presenting symptom in pregnant patients with infection, especially as their altered immune response during pregnancy makes them more susceptible to infectious pathogens.

While rare, meningitis should be considered in pregnant patients who present with headache, especially if accompanied by other crucial diagnostic indicators such as altered mental status or fever. One study in the Netherlands demonstrated that 4.4% of all maternal deaths were due to meningitis, with 80% of these women presenting during pregnancy. The most common presenting symptoms were headache (87%), altered mental status (73%), fever (60%), and nuchal rigidity (33%).[53] A specific bacterial pathogen of interest is *Listeria monocytogenes* due to its associated risk of congenital infection. Women are at higher risk of *listeria* infection than the general population, and prevention of this infection includes counseling pregnant patients to avoid unpasteurized cheeses, hot dogs, and lunch meats.

Pituitary apoplexy

An acute hemorrhage into the pituitary gland causes pituitary apoplexy. Predisposing factors for pituitary apoplexy during pregnancy include the physiologic enlargement of the pituitary gland, a known history of micro- or macroadenoma, and anticoagulation therapy. A patient with pituitary apoplexy will present with severe headache, associated visual defects, and symptoms associated with deficiencies of the hypopituitary gland. The most life-threatening pituitary hormone deficiency is cortisol deficiency, which may cause hypotension; thus, this diagnosis requires a high index of suspicion and prompt treatment.

Posterior reversible encephalopathy syndrome (PRES) and reversible cerebral vasoconstriction syndrome (RCVS)

PRES and RCVS, both associated with preeclampsia, may present with headache and accompanying symptoms such as altered mental status, seizure, nausea/vomiting, focal neurologic signs, and visual disturbances (e.g., blurred vision, homonymous hemianopsia, and cortical blindness due to involvement of the occipital lobe).

PRES is commonly diagnosed by radiologic findings of vasogenic edema within the posterior circulation, primarily affecting the subcortical white matter of the parieto-occipital lobes. PRES may be associated with hypertensive encephalopathy, renal failure, immunosuppressive therapy or chemotherapy, and preeclampsia or eclampsia.[54] The mainstay of treatment for PRES associated with concomitant preeclampsia or eclampsia is blood pressure management and seizure treatment with intravenous magnesium sulfate therapy.

Patients with RCVS frequently present with a thunderclap headache. Additional findings may include focal neurologic deficits due to edema, stroke, seizure, or angiographic reversible multifocal narrowing of the cerebral vessels. Patients with thunderclap headaches should undergo rapid imaging to rule out conditions that need emergent intervention, including subarachnoid hemorrhage, ruptured brain aneurysm, and cervical artery dissection. Many patients with RCVS will have normal initial brain imaging on CT or MRI, so the addition of cerebral angiography is paramount to detect the primary diagnostic features of RCVS. The mainstay of treatment for RCVS is supportive measures, including pain control and blood pressure management.

The Approach to Headache Postpartum

CASE STUDY #2 CLINICAL CASE SCENARIO: HEADACHE IN A POSTPARTUM PATIENT

History: 24-year-old primigravida with no significant medical or surgical history presented in active labor at 40 weeks gestation. Her prenatal course was uncomplicated. She received an epidural for pain control and proceeded to have a normal spontaneous vaginal delivery of a healthy infant.

Clinical Presentation: On postpartum day #1, the patient developed a persistent and severe headache. She described the headache as throbbing and located at the front of her head. The pain worsened when she sat upright and improved lying flat. She also reported neck stiffness and low back pain but denied nausea, vomiting, fever, chills, vertigo, vision changes, weakness, and paresthesia.

Physical Examination: *Vital signs*: Blood pressure: 124/78 mmHg, pulse rate: 82 beats per minute, temperature: 98.6°F (37°C), respiratory rate: 16 breaths per minute.

Neurological examination: Cranial nerves were intact, and no focal neurological deficits observed.

Physical exam: Patient was alert and in no acute distress. Cardiac and respiratory exams were normal. Her uterine fundus was firm and below the umbilicus. No calf tenderness or excess edema.

Laboratory Results: CBC, including platelets, liver function tests, serum creatinine, and urine protein, were within normal limits.

Assessment: Based on the clinical presentation, examination, and laboratory results, she was diagnosed with a postdural puncture headache (PDPH).

Postpartum Postdural Puncture Headache

PDPH may occur following dural puncture either inadvertently during attempted epidural analgesia for labor or from deliberate dural puncture during spinal anesthesia for operative interventions.[55] The occurrence of PDPH shows considerable variability, influenced by patient and procedural risk factors, with reported incidences of up to 9% and 6% following spinal and epidural anesthesia, respectively.[56] In the postpartum setting, mothers may experience PDPH, which can significantly impact their recovery and bonding with their newborn. Understanding the pathophysiology, clinical presentation, and appropriate treatment strategies for PDPH is crucial for obstetricians and health-care providers caring for postpartum patients.

PDPH is primarily thought to be caused by cerebrospinal fluid (CSF) leakage from the dural puncture site, resulting in decreased CSF volume around the brain and spinal cord. The resultant traction on pain-sensitive structures and reactive venodilation leads to the characteristic symptoms of PDPH.[55–57]

Most PDPH manifests within 72 hours after a dural puncture, but symptoms can be delayed up to two weeks.[58, 59] The headache is described as a severe, throbbing occipitofrontal pain that worsens when the patient is upright and improves when lying down.[55–57] This positional component is a hallmark feature of PDPH that is useful to distinguish it from other headache types. PDPH is often accompanied by neck and shoulder stiffness, although nausea, vomiting, vertigo, vision changes, tinnitus, and photophobia have been reported.[55–57] Neurological examination usually reveals no focal deficits.

PDPH is a clinical diagnosis. Neuroimaging and other diagnostics tests are generally not required to make this diagnosis; however, imaging may be indicated if symptoms are atypical and other causes need to be ruled out. The differential diagnosis for PDPH includes other primary headache disorders, preeclampsia/eclampsia, idiopathic intracranial hypotension, RCVS, subdural hematoma, and CVT.

Treatment strategies for PDPH range from conservative management (e.g., bed rest, oral and IV hydration, caffeine, and over-the-counter analgesics such as acetaminophen and NSAIDs) to more invasive measures such as an epidural blood patch. Some medications should be avoided during lactation as they can inadvertently impair milk supply, including decongestants such as diphenhydramine and phenylephrine. Some narcotic analgesics, such as codeine-containing products, should be avoided due to the risk of neonatal sedation. Communication and shared decision-making between the obstetrician and the patient are essential to achieve the best possible outcome while prioritizing both the mother's recovery and the well-being of the newborn.

Epidural blood patches can provide immediate relief and be long-lasting. Sometimes, a second procedure may be necessary, or a patient may fail to benefit from the procedure(s). Additional therapies such as nerve blocks (e.g., transnasal sphenopalatine block or greater occipital nerve block) have been used; however, data is limited on efficacy. PDPH can be distressing for postpartum patients, affecting their overall well-being and ability to care for their newborns. Early recognition and appropriate treatment are vital to ensuring a prompt recovery.

MIGRAINE TREATMENT AND CONTRACEPTION

CASE STUDY #3

Clinical Scenario: A patient with migraine with aura who is interested in contraception options

History: 24-year-old G1 P1 patient presents for contraceptive counseling. Past medical history is significant for migraine with aura initially diagnosed at the age of 12 years. Headache triggers include menses, dehydration, sleep deprivation, and alcohol. Most recently, she notes reasonable control of her headaches with lifestyle modifications and topiramate, rarely requiring triptans for abortive therapy. She has had one prior vaginal delivery and reports regular but heavy menstrual cycles. The patient is in a monogamous relationship and is not planning on pregnancy in the near future. She is concerned about potential weight gain and the effects on her current headache regimen when discussing contraceptive options. When asked about cycle control, she desires lighter or absent menses.

Physical Examination: BP 110/70, Pulse 65, BMI 24

The patient is well appearing, breast and pelvic exam are normal

Laboratory Results: Pap smear negative for intraepithelial lesion of malignancy

Gonorrhea and chlamydia testing negative

Assessment: The described patient has a history of migraine with aura and is otherwise healthy with normal blood pressure and BMI. The patient is counseled on contraceptive options, including hormonal and nonhormonal methods. With an aura diagnosis, estrogen-containing contraception should be avoided, as it is a medical eligibility criteria (MEC) risk of four. The patient is also interested in highly effective long-acting reversible contraception that will improve menstrual bleeding and will not interfere with her headache regimen or lead to weight gain. Therefore, the patient chose a levonorgestrel intrauterine device (IUD) to support all of these goals.

TABLE 17.1   MEC categories

MEC CATEGORY	RECOMMENDATION
1	No restrictions on contraceptive method
2	Advantages of the method generally outweigh the theoretical or proven risk
3	Theoretical or proven risks usually outweigh the advantages of the method
4	Unacceptable health risk

Source: CDC, US Medical Eligibility Criteria for Contraceptive Use, 2016.

When counseling patients regarding contraceptive options, various factors, including a history of headaches, must be considered. First, the patient's medical history should be queried to determine any potential contraindications or risk factors for contraception. The Centers for Disease Control and Prevention (CDC) provides updated MEC to assist in counseling patients regarding the risks of the contraceptive option with numerous medical conditions, as shown in Table 17.1.[60]

Patient preferences concerning potential benefits, delivery methods, and efficacy should be reviewed. Additionally, prior experiences with contraceptive methods should be assessed, including satisfaction. In patients with migraine, decisions regarding contraception should include the risks related to the presence of aura and the potential positive or negative effects of contraception on menstrual migraine headaches. Providers also need to consider the potential interactions between common headache therapies and contraception and the potential for teratogenicity in pregnancy if the contraceptive method fails.

Migraine is a common concern during the female reproductive years. Female patients with migraine often report that their headaches began during adolescence with the onset of menarche and note that menses are a trigger. Menstrual migraine symptoms typically begin one to two days before the onset of menstrual bleeding and may last for several days.[61] Menstrual headaches are less likely to respond to typical therapies and are often more frequent and intense than headaches experienced during other times of the month. For many women, the symptoms of menstrual migraine headaches can lead to loss of work,[62] increased strain on relationships,[63] and decreased quality of life.[13]

A direct correlation has been demonstrated between the onset of migraine symptoms and the rapid decline in estradiol levels before the onset of menstrual bleeding. A study by Somerville noted that migraine headaches were deferred in patients who received estrogen depot injections.[64] Additional studies have reported that women with migraine have a faster late luteal phase decline in estrogen levels.[65] Both patients on cyclic combined oral contraceptive pills (those with inert or placebo pills) and those with natural menstrual cycles can experience the described effects. Missed contraceptive pills have been shown to initiate headache and decrease contraceptive efficacy.

Perimenopause is a time of significant hormone fluctuation. As ovarian reserves decline, the hypothalamic-pituitary-ovarian axis is activated to increase estrogen production by the ovary. Perimenopause typically lasts several years before the cessation of menses and the start of menopause. During the perimenopausal transition, there is inconsistent and progressively waning ovulation in women who do not take hormonal contraceptives. Estradiol levels can vary greatly, with some months notable for elevated levels. Common symptoms of perimenopause include menstrual irregularities, hot flashes, night sweats, and mood swings. Additionally, the fluctuation in estradiol levels can lead to increased headaches. Perimenopause is a common time for women with estrogen-associated headaches to report increased frequency and severity of symptoms. Once patients enter early menopause (the first three to five years), vasomotor symptoms and headaches can be highly variable but typically decrease with time. Patients for whom estrogen changes can exacerbate headache may find that these improve or resolve once they transition into the later stages of menopause.

Continuous combined oral contraceptive pills have been shown to decrease both the frequency and severity of menstrually associated headache in reproductive-age and perimenopausal women by establishing consistent, low estrogen levels.[66, 67] However, data regarding optimal estradiol dosing, progestin type, or delivery system (oral versus transdermal versus vaginal) is lacking. Triphasic contraceptive pills, in which the hormonal dosing is adjusted weekly, will often increase the occurrence of headache. Additionally, for those with menstrually related migraine on monophasic contraceptive pills, headaches often occur during the first two days of the placebo week. While transdermal and transvaginal combination contraception provides more stable dosing than daily oral medications, they are unavailable in varying doses. Additionally, the transdermal contraceptive patch has been shown to deliver higher estrogen levels; therefore, continuous usage is not currently recommended.[68]

Estrogen therapy increases the risk of venous thromboembolism (VTE) and stroke, particularly at high doses. Historically, oral contraceptive pills contained 50–100 micrograms (mcg) of ethinyl estradiol (EE). Currently, hormonal contraceptive methods contain 10–35 mcg EE. Low-dose estrogen preparations minimize the risk of VTE and stroke without lowering the efficacy of contraceptive benefits. Side effects such as nausea, vomiting, weight gain, and secondary headaches are less likely with the lower dose preparations.

Initial studies evaluating the effects of higher dose oral estrogen (50–100 mcg EE) demonstrated an increased risk of stroke in women with migraine headaches.[67] The risk of stroke was found to be greater in women suffering from migraine with aura. More recent studies evaluating low-dose and ultra-low-dose estrogen contraception have demonstrated a decreased risk of thromboembolism and stroke. Subsequently, the World Health Organization (WHO) and CDC categorized combination hormonal contraception as acceptable (category 2) for women with migraine without aura. The International Headache Society (IHS) recommends that patients who are otherwise low risk may benefit from combined hormonal contraception and that treatment should be individualized regardless of the presence of aura.

Providers should query their female patients on the timing and severity of their headaches compared to their menstrual cycle. The diagnosis can be easily overlooked if a menstrual history is not solicited. Providers should also ask their patients about the timing of the onset of headache with menarche and menses. Patients should be instructed to maintain a headache log to track the occurrence, severity, medication usage, menstrual cycle, and other potential triggers. The initial evaluation and treatment of menstrual headaches do not differ from nonmenstrual headaches. However, patients at low risk for hormone therapy and who do not respond to standard headache treatments may benefit from hormonal suppression.

Various hormonal regimens exist for the prevention of menstrual migraine headaches. Extended-cycle estrogen/progestin contraception appears to have the greatest efficacy, and various regimens are available (Table 17.2). Many of these regimens can be prescribed using standard monophasic contraceptive pills, providing the patient with detailed instructions on eliminating the inert pills. The contraceptive vaginal ring can be placed for 21 days and then immediately replaced with a new ring upon removal to provide continuous monophasic treatment. The ring releases 15 mcg/day of EE and 0.12mg/day of etonogestrel.

TABLE 17.2 Continuous combined oral hormonal contraception regimens and potential effect on menstrual migraine symptoms

TIMING (ACTIVE/ INERT)	ACTIVE MEDICATION	INACTIVE MEDICATION	EFFECT ON MENSTRUAL HEADACHE
84/7 days	30 mcg EE 0.15 mg levonorgestrel	7 days of inert	Overall decrease, headaches with inert
84/7 days	30 mcg EE 0.15 mg levonorgestrel	10 mcg EE	Decrease
84/7 days	20 mcg EE 0.1 mg levonorgestrel	10 mcg EE	Decrease
365/0 days	20mcg EE 0.09mg levonorgestrel	N/A	Decrease
21/0 days	Vaginal ring used continuously for 21 days and then immediately replaced	N/A	Decrease

In a small pilot study, continuous use of the vaginal ring was shown to be successful in decreasing menstrual migraine headaches.[69]

An alternative treatment is to prescribe supplemental low-dose estrogen starting approximately two days before anticipated menses in those with regular menstrual cycles. This treatment is an option for women who do not need or want contraception or have an alternative nonhormonal form, such as sterilization. This process is often called *menstrual supplementation* and can be delivered with either an oral or transdermal formulation. Typically, 10–20 mcg of EE or an equivalent is needed to minimize symptoms of estrogen withdrawal. Menstrual supplementation should be reserved for those with predictable menses to reliably prevent the decline in estrogen before the onset of menstrual bleeding. For women already on combined cyclical hormonal contraception, using supplemental estrogen during the placebo week has decreased the frequency and severity of headaches.

For patients with migraine with aura, the CDC lists combined hormonal contraceptives such as the estrogen-containing pill, patch, or ring as a category 4 (risks outweigh benefits) given the potential risk of stroke. However, all non-estrogen-containing contraceptive methods, such as the copper IUD, progestin IUD, implants, and injectable or oral progestin medications, are category 1. Non-estrogen-containing options are included in Table 17.3.

Norethindrone contraceptive pills, often referred to as the minipill, have a lower contraceptive efficacy as it is highly dependent on the timing of the medication. Norethindrone-only contraceptive pills only suppress ovulation approximately 50% of the time. The contraceptive benefit results from increased cervical mucous thickness, thinning of the endometrium, and decreased fallopian tube motility. Norethindrone pills are unlikely to decrease menstrual migraine attacks but have been shown to decrease the occurrence of aura symptoms. Desogestrel-only pills have effectively decreased menstrual migraine symptoms; however, the regimen is not currently available in the United States. More recently, an alternative oral progestin-only medication, drospirenone, has become available. It has a higher contraceptive effectiveness through

TABLE 17.3   Reversible contraceptive options for patients with migraine with aura

METHOD	CONTRACEPTIVE EFFICACY WITH TYPICAL USE (%)	COMMENTS	BLEEDING PATTERN
Copper IUD	99	Can be used for emergency contraception	Often heavier and longer menses
Levonorgestrel IUD	99		Decreased flow over time, amenorrhea
Etonogestrel Subdermal Implant	99		Irregular bleeding most common reason for removal, amenorrhea
Depot Medroxyprogesterone Injections	94–96	Weight gain is common, requires q 3 month injection	Initially increased irregularity and then amenorrhea
Norethindrone Pills	90	Time sensitive, Can increase acne and hirsutism	Variable bleeding patterns
Drospirenone Pills	91–94	Decreased acne and hirsutism, may increase potassium levels	Variable bleeding patterns
Male Condom	82	Protects against STIs	n/a
Female Condom	79	Protects against STIs	n/a
Sponge	76–88		n/a
Spermicide	72		n/a

Source: IUD = intrauterine device, STIs = sexually transmitted infections.

reliably suppressing ovulation and stabilizing hormone levels. Drospirenone pills have approximately a 30-hour half-life compared to only 9 hours with norethindrone. Although not yet studied in clinical trials, the drospirenone oral contraceptive pill has the potential to minimize estrogen decline when used continuously. Similarly, data is lacking in regard to using other progestin-only methods for the suppression of estrogen-related headaches.

SUMMARY

- Headaches impact women more frequently than men with special considerations taken of the unique life phases of women including menstruation, pregnancy, lactation, family planning, and menopause
- In pregnancy, women may be affected by primary diagnosis of headaches in addition to secondary causes that may be specific to or exacerbated by pregnancy such as preeclampsia, stroke, or postpartum post-dural puncture headache
- Women with migraine require special consideration if the headaches are related to the menstrual cycle or if aura is present in regards to contraception

REFERENCES

1. Burch R, Rizzoli P, Loder E. The prevalence and impact of migraine and severe headache in the United States: Figures and trends from government health studies. *Headache: The Journal of Head and Face Pain.* 2018;*58*(4):496–505. https://doi.org/10.1111/head.13281.
2. Smitherman TA, Burch R, Sheikh H, Loder E. The prevalence, impact, and treatment of migraine and severe headaches in the United States: A review of statistics from national surveillance studies. *Headache: The Journal of Head and Face Pain.* 2013;*53*(3):427–436. https://doi.org/10.1111/head.12074.
3. Radtke A, Neuhauser H. Prevalence and burden of headache and migraine in Germany. *Headache: The Journal of Head and Face Pain.* 2009;*49*(1):79–89. https://doi.org/10.1111/j.1526-4610.2008.01263.x.
4. Granella F, Sances G, Pucci E, Nappi R, Ghiotto N, Nappi G. Migraine with aura and reproductive life events: A case control study. *Cephalalgia* 2000;*20*(8):701–707. https://ezproxy.lib.uconn.edu/login?url=https://search.ebscohost.com/login.aspx?direct=true&db=aph&AN=5466336&site=ehost-live. Accessed Sep 10, 2023. doi: 10.1046/j.1468-2982.2000.00112.x.
5. Aegidius K, Zwart J, Hagen K, Stovner L. The effect of pregnancy and parity on headache prevalence: The head-HUNT study. *Headache: The Journal of Head and Face Pain.* 2009;*49*(6):851–859. https://doi.org/10.1111/j.1526-4610.2009.01438.x.
6. Marcus DA, Scharff L, Turk D. Longitudinal prospective study of headache during pregnancy and postpartum. *Headache.* 1999;*39*(9):625–632. doi: 10.1046/j.1526-4610.1999.3909625.x.
7. Brandes JL. The influence of estrogen on MigraineA systematic review. *Journal of the American Medical Association* 2006;*295*(15):1824–1830. https://doi.org/10.1001/jama.295.15.1824. Accessed 9/16/2023
8. Somerville BW. Estrogen-withdrawal migraine: I. duration of exposure required and attempted prophylaxis by premenstrual estrogen administration. *Neurology.* 1975;*25*(3):239.
9. Charles A, Brennan KC. The neurobiology of migraine. *Handbook of Clinical Neurology* 2010;*97*:99–108. doi: 10.1016/S0072-9752(10)97007-3.
10. Chen Z, Yuhanna IS, Galcheva-Gargova Z, Karas RH, Mendelsohn ME, Shaul PW. Estrogen receptor α mediates the nongenomic activation of endothelial nitric oxide synthase by estrogen. *The Journal of Clinical Investigation* 1999;*103*(3):401–406.

11. Macgregor EA, Rosenberg JD, Kurth T. Sex-related differences in epidemiological and clinic-based headache studies. *Headache* 2011;*51*(6):843–859. doi: 10.1111/j.1526-4610.2011.01904.x.

12. Turner SB, Szperka CL, Hershey AD, Law EF, Palermo TM, Groenewald CB. Association of headache with school functioning among children and adolescents in the United States. *JAMA Pediatrics*. 2021;*175*(5):522–524. https://doi.org/10.1001/jamapediatrics.2020.5680. Accessed 9/16/2023.

13. Norazah AB, Tanprawate S, Lambru G, Torkamani M, Jahanshahi M, Matharu M. Quality of life in primary headache disorders: A review. *Cephalalgia* 2016;*36*(1):67–91. https://doi.org/10.1177/0333102415580099.

14. Hu XH, Markson LE, Lipton RB, Stewart WF, Berger ML. Burden of migraine in the United States: Disability and economic costs. *Archives of Internal Medicine*. 1999;*159*(8):813–818. doi: 10.1001/archinte.159.8.813.

15. Celentano DD, Linet MS, Stewart WF. Gender differences in the experience of headache. *Social Science & Medicine* 1990;*30*(12):1289–1295. https://www.sciencedirect.com/science/article/pii/027795369090309G. doi: 10.1016/0277-9536(90)90309-G.

16. Maggioni F, Alessi C, Maggino T, Zanchin G. Headache during pregnancy. *Cephalalgia* 1997;*17*(7):765–769.

17. Goldszmidt E, Kern R, Chaput A, Macarthur A. The incidence and etiology of postpartum headaches: A prospective cohort study. *Canadian Journal of Anaesthesia= Journal Canadien D'anesthesie*. 2005;*52*(9):971–977.

18. Matthews TJ, Hamilton BE. First births to older women continue to rise. *NCHS Data Brief*. 2014;*152*:1–8.

19. Raffaelli B, Neeb L, Israel-Willner H, et al. Brain imaging in pregnant women with acute headache. *Journal of Neurology* 2018;*265*(8):1836–1843. doi: 10.1007/s00415-018-8924-6.

20. Jain C. ACOG committee opinion no. 723: Guidelines for diagnostic imaging during pregnancy and lactation. *Obstetrics & Gynecology*. 2019;*133*(1):186.

21. Miller RW. Discussion: Severe mental retardation and cancer among atomic bomb survivors exposed in utero. *Teratology* 1999;*59*(4):234–235.

22. Gjelsteen AC, Ching BH, Meyermann MW, et al. CT, MRI, PET, PET/CT, and ultrasound in the evaluation of obstetric and gynecologic patients. *The Surgical Clinics of North America* 2008;*88*(2):361–390.

23. Tremblay E, Thérasse E, Thomassin-Naggara I, Trop I. Quality initiatives: Guidelines for use of medical imaging during pregnancy and lactation. *Radiographics* 2012;*32*(3):897–911.

24. Rosa FW. Spina bifida in infants of women treated with carbamazepine during pregnancy. *The New England Journal of Medicine* 1991;*324*(10):674–677.

25. Robert E, Guibaud P. Maternal valproic acid and congenital neural tube defects. *The Lancet*. 1982;*320*(8304):937.

26. Rasmussen BK. Migraine and tension-type headache in a general population: Precipitating factors, female hormones, sleep pattern and relation to lifestyle. *Pain* 1993;*53*(1):65–72. doi: 10.1016/0304-3959(93)90057-V.

27. Bahra A, May A, Goadsby PJ. Cluster headache: A prospective clinical study with diagnostic implications. *Neurology* 2002;*58*(3):354–361. doi: 10.1212/wnl.58.3.354.

28. Sances G, Granella F, Nappi RE, et al. Course of migraine during pregnancy and postpartum: A prospective study. *Cephalalgia* 2003;*23*(3):197–205.

29. Allais G, Chiarle G, Sinigaglia S, Mana O, Benedetto C. Migraine during pregnancy and in the puerperium. *Neurological Sciences* 2019;*40*:81–91.

30. MacGregor EA. Headache in pregnancy. *Neurologic Clinics* 2012;*30*(3):835–866. doi: 10.1016/j.ncl.2012.04.001.

31. Aukes AM, Yurtsever FN, Boutin A, Visser MC, De Groot CJ. Associations between migraine and adverse pregnancy outcomes: Systematic review and meta-analysis. *Obstetrical & Gynecological Survey* 2019;*74*(12):738–748.

32. Facchinetti F, Allais G, Nappi RE, et al. Migraine is a risk factor for hypertensive disorders in pregnancy: A prospective cohort study. *Cephalalgia* 2009;*29*(3):286–292.

33. Chen HM, Chen SF, Chen YH, Lin HC. Increased risk of adverse pregnancy outcomes for women with migraines: A nationwide population-based study. *Cephalalgia* 2010;*30*(4):433–438.

34. Informed consent and shared decision making in obstetrics and gynecology: ACOG committee opinion, number 819. *Obstetrics and Gynecology*. 2021;*137*(2):e34–e41. https://www.ncbi.nlm.nih.gov/pubmed/33481530. doi: 10.1097/AOG.0000000000004247.

35. Peretz A, Stark-Inbar A, Harris D, et al. Safety of remote electrical neuromodulation for acute migraine treatment in pregnant women: A retrospective controlled survey-study. *Headache: The Journal of Head and Face Pain*. 2023.

36. Govindappagari S, Grossman TB, Dayal AK, Grosberg BM, Vollbracht S, Robbins MS. Peripheral nerve blocks in the treatment of migraine in pregnancy. *Obstetrics & Gynecology* 2014;*124*(6):1169–1174.

37. Moir C, Dale HH. The action of ergot preparations on the puerperal uterus: A clinical investigation with special reference to an active constituent of ergot as yet unidentified. *British Medical Journal* 1932;*1*(3728):1119.

38. Headaches in pregnancy. *Obstetrics and Gynecology (New York. 1953)*. 2022;*139*(5):944–972. https://www.ncbi.nlm.nih.gov/pubmed/35576364. doi: 10.1097/AOG.0000000000004766.

39. Beckert RH, Baer RJ, Anderson JG, Jelliffe-Pawlowski L, Rogers EE. Maternal anemia and pregnancy outcomes: A population-based study. *Journal of Perinatology* 2019;*39*(7):911–919. doi: 10.1038/s41372-019-0375-0.

40. Gestational hypertension and preeclampsia: ACOG practice bulletin, number 222. *Obstetrics and Gynecology (New York. 1953)*. 2020;*135*(6):e237–e260. http://ovidsp.ovid.com/ovidweb.cgi?T=JS&NEWS=n&CSC=Y&PAGE=fulltext&D=ovft&AN=00006250-202006000-00046. doi: 10.1097/AOG.0000000000003891.

41. Cooray SD, Edmonds SM, Tong S, Samarasekera SP, Whitehead CL. Characterization of symptoms immediately preceding eclampsia. *Obstetrics & Gynecology* 2011;*118*(5):995–999.

42. James AH, Bushnell CD, Jamison MG, Myers ER. Incidence and risk factors for stroke in pregnancy and the puerperium. *Obstetrics & Gynecology* 2005;*106*(3):509–516.

43. Ros HS, Lichtenstein P, Bellocco R, Petersson G, Cnattingius S. Increased risks of circulatory diseases in late pregnancy and puerperium. *Epidemiology* 2001:456–460.

44. Kittner SJ, Stern BJ, Feeser BR, et al. Pregnancy and the risk of stroke. *The New England Journal of Medicine* 1996;*335*(11):768–774.

45. Feske SK, Singhal AB. Cerebrovascular disorders complicating pregnancy. *Continuum: Lifelong Learning in Neurology*. 2014;*20*(1):80–99.

46. Moatti Z, Gupta M, Yadava R, Thamban S. A review of stroke and pregnancy: Incidence, management and prevention. *European Journal of Obstetrics, Gynecology, and Reproductive Biology* 2014;*181*:20–27.

47. James AH, Bushnell CD, Jamison MG, Myers ER. Incidence and risk factors for stroke in pregnancy and the puerperium. *Obstetrics & Gynecology* 2005;*106*(3):509–516.

48. Saposnik G, Barinagarrementeria F, Brown Jr RD, et al. Diagnosis and management of cerebral venous thrombosis: A statement for healthcare professionals from the American Heart Association/American Stroke Association. *Stroke* 2011;*42*(4):1158–1192.

49. Ferro JM, Canhão P, Stam J, Bousser M, Barinagarrementeria F. Prognosis of cerebral vein and dural sinus thrombosis: Results of the international study on cerebral vein and dural sinus thrombosis (ISCVT). *Stroke* 2004;*35*(3):664–670.

50. Thaller M, Homer V, Mollan SP, Sinclair AJ. Disease course and long-term outcomes in pregnant women with idiopathic intracranial hypertension: The IIH prospective maternal health study. *Neurology* 2023;*100*(15):e1598–e1610.

51. Falardeau J, Lobb BM, Golden S, Maxfield SD, Tanne E. The use of acetazolamide during pregnancy in intracranial hypertension patients. *Journal of Neuro-Ophthalmology* 2013;*33*(1):9–12.

52. Bedson CR, Plaat F. Benign intracranial hypertension and anaesthesia for caesarean section. *International Journal of Obstetric Anesthesia* 1999;*8*(4):288–290.

53. Schaap TP, Schutte JM, Zwart JJ, Schuitemaker N, Van Roosmalen J, Dutch maternal mortality committee. Fatal meningitis during pregnancy in the Netherlands: A nationwide confidential enquiry. *BJOG: An International Journal of Obstetrics & Gynaecology*. 2012;*119*(13):1558–1563.

54. Hinchey J, Chaves C, Appignani B, et al. A reversible posterior leukoencephalopathy syndrome. *The New England Journal of Medicine* 1996;*334*(8):494–500.

55. FitzGerald S, Salman M. Postdural puncture headache in obstetric patients. *The British Journal of General Practice* 2019;*69*(681):207–208. https://www.ncbi.nlm.nih.gov/pubmed/30923161. doi: 10.3399/bjgp19X702125.

56. Bateman, B., Cole, N., Sun-Edelstein, C., Lay, C. Post dural puncture headache. UpToDate Web site.

57. Gaiser RR. Postdural puncture headache: An evidence-based approach. *Anesthesiology Clinics* 2017;*35*(1):157–167.

58. Vilming ST, Schrader H, Monstad I. The significance of age, sex, and cerebrospinal fluid pressure in post-lumbar-puncture headache. *Cephalalgia* 1989;*9*(2):99–106. doi : 10.1046/j.1468-2982.1989.0902099.x.

59. Kuntz KM, Kokmen E, Stevens JC, Miller P, Offord KP, Ho MM. Post-lumbar puncture headaches: Experience in 501 consecutive procedures. *Neurology* 1992;*42*(10):1884. https://www.ncbi.nlm.nih.gov/pubmed/1407567. doi: 10.1212/wnl.42.10.1884.

60. US medical eligibility criteria for contraceptive use, 2016 (US MEC) | CDC. https://www.cdc.gov/reproductivehealth/contraception/mmwr/mec/summary.html Web site. https://www.cdc.gov/reproductivehealth/contraception/mmwr/mec/summary.html. Updated 2023. Accessed Oct 7, 2023.

61. Martin VT, Lipton RB. Epidemiology and biology of menstrual migraine. *Headache: The Journal of Head and Face Pain*. 2008;*48*:S124–S130.

62. Lipton RB, Stewart WF, Diamond S, Diamond ML, Reed M. Prevalence and burden of migraine in the United States: Data from the American migraine study II. *Headache* 2001;*41*(7):646–657. https://api.istex.fr/ark:/67375/WNG-XVMTK15R-5/fulltext.pdf. doi: 10.1046/j.1526-4610.2001.041007646.x.

63. Buse DC, Fanning KM, Reed ML, et al. Life with migraine: Effects on relationships, career, and finances from the chronic migraine epidemiology and outcomes (CaMEO) study. *Headache: The Journal of Head and Face Pain*. 2019;*59*(8):1286–1299.

64. Somerville BW. The role of estradiol withdrawal in the etiology of menstrual migraine. *Neurology* 1972;*22*(4):355. https://www.ncbi.nlm.nih.gov/pubmed/5062827. doi: 10.1212/wnl.22.4.355.

65. Pavlović J, Allshouse A, Santoro N, et al. Sex hormones in women with and without migraine: Evidence of migraine-specific hormone profiles. *Neurology* 2016;*87*(1):49–56. https://www.ncbi.nlm.nih.gov/pubmed/27251885. doi: 10.1212/WNL.0000000000002798.

66. Sulak P, Willis S, Kuehl T, Coffee A, Clark J. Headaches and oral contraceptives: Impact of eliminating the standard 7-day placebo interval. *Headache: The Journal of Head and Face Pain*. 2007;*47*(1):27–37.

67. Martin VT, Behbehani M. Ovarian hormones and migraine headache: Understanding mechanisms and pathogenesis-part 2. *Headache* 2006;*46*(3):365–386. https://api.istex.fr/ark:/67375/WNG-S8823K4G-T/fulltext.pdf. doi: 10.1111/j.1526-4610.2006.00370.x.

68. Lopez LM, Grimes DA, Gallo MF, Stockton LL, Schulz KF, Lopez LM. Skin patch and vaginal ring versus combined oral contraceptives for contraception. *Cochrane Database of Systematic Reviews* 2013;*2013*(4):CD003552. doi: 10.1002/14651858.CD003552.pub4.

69. Calhoun A, Ford S, Pruitt A. The impact of extended-cycle vaginal ring contraception on migraine aura: A retrospective case series. *Headache: The Journal of Head and Face Pain*. 2012;*52*(8):1246–1253.

70. Sacco S, Ricci S, Degan D, Carolei A. Migraine in women: The role of hormones and their impact on vascular diseases. *The Journal of Headache and Pain*. 2012;*13*(3):177–189.

Perioperative Management of Migraine

18

Vamsi Aribindi and Shanthi Aribindi

TEACHING POINTS

1. Postoperative readmissions are higher in migraine patients, and good control of migraine symptomatology is important to reduce readmissions
2. Many drugs have unique interactions and considerations in the postoperative period, which may result in negative outcomes; pharmacotherapy must be chosen to take into account the patient's surgery and unique medical risk factors
3. Opiate therapy should not be considered first-line therapy to reduce migraine symptoms, even if it is used to control postoperative pain, and many anti-migraine medications also have roles in multimodal pain medications to reduce postoperative pain

---

INTRODUCTION

Postoperative readmissions are a marker of quality and perioperative performance.[1] Patients with migraine are established to have higher rates of readmission relative to patients who do not.[2] This increase is multifactorial, and reducing incidence would greatly benefit patients undergoing surgical procedures. In addition, patients with migraine often require additional therapies while inpatient if they suffer from migraine attacks in the perioperative period.

Medications commonly used in the treatment of migraine may be continued in the perioperative period, though interestingly, the continuation of perioperative migraine medications as migraine prevention did not have an independent positive effect on the prevention of pain-related readmissions relative to prescription of acute migraine therapy on discharge.[3]

Many medications commonly used in the treatment of migraine have significant side effects that should be considered by providers managing patients in the perioperative period. Also of note, there is little to no role for opiates in the acute treatment of migraine, and the use of these medications to treat migraine in the postoperative period has the potential to subject the patient to the harms of opiate therapy

DOI: 10.1201/b23330-18

for little to no benefit.[4] Clinicians must avoid the trap of relying on this class of drugs, commonly prescribed to post-op patients, to effectively treat patients' migraine symptoms.

A broad overview of medications used to treat migraine and considerations in the perioperative period follows.

Nonsteroidal Anti-inflammatory Drugs (NSAIDs)

NSAIDs have been a mainstay of migraine treatment for many years. Ketorolac in particular has been found to be an effective treatment for migraines,[5] and as an added bonus, NSAIDs are commonly part of many multimodal pain pathways, which are rapidly becoming part of national guidelines and quality metrics.[6] However, while commonly prescribed and used, NSAIDs do have many relative contraindications, including patients with ulcers, kidney disease, coronary artery disease, inflammatory bowel disease and many more. While commonly reported, the association between NSAIDs and bleeding in the perioperative period is heavily disputed, and many surgeons do not consider NSAIDs as a culprit.[7] Overall, these drugs have a long history and well-known risks and can form a mainstay of treatment.

Tricyclic Antidepressants

Amitriptyline has proven efficacy in preventing migraine, with known side effects of sedation, confusion, tachycardia, and weight gain.[8] This class of medications has been known and used for many years for both depression and pain, and has a role in the treatment of migraine, albeit with known side effects. While multiple medications in this class have been used for migraine, only amitriptyline has been specifically studied and proven to have efficacy in the treatment of this etiology. Nonetheless, many clinicians extrapolate to other drugs in the class, such as nortriptyline. This class of drugs is often continued in the perioperative period due to concerns of severe withdrawal symptoms if stopped.[9] However, the Food and Drug Administration and other authorities have recommended cessation of this drug, if possible, well before the operating room due to concerns of interactions with anesthetics and seizures.[10]

Triptans

Another class of drugs with a long history and safety profile forms a mainstay of acute migraine treatment. There is a theoretical risk of vasoocclusive events which arise from the drug's potential vasoconstriction, though no study has demonstrated such a risk.[11] Nonetheless, caution is suggested under the precautionary principle when using such drugs in surgical patients at high risk of vasoocclusive events, including those undergoing neurosurgical procedures as well as patients with cerebrovascular, coronary, and peripheral vascular disease. But it should be noted that all risks must be weighed against benefits. A patient with severe migraine in the post-op period after an open coronary artery bypass procedure may benefit greatly from the prompt termination of migraine, as the sympathetic stimulation from pain may push the patient into an abnormal heart rhythm. As with any drug, risks and benefits must be taken into account.

Antiemetics

This is a broad class of medications with multiple mechanisms of action. Two drugs are most well studied in migraine: prochlorperazine[12] and metoclopramide.[13] It should be noted that drugs were commonly given in conjunction with diphenhydramine in most studies in order to reduce tardive dyskinesia effects, resulting in difficulty in separating the effect of the antiemetics alone. Nonetheless, these drugs have been shown to be as effective, if not more so, than triptans and certainly more effective than opiates.

In the perioperative period, metoclopramide should be used with caution in patients with small bowel obstruction, as the increase in gastrointestinal motility from this drug can theoretically exacerbate the risk of small bowel perforation.

Finally, the most commonly used perioperative antiemetic in the United States is undoubtedly ondansetron. This drug does not have a track record of efficacy in migraine treatment comparable to other antiemetics, and it may even cause headaches,[14] though case reports of its use to treat migraines exist.[15] Given the superiority of other drugs above and the risks of stacking effects of QT prolongation if multiple drugs are used, it may be preferable in perioperative patients to preferentially prescribe metoclopramide or prochlorperazine over ondansetron as first-line antiemetic therapy.

Ergots

While long used in the treatment of migraine, these drugs lack the safety profile of triptans and have been associated with vascular ischemic complications.[16] All patients undergoing surgery have a hypercoagulable state by definition, one of the key elements of thrombosis according to Virchow's triad, and thus are at elevated risk of vascular events. This risk is likely compounded by the use of this class of drugs. Thus, ergots should be avoided in perioperative patients in general, and especially in cardiac and vascular patients who take cardiovascular drugs. Patients taking such drugs were found to be at nearly eightfold increased risk of ischemic complications if overusing ergotamine.

Lasmiditan

A newer drug approved for the acute treatment of migraine[17], without the theoretical risks of vascular occlusive complications of triptans, these drugs are a promising option in the treatment of perioperative migraine. However, caution is still warranted: the most commonly reported side effect of these drugs was dizziness. Thus, post-op patients should be mobilized with caution after the use of this drug, as patients may be at elevated risk for falls.

Calcitonin Gene-Related Peptide Monoclonal Antibodies

Drugs in this class include galcanezumab and erenumab. These monoclonal antibodies are emerging as a promising therapy in the treatment of migraine. However, their use in the perioperative period should take into account several possibly deleterious effects.[18] These include possible reductions in gastrointestinal motility, which may prolong postoperative ileus. This suggests caution in use in patients undergoing small bowel or large bowel resections. Possible wound-healing effects have been documented in case reports.[19] And finally, the common contraindication patients with cerebrovascular or coronary vascular occlusive disease, where reduced blood supply may lead to ischemia.

Valproate

Valproate is another well-established medication in the treatment of migraine, in addition to being a well-known and commonly used anti-epileptic medication.[20] It has some potential for dizziness and nausea in the perioperative period; however, in its anti-epileptic role, it is almost universally continued in the perioperative period and can likely be continued as an anti-migraine agent as well without significant concerns.

Gabapentin

Gabapentin is commonly used in the perioperative period as a part of multimodal pain control strategies.[21] These strategies have been shown overall to significantly reduce opioid pain medical usage. However, a recent study showed an association between gabapentin use in the perioperative period and delirium and pneumonia in the elderly.[22] Any drug that reduces alertness has the potential to increase micro-aspirations and large aspirations, a risk that may be compounded by gastrointestinal surgeries with prolonged ileus. In such patients, caution is advised.

Serotonin and Norepinephrine Reuptake Inhibitors

Serotonin and norepinephrine reuptake inhibitors (SNRIs) such as venlafaxine and duloxetine are commonly used to treat migraine, particularly in the setting of comorbid depression.[23] The older selective serotonin reuptake inhibitors have a well-known mild increase in bleeding due to the role of serotonin in the clotting cascade, though the clinical effect of this is uncertain, with studies inconsistently suggesting an increase in transfusion requirements and others noting increased mortality of unclear etiology.[24, 25] This data is often extrapolated to guide management of the less well-studied SNRI class of medications. In patients with a high risk of bleeding and who are undergoing critical procedures, such as intracranial operations, it is not unreasonable to withhold SNRIs used to treat migraine, particularly if other antiplatelet agents are required to be continued. However, barring these scenarios, the significant withdrawal symptoms of holding SNRIs may argue in favor of generally continuing these drugs if possible.[26]

Topiramate

Topiramate is a well-known medication that is used to treat migraine and seizures. Its side effect profile includes nausea, taste perversion, paresthesias, and weight loss.[27] The weight loss is a relatively unique side effect of this drug. In patients with cachexia or malnutrition in whom weight and strength gain in the perioperative period is a goal, such as patients with weight loss secondary to obstructive esophageal or gastric malignancies, alternate agents may be preferred.

Angiotensin Converting Enzyme Inhibitors/Angiotensin II Receptor Blockers

These classes of medications are widely used and well studied for the treatment of hypertension, and guidelines regarding their perioperative continuation can be used to guide their use for migraine in the perioperative period as well. Lisinopril and Candesartan have both been shown to have efficacy in migraine prevention. Overall, the data on their perioperative safety is highly conflicting. Some studies point to significant blunting of the renin-angiotensin system, resulting in significant perioperative hypotension in patients who continue this drug in the perioperative period.[28] However, other studies suggested a protective effect of ACEi/ARBs in the postoperative period after coronary artery bypass grafting and increased ischemic events if they were held.[29] Thus, the decision to continue/initiate these drugs for migraine in the perioperative period must be individualized, though in general, these medications are held until just prior to discharge in order to avoid diagnostic confusion. These drugs can cause electrolyte abnormalities and alterations in kidney function that can be difficult to parse out from acute changes in the perioperative period. For example, a rise in creatinine may often represent new urinary retention after the removal of a perioperative foley, over diuresis, and a prerenal injury, or allergic interstitial nephritis in response to an antibiotic. But an ACEi/ARB being initiated at the same time may create confusion and make interpretation of these laboratory changes difficult.

Beta-Blockers

Beta-blockers have a long and well-documented safety profile. Their use in migraine is also long-standing and well evaluated, although it may take several weeks, if not months, for the effects to become known.[30] The management of beta-blockers given for heart failure and angina is well established. Based on multiple studies showing increased mortality in patients in whom beta-blockers prescribed for angina are discontinued in the perioperative period, current guidelines recommend continuing them throughout the perioperative period.[31] Though this recommendation does not technically apply to beta-blockers prescribed for migraine, it is reasonable to continue beta-blockers throughout the perioperative period as would normally be done if they were prescribed for other indications. Indeed, under the Surgical Care Improvement Project guidelines, not continuing a home beta-blocker that the patient is taking for any reason in the perioperative period may be penalized under quality metrics. If the patient requires pressors postoperatively, beta-blockers are, of course, held while the patient is resuscitated. Initiating beta-blockers in the perioperative period is controversial even for heart failure patients, and given the prolonged time to effect and potential masking of acute postsurgical complications such as bleeding and sepsis, it is likely not wise to initiate beta-blockers as a new therapy for acute migraine treatment in the perioperative period, unless they are indicated for other reasons such as non-ST-elevation myocardial infarction.[32]

Steroids

A single dose of dexamethasone has been shown to reduce the recurrence of migraine, with modest but significant benefits.[33] While steroids have known effects on wound healing, and chronic steroid use is likely deleterious, a single dose of steroids in the postoperative period has long been used to reduce postoperative nausea and vomiting and has been shown to be safe.[34] Nonetheless, caution should be exercised in patients at elevated risk of wound-healing complications or hyperglycemia, such as patients on immunosuppressive medications and with diabetes, as these patients were often excluded from studies establishing dexamethasone's safety profile in the perioperative period.

SCENARIOS

Case 1

A 45-year-old woman with no significant past medical history apart from obesity presents with acute cholecystitis and is planned for a laparoscopic cholecystectomy. She is on nortriptyline and rizatriptan for prevention of episodic migraine.

Considerations: The nortriptyline represents a treatment to prevent migraine from occurring. It should be continued in the perioperative period, with the added benefit of additional pain control. However, its sedating effect should be monitored. In conjunction with commonly used opiates and the patient's possibly undiagnosed but present obesity hypoventilation syndrome and/or obstructive sleep apnea, the patient may suffer respiratory depression in the perioperative period. Consequently, placing the patient on continuous pulse-oximetry or otherwise monitoring the patient may be warranted.

The rizatriptan represents a treatment to terminate acute migraine attacks. This may be written as a PRN or held unless the patient develops migraine symptoms. While triptans have theoretical concerns around ischemia due to vasoconstriction, such concerns are less of a consideration in a relatively young patient, particularly one who has been prescribed and is using triptans in the outpatient environment.

Case 2

A 25-year-old woman with chronic migraine on galcanezumab presents with appendicitis and requires an appendectomy.

Considerations: This patient is on prophylactic therapy against migraines. This class of medications is relatively new, with less well-known risks and benefits. While there is a theoretical risk of worsening cerebral and coronary ischemia, these would not be concerns in an otherwise healthy 25-year-old. However, this class of medications may interfere with wound healing. It is not unreasonable therefore to hold the medication in the perioperative period, after a discussion with the patient of risks and benefits. However, it is also reasonable to continue the medication if the patient reports devastating migraines that would prevent her from adequately mobilizing in the postoperative period, exposing the patient to a longer hospital stay as well as the risk of blood clots from lack of sufficient time spent out of bed.

However, this scenario is an appendectomy, which is an operation that does not require an anastomosis. Should this patient be an inflammatory bowel disease patient undergoing a resection and anastomosis, especially a patient on steroids, the balance of risks may tilt toward discontinuing the medication or choosing an operative approach (diverting ostomies) that reduces the risk of anastomotic leak.

Case 3

A 65-year-old man with diabetes, hypertension, coronary artery disease as well as episodic migraine undergoes an uncomplicated coronary artery bypass graft (CABG) operation. In the postoperative period, he develops severe headaches.

Considerations: This scenario is notable for a relatively older and less healthy patient, for whom concerns about vasoocclusive events may lead to caution with many otherwise effective options. However, prior to considering medications, the diagnosis must be confirmed. While patients may well have migraine flares in the postoperative period, surgeries such as CABG carry unique risks: the full heparinization during the operation places the patient at risk for intracranial hemorrhage, and the relative hypotension of the bypass run places the patient at risk for rare causes of headache such as pituitary apoplexy.[35] Furthermore, rarely, headache may be the first sign of serious pathologies such as developing tamponade[36] or compression of the superior vena cava due to postoperative mediastinal bleeding.[37] In addition, hypoxia from pneumonia or fluid overload, as well as unrevascularized territory or early graft failure resulting in cardiac cephalgia, must be considered.[38]

Provided these alternate explanations for headache have been ruled out, and migraine is the most likely diagnosis, the next question is what treatment to employ. Given the patient's coronary artery disease and recent bypass run, NSAIDs such as ibuprofen or ketorolac should be used only with extreme caution or as a last resort, as they may worsen/cause acute kidney injury and lead to thrombosis and/or bleeding. Triptans and Ergots have theoretical vasoocclusive risks. While they would be less favored in this scenario, it should be remembered that no definitive study has ever shown increased risks of stroke or thrombosis with triptans, though ergots do have increased risks of ischemia and should be avoided. Acetaminophen would be relatively safe, and other good choices would be antiemetics and lasmiditan.

CONCLUSION

There are many options for the acute treatment of migraine in the perioperative period, and long-term maintenance therapy for migraine can often be safely continued. Nonetheless, important exceptions exist, and the use of any of these drugs must take into account both risks and benefits, as oftentimes, the benefits of successful perioperative migraine control may outweigh theoretical or rare risks.

REFERENCES

1. Krumholz, et al. Hospital readmission risk: Isolating hospital from patient effects. *N Engl J Med.* 2017 Sep 14; *377*(11): 1055–1064.
2. Platzbecker et al. The association between migraine and hospital readmission due to pain after surgery: A hospital registry study. *Cephalalgia.* 2019 Feb;*39*(2):286–295.
3. Platzbecker et al. Migraine treatment and the risk of postoperative, pain-related hospital readmissions in migraine patients. *Cephalalgia.* 2020 Dec;*40*(14):1622–1632.
4. Langer-Gould et al. The American Academy of Neurology's top five choosing wisely recommendations. *Neurology.* 2013 Sep 10;*81*(11):1004–11.
5. Taggart et al. Ketorolac in the treatment of acute migraine: a systematic review. *Headache.* 2013 Feb;*53*(2):277–87.
6. American Society of Anesthesiologists Task Force on Acute Pain Management. Practice guidelines for acute pain management in the perioperative setting: an updated report by the American Society of Anesthesiologists Task Force on Acute Pain Management. *Anesthesiology.* 2012 Feb;*116*(2):248–73.
7. Bongiovanni et al. Systematic review and meta-analysis of the association between non-steroidal anti-inflammatory drugs and operative bleeding in the perioperative period. *J Am Coll Surg.* 2021 May;*232*(5): 765–790.
8. Silberstein et al. Migraine: preventative treatment. *Cephalalgia.* 2002 Sep;*22*(7):491–512.
9. Kroenke et al. Chronic medications in the perioperative period. *South Med J.* 1998 Apr;*91*(4):358–64.
10. Huyse et al. Psychotropic drugs and the perioperative period: a proposal for a guideline in elective surgery. *Psychosomatics.* 2006 Jan-Feb;*47*(1):8–22.
11. Roberto et al. Adverse cardiovascular events associated with triptans and ergotamines for treatment of migraine: systematic review of observational studies. *Cephalalgia.* 2015 Feb;*35*(2):118–31.
12. Kostic et al. A prospective, randomized trial of intravenous prochlorperazine versus subcutaneous sumatriptan in acute migraine therapy in the emergency department. *Ann Emerg Med.* 2010 Jul;*56*(1):1–6.
13. Colman et al. Parenteral metoclopramide for acute migraine: meta-analysis of randomised controlled trials. *BMJ.* 2004 Dec 11;*329*(7479):1369–73.
14. Veneziano et al. Ondansetron-induced headache. Our experience in gynecological cancer. *Eur J Gynaecol Oncol.* 1995;*16*(3):203–7.
15. Bachur et al. A comparison of acute treatment regimens for migraine in the emergency department. *Pediatrics.* 2015 Feb;*135*(2):232–8.
16. der Heijden et al. Risk of ischemic complications related to the intensity of triptan and ergotamine use. *Neurology.* 2006 Oct 10;*67*(7):1128–34.
17. Goadsby et al. Phase 3 randomized, placebo-controlled, double-blind study of lasmiditan for acute treatment of migraine. *Brain.* 2019 Jul 1;*142*(7):1894–1904.
18. Schoenen et al. Ten open questions in migraine prophylaxis with monoclonal antibodies blocking the calcitonin-gene related peptide pathway: a narrative review. *J Headache Pain.* 2023;*24*(1):99.
19. Wurthmann et al. Impaired wound healing in a migraine patient as a possible side effect of calcitonin gene-related peptide receptor antibody treatment: A case report. *Cephalalgia.* 2020 Oct;*40*(11):1255–1260.
20. Linde et al. Valproate (valproic acid or sodium valproate or a combination of the two) for the prophylaxis of episodic migraine in adults. *Cochrane Database Syst Rev.* 2013 Jun 24;*2013*(6):CD010611.
21. Wick et al. Postoperative multimodal analgesia pain management with nonopioid analgesics and techniques: A review. *JAMA Surg.* 2017 Jul 1;*152*(7):691–697.
22. Park et al. Perioperative gabapentin use and in-hospital adverse clinical events among older adults after major surgery. *JAMA Intern Med.* 2022 Nov 1;*182*(11):1117–1127.
23. Burch R. Antidepressants for preventive treatment of migraine. *Curr Treat Options Neurol.* 2019 Mar 21;*21*(4):18.
24. Sajan et al. Association of selective serotonin reuptake inhibitors with transfusion in surgical patients. *Anesth Analg.* 2016 Jul;*123*(1):21–8.
25. Tully et al. Selective serotonin reuptake inhibitors, venlafaxine and duloxetine are associated with in hospital morbidity but not bleeding or late mortality after coronary artery bypass graft surgery. *Heart Lung Circ.* 2012 Apr;*21*(4):206–14.

26. Fava et al. Withdrawal symptoms after serotonin-noradrenaline reuptake inhibitor discontinuation: Systematic review. *Psychother Psychosom.* 2018;*87*(4):195–203.
27. Silberstein et al. Topiramate in migraine prevention: results of a large controlled trial. *Arch Neurol.* 2004 Apr;*61*(4):490–5.
28. Shiffermiller et al. Prospective randomized evaluation of preoperative angiotensin-converting enzyme inhibition (PREOP-ACEI). *J Hosp Med.* 2018 Sep;*13*(10):661–667.
29. Drenger et al. Patterns of use of perioperative angiotensin-converting enzyme inhibitors in coronary artery bypass graft surgery with cardiopulmonary bypass: effects on in-hospital morbidity and mortality. *Circulation.* 2012 Jul 17;*126*(3):261–269.
30. Rosen JA. Observations on the efficacy of propranolol for the prophylaxis of migraine. *Ann Neurol.* 1983 Jan;*13*(1):92–3.
31. Kertai et al. Is compliance with surgical care improvement project cardiac (SCIP-Card-2) Measures for perioperative β-blockers associated with reduced incidence of mortality and cardiovascular-related critical quality indicators after noncardiac surgery? *Anesth Analg.* 2018 Jun;*126*(6):1829–1838.
32. American College of Cardiology Foundation/American Heart Association Task Force on Practice Guidelines. 2009 ACCF/AHA focused update on perioperative beta blockade. *J Am Coll Cardiol.* 2009 Nov 24;*54*(22):2102–2128.
33. Singh et al. Does the addition of dexamethasone to standard therapy for acute migraine headache decrease the incidence of recurrent headache for patients treated in the emergency department? A meta-analysis and systematic review of the literature. *Acad Emerg Med.* 2008 Dec;*15*(12):1223–1233.
34. Polderman et al. Adverse side effects of dexamethasone in surgical patients. Cochrane Database *Syst Rev.* 2018 Nov 23;*11*(11):CD011940.
35. Semenov et al. Pituitary apoplexy following coronary bypass surgery: A case report and literature review. *Rev Med Interne.* 2020 Dec;*41*(12):852–857.
36. Dulam et al. Cardiac tamponade masquerading as headache: A diagnostic conundrum. *J Card Surg.* 2020 Aug;*35*(8):2081–2083.
37. Ibrahim et al. Superior Vena Cava syndrome due to right anterior mediastinal hematoma: A case report. *Cureus.* 2022 Jul 18;*14*(7):e26994.
38. Shankar et al. Cardiac cephalgia: A diagnostic headache. *Intern Med J.* 2016 Oct;*46*(10):1219–1221.

Special Considerations for Headache Diagnosis and Treatment in the Geriatric Patient

19

Angela Primbas

LEARNING OBJECTIVES

1. Distinguish common ways that headaches present differently in older populations
2. Identify the increased risk of secondary headache causes in older adults and related comorbid conditions
3. Understand how polypharmacy and multimorbidity impact treatment of headaches in older adults
4. Recognize adverse effects of common headache therapies in older adults

---

INTRODUCTION

Headache is a common medical complaint in the outpatient setting, with an estimated lifetime prevalence of at least 46%.[1] Incidence of new-onset headache decreases with advancing age, though primary headaches can and do present de novo in older populations. Studies vary, but the incidence of new headache in older patients can reach up to 24%.[2] While the incidence of new primary headache decreases with age, prevalence of comorbid conditions potentially leading to secondary causes of headache increases. As such, consideration of secondary causes of headache is much more pertinent when assessing causes of headache among older adults. Diagnosing and treating headaches in older adults also involves knowledge of differing presentations of common headache types that occur with older age. Additionally, there are limitations

DOI: 10.1201/b23330-19

on treatment options due to age and comorbid conditions that can change standard approaches to symptom management. This chapter focuses on the types of headaches that occur in older adults and how their presentations may differ from younger adult populations. We will also cover comorbid conditions that should be considered in diagnosing and treating headache in older patients.

Clinical Case 1

The patient is a 78-year-old male with a history of hypertension, well controlled on lisinopril, and dyslipidemia, well controlled on rosuvastatin, who presents for evaluation of new-onset visual and language symptoms. He notes that three months ago, he began to have recurrent episodes of an arc of shimmering lights in his vision that would slowly grow over about 20 minutes before resolving. He notes that during this time, he can also have a bit of difficulty speaking the words he would like and can be a bit more sensitive to light during that time. While he denies any previous history of migraine, he does state that he has a history of motion sickness and that his sister has episodic migraine with aura. He initially presented to his geriatrician, who ordered a magnetic resonance imaging (MRI) brain with contrast. This showed some mild chronic microvascular ischemia appropriate for age but no acute intracranial abnormalities. A diagnosis of typical aura without headache was made. The patient was reassured by the MRI results, and since he was only having one to two episodes per month, preventive medications are not indicated, and the patient is encouraged to follow up if anything changes, including if he has an increased frequency of visual symptoms.

Primary Headache Disorders

Tension-type headache (TTH) is the most common form of primary headache for persons of all ages and has an estimated prevalence of 35.8% in older adults. Migraine is the next most common, with an estimated prevalence of approximately 6% in older adults.[3] It is important to distinguish differences in primary headache presentation that are common among older adults compared to younger populations, as well as identify when to be concerned for secondary causes.

Tension-Type Headache

TTH are bilateral mild to moderate, dull, achy headache attacks that lack features classically attributed to migraines (photo- and phonophobia, nausea, autonomic symptoms).[4] The presentation of TTH in patients older than 65 years generally does not differ from younger patients. While TTH remains the most common headache in older adults, a detailed history is important to distinguish TTH from secondary causes, as they are much more common in older patients. Most older patients with TTH will have had headache from a younger age (usually beginning before age 50). If headaches are new onset after age 50 or changing in quality, severity, or frequency, generally, workup for secondary headache is warranted.[5]

Migraine

Migraine is generally defined by moderate to severe, usually throbbing, headache attacks that may be associated with nausea, light, and sound sensitivity, with symptoms lasting between 4 and 72 hours. Auras can often be characteristic of a migraine and are visual, sensory, language, or speech changes that precede headache symptoms.

In older adults, migraine without aura or aura without migraine are more common than migraine with auras. In particular, older adults with a prior history of migraine are more prone to aura without headaches as they age. The frequency of aura increases while the painful headache attacks generally become less severe and/or less frequent.[6] These episodic auras were sometimes referred to as "acephalgic migraine," "migraine equivalent," and "complicated migraine." Of note, the decrease in incidence and frequency of headache associated with migraine after menopause results in a narrowing of the prevalence gap between men and women (women typically have a higher prevalence prior to menopause).

The presence of aura in older adults is noted as a vascular risk factor, and thus comorbidities and other vascular risk factors should be assessed in older adults presenting with auras. This is especially important, as episodic aura in older adults can mimic transient ischemic attacks (TIAs). While auras in later life usually present with visual symptoms, they can also have a dysphasic (speech) or sensory presentation that can be concerning for an ischemic event.[7]

DISTINGUISHING MIGRAINE AURAS FROM ISCHEMIC ATTACKS IN OLDER PATIENTS

There are a few strategies to distinguish neurologic symptoms associated with migraine (especially aura) from ischemic events in older patients. In general, migraine aura symptoms last longer than 15 minutes (usually 15–60 minutes), and TIAs are shorter in duration, usually less than 15 minutes.[8] Visual symptoms associated with migraine aura tend to evolve slowly, enlarge, grow, or move across a visual field before subsiding. They tend to be "bright" and sometimes "shimmering" and be homonymous. In comparison, visual symptoms associated with ischemic attacks tend to be dark, dim, and unchanging, usually unilateral.

Migraine-related paresthesias also evolve gradually and tend to spread slowly up or down the extremities. The sensation is mostly tingling, lasts for 20 to 30 minutes, and then resolves gradually. The area involved first tends to clear of symptoms last. By contrast, ischemic paresthesias arise suddenly, last 5 to 10 minutes, and resolve in the same order that the body parts were affected (opposite pattern to migrainous paresthesias).[9]

To further complicate matters, new-onset migraine in older adults often presents atypically, especially at symptom onset. Traveling paresthesias, homonymous visual field defects, or speech disturbances are more common as presenting symptoms of migraine in older adults compared to younger patients.[3] Additionally, older adults can also present with a rare form of aura that manifests as motor symptoms, specifically hemiplegia (hemiplegic migraine).[10] These symptoms can easily mimic TIA symptoms, especially as actual headaches are often absent among older adults experiencing migraines, as mentioned.

A thorough history, neurologic examination, and clinical correlation are necessary to appropriately distinguish migraine and ischemic symptoms. In older adults who have had migraine since they were younger than age 50, a history of current symptoms of aura as they compare to prior is crucial. If symptoms are consistent with prior symptoms across a lifetime, imaging and emergency workups can be potentially avoided. If potential migrainous symptoms are new onset, different from prior symptoms, associated with objective neurologic deficit on exam, or meet any aforementioned description for potential ischemic symptoms, there should be emergent evaluation for ischemia and neuroimaging (computed tomography [CT] or MRI brain).

Hypnic Headache

Hypnic headaches are rare headaches that almost exclusively occur in older adults. Also called the "alarm clock headache," it is estimated that 92% of hypnic headaches occur in adults aged 50 and older[11] with a mean age of onset of 61 years.[12] They are recurrent primary headaches that happen during sleep and wake the sufferer about three to five hours after falling asleep. Duration is usually around 15 minutes to 3–4 hours, and they occur at least 10 days per month.[3] The parasympathetic symptoms (lacrimation, conjunctival injection, rhinorrhea) that commonly accompany cluster headache are absent.[9] In part due to the rarity of this disorder (estimated 0.2% to 0.3% of headache outpatients), this condition has not been systematically studied.[12] These headaches are usually self-limited and ease in frequency and intensity after several months. Nocturnal headaches that mimic hypnic headache can occur in people with intracranial masses, obstructive sleep apnea, hypertension or hypoglycemia, and medication overuse or withdrawal.[13] Given these are usually new-onset headaches in older patients and potentially serious secondary conditions can mimic symptoms, patients usually undergo evaluation for secondary headache causes, as well as neuroimaging.

Trigeminal Autonomic Cephalalgias (Cluster Headache)

Trigeminal autonomic cephalalgias (TACs) are characterized by unilateral headache attacks in the V1 distribution of the trigeminal nerve, associated with ipsilateral autonomic features, such as lacrimation, ptosis, and pupillary irregularities. The most common TACs are cluster headaches: people experience a minimum of 5 attacks of severe unilateral orbital, supraorbital, or temporal pain lasting 15 to 180 minutes with a sense of agitation and/or ipsilateral autonomic features. Attacks typically occur in series lasting weeks or months (cluster periods) followed by periods of remission that can last several years.

Cluster headache is estimated to be four times more common in men than women,[14] and studies on peak age of incidence vary. Some studies describe trends of later onset; for instance, a study in Minnesota found that peak incidence for onset in men was between the ages of 40 to 49 years, while peak incidence for onset in women was between the ages of 60 and 69 years.[15] Most older literature suggests a younger age of onset, usually between 20 and 50 years.[16] There have been reports of new-onset cluster headaches in individuals in their eighth, ninth, and tenth decades.[14] Hemicrania continua is another form of TAC where patients experience constant unilateral headache with intermittent ipsilateral autonomic features that uniquely respond to indomethacin. The incidence of rare TACs in older adults is unknown but has been described.[3]

As with migraine, cluster headache tends to become less frequent and severe with age in patients who began having symptoms at younger ages.[9] New-onset cluster headache after age 50 should prompt evaluation for secondary causes. In particular, consideration of glaucoma (that can present with severe orbital headache, pupillary irregularities, and conjunctival injection), ischemic events, and temporal arteritis are crucial, as the prevalence of these conditions increases with age and can mimic TACs. Neuroimaging, blood work (including inflammatory markers), and appropriate ophthalmic evaluation are usually warranted.

Chronic Daily Headache

Chronic daily headache (CDH) is an umbrella term referring to headaches that occur 15 or more days per month. There are multiple types of CDH, the most common being chronic migraine and chronic tension-type headache (CTTH).

The prevalence of CDH in the general population is consistently cited as between 3% and 4% in multiple studies. When looking specifically at older adults, prevalence was demonstrated to be 4.4%, with higher prevalence in women (6%) compared to men (2.5%). Within the population of patients suffering from CDH, chronic migraines occurred in 2.5% of patients, while CTTH occurred in 1.5% of patients.[17]

In older patients with CDH, careful review of medications is indicated, as medication overuse and adverse effects of common medications in older adults can lead to chronic headache.

SECONDARY HEADACHES

Evaluation for secondary causes of headache is especially pertinent in older adults, as age alone is a significant risk factor for secondary etiologies. It is estimated that the risk of a potentially life-threatening secondary headache is increased tenfold in patients aged 65 and above. In one study assessing patients with new-onset headache, 15% of those above age 65 had a secondary headache cause compared to 1.6% of younger patients.[18] Several studies have found a higher proportion of secondary headaches among older patients, with prevalence ranging from 10% to 30%.[19, 20]

A detailed history and neurologic examination are indicated in every patient with a new-onset headache, and this initial approach is similar for older adults. Suspicion for secondary causes should be higher in older adults, as mentioned, with a lower threshold to pursue neuroimaging, especially if a patient has vascular comorbidities. In a study investigating causes of sudden death after new-onset headache, a majority were secondary to vascular events (aneurysm, hemorrhage, cervical artery dissection).[21]

It can be challenging to determine when to pursue further workup for secondary causes, especially among older patients, a majority of whom will have at least one comorbid condition. While there is no universal guideline, monitoring for "red flag" symptoms is helpful in clinical decision-making. SNOOP4 is a previously published pneumonic that characterizes concerning symptoms in headache evaluation (Table 19.1). Diagnostic testing depends on the red flag symptoms identified but usually includes blood tests, testing for inflammatory markers (e.g., erythrocyte sedimentation rate [ESR], C reactive protein [CRP]), and neurovascular imaging.[22] The American College of Radiology considers any new headache in people above the age of 50 years to be appropriate for neuroimaging.[23]

In this section, we will detail common causes of secondary headaches linked to comorbid conditions common in older adults, as well as the workup warranted if history and exam are suspicious for one of these secondary causes. Table 19.2 summarizes relevant secondary causes of headache and distinguishing symptoms, and Table 19.3 summarizes imaging recommendations for suspected secondary causes of headache.

Medication-Induced and -Overuse Headache

Medication-overuse headaches (MOH) are headaches that occur 15 or more days per month in the setting of taking a pain medication 15 or more days per month (defined as overuse). The culprit medications are typically over-the-counter analgesics, usually recommended to patients for other forms of pain (e.g., back

TABLE 19.1 Headache red flags

HEADACHE HISTORY RED FLAGS – SNOOP4		POSSIBLE CONDITIONS
S	Systemic symptoms, fevers, chills, myalgias, weight loss	Meningitis, vasculitis, cancer, infection
N	Neurologic deficit (focal)	Neoplasm, stroke, TIA
O	Older age at onset (>50 years)	GCA, neoplasm
O	Sudden onset	Subarachnoid hemorrhage, cerebrovascular, CSF leak
P	Pattern change/progression	Neoplasm
P	Positional aggravation	High or low blood pressure
P	Precipitated by Valsalva maneuver	Posterior fossa lesion
P	Papilledema	Increased intracranial pressure

TABLE 19.2   Secondary headaches in older adults

DISORDER	CHARACTERISTIC SIGNS AND SYMPTOMS
Medication Overuse	Use of analgesic medications, polypharmacy, other areas of chronic pain
Cervicogenic Headache	Exacerbated by neck movement, history of arthritis or disorders of spine Often associated with neck pain or stiffness Often unilateral
Sleep Apnea	Chronic morning headache, OSA risk factors Excessive daytime sleepiness, history of interrupted sleep
Cardiac Cephalalgia	Precipitated by exertion, vascular risk factors May be associated with nausea, diaphoresis, chest discomfort Improves with nitrates
Subdural Hematoma	Dull, aching, associated with drowsiness, mood changes, or confusion. Use of anticoagulation
Subarachnoid Hemorrhage	Thunderclap headache, severe Depressed level of consciousness Use of anticoagulation
Subacute Glaucoma	Headache in dim light May be associated with photophobia, nausea or vomiting Visual blurring Mid-dilated pupil, conjunctival injection
Trigeminal Neuralgia	Paroxysmal, severe, neuropathic quality Trigeminal nerve territory Triggered by innocuous stimuli to trigeminal nerve
GCA	Scalp tenderness, jaw claudication Systemic symptoms (fever, fatigue, weight loss) Loss of temporal artery pulse on examination
Cerebral Neoplasm	Subacute onset of focal neurologic deficits, papilledema, new or changing headache
TIA/Stroke	Sudden onset of focal neurologic deficits
Hypertension	Bilateral, throbbing Often rapid onset Acute, severe rise in blood pressure

TABLE 19.3   Secondary causes of headache and imaging recommendations

CLINICAL FEATURES/RED FLAGS	SUSPECTED CONDITION	RECOMMENDED IMAGING
New neurologic deficit	Neoplasm, vascular malformation, ischemic event	CT brain, MRI brain
Severe, sudden onset (thunderclap)	Subarachnoid Hemorrhage Bleed	CT brain without contrast MRI brain without gadolinium MRA head and neck
Sudden unilateral and/or pain radiating to the neck	Vascular (e.g., arterial dissection)	CTA head and neck or MRA head and neck
Positional pain	Intracranial hypertension CSF leak	MRI brain with/without gadolinium
Head trauma	Bleed	CT head without contrast
New onset in patient >50 years	Neoplasm, GCA	MRI brain with/without gadolinium
Jaw claudication, temporal pain	GCA	MRI brain with/without gadolinium

pain). Some studies indicate that up to 15% of headaches in patients 65 and over are the result of overuse of medications.[20]

Additionally, many medications commonly prescribed to older adults can be associated with headache, including but not limited to nitroglycerin, calcium channel blockers, proton pump inhibitors, and selective serotonin reuptake inhibitors.[24] New-onset or worsening headache after a recently initiated medication should prompt suspicion for a medication-induced headache.

Vascular Events

Vascular risk factors are more common in older adults, and age is an independent risk factor for cerebrovascular ischemic events. Generally, strokes and TIAs result in focal neurologic deficits (weakness, sensory loss, ataxia, difficulty with speech or vision). As alluded to previously, ischemic events and primary headache symptoms (especially migrainous) can present similarly. There should be a low threshold for prompt emergency evaluation if an older adult presents with any neurologic features potentially consistent with an ischemic event.

Subdural Hematoma and Subarachnoid Hemorrhage

Subdural hematomas (SDH) occur much more frequently in older adults compared to younger populations. SDH can develop with motions as limited as coughing or sneezing, or even falling *without* head trauma can cause rupture of bridging veins, leading to a bleed. In addition to the fragility of intracranial blood vessels, older adults are at higher risk of SDH due to increased use of anticoagulation and higher incidence of falls and gait instability. The combination of increased risk of falls, use of anticoagulation, and fragile blood vessels places older adults at much higher risk with even minimal injury or trauma to the head.

Headaches from SDH are usually dull, mild, and generalized, often mistaken for TTHs. Other symptoms may include drowsiness, confusion, or increased irritability, but there are rarely focal neurologic deficits.[25] If an older patient presents with a headache after even a minor trauma or the headache is associated with confusion, grogginess, brain fog, or mood changes, there should be a low threshold to obtain a CT scan for an SDH.

Just as older adults are more susceptible to subdural hematomas, they are also at higher risk of subarachnoid bleeds, which are severe, sudden-onset headaches that reach peak intensity within 60 seconds. Any sudden-onset and severe headache in an older patient should be evaluated by emergency services immediately for hemorrhage.

Cervicogenic Headache

Cervicogenic headaches are caused by disorders of the cervical spine and neck, where pain from the neck is referred to the head. Referral pain tends to be occipital but can also be frontal, around the eye, and periauricular. Pain typically starts in the neck and radiates anteriorly, often involving ipsilateral shoulder or arm, often accompanied by limited neck range of motion. Referral patterns tend to be from abnormalities in C1–C3; lower cervical disease is less likely to cause symptoms.[26] Trauma (whiplash injury), muscle strain, and cervical arthropathy are all risk factors. Cervicogenic headaches should be suspected in older adults in general as cervical arthropathy, disorders of the cervical spine, and muscle strain are common in this population. Despite the increased prevalence of neck and upper back disorders, cervicogenic headaches are actually more prevalent in younger populations (ages 30–44 years),[27] and some studies have found that neck pain actually decreases with age.[28] Presence of radiographic degenerative disc disease of the cervical spine increases with age but is not independently a risk factor for cervicogenic headaches.[28]

A careful exam and history are important to determine if headache pain is truly radiating from the neck and back. If cervicogenic headache is suspected, imaging is often not required unless symptoms are severe or associated with marked limitation in motion. A trial of treatment and conservative management is often sufficient.

Trigeminal Neuralgia

Trigeminal neuralgia (unilateral, paroxysmal severe pain in the trigeminal nerve distribution) is more common in older populations; the average age of onset varies but is generally after age 50. Pain is often triggered by innocuous activity involving the distribution of the trigeminal nerve (chewing, talking, light touch, etc.). In patients refractory to initial medical treatments, an MRI of the brain is indicated to rule out secondary causes (e.g., tumor) unless contraindicated, especially in older adults with consistent symptoms.[9]

For elder patients, it is particularly important to distinguish dental etiologies and temporal mandibular joint (TMJ) pain from trigeminal neuralgia. Cracked or injured teeth, dental infection, and ill-fitting dentures are very common among older adults and can mimic episodic, severe, unilateral pain associated with trigeminal neuralgia. Dental irregularities can also lead to TMJ pain, which can be unilateral or bilateral, and mimic aforementioned symptoms. A thorough dental examination is important for all patients but crucial for older adults with a potential trigeminal neuralgia presentation as it could potentially avoid expensive and cumbersome brain imaging and workup.

Postherpetic Neuralgia and Herpes Zoster

Reactivation of dormant varicella virus is far more common in older adults due to suppressed immunity associated with age, as well as an increased likelihood of comorbidities associated with immune suppression (e.g., diabetes). Pain may precede vesicular lesions by several days and can be severe over the eye and face. Postherpetic neuralgia can mimic trigeminal neuralgia—allodynia and hyperalgesia, and pain that can be burning, sharp, or shooting.[29] Thorough medical history, including of the prior zoster infection in the affected area, is vital, as pain from postherpetic neuralgia generally does not require the same neuro-imaging workup as trigeminal neuralgia. Postherpetic neuralgia generally resolves within a few weeks to months, whereas trigeminal neuralgia is likely to persist.

Obstructive Sleep Apnea

Sleep-related complaints are very common in older adults, with over 50% of people over age 65 reporting some form of chronic sleep-related issue.[30] The prevalence of obstructive sleep apnea (OSA) also increases with age. Estimated prevalence varies, but epidemiologic studies consistently show increased prevalence with increasing age. In a sample of men from the United States, the prevalence of OSA increased from 11.3% of men between ages 44 and 64 years to 18.1% of men above 65 years.[31]

Headache is one of the common problems associated with untreated OSA and should be suspected in most older adults presenting with chronic headache (more than 15 days per month), especially in the morning. The headache is typically bilateral, pressing in quality, and lasts for several hours upon waking up in the morning. Morning headache occurs in 12% to 18% of patients with OSA and improves with appropriate treatment of sleep apnea. CPAP treatment is associated with complete resolution of headache treatment in 45% to 90% of patients.[32] Any older patients with chronic morning headache should be screened for sleep apnea and offered a sleep study.[22] If the headache is new, appropriate assessment for red flags and the need for neuro-imaging should be done prior to sleep study.

It is important to note that older patients with OSA often do not fit the same "classic" presentation of younger patients with OSA. Many older patients with OSA are not obese or overweight, nor do they have increased neck circumference. As a result, older adults with sleep apnea are often underdiagnosed—the American Academy of Sleep Medicine estimates that up to 56% of patients above age 65 have sleep apnea, many of whom have atypical risk factors.[33] This emphasizes the importance of obtaining a sleep study in older patients with chronic headache, as OSA is often a missed cause.

Cardiac Cephalalgia

While rare, headache can be associated with cardiac vascular disease, and this type of headache is almost exclusively present in older adults. Cardiac cephalalgia is characterized by headache precipitated and worsened by exertion and activity, and subsequently relieved with rest. The headache itself is a symptom of myocardial ischemia and sometimes can be the only manifestation (absent chest pain).[34] They are generally moderate to severe in intensity and can be associated with nausea or emesis. Cardiac cephalalgia is often mistaken for migraine given the moderate to severity intensity and association with nausea. Distinguishing the two is important, as treatment of cardiac cephalalgia with triptans can worsen myocardial ischemia. In a similar vein, nitroglycerin improves symptoms of cardiac cephalalgia, while it can precipitate a migraine attack or worsening of symptoms of existing migraine.[35] Photophonia and phonophobia are not usually associated with cardiac cephalalgia, and while activity may worsen a migraine, it generally doesn't trigger the initial symptoms. These headaches should be suspected in older patients with cardiovascular risk factors, especially without a prior history of migraine, and electrocardiogram (ECG), cardiac stress test, and neuroimaging should be pursued in most cases.

Subacute Glaucoma

Glaucoma is a multifactorial condition characterized by progressive optic neuropathy and peripheral visual field loss. Prevalence increases with age, with an estimated 76 million people globally living with the disease, a number that is expected to increase to 111 million with a globally aging population.[36] Subacute glaucoma can cause headache symptoms — intermittent dull headache that is often associated with visual blurring. Glaucoma should be suspected in older patients with dull headache associated with visual blurring/changes and triggered by low light conditions. Visual symptoms can be distinguished from migraine as blurring in the peripheral vision is generally different than the spots, lights or patterns associated with visual migraine auras. Additionally, migraine aura does not generally worsen in low light conditions, while symptoms of glaucoma do worsen. Often, older patients will have an already diagnosed history of glaucoma. Usually, the duration of subacute glaucoma is less than 4 hours, and mean age of onset is 60 years.[37] In patients with headache related to suspected glaucoma, urgent ophthalmologic evaluation is indicated, as untreated subacute glaucoma can result in optic nerve damage and loss of vision.

Giant Cell Arteritis

Giant cell arteritis (GCA) should be considered in anyone over the age of 50 presenting with a new or changing/worsening headache. Headache is the primary symptom for over 85% of GCA patients, and scalp tenderness and jaw claudication are often associated features.[38] Jaw claudication is the most specific predictor of a positive temporal artery biopsy but is not always present. There is a strong association with polymyalgia rheumatica (40%–60% of cases are co-occurring), so assessing for pain and stiffness of shoulders and hips can be helpful clues. While these are well-known symptoms of GCA, in the clinical setting they can be challenging to distinguish from other secondary causes of headaches in older adults (especially cervicogenic and medication overuse). Missing GCA can have devastating consequences; in one study, 8.2% of GCA patients suffered permanent vision loss because of delayed diagnosis.[39] Because of this, some experts recommend obtaining an ESR and CRP in all patients over age 50 presenting with a new or different headache, regardless of the presence of classic GCA features.[40] While inflammatory markers are often elevated in GCA, they can be normal in up to 4% of patients; thus, if clinical suspicion is high despite normal markers, the patient should be started on steroids, and further workup should be pursued.[41]

Hypertensive Headache

Hypertension is often associated with headache—namely, migraine and TTH, and has a higher prevalence among older adults (similar to almost all chronic conditions). Malignant hypertension (identified as hypertension with evidence of end-organ damage) was associated with headache in the past, namely due to a lack of effective antihypertensive treatment. Now, headache is still thought of as a warning symptom for a potential hypertensive emergency, though prognostic significance remains murky at best. It is believed that headache may be attributed to hypertension only if blood pressure values are very high or rise very quickly, though some studies have found an inverse association (lower blood pressure is more associated with headaches). Hypertensive headache is usually throbbing, generalized, worse with awakening, and tends to ease with activity.[9]

CONSIDERATIONS IN TREATMENT OF HEADACHE DISORDERS IN OLDER ADULTS

Clinical Case 2

The patient is a 75-year-old male with a history of benign prostatic hyperplasia, hypertension, and pre-diabetes who presents for follow-up after last being seen six months prior. At the patient's last visit, he was diagnosed with chronic migraine, which he had previously had for 30 years but had not previously seen a provider for. At that time, he was taking daily tamsulosin, carvedilol, losartan, atorvastatin, and metformin. Starting onabotulinumtoxinA had been discussed as the best next step for both efficacy and limiting the number of possible side effects as well as drug-drug interactions. However, the patient wanted to start amitriptyline because he had read on the internet that it could fix migraine. The inclusion of this medication on the BEERS Criteria as a medication to avoid in older adults due to strong anticholinergic properties, including urinary retention, was discussed. The patient ultimately left the visit early when amitriptyline would not be prescribed for him.

One month later, the patient returns to clinic; he has now read more about onabotulinumtoxinA and is interested in starting it.

Multimorbidity and polypharmacy

Multimorbidity is defined as the presence of two or more medical conditions requiring medical treatment. Multimorbidity is highly prevalent among older adults—approximately 84% of adults above the age of 60 in the United States had two or more medical conditions, with the prevalence increasing to 90% for individuals above the age of 80.[42] A high prevalence of multiple medical conditions means the majority of older patients are taking several medications simultaneously. These medications could potentially interact with standard headache treatments and should be carefully considered prior to initiating a new therapy.

Polypharmacy is standardly defined as the concurrent use of five or more medications,[43] extreme polypharmacy is sometimes defined as taking ten or more medications.[44] Studies on the prevalence of polypharmacy among older adults vary; several have found a prevalence of 30%–40% of persons over 65 years taking five or more medications.[45] Upwards of 10% of older adults take ten or more medications. The prevalence increases with increasing age.[46]

TABLE 19.4 Comorbid conditions and potential complications from headache medications

CLINICAL CONDITION	POTENTIAL COMPLICATION	MEDICATIONS
Benign Prostatic Hyperplasia	Severe urinary retention with anticholinergic medications	TCAs Opioids
Cognitive Impairment	Higher risk of falls and delirium with sedating medications	Opioids Barbiturates TCAs
Cardiac Arrhythmia	Risk of heart block and QTc prolongation	Antiemetics Beta-blockers CCBs
Cardiovascular Disease	Theoretical risk of inducing ischemia	Triptans
Peptic Ulcer Disease	Increased risk of gastrointestinal bleeding	NSAIDs
Chronic Kidney Disease	Acute kidney injury or renal failure	NSAIDs
Use of anticoagulation	Increased risk of gastrointestinal bleeding	NSAIDs

Treating headache disorders is complicated in older adults because of multimorbidity and polypharmacy (increased risk of drug-drug interactions). This section will highlight common medications used in headache and considerations pertinent to older adults with multiple comorbid conditions and high risk of drug interactions.

Pharmacologic treatment of headache disorders will be placed into two categories: acute (abortive) and preventative (prophylactic) treatment. Table 19.4 summarizes common comorbid conditions in older adults and potential complications from different headache treatments.

Clinical Case 3

The patient is an 81-year-old female with a history of chronic migraine and a remote history of myocardial infarction currently well controlled on daily magnesium, memantine, and quarterly onabotulinumtoxinA who presents for urgent follow-up for an episode of intractable migraine. Prior to two weeks ago, she reported having roughly eight headache days per month, including four migraine days; however, two weeks prior to the visit, she noted the onset of a severe headache episode that did not respond to her usual lasmiditan and transcutaneous supraorbital nerve stimulator. The headache was sufficiently severe that she presented on the third day to the emergency department, where a CT head without contrast showed no evidence of a bleed, and follow-up MRI brain confirmed no new abnormalities.

A diagnosis of status migrainosus is made, and the patient is scheduled for a peripheral nerve block of the bilateral occipital, supraorbital, supratrochlear, and auriculotemporal nerves. Two days after receiving the peripheral nerve block, the patient sends a message through the electronic health record that her headache has resolved.

ACUTE TREATMENTS

Nonsteroidal Anti-inflammatory Drugs and Analgesics

Acetaminophen and nonsteroidal anti-inflammatory drugs (NSAIDs) are considered first line among simple, readily available analgesics for headache treatment in older adults. NSAIDs in particular are effective for treatment of moderate to severe headaches, including migraine. There is no clear evidence for using one NSAID over another for efficacy in headache treatment, particularly in TTH.[47] Despite their efficacy, they are generally not preferred over the use of acetaminophen in older adults due to their adverse risk profile. Older adults are more likely to have peptic ulcer disease or gastric irritation that could be aggravated by the use of NSAIDs. According to the American Geriatrics Society, upper gastrointestinal ulcers, gross bleeding, or gastric perforation occur in approximately 1% of older patients using NSAIDs regularly for three to six months and 2%–4% of patients using NSAIDs regularly for one year. These trends worsen with advancing age and long-term, regular use.[48]

Additionally, older adults are far more likely than younger adults to be using anticoagulants given higher rates of cardiac and vascular comorbidities (cardiac arrhythmias, blood clots, and cardiovascular procedures such as stenting). NSAIDs should not be used in older adults taking blood thinners due to the increased risk of bleeding.[49] Older adults are also far more likely to take aspirin for cardiovascular indications, which can interact with COX-2 inhibitors used for the treatment of headache.[50]

Renal dysfunction is also important to consider in this population – estimates vary, but most cite that over 10% of the global adult population has chronic kidney disease,[51] with prevalence steadily increasing with age. Some estimates cite the worldwide prevalence of chronic kidney disease at 47% among persons 70 years or older.[52] NSAID use in patients with even mild renal dysfunction can cause acute renal failure, interstitial nephritis, proteinuria, and fluid retention.[53] As such, NSAIDs should generally be avoided as a primary headache treatment in older adults; acetaminophen should generally be tried first. When NSAIDs are the most appropriate option for treatment of headache (e.g., for a patient with liver dysfunction, acetaminophen is ineffective), prescribed courses should be short (days to weeks), and consideration of taking NSAIDs in conjunction with an H2 blocker (e.g., famotidine) for gastric protection is warranted.[48]

Antiemetics

Antiemetic medications such as metoclopramide, promethazine, prochlorperazine, and chlorpromazine are useful in the treatment of migraine. The majority of these medications can cause anticholinergic side effects, to which older adults are particularly susceptible, and can especially cause issues with urinary retention. Older adults are also more prone to parkinsonism with repeated use.[54] These medications should be used with caution in older adults—treatment regimens should avoid reliance on repeated use or high doses of antiemetic medications. Prochlorperazine and promethazine in particular have strong anticholinergic properties and should be avoided.[48]

Close monitoring of the QT interval is also warranted with use of antiemetics in older patients, particularly with repeated use. Most antiemetics can cause QT prolongation, another risk that is higher in older patients compared to younger headache sufferers. Antiemetics should be avoided in older adults taking other medications that prolong the QT interval, including SSRIs, SNRIs, and atypical/typical antipsychotic medications.[55]

Caffeine

Caffeine has acute analgesic effects on its own and is often used in combination with other analgesics (especially acetaminophen) for treatment of migraine, TTH, and hypnic headache. Caffeine should be used cautiously in older adults, as older patients are more sensitive to the effects of caffeine. Caffeine is also a known cause of withdrawal headache, and excessive caffeine intake is a known risk factor for chronic headache.[56] Caffeine use should be limited in headache patients—some experts recommend a limit of 100 mg per day in patients with a high frequency of migraine or TTH.[57] For adult patients without frequent headaches, 200–400 mg of caffeine daily is generally considered safe. In older adults, however, even these doses of caffeine can lead to increased symptoms of anxiety and sleep disruption. Caffeine sensitivity increases as patients age—one study predicted that coffee drinkers between ages 65 and 70 take approximately 33% longer to metabolize caffeine compared to younger participants.[58] In general, daily doses of caffeine between 50 and 100 mg are well tolerated, which translates to approximately one cup of coffee per day. Doses in over-the-counter combination medications for headache usually have between 30 and 65 mg per pill, and taking two tablets is often common practice.[57] When caffeine is used for headache treatment in older adults, a general principle is to begin with lower doses and cautiously increase as tolerated, monitoring for sleep disruption and anxiety.

Serotonin 5-HT Receptor Agonists (Triptans)

Triptans are first-line acute therapies for most cluster and migraine headaches and are widely used in patients of all ages. The mechanism impacts the meningeal blood vessels and the trigeminal nerve endings that innervate these vessels.[59] Triptans are contraindicated in patients with a history of coronary artery disease, coronary artery vasospasm, peripheral artery disease, stroke, uncontrolled hypertension, and ischemic bowel disease because of their potential for vasoconstriction. They are considered safe in patients with no cardiovascular risk factors. Because of their capacity for vasoconstriction, they are considered to increase the risk of serious ischemic events in patients with vascular disease.[60] This is especially pertinent to older adults, as data consistently indicate that the prevalence of cardiovascular diseases, ischemic stroke, and peripheral artery disease increases with age. An analysis in the *Journal of the American College of Cardiology* found that the prevalence of vascular disease steadily increased from 2% for patients between 40 and 50 years old to 32.5% for patients 91 to 100 years old.[61] As such, triptan use is generally recommended against as first-line treatment for older patients with unknown cardiovascular risk factors given the high risk of cardiovascular disease. If older adults have been taking triptans for migraine since they were younger, it is generally safe to continue if they are not having symptoms consistent with ischemia.

Triptans are indicated in some older patients, especially with severe headache symptoms associated with migraine that cannot be managed with simple analgesics. Assessing cardiovascular risk in older patients prior to starting a triptan can be challenging, especially if they have atypical symptoms or potentially experience "silent myocardial ischemia." A reasonable approach is to try and stratify patients into low, intermediate, or high risk of coronary disease and ischemic stroke. There are several tools, including the adult treatment panel report of the National Cholesterol Education Program. Patients with only one risk factor are considered low risk, while those with two or more risk factors are considered intermediate. An important consideration is that age (>45 years for men and >55 years for women) is a risk factor in and of itself.[62] For patients with intermediate and high risk of vascular disease, it is generally recommended to avoid starting triptans when possible. In general, it is not recommended that asymptomatic patients undergo workup for coronary artery disease prior to initiating triptan therapy, but it should be considered in cases where a patient has concerning or even vague but suspicious symptoms.

Opioids and Barbiturates

Opiate and barbiturate derivatives are used in the management of headaches, especially migraine, despite a lack of evidence of their efficacy and safety.[63] Medications containing butalbital are no longer available in Europe but are still used in the United States. These classes are most commonly used in combination pills that include acetaminophen or aspirin with caffeine and butalbital. These medications should only be used rarely and with extreme caution in older adults for several reasons. First, these medications carry the risk of renal and hepatic toxicity, to which older adults are more susceptible. Second, they carry risks of tolerance and dependence, meaning that older adults are at risk of needing to use them more frequently, further raising the risk of developing toxicity.[64] Third, overuse of barbiturates and opiates is one of the leading causes of the transformation of episodic to chronic migraine.[65] Further, there is an increased risk of sedation, falls, and adverse cognitive effects for older adults taking these therapies.[66] As such, opioids and barbiturates should be avoided.[3]

Corticosteroids

Corticosteroids are sometimes used in transitional or bridging treatment of primary headache disorders (especially cluster headaches)—meaning a therapy to rapidly suppress headache attacks while the use of long-term maintenance prophylactic agents is increased. Prednisone, prednisolone, and dexamethasone have all been used for this purpose, usually with a two- to three-week taper regimen. Corticosteroids should be used cautiously in older adults due to the higher prevalence of osteoporosis, diabetes, and hypertension, all of which can be worsened with steroid use, especially over long periods of time.[33] If corticosteroids need to be used for transitional treatment of primary headache disorders, low doses should be initiated, with short durations of use. For GCA, 40–60 mg of prednisone daily should be started in older patients, barring an absolute contraindication due to the risk of vision loss. If patients have diabetes, hypertension, or osteoporosis, close monitoring during the treatment course is warranted.

Peripheral Nerve Blocks

Peripheral nerve blocks are sometimes used for immediate relief of multiple forms of headache. They are generally safe, with few contraindications, and are well tolerated. Peripheral nerve blocks are fairly widely used despite few studies demonstrating efficacy. The technique involves local anesthetic blockade to the greater occipital nerve. There is better evidence for cluster and cervicogenic headaches, but this technique is also used for TTH and migraines.[67] As they are generally well tolerated with few contraindications, peripheral nerve blockades are a reasonable choice for older patients who may have comorbid conditions contraindicating standard therapies or who cannot tolerate therapeutic doses of systemic medications due to adverse effects.

PREVENTATIVE TREATMENTS

Tricyclic Antidepressants (TCAs)

TCAs are used for the prevention of both migraine and TTH. Amitriptyline has the best evidence for TTH, usually doses between 10 mg to 75 mg every evening.[68] There is evidence that amitriptyline helps with reducing myofascial tenderness, which is helpful in addressing symptoms of CTTH.[69] Amitriptyline is also the best-studied TCA for migraine prophylaxis, used at similar doses for treating TTH. Other TCAs that may be effective are nortriptyline, protriptyline, and doxepin, though they are less studied.

TCAs should be generally avoided in older adults as headache treatment. The anticholinergic adverse effects of TCAs (sedation, dry mouth, constipation, and urinary retention) are common and more pronounced in older patients.[70] Sedation is very common with TCAs (as such, they are usually administered at bedtime), which can be helpful in patients with comorbid insomnia. This impact in older adults puts patients at higher risk of falls and delirium with increased sedation. Urinary retention is a significant risk with TCAs, especially in older men with benign prostatic hyperplasia who may experience some degree of retention at baseline. TCAs can dramatically worsen symptoms of BPH and retention in older men.[71] The American Geriatrics Society recommends against use of TCAs (and most anticholinergic medications) in patients with cognitive impairment or dementia due to higher risk of sedation, falls, and urinary retention in these patients.[33]

If necessary, initiating TCAs for migraines and TTH in older adults should start with low doses (usually 10 mg) and uptitrat slowly for desired effect while monitoring for symptoms. Of note, many older adults are on serotonin reuptake inhibitors—the Centers for Disease Control and Prevention found 19% of older adults were on antidepressant medication compared with 8% of those 18–39 years and 14% of people 40–59 years.[72] Concomitant use of these medications can reduce the metabolism of TCAs, which can significantly increase the risk of side effects.[73] TCAs should be avoided in older adults taking serotonin reuptake inhibitors unless other options are not available.

Topiramate

Topiramate is a second-generation, anti-epileptic medication that is commonly used as a preventative treatment for migraine and cluster headaches. Doses between 100 and 200 mg have been found to significantly reduce monthly headache frequency in chronic migraine patients.[74] While there are no direct contraindications for use in older adults, a distinctive adverse effect profile warrants careful consideration prior to recommending it to older adults. Topiramate can cause anorexia, weight loss, and altered taste. Older adults are particularly susceptible to this side effect (reduction in appetite is common as people age, with an estimated prevalence of poor appetite between 15% and 30% of older adults).[75] Additionally, topiramate can also cause dose-related and reversible cognitive effects, including language difficulties and issues with short-term memory. Older patients are more susceptible to these effects, especially if they have any degree of underlying cognitive impairment.[71] When used in combination with other central nervous system (CNS)-active drugs that may be prescribed to older adults for different indications, there is an increased risk of falls and potential fractures (specifically three or more CNS-active medications).[33] Topiramate has also been shown to increase plasma levels of serotonin[76] and should be used with caution in older adults taking other serotinergic medications (e.g., antidepressants). As such, a thorough review of current medications is important prior to initiating treatment with topiramate as a crucial first step. As with most medications, uptitration of topiramate is best done slowly in older patients, with some recommendations suggesting starting as low as 12.5 mg daily and increasing by 12.5 mg every two to three weeks while monitoring for side effects. Doses above 100 mg daily are rarely used in older patients. Older patients with chronic kidney disease should have topiramate doses renally adjusted.[71]

Beta-Blockers

Despite an uncertain mechanism of action, beta-blockers are commonly used for migraine prophylaxis. Propranolol and timolol have the most evidence, though other beta-blockers such as metoprolol and atenolol are often used. In older adults, beta-blockers can cause sedation, lethargy, and exercise intolerance, which can potentially worsen falls and confusion. While the adverse effects of beta-blockers are not thoroughly studied in older populations, one study demonstrated that beta-blockers are associated with an increased risk of functional decline in older patients with moderate to severe dementia (patients with no or mild cognitive impairment did not have increased risk).[77] Moreover, beta-blockers (especially nonselective ones) should be avoided in patients with chronic obstructive pulmonary disease and used with caution in older adults with diabetes, as they can blunt the sympathetic response to hypoglycemia. Beta-blockers should be started at low doses in older patients and titrated up slowly. Ideally, they should be used in patients with another indication (coronary artery disease, hypertension) to reduce the likelihood of polypharmacy.[71]

Calcium Channel Blockers

Calcium channel blockers (CCBs) are used in migraine prophylaxis, and verapamil is the prophylactic agent of choice for cluster headaches. Verapamil is associated with a number of adverse effects, including constipation, dizziness, hypotension, and bradycardia, all of which are more common in older adults.

One study found that 19% of cluster headache patients on verapamil had ECG abnormalities as a result, predominantly first-degree heart block and junctional heart rhythm.[78] Older adults are more likely to have underlying cardiac arrhythmia and/or be taking other medications that can cause bradycardia, so close monitoring for symptoms such as dizziness, fatigue, and exercise intolerance is warranted. Verapamil is usually recommended at higher doses for cluster headache prophylaxis than those used for the treatment of hypertension; however, given the higher risk of side effects in older adults, the increase of verapamil should not be faster than 80 mg weekly. Starting dose for migraine prophylaxis is often recommended at 240 mg (up to 1,200 mg daily), but beginning at a lower dose in older patients is often practiced to assess for tolerance.[71]

Valproic Acid

Valproic acid is an anti-epileptic medication used for migraine and cluster headache prophylaxis. It has been demonstrated as effective in migraine prophylaxis[79] and prophylaxis of cluster headaches.[80] Similar to topiramate, valproic acid can be used in older adults but with conscious attention paid to the side effect profiles. Nausea, anorexia, and diarrhea are common side effects, and are more likely to have a pronounced effect on frail older adults. Sedation and ataxia are also known side effects—older adults are more likely to also be taking other medications, which can amplify the cognitive side effects of valproic acid and place older adults at risk of falls and confusion. Starting with lower doses (suggestions generally start with 250 mg daily in the evening) and increasing slowly to a target dose of 500 mg to 750 mg over the course of several weeks allows for closer monitoring of side effects.[71]

SUMMARY

Primary and secondary headache disorders present differently in older adults compared to younger patients, and older adults are more susceptible to side effects from common medications used in the management of headache symptoms. Diagnosis of headache disorders in older adults is complicated due to the higher prevalence of comorbidities and the risk of secondary causes of headache symptoms. Beginning with a careful headache history and inventory of comorbid conditions and current medications is a good starting point in headache assessment for older patients. A lower threshold for head imaging and workup of secondary causes is crucial, as is consideration of medications and interactions that could be contributing to symptoms. Finally, when determining headache treatment, there are some therapies that should be avoided in older adults that are safer in younger patients. In general, a strategy of starting with lower doses of both therapeutic and prophylactic medications and increasing as slowly as tolerated is more important for older adults given increased sensitivity to common headache therapies.

- Presentations of primary headache disorders differ in older adults
- Higher suspicion of secondary causes of headache is warranted in older adults due to comorbidities
- Polypharmacy and multimorbidity complicate headache treatment in older adults
- Older adults are at higher risk of adverse effects from common headache therapies
- Most medication regimens should start at lower doses for older adults and be increased slowly while assessing for tolerance and side effects

REFERENCES

1. Stovner L, Hagen K, Jensen R, et al. The global burden of headache: A documentation of headache prevalence and disability worldwide. *Cephalalgia* 2007;*27*(3):193–210. doi:https://doi.org/10.1111/j.1468-2982.2007.01288.x

2. Franceschi M, Colombo B, Rossi P, Canal N. Headache in a population-based elderly cohort. An ancillary study to the Italian longitudinal study of aging (ILSA). *Headache: J Head Face Pain* 1997;*37*(2):79–82. doi:https://doi.org/10.1046/j.1526-4610.1997.3702079.x

3. Schwaiger J, Kiechl S, Seppi K, et al. Prevalence of primary headaches and cranial neuralgias in men and women aged 55–94 Years (Bruneck Study). *Cephalalgia* 2009;*29*(2):179–187. doi:https://doi.org/10.1111/j.1468-2982.2008.01705.x

4. Schwartz BS. Epidemiology of tension-type headache. *JAMA* 1998;*279*(5):381. doi:https://doi.org/10.1001/jama.279.5.381

5. Ready, M. *When Does a Patient with Headache Need a Workup?* 2022. Accessed September 5, 2023. https://americanheadachesociety.org/wp-content/uploads/2022/05/AHS-First-Contact-Headache-WorkUp.pdf

6. Berk T, Ashina S, Martin V, Newman L, Vij B. Diagnosis and Treatment of Primary Headache Disorders in Older Adults. *J Am Geriatr Soc* 2018;*66*(12):2408–2416. doi:https://doi.org/10.1111/jgs.15586

7. Vongvaivanich K, Lertakyamanee P, Silberstein SD, Dodick DW. Late-life migraine accompaniments: A narrative review. *Cephalalgia* 2014;*35*(10):894–911. doi:https://doi.org/10.1177/0333102414560635

8. Hershey LA, Bednarczyk EM. Treatment of Headache in the Elderly. *Curr Treat Options Neurol* 2012;*15*(1):56–62. doi:https://doi.org/10.1007/s11940-012-0205-6

9. Kunkel RS. Headaches in older patients: special problems and concerns. *Cleve Clin J Med* 2006;*73*(10):922–928. doi:https://doi.org/10.3949/ccjm.73.10.922

10. Fisher CM. Late-life migraine accompaniments--further experience. *Stroke* 1986;*17*(5):1033–1042. doi:https://doi.org/10.1161/01.str.17.5.1033

11. Liang JF, Wang SJ. Hypnic headache: a review of clinical features, therapeutic options and outcomes. *Cephalalgia* 2014 Sep;*34*(10):795–805.

12. Evers S, Goadsby PJ. Hypnic headache: Clinical features, pathophysiology, and treatment. *Neurology* 2003;*60*(6):905–909. doi:https://doi.org/10.1212/01.wnl.0000046582.21771.9c

13. Lindner D, Scheffler A, Nsaka M, Holle-Lee D. Hypnic Headache – What do we know in 2022? *Cephalalgia* 2023;*43*(3). doi:10.1177/03331024221148659

14. Fischera M, Marziniak M, Gralow I, Evers S. The incidence and prevalence of cluster headache: a meta-analysis of population-based studies. *Cephalalgia* 2008 Jun;*28*(6):614–8. doi: 10.1111/j.1468-2982.2008.01592

15. Swanson JW, Yanagihara T, Stang PE, et al. Incidence of cluster headaches. *Neurology* 1994;*44*(3 Part 1): 433–433. doi:https://doi.org/10.1212/wnl.44.3_part_1.433

16. Matharu MS, Goadsby PJ. Trigeminal autonomic cephalalgias: diagnosis and management. In: Silberstein SD, Lipton RB, Dodick DW, editors. *Wolff's headache and other head pain*. 8th ed. New York: Oxford University Press, Inc USA, 2008: 379–430.

17. Prencipe M. Prevalence of headache in an elderly population: attack frequency, disability, and use of medication. *J Neurol Neurosurg Psychiatry* 2001;*70*(3):377–381. doi:https://doi.org/10.1136/jnnp.70.3.377

18. Pascual J, Berciano J. Experience in the diagnosis of headaches that start in elderly people. *J Neurol Neurosurg Psychiatry* 1994;*57*(10): 1255–1257.

19. Ward TN. Headache disorders in the elderly. *Curr Treat Options Neurol* 2002;*23*(2): 291–305

20. Ruiz M, Pedraza MI, de la Cruz C, Baron J, Munoz I, Rodriguez C, et al. Headache in the elderly: a series of 262 patients. *Neurologia* 2014;*29*(6): 321–6.

21. Lynch KM, Brett F. Headaches that kill: a retrospective study of incidence, etiology and clinical features in cases of sudden death. *Cephalagia* 2012;*32* (13): 972–978.

22. Starling, A. Diagnosis and management of headache in older adults. *Mayo Clin Proc* 2018;*93*(2): 252–262

23. Expert Panel on Neurologic Imaging. ACR Appropriateness Criteria headache. *J Am Coll Radiol* 2019;*16*: S364–S377.

24. Toth, C. Medications and substances as cause of headache: a systematic review of the literature. *Clin Neuropharmacol* 2003;*26* (3): 122–136.

25. Auers, LM. Epidural and Subdural Hematomas. In Vinken PJ, Bruyn GW, Klawans HL, editors. *Vascular Diseases. Handbook of Clinical Neurology*, part II, vol *54*, Amsterdam; Elsevier, 1989: 345–360.

26. Bogduk N, Govind J. Cervicogenic headache: an assessment of the evidence on clinical diagnosis, invasive tests, and treatment. *Lancet Neurol* 2009;*8*(10):959–968. doi:https://doi.org/10.1016/s1474-4422(09)70209-1

27. Sjaastad O. Cervicogenic headache: comparison with migraine without aura; Vågå study. *Cephalalgia* 2008 Jul;*28* Suppl 1:18–20.

28. Hogg-Johnson S, van der Velde G, Carroll LJ, et al. The burden and determinants of neck pain in the general population. *Spine* 2008;*33*(Supplement):S39–S51. doi:https://doi.org/10.1097/brs.0b013e31816454c8

29. Wasner G, Kleinert A, Binder A, Schattschneider J, Baron R Postherpetic neuralgia: Topical lidocaine is effective in nociceptor-deprived skin. *J Neurol* 2005;*252*(6):677–686.

30. Foley DJ, Monjan AA, Brown SL, Simonsick EM, Wallace RB, Blazer DG. Sleep complaints among elderly persons: An epidemiologic study of three communities. *Sleep* 1995;*18*(6):425–432. doi:https://doi.org/10.1093/sleep/18.6.425

31. Bixler EO, Vgontzas AN, Ten Have T, Tyson K, Kales A. Effects of age on sleep apnea in men: I. Prevalence and severity. *Am J Respir Crit Care Med* 1998;*157*(1):144–148. doi:https://doi.org/10.1164/ajrccm.157.1.9706079

32. Johnson, KG, Ziemba AM, Garb JL. Improvement in headaches with continuous positive airway pressure for obstructive sleep apnea syndrome: a retrospective analysis. *Headache* 2013;*53*(2): 333–343.

33. American Academy of Sleep Medicine. Study Finds High Rate of Undiagnosed Sleep Apnea in Older Adults. May 11, 2018. Found on the internet at https://foundation.aasm.org/aasm-foundation-study-published-jags/

34. Lipton RB, Lowenkopf T, Bajwa ZH, et al. Cardiac cephalagia: a treatable form of exertional headache. *Neurology* 1997;*49* (3): 813–816.

35. Bini A, Evangelista A, Castellini P. Cardiac Cephalgia. *J Headache Pain* 2009;*10*(1): 3–9.

36. Tham Y, Li X, Wong T, Quigley H, Aung T, Cheng C. Global Prevalence of Glaucoma and Projections of Glaucoma Burden through 2040. *Ophthalmology* 2014;*121*(11): 2081–2090.

37. Nesher R, Epstein E, Stern Y, Assia E, Nesher G. Headaches as the main presenting symptom of subacute angle closure glaucoma. *Headache* 2005;*45* (2):172–176.

38. Gonzalez-Gay MA, Barros S, Lopez-Diaz MJ, Garcia-Porrua C, Sanchez-Andrade A, Llorca J. Giant cell arteritis: disease patterns of clinical presentation in a series of 240 patients. *Medicine* 2005;*84*:269–276.

39. Chen JJ, Leavitt JA, Fang C, Crowson CS, Matteson EL, Warrington KJ. Evaluating the incidence of arteritic ischemic optic neuropathy and other causes of vision loss from giant cell arteritis. *Ophthalmology* 2016;*123*:1999–2003.

40. Stern J, Anderson C, Robertson C, Halker Singh R. *Headache in Older Adults*. Practical Neurology. May 2023.

41. Kermani TA, Schmidt J, Crowson CS, Ytterberg SR, Hunder GG, Matteson EL, Warrington KJ. Utility of erythrocyte sedimentation rate and C-reactive protein for the diagnosis of giant cell arteritis. *Semin Arthritis Rheum* 2012 Jun;*41*(6):866–871.

42. Mossadeghi, B, Caxieta R, Ondarsuhu D et al. Multimorbidity and social determinants of health in the US prior to the COVID -19 pandemic and implications for health outcomes: a cross-sectional analysis based on NHANES 2017-2018. *BMC Public Health* 2023;*23* (1): 887.

43. Van Wilder L, Devleesschauwer B, Clays E, Pype P, Vandepitte S, De Smedt D. Polypharmacy and health-related quality of life/psychological distress among patients with chronic disease. *Prev Chronic Dis* 2022;*19*:220062. DOI: http://dx.doi.org/10.5888/pcd19.220062

44. Morin L, Johnell K, Laroche ML, Fastbom J, Wastesson JW. The epidemiology of polypharmacy in older adults: register-based prospective cohort study. *Clin Epidemiol* 2018;*12* (10):289–298.

45. Kurczewska-Michalak M, Lewek P, Jankowska-Polańska B, Giardini A, Granata N, Maffoni M, Costa E, Midão L, Kardas P. Polypharmacy management in the older adults: A scoping review of available interventions. *Front Pharmacol* 2021;*26*(12):734045

46. Barnett K, Mercer SW, Norbury M, Watt G, Wyke S, Guthrie B. Epidemiology of multimorbidity and implications for health care, research, and medical education: a cross-sectional study. *Lancet* 2012;*380*(9836):37–43

47. Bigal M, Rapoport A, Hargreaves R. Advances in the pharmacologic treatment of tension-type headache. *Curr Pain Headache Rep* 2008;*12*(6): 442–6.

48. American Geriatrics Society. American Geriatrics Society 2023 updated AGS Beers Criteria® for potentially inappropriate medication use in older adults. *J Am Geriatr Soc* 2023;*71*(7). doi:https://doi.org/10.1111/jgs.18372

49. Griffin MR, Piper JM, Daugherty JR et al. Nonsteroidal anti-inflammatory drug use and increased risk for peptic ulcer disease in elderly persons. *Ann Intern Med* 1991;*114* (4) 257–263.

50. Farkouh M, Greenberg B. An evidence based review of the cardiovascular risks of non-steroidal anti-inflammatory drugs. *Am J Cardiol* 2009;*103*(9): 1227–1237.

51. Kovesdy C. Epidemiology of chronic kidney disease: an update 2022. *Kidney Int Suppl* 2022;*12*(1): 7–11.

52. Xie Y, Bowe B, Mokdad AH, et al. Analysis of the global burden of disease study highlights the global, regional and national trends of chronic kidney disease epidemiology from 1990 to 2016. *Kidney Int* 2018;*94*(3): 567–581.

53. Suleyman H, Demircan B, Karagoz Y. Anti-inflammatory and side effects of cyclooxygenase inhibitors. *Pharmacol Rep* 2007;*59* (3) 247–258.
54. Savica R, Grossardt BR, Bower JH et al. Incidence and time trends of drug-induced parkinsonism: A 30 year population based study. *Mov Disord* 2017;*32*(2): 227–234.
55. Gladstone JP, Eross EJ, Dodick DW. Migraine in special populations. Treatment Strategies for children and adolescents, pregnant women and the elderly. *Postgrad Med* 2004;*115*(4): 39–44, 47–50.
56. Scher AI, Stewart WF, Lipton RB. Caffeine as a risk factor for chronic daily headache: a population-based study. *Neurology* 2004;*63*(11): 2022–7.
57. Shapiro, R. Caffeine and headaches. *Curr Pain Headache Rep* 2008;*12*(4): 311–315
58. Polasek T, Patel F, Jensen B et al. Predicted metabolic drug clearance with increasing adult age. *Br J Clin Pharmacol* 2013;*75*(4): 1019–1028.
59. Rapaport AM, Tepper SJ, Sheftell FD, et al. Which Triptan for which patient? *Neurol Sci* 2006;*27* Suppl 2: S123–9.
60. Dodick D, Shewale A, Lipton R et al. Migraine patients with cardiovascular disease and contraindications: an analysis of real-world claims. *J Prim Care Community Health* 2020; doi:10.1177/2150132720963680
61. Savji N, Rockman C, Skolnick A et al. Association between advanced age and vascular disease in different arterial territories: a population database of over 3.6 million subjects. *J Am Coll Cardiol* 2013;*61*(16): 1736–1743.
62. Expert Panel on Detection, Evaluation and Treatment of High Blood Cholesterol in Adults. Executive Summary on the Third Report of the National Cholesterol Education Program (NCEP) Panel on Detection, Evaluation and Treatment of High Blood Cholesterol in Adults (Adult Treatment Panel III). *JAMA* 2001;*285*(19):2486–2497.
63. Bigal ME, Borucho S, Serrano D et al. The acute treatment of episodic and chronic migraine in the USA. *Cephalalgia* 2009;*29* (8): 891–897.
64. Loder, E. Fixed drug combinations for the acute treatment of migraine: place in therapy. *CNS Drugs* 2005;*19*(9): 769–784.
65. Bigal ME, Serrano D, Buse D et al. Acute migraine medications and the evolution from episodic to chronic migraine: A longitudinal population-based study. *Headache* 2008;*48* (8): 1157–1168.
66. Fick DM, Cooper JW, Wade WE et al. Updating the Beers criteria for potentially inappropriate medication use in older adults: results of a US consensus panel of experts. *Arch Intern Med* 2003;*163* (22): 2716–2724.
67. Tobin J, Flitman S. Occipital nerve blocks: when and what to inject? *Headache* 2009;*49*(10): 1521–1533
68. Mathew NT, Bendtsen L. In: *Prophylactic pharmacotherapy of tension-type headache. The Headaches.* 2nd ed. Olesen J, Tfelt-Hansen P, Welch KMA, editors. Lippincott Williams & Wilkins; Philadelphia, Pa: 2000. pp. 667–774.
69. Bendsten L, Jensen R. Amitryptiline reduces myofascial tenderness in patients with chronic tension type headache. *Cephalalgia* 2000;*20*(6): 603–610.
70. Buchanan T, Ramadan N. Prophylactic pharmacotherapy for migraine headaches. *Semin Neruol* 2006; *26*(2):188–198.
71. Robbins M, Lipton R. Management of Headache in the Elderly. *Drugs Aging* 2010;*27*(5): 377–398.
72. Brody, D., Gu Q. Antidepressant Use Among Adults: United States 2015–2018.
73. Taylor, D. Selective Serotonin reuptake inhibitors and tricyclic antidepressants in combination. Interactions and therapeutic uses. *Br J Psychiatry* 1995;*167*(5): 575–580.
74. Silberstein S, Neto W, Schmitt J. Topiramate in Migraine Prevention: Results of a Large Controlled Trial. *JAMA Neurol* 2004;*61*(4): 490–495.
75. Malafarina V, Uriz-Otano F, Gil-Guerrero L, et al. The anorexia of ageing: physiopathology, prevalence, associated comorbidity and mortality. A systematic review. *Maturitas* 2013;*74*:293–302.
76. Reife R, Pledger G, Wu SC. Topiramate as add-on therapy: pooled analysis of randomized controlled trials in adults. *Epilepsia* 2000;*41*:66–71.
77. Steinman MA, Zullo AR, Lee Y, et al. Association of β-Blockers with functional outcomes, death, and rehospitalization in older nursing home residents after acute myocardial infarction. *JAMA Intern Med* 2017;*177*(2):254–262. doi:10.1001/jamainternmed.2016.7701
78. Cohen AS, Matharu MS, Goadsby PJ. Electrocardiographic abnormalities in patients with cluster headache on verapamil therapy. *Neurology* 2007;*69*(7): 668–675.
79. Silberstein SD. Divalproex sodium in headache: literature review and clinical guidelines. *Headache* 1996;*36*(9):547–555.
80. Freitag FG, Diamond S, Diamond ML, et al. Divalproex sodium in the preventative treatment of cluster headache. *Headache* 2000;*40*:408.

Index

Pages in *italics* refer to figures and pages in **bold** refer to tables.

For Product Safety Concerns and Information please contact our EU
representative GPSR@taylorandfrancis.com
Taylor & Francis Verlag GmbH, Kaufingerstraße 24, 80331 München, Germany

www.ingramcontent.com/pod-product-compliance
Lightning Source LLC
Chambersburg PA
CBHW080917220326
41598CB00034B/5602